Cardiac Pacing and ICDs
Fourth Edition

Cardiac Pacing and ICDs

Fourth Edition

Kenneth A. Ellenbogen, MD
Kontos Professor of Medicine
Director, Electrophysiology and Pacing Laboratory
Virginia Commonwealth University Medical Center
Richmond, Virginia

Mark A. Wood, MD
Professor of Medicine
Assistant Director, Electrophysiology and Pacing Laboratory
Virginia Commonwealth University Medical Center
Richmond, Virginia

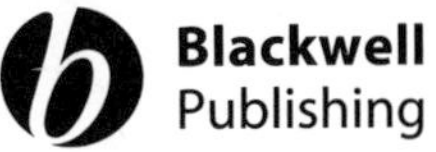

Blackwell Publishing, Inc., 350 Main Street, Malden, Massachusetts 02148-5018, USA
Blackwell Publishing Ltd, 9600 Garsington Road, Oxford OX4 2DQ, UK
Blackwell Publishing Asia Pty Ltd, 550 Swanston Street, Carlton, Victoria 3053, Australia

06 07 08 09 10 8 7 6 5 4 3

ISBN-13: 978-1-4051-0447-0
ISBN-10: 1-4051-0447-3

Library of Congress Cataloging-in-Publication Data

Cardiac pacing and ICDs / [edited by] Kenneth A. Ellenbogen, Mark A. Wood.—4th ed.
p. ; cm.
Includes bibliographical references and index.
ISBN-13: 978-1-4051-0447-0 (pbk.)
ISBN-10: 1-4051-0447-3 (pbk.)
1. Cardiac pacing. 2. Implantable cardioverter-defibrillators. [DNLM: 1. Cardiac Pacing, Artificial. 2. Defibrillators, Implantable. 3. Pacemaker, Artificial. WG 168 C26333 2005] I. Ellenbogen, Kenneth A. II. Wood, Mark A.
RC684.P3C29 2005
617.4′120645—dc22

2004026975

A catalogue record for this title is available from the British Library

Acquisitions: Nancy Duffy
Development: Selene Steneck
Production: Debra Murphy
Cover design: Electronic Illustrators Group
Typesetter: SNP Best-set Typesetter Ltd., Hong Kong
Printed and bound by Sheridan Books, Inc., Chelsea, MI

For further information on Blackwell Publishing, visit our website: www.blackwellmedicine.com

Notice: The indications and dosages of all drugs in this book have been recommended in the medical literature and conform to the practices of the general community. The medications described do not necessarily have specific approval by the Food and Drug Administration for use in the diseases and dosages for which they are recommended. The package insert for each drug should be consulted for use and dosage as approved by the FDA. Because standards for usage change, it is advisable to keep abreast of revised recommendations, particularly those concerning new drugs.

The publisher's policy is to use permanent paper from mills that operate a sustainable forestry policy, and which has been manufactured from pulp processed using acid-free and elementary chlorine-free practices. Furthermore, the publisher ensures that the text paper and cover board used have met acceptable environmental accreditation standards.

To my wife, Phyllis, whose support and encouragement helped make this project successful, and to my children, Michael, Amy, and Bethany for their patience and love.

—Kenneth A. Ellenbogen, MD

To my wife, Helen E. Wood, PhD, for her unquestioning love and support, and to my parents, William B. Wood, PhD, and Donna S. Wood, EdD, for their enduring examples of scholarship.

—Mark A. Wood, MD

Contents

Contributors viii
Preface x

1. Indications for Permanent and Temporary Cardiac Pacing 1
   Pugazhendhi Vijayaraman, Robert W. Peters, and Kenneth A. Ellenbogen
2. Basic Concepts of Pacing 47
   G. Neal Kay
3. Hemodynamics of Cardiac Pacing 122
   Richard C. Wu and Dwight W. Reynolds
4. Temporary Cardiac Pacing 163
   Mark A. Wood and Kenneth A. Ellenbogen
5. Techniques of Pacemaker Implantation and Removal 196
   Jeffrey Brinker and Mark G. Midei
6. Pacemaker Timing Cycles 265
   David L. Hayes and Paul A. Levine
7. Evaluation and Management of Pacing System Malfunctions 322
   Paul A. Levine
8. The Implantable Cardioverter Defibrillator 380
   Michael R. Gold
9. Cardiac Resynchronization Therapy 415
   Michael O. Sweeney
10. ICD Follow-up and Troubleshooting 467
    Henry F. Clemo and Mark A. Wood
11. Follow-up Assessments of the Pacemaker Patient 500
    Mark H. Schoenfeld and Mark L. Blitzer

Index 545

Contributors

Mark L. Blitzer, MD
Instructor in Medicine
Yale University School of Medicine
Hospital of Saint Raphael
New Haven, Connecticut

Jeffrey Brinker, MD
Professor of Medicine
Johns Hopkins University School of Medicine
Johns Hopkins Hospital
Baltimore, Maryland

Henry F. Clemo, MD, PhD
Associate Professor of Medicine
Virginia Commonwealth
University School of Medicine
Richmond, Virginia

Michael R. Gold, MD, PhD
Michael E. Assey Professor of Medicine
Chief, Division of Cardiology
Medical Director, Heart and Vascular Center
Medical University of South Carolina
Charleston, South Carolina

David L. Hayes, MD
Chair, Cardiovascular Diseases
Mayo Clinic
Professor of Medicine
Mayo Clinic College of Medicine
Rochester, Minnesota

G. Neal Kay, MD
Professor of Medicine
University of Alabama at Birmingham
University of Alabama Hospital
Birmingham, Alabama

Paul A. Levine, MD
Clinical Professor of Medicine
Loma Linda University School of Medicine
Loma Linda University Medical Center
Loma Linda, California
Vice President and Medical Director
St. Jude Medical CRMD
Sylmar, California

Mark G. Midei, MD
Assistant Professor of Medicine
Johns Hopkins University School of Medicine
Midatlantic Cardiovascular Associates
Baltimore, Maryland

Robert W. Peters, MD
Professor of Medicine
University of Maryland School of Medicine
Chief of Cardiology
Veterans Administration Medical Center
Baltimore, Maryland

Dwight W. Reynolds, MD
Professor of Medicine and
Chief, Cardiovascular Section
The University of Oklahoma Health Sciences Center
Chief of Staff
OU Medical Center
Oklahoma City, Oklahoma

Mark H. Schoenfeld, MD
Clinical Professor of Medicine
Yale University School of Medicine
Director, Cardiac Electrophysiology and Pacer Laboratory
Hospital of Saint Raphael
New Haven, Connecticut

Michael O. Sweeney, MD
Assistant Professor
Harvard Medical School
Cardiac Arrhythmia Service
Brigham and Women's Hospital
Boston, Massachusetts

Pugazhendhi Vijayaraman, MD
Assistant Professor of Medicine
Virginia Commonwealth
University School of Medicine
Co-Director, Cardiac Electrophysiology Lab
McGuire VA Medical Center
Richmond, Virginia

Richard C. Wu, MD
Attending Physician, Clinical Electrophysiology Laboratory
Assistant Professor of Medicine
Cardiac Arrhythmia Research Institute
The University of Oklahoma Health Sciences Center
Oklahoma City, Oklahoma

Preface

It has been almost five years since our last edition was published. Much has happened in the world of cardiology and especially device therapy since then. A major advance has been the development of cardiac resynchronization therapy as heralded by the development of biventricular pacemakers and implantable cardioverter defibrillators (ICDs). Cardiac resynchronization therapy represents an important new device therapy for patients with congestive heart failure. Its impact on the care of large numbers of patients requires that cardiologists become familiar with the physiology, and implantation and follow-up of these new devices. Additionally, several recent clinical trials of ICDs has led to a marked increase in defibrillator implantation. It is important that cardiologists and other healthcare providers become familiar with the results of these clinical trials.

These exciting new developments have been the stimulus for Dr. Mark A. Wood and I to prepare the fourth edition. Like our previous editions, we have focused on providing a "clinician" friendly book. We have strived to continue our tradition of providing numerous tables, examples and figures that illustrate important teaching points. We have gone through the entire book and replaced "old" figures, or "poorly reproduced figures" with newer more relevant figures. We have added numerous tables and updated each chapter thoroughly to keep the healthcare provider, at whatever level, current with the latest developments in clinical device therapy. There is a new comprehensive chapter on cardiac resynchronization therapy, and the information on ICDs has been increased greatly throughout the text to emphasize their increasing importance. The bibliographies have been shortened and we have made every attempt to include recent references through 2004. This edition promises to provide a thoroughly readable textbook for individuals at all levels caring for device patients.

Finally, this revision was once again made possible because of the hard work of many people. I want to thank the new authors and co-authors who helped with this edition. It is really the contributors who have made this book so successful. We are indebted to them for taking time from their busy clinical commitments to continue their contributions to this edition. My co-editor, Dr. Mark A. Wood, toiled over each chapter making sure the tables and figures were updated and did not rest until each figure was as close to perfect as possible. His commitment to scholarship is a constant reminder to me about the importance of academic medicine. We are also indebted to Dr. George W. Vetrovec, Chairman of Cardiology who has provided unquestioning support and encouragement for all our academic and scholarly activities.

Kenneth A. Ellenbogen, M.D.

Indications for Permanent and Temporary Cardiac Pacing

Pugazhendhi Vijayaraman, Robert W. Peters, and Kenneth A. Ellenbogen

1

ANATOMY

To understand the principles and concepts involved in cardiac pacing more completely, a brief review of the anatomy and physiology of the specialized conduction system is warranted (Table 1.1).[1]

Sinoatrial Node

The sinoatrial (SA) node is a subepicardial structure located at the junction of the right atrium and superior vena cava. It has abundant autonomic innervation and a copious blood supply; it is often located within the adventitia of the large SA nodal artery, a proximal branch of the right coronary artery (55%), or the left circumflex coronary artery. Histologically, the SA node consists of a dense framework of collagen that contains a variety of cells, among them the large, centrally located P cells, which are thought to initiate impulses; transitional cells, intermediate in structure between P cells and regular atrial myocardial cells; and Purkinje-like fiber tracts, extending through the perinodal area and into the atrium.

Atrioventricular Node

The atrioventricular (AV) node is a small subendocardial structure within the interatrial septum located at the convergence of the specialized conduction tracts that course through the atria. Like the SA node, the AV node has extensive autonomic innervation and an abundant blood supply from the large AV nodal artery, a branch of the right coronary artery in 90% of cases, and also from septal branches of the left anterior descending coronary artery. Histologic examination of the AV node reveals a variety of cells embedded in a loose collagenous network including P cells (although not nearly as many as in the SA node), atrial transitional cells, ordinary myocardial cells, and Purkinje cells.

His Bundle

Purkinje fibers emerging from the area of the distal AV node converge gradually to form the His bundle, a narrow tubular structure that runs through the

Table 1.1. The Specialized Conduction System

Structure	Location	Histology	Arterial Blood Supply	Autonomic Innervation	Physiology
SA node	Subepicardial; junction of SVC and HRA	Abundant P cells	SA nodal artery from RCA 55% or LCX 45%	Abundant	Normal impulse generator
AV node	Subendocardial; interatrial septum	Fewer P cells, Purkinje cells, "working" myocardial cells	AV nodal artery from RCA 90%, LCX 10%	Abundant	Delays impulse, subsidiary pacemaker
His bundle	Membranous septum	Narrow tubular structure of Purkinje fibers in longitudinal compartments; few P cells	AV nodal artery, branches of LAD	Sparse	Conducts impulses from AV node to bundle branches
Bundle branches	Starts in muscular septum and branches out into ventricles	Purkinje fibers; highly variable anatomy	Branches of LAD, RCA	Sparse	Activates ventricles

Abbreviations: AV node = atrioventricular node; LAD = left anterior descending coronary artery; LCX = left circumflex coronary artery; RCA = right coronary artery; SA node = sinoatrial node.

membranous septum to the crest of the muscular septum, where it divides into the bundle branches. The His bundle has relatively sparse autonomic innervation, although its blood supply is quite ample, emanating from both the AV nodal artery and septal branches of the left anterior descending artery. Longitudinal strands of Purkinje fibers, divided into separate parallel compartments by a collagenous skeleton, can be discerned by histologic examination of the His bundle. Relatively sparse P cells can also be identified, embedded within the collagen.

Bundle Branches

The bundle branch system is an enormously complex network of interlacing Purkinje fibers that varies greatly among individuals. It generally starts as one or more large fiber bands that split and fan out across the ventricles until they finally terminate in a Purkinje network that interfaces with the myocardium. In some cases, the bundle branches clearly conform to a trifascicular or quadrifascicular system. In other cases, however, detailed dissection of the conduction system has failed to delineate separate fascicles. The right bundle is usually a single, discrete structure that extends down the right side of the interventricular septum to the base of the anterior papillary muscle, where it divides into three or more branches. The left bundle more commonly originates as a very broad band of interlacing fibers that spread out over the left ventricle, sometimes in two or three distinct fiber tracts. There is relatively little autonomic innervation of the bundle branch system, but the blood supply is extensive, with most areas receiving branches from both the right and left coronary systems.

PHYSIOLOGY

The SA node has the highest rate of spontaneous depolarization (automaticity) in the specialized conduction system, and under ordinary circumstances, it is the major generator of impulses. Its unique location astride the large SA nodal artery provides an ideal milieu for continuous monitoring and instantaneous adjustment of heart rate to meet the body's changing metabolic needs. The SA node is connected to the AV node by several specialized fiber tracts, the function of which has not been fully elucidated. The AV node appears to have three major functions: It delays the passing impulse for approximately 0.04 seconds under normal circumstances, permitting complete atrial emptying with appropriate loading of the ventricle; it serves as a subsidiary impulse generator, as its concentration of P cells is second only to that of the SA node; and it acts as a type of filter, limiting ventricular rates in the event of an atrial tachyarrhythmia.

The His bundle arises from the convergence of Purkinje fibers from the AV node, although the exact point at which the AV node ends and the His bundle begins has not been delineated either anatomically or electrically. The separation of the His bundle into longitudinally distinct compartments by the collagenous framework allows for longitudinal dissociation of electrical impulses. Thus a localized lesion below the bifurcation of the His bundle (into the bundle branches) may cause a specific conduction defect (e.g., left anterior fascicular block). The bundle branches arise as a direct continuation of the His bundle fibers. Disease within any aspect of the His bundle branch system may cause conduction defects that can affect AV synchrony or prevent synchronous right and left ventricular activation. The accompanying hemodynamic consequences have considerable clinical relevance. These consequences have provided the impetus for some of the advances in pacemaker technology, which will be addressed in later chapters of this book.

Although a detailed discussion of the histopathology of the conduction system is beyond the scope of the present chapter, it is worth noting that conduction system disease is often *diffuse*. For example, normal AV conduction cannot necessarily be assumed when a pacemaker is implanted for a disorder seemingly localized to the sinus node. Similarly, normal sinus node function cannot be assumed when a pacemaker is implanted in a patient with AV block.

Indications for Permanent Pacemakers

The decision to implant a permanent pacemaker is an important one and should be based on solid clinical evidence. A joint committee of the American College of Cardiology and the American Heart Association was formed in the 1980s to provide uniform criteria for pacemaker implantation. These guidelines were first published in 1984 and most recently revised in 2002.[2,3] It must be realized, however, that medicine is a constantly changing science, and absolute and relative indications for permanent pacing may change as a result of advances in the diagnosis and treatment of arrhythmias. It is useful to keep the ACC/AHA guidelines in mind when evaluating a patient for pacemaker implantation. When approaching a patient with a documented or suspected bradyarrhythmia, it is important to take the clinical setting into account. Thus, the patient's overall general medical condition must be considered as well as his or her occupation or desire to operate a motor vehicle or equipment where the safety of other individuals may be at risk.

In the ACC/AHA classification, there are three classes of indications for permanent pacemaker implantation, defined as follows:

Class I

Conditions for which there is evidence and/or general agreement that a pacemaker implantation is beneficial, useful, and effective.

Class II

Conditions for which there is conflicting evidence and/or a divergence of opinion about the usefulness/efficacy of pacemaker implantation.

Class IIa: Weight of evidence/opinion in favor of efficacy

Class IIb: Usefulness/efficacy less well established by evidence/opinion

Class III
Conditions for which there is evidence and/or general agreement that a pacemaker is not useful/effective and in some cases may be harmful.

Level of Evidence

Additionally, the ACC/AHA Committee ranked evidence supporting their recommendations by the following criteria.

Level A: Data derived from multiple randomized trials involving a large number of patients.
Level B: Data derived from a limited number of trials involving a relatively small number of patients or from well-designed analyses of nonrandomized studies or data registries.
Level C: Recommendations derived from the consensus of experts.

ACQUIRED ATRIOVENTRICULAR BLOCK

Acquired atrioventricular block with syncope (e.g., Stokes-Adams attacks) was historically the first indication for cardiac pacing. The site of AV block (e.g., AV node, His bundle, or distal conduction system) will to a great extent determine the adequacy and reliability of the underlying escape rhythm (Figs. 1.1–1.3). It is worth noting that, in the presence of symptoms documented to be due to AV block, permanent pacing is *indicated*, regardless of the site of the block (e.g., above the His bundle as well as below the His bundle). Because of different indications for permanent pacing heart block due to acute myocardial infarction, congenital AV block and increased vagal tone are discussed in other sections.

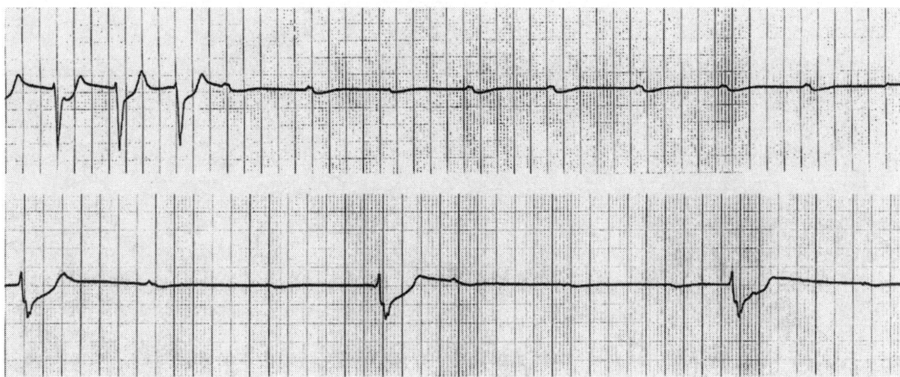

Figure 1.1. An elderly man with underlying left bundle branch block was prescribed propafenone for prevention of atrial fibrillation. He was admitted to the hospital because of syncopal episode and the following rhythm strip was obtained, demonstrating development of complete heart block. Propafenone is a class IC antiarrhythmic drug that has the potential to cause AV block in patients who have a conduction system disease.

Rate of Escape Rhythm vs. Site of Block

INFRA — HIS

INTRA — HIS

AVN

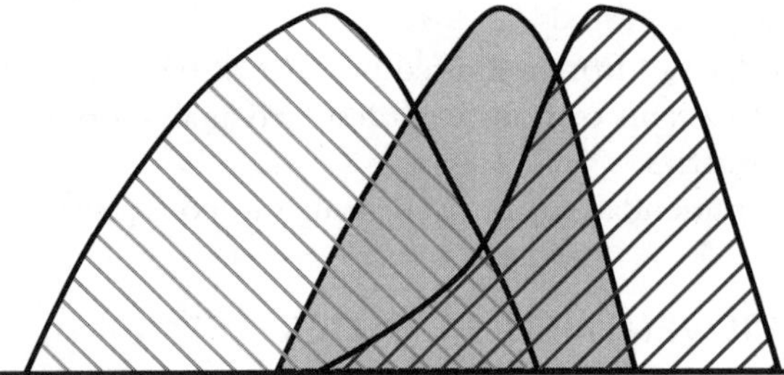

Figure 1.2. A diagram outlining the rate of the escape rhythm in patients with high-grade AV block. As can be seen, the escape rate in a patient with block at the AV node is usually considerably faster than in individuals with intra-Hisian or infra-Hisian block, although there is considerable overlap between groups.

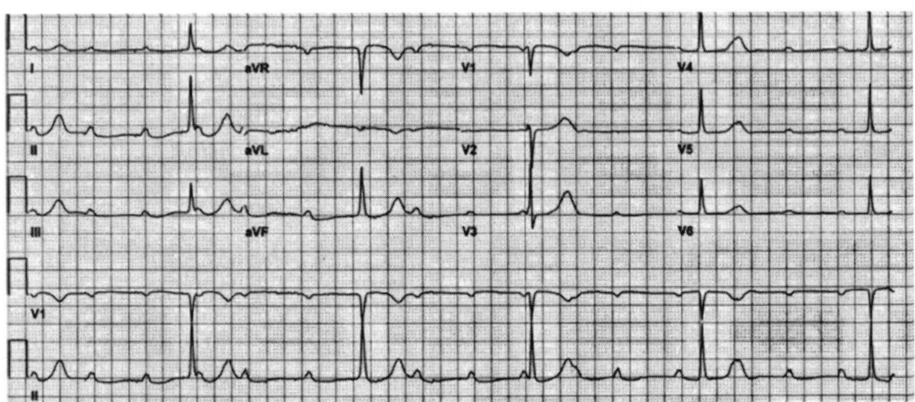

Figure 1.3. A 70-year-old man was admitted to the hospital complaining of weakness and presyncopal episodes. A 12-lead electrocardiogram revealed complete AV block and a slow junctional escape rhythm with narrow QRS complexes. He received a permanent dual-chamber pacemaker, which completely relieved his symptoms.

The indications for permanent pacing with AV block follow.

Class I

1. Third-degree and advanced second-degree AV block at any anatomic level, associated with any one of the following conditions:
   a. Bradycardia with symptoms (including heart failure) presumed to be due to AV block. (Level of evidence: C.)
   b. Arrhythmias and other medical conditions requiring drugs that result in symptomatic bradycardia. (Level of evidence: C.)
   c. Documented periods of asystole greater than or equal to 3.0 seconds or any escape rate less than 40 bpm in awake, symptom-free patients. (Levels of evidence: B, C.)
   d. After catheter ablation of the AV junction. (Levels of evidence: B, C.) There are no trials to assess outcome without pacing, and pacing is virtually always planned in this situation unless the operative procedure is AV junction modification.
   e. Postoperative AV block that is not expected to resolve after cardiac surgery. (Level of evidence: C.)
   f. Neuromuscular diseases with AV block, such as myotonic muscular dystrophy, Kearns-Sayre syndrome, Erb's dystrophy, and peroneal muscular atrophy, with or without symptoms, because there may be unpredictable progression of AV conduction disease. (Level of evidence: B.)
2. Second-degree AV block regardless of type or site of block, with associated symptomatic bradycardia. (Level of evidence: B.)

Class IIa

1. Asymptomatic third-degree AV block at any anatomic site with average awake ventricular rates of 40 beats per minute or faster, especially if cardiomegaly or left ventricular dysfunction is present. (Levels of evidence B, C.)
2. Asymptomatic type II second-degree AV block with a narrow QRS. When type II second-degree AV block occurs with a wide QRS, pacing becomes a class I recommendation. (Level of evidence: B.)
3. Asymptomatic type I second-degree AV block at intra- or infra-His levels found at electrophysiology study performed for other indications. (Level of evidence: B.)
4. First- or second-degree AV block with symptoms similar to those of pacemaker syndrome. (Level of evidence: B.)

Class IIb

1. Marked first degree-AV block (more than 0.30 seconds) in patients with left ventricular (LV) dysfunction and symptoms of congestive heart failure in whom a shorter AV interval results in hemodynamic improvement, presumably by decreasing left atrial filling pressure. (Level of evidence: C.)

2. Neuromuscular diseases such as myotonic muscular dystrophy, Kearns-Sayre syndrome, Erb's dystrophy, and peroneal muscular atrophy with any degree of AV block (including first-degree AV block) with or without symptoms, because there may be unpredictable progression of AV conduction disease. (Level of evidence: B.)

Class III

1. Asymptomatic first-degree AV block. (Level of evidence: B.)
2. Asymptomatic type I second-degree AV block at the AV nodal level or not known to be intra- or infra-Hisian. (Levels of evidence B, C.)
3. AV block expected to resolve and/or unlikely to recur (e.g., drug toxicity, Lyme disease, or during hypoxia in sleep apnea syndrome in absence of symptoms). (Level of evidence: B.)

The majority of these diagnoses can be made from the surface electrocardiogram. Invasive electrophysiology studies are only rarely necessary but may be helpful or of interest in elucidating the site of AV block (Figs. 1.4–1.6). Regarding the first two items in class II, it is likely that permanent pacemakers are more frequently implanted in patients with wide QRS complexes and/or documented infranodal block than in patients with narrow QRS complex escape rhythms.

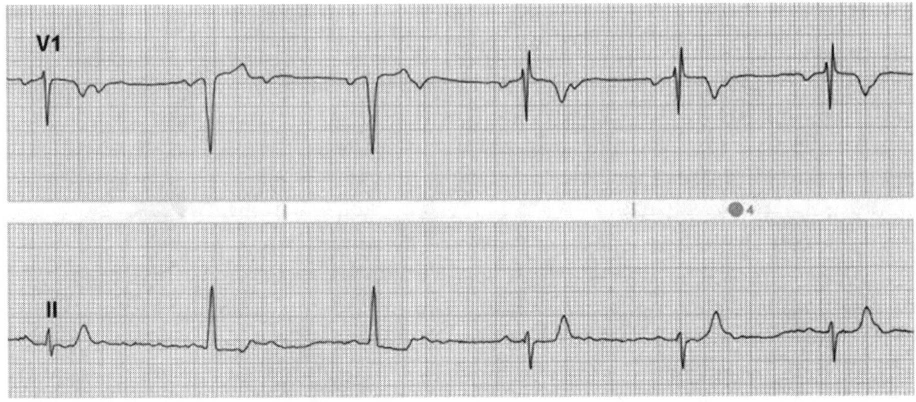

Figure 1.4. This 12-lead electrocardiogram showing 2:1 AV block was obtained as part of a routine preoperative evaluation from an asymptomatic 75-year-old woman who was scheduled to undergo surgery for severe peripheral vascular disease. The site of block is uncertain but the presence of alternating left bundle branch block and right bundle branch block suggests that the block is infranodal. The electrophysiologic study confirmed an infranodal block and this patient underwent permanent pacemaker implantation. Although this is a class IIa indication for pacing, it was decided that the patient could not truly be considered asymptomatic because her activity was limited by severe intermittent claudication.

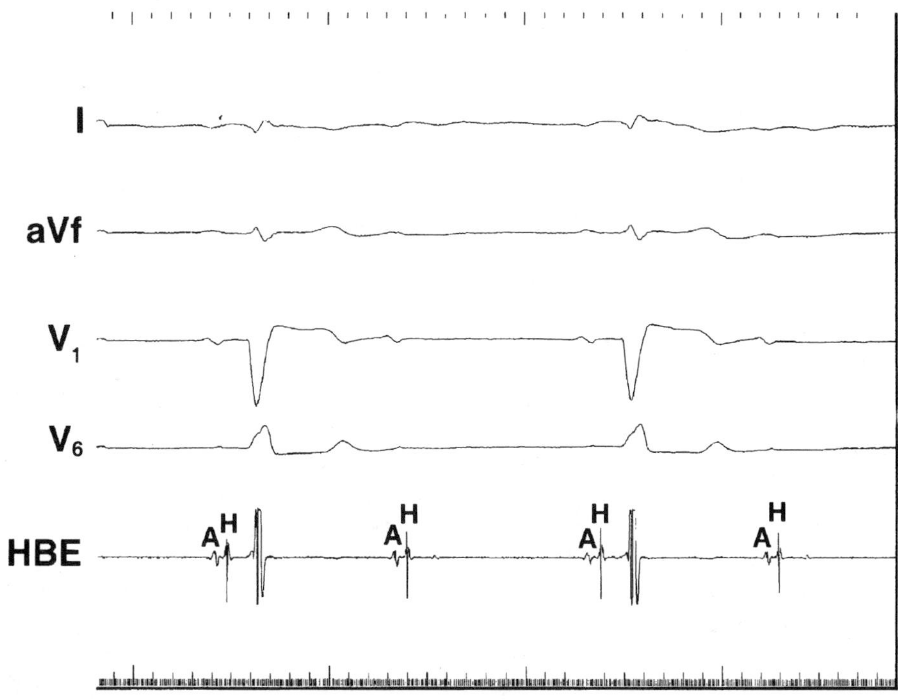

Figure 1.5. An example of 2:1 AV block with the level of block occurring within the His-Purkinje system. In the presence of a narrow QRS complex, 2:1 AV block is usually situated at the AV node whereas a wide QRS complex in the conducted beats often indicates infranodal block. Note that every other P wave is blocked below the His bundle. The paper speed is 100 mm/sec. From top to bottom: I, aVf, V_1, and V_6 are standard ECG leads; HBE is the intracardiac recording of the His bundle electrogram. Abbreviations: A = atrial electrogram, H = His bundle electrogram.

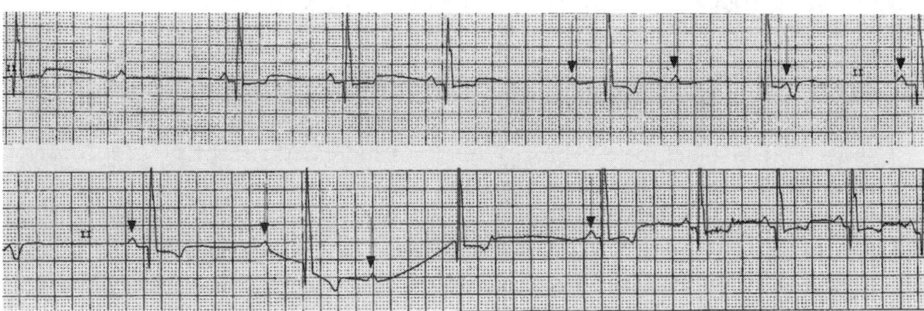

Figure 1.6. An example of "vagotonic" block. P waves are indicated by the arrows. The simultaneous occurrence of AV block and slowing of the sinus rate is diagnostic of hypervagotonia. This type of block is located at the level of the AV node. It is generally considered benign and does not warrant a permanent pacemaker unless the patient is very symptomatic with medically refractory recurrences.

Table 1.2. Differential Diagnosis of 2:1 AV Block

Condition	Block above AV Node	Block below AV Node
Exercise	+	+/− or −
Atropine	+	+/− or −
Carotid sinus massage	−	+ or +/−
Isoprenaline	−	+ or +/−

+ Represents improved AV conduction.
− Represents worsened AV conduction.

It is worth emphasizing that 2:1 AV block may be either type I or type II, but this cannot always be discerned from the surface electrocardiogram (ECG) (Table 1.2). As a rough approximation, if the QRS complex is narrow, the block is most likely localized to the AV node and considered type I. If the QRS complex is wide, the level of block may be in the AV node or His bundle, and the site of the block can best be determined from an invasive electrophysiologic study (His bundle recording). The causes of acquired high-grade AV block are listed in Box 1.1.

The class I indication for permanent pacing after catheter ablation of the AV junction for refractory supraventricular tachycardia is also deserving of comment. Many of these patients will have an apparently stable escape rhythm, some with a narrow QRS complex. Nevertheless, until more is known about the long-term reliability of these escape rhythms, permanent pacemaker implantation is mandatory. In contrast, patients who undergo selective ablation of a "slow" pathway (AV nodal modification) may have no interruption of AV conduction and should not be considered for permanent pacemakers unless AV block develops.

CHRONIC BIFASCICULAR OR TRIFASCICULAR BLOCK

Patients with chronic bifascicular block (right bundle branch block and left anterior hemiblock, right bundle branch block and left posterior hemiblock, or complete left bundle branch block) and patients with trifascicular block (any of the above and first-degree AV block) are at an increased risk of progression to complete AV block.

In the 1980s, the results of several prospective studies of the role of His bundle recordings in *asymptomatic* patients with *chronic* bifascicular block were published.[2–7] In these studies, more than 750 patients were observed for 3 to 5 years. The incidence of progression from bifascicular to complete heart block varied from 2% to 5%. Most important, the total cardiovascular mortality was 19% to 25%, and the mortality from sudden cardiac death was 10% to 20%. In these patients, the presence of bifascicular block on the ECG should be taken as a sign of coexisting organic heart disease. These studies concluded that patients

Box 1.1. Causes of Acquired High-Grade AV Block

- Ischemic
  - Acute myocardial infarction
  - Chronic ischemic heart disease
- Nonischemic cardiomyopathy
  - Hypertensive
  - Idiopathic dilated
- Fibrodegenerative
  - Lev's disease
  - Lenègre's disease
- After cardiac surgery
  - Coronary artery bypass grafting
  - Aortic valve replacement
  - Ventricular septal defect repair
  - Septal myomectomy (for IHSS surgery)
- Other iatrogenic
  - After His bundle (AV junction) ablation
  - After ablation of septal accessory pathways, AV nodal reentry
  - After radiation therapy (e.g., lung cancer, Hodgkin's lymphoma)
- Infectious
  - Bacterial endocarditis
  - Chagas' disease
  - Lyme disease
  - Other (viral, rickettsial, fungal, etc.)
- Neuromuscular disease
  - Myotonic dystrophy
  - Muscular dystrophies (fascioscapulohumeral)
  - Kearns-Sayre syndrome
  - Friedreich's ataxia
- Infiltrative disease
  - Amyloid
  - Sarcoid
  - Hemochromatosis
  - Carcinoid
  - Malignant
- Connective tissue disease
  - Rheumatoid arthritis
  - Systemic lupus erythematosus
  - Systemic scleroderma
  - Ankylosing spondylitis

with *chronic asymptomatic bifascicular block* and a prolonged HV interval (HV interval represents the shortest conduction time from the His bundle to the endocardium over the specialized conduction system) have more extensive organic heart disease and an increased risk of sudden cardiac death. The risk of spontaneous progression to complete heart block is small, although it is probably slightly greater in patients who have a prolonged HV interval. Permanent pacing appears to prevent recurrent syncope in these patients but does not reduce the frequency of sudden death, which is often due to heart failure or ventricular arrhythmias.[2] Routine His bundle recordings are therefore of little value in evaluating patients with chronic bifascicular block and *no* associated symptoms (e.g., syncope or presyncope) (Fig. 1.7).

In patients with bifascicular or trifascicular block and associated *symptoms* of syncope or presyncope, electrophysiologic testing is useful.[8] A high incidence of sudden cardiac death and inducible ventricular arrhythmias is noted in this group of patients. Electrophysiologic testing is useful for identifying the disorder responsible for syncope, and potentially avoiding implantation of a pacemaker (Fig. 1.8). In patients who have a markedly prolonged HV interval (>100 milliseconds) and syncope not attributable to other causes, there is a high incidence of subsequent development of complete heart block, and permanent pacing is warranted. However, these patients comprise a relatively small percentage of patients undergoing electrophysiologic testing with cardiac symptoms and bifascicular block. In the majority of patients, the HV interval is normal (HV: 35 to 55 milliseconds) or only *mildly* prolonged, and His bundle recording does not effectively separate out high-risk and low-risk subpopulations with bifascicular block who are likely to progress to complete heart block. Electrophysiologic testing will often provoke sustained ventricular arrhythmias, which are the cause of syncope in many of these patients. In patients with left ven-

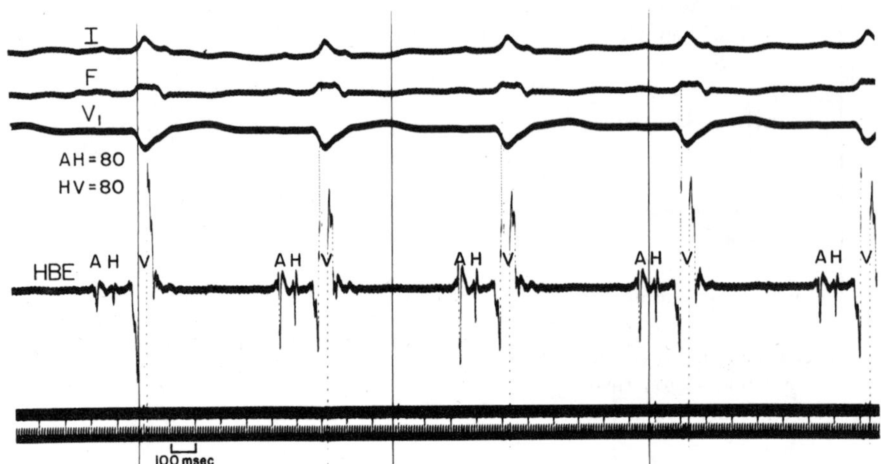

Figure 1.7. An intracardiac recording in a patient with left bundle branch block. The prolonged HV interval (80 milliseconds) is indicative of infranodal conduction disease, but in the absence of transient neurologic symptoms (syncope, dizzy spells, etc.), no specific therapy is indicated. From top to bottom: I, F, and V_1 are standard ECG leads; HBE is the intracardiac recording of the His bundle electrogram. Abbreviations: A = atrial depolarization, H = His bundle depolarization, V = ventricular electrogram. Paper speed is 100 mm/sec.

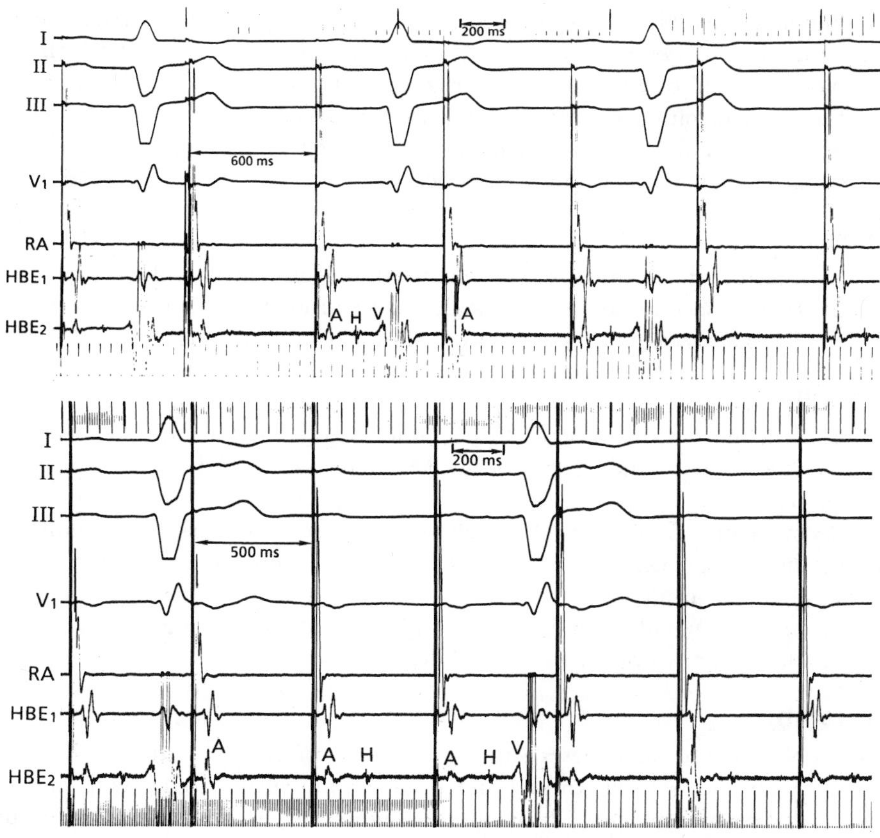

Figure 1.8. A 68-year-old man was admitted complaining of recurrent dizziness and syncope. His baseline 12-lead ECG showed a PR interval of 0.20 seconds and a right bundle block QRS morphology. During the electrophysiologic study, the patient's baseline HV interval was 90 milliseconds. Top: During atrial pacing at a cycle length of 600 milliseconds (100 ppm), there is block in the AV node. Bottom: During pacing at 500 milliseconds (120 ppm), there is block below the His bundle. These findings are indicative of severe diffuse conduction system disease. A permanent dual-chamber pacemaker was implanted, and the patient's symptoms resolved. From top to bottom: I, II, III, and V_1 are standard ECG leads; intracardiac recording from the right atrial appendage (RA) and His bundle (HBE_1 for the proximal His bundle and HBE_2 for the distal His bundle). Abbreviations: A = atrial depolarization, H = His bundle depolarization, V = ventricular depolarization.

tricular systolic dysfunction, advanced heart failure, and bundle branch block, especially left bundle branch block and QRS interval greater than 120 milliseconds, defibrillators with biventricular pacing have been shown to improve symptoms from heart failure and reduce mortality.[9]

Barold has pointed out that the standard definition of trifascicular block is often too loosely applied.[10] Thus, in patients with right bundle branch block and either left anterior or left posterior fascicular block or in patients with left bundle branch block and first-degree AV block, the *site* of block could be located either in the His-Purkinje system *or* in the AV node. The term "trifascicular block" should be reserved for alternating right and left bundle branch block or for block of either bundle in the setting of a prolonged HV interval.

The indications for pacing in the setting of chronic bifascicular/trifascicular block are listed subsequently.

Class I

1. Intermittent third-degree AV block. (Level of evidence: B.)
2. Type II second-degree AV block. (Level of evidence: B.)
3. Alternating bundle-branch block. (Level of evidence: C.)

Class IIa

1. Syncope not demonstrated to be due to AV block when other likely causes have been excluded, specifically ventricular tachycardia. (Level of evidence: B.)
2. Incidental finding at electrophysiology study of markedly prolonged HV interval (greater than or equal to 100 milliseconds) in asymptomatic patients. (Level of evidence: B.)
3. Incidental finding at electrophysiology study of pacing induced infra-His block that is not physiologic. (Level of evidence: B.)

Class IIb

1. Neuromuscular diseases such as myotonic muscular dystrophy, Kearn-Sayre syndrome, Erb's dystrophy, and peroneal muscular atrophy with any degree of fascicular block with or without symptoms, because there may be unpredictable progression of AV conduction disease. (Level of evidence: C.)

Class III

1. Fascicular block without AV block or symptoms. (Level of evidence: B.)
2. Fascicular block with first-degree AV block without symptoms.

SINUS NODE DYSFUNCTION

Sinus node dysfunction, or sick sinus syndrome and its variants, is a heterogeneous clinical syndrome of diverse etiologies.[11] This disorder includes sinus bradycardia, sinus arrest, sinoatrial block, and various supraventricular tachycardias (atrial or junctional) alternating with periods of bradycardia or asystole. Sinus node dysfunction is quite common and its incidence increases with advancing age. In patients with sinus node dysfunction, the correlation of symptoms with the bradyarrhythmia is critically important. This is because there is a great deal of disagreement about the absolute heart rate or length of pause required before pacing is indicated. If the symptoms of sinus node disease are dramatic (e.g., syncope, recurrent dizzy spells, seizures, or severe heart failure), then the diagnosis may be relatively easy. Often, however, the symptoms are extremely nonspecific (e.g., easy fatigability, depression, listlessness, early signs of dementia) and in the elderly may be easily misinterpreted.[12] Instead, many of these patients have symptoms as a result of an abrupt change in heart rate (e.g., termination of tachycardia with a sinus pause or sinus bradycardia) (Fig. 1.9). It is important to realize that the degree of bradycardia that may produce symptoms will vary depending on the patient's physiologic status, age, and activity at the time of bradycardia (e.g., eating, sleeping, or walking) (Fig. 1.10). In patients

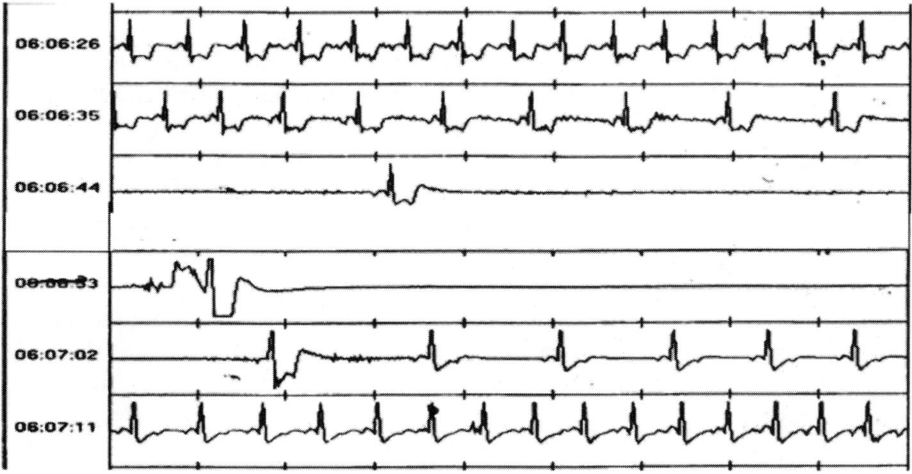

Figure 1.9. A dramatic example of sinus node dysfunction manifested by 7 and 10 seconds of asystole as documented by an implantable loop monitor in a patient with recurrent undiagnosed syncope. He underwent permanent pacemaker implantation.

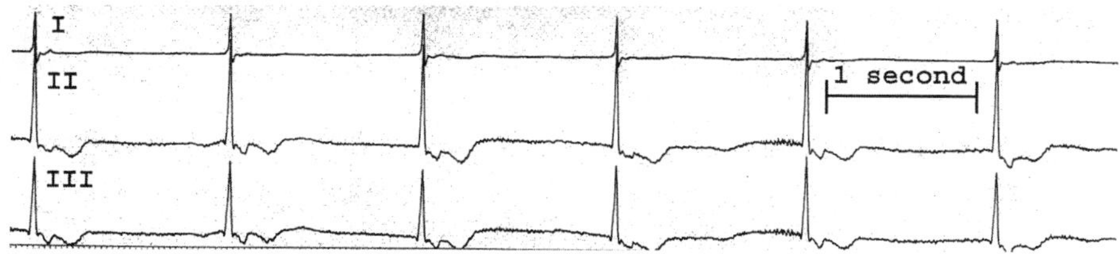

Figure 1.10. ECG recording from a 50-year-old woman with progressive fatigue and exercise intolerance. During extended treadmill exercise, her heart rate did not exceed 80 bpm. This tracing at rest shows junctional rhythm at approximately 50 bpm. Her exercise capacity improved dramatically after implantation of an AAIR pacing system for sinus node dysfunction.

with sinus node dysfunction whose symptoms have not been shown to correlate with electrocardiographic abnormalities, a simple exercise test may be helpful (to assess the degree of chronotropic incompetence, especially in the individual with vague symptoms) or an electrophysiologic study may be considered.

More permanent pacemakers are implanted for sinus node disease than for any other indication in the United States. Patients with alternating periods of bradycardia and tachycardia (i.e., tachy-brady syndrome) are especially likely to require permanent pacing because medical treatment of the tachycardia often worsens the bradycardia and vice versa (Fig. 1.11). Up to 30% of patients with sinus node disease will also have distal conduction system disease. Thus, atrial fibrillation, which is a common complication of sinus node disease, may be accompanied by a slow ventricular response, even in the absence of medications that depress AV conduction. Other important complications of sinus node disease include systemic emboli, especially in the setting of alternating periods of bradycardia and tachycardia, and congestive heart failure, usually related to the slow heart rate. In addition, many commonly used medications may exacerbate sinus node dysfunction (Box 1.2). For many patients, an acceptable alternative cannot be found, and pacing is necessary so the patient can continue their medications.

A group of patients has been identified who have a relatively fixed heart rate during exercise; this condition is referred to as chronotropic incompetence. These patients frequently have other symptoms of sinus node dysfunction. Some of these patients may have symptoms at rest (generally nonspecific), but most will note symptoms such as fatigue or shortness of breath with exercise. In some cases, the diagnosis is straightforward; there is no or only a very slight increase in heart rate with exercise. In other cases, the diagnosis is difficult and will

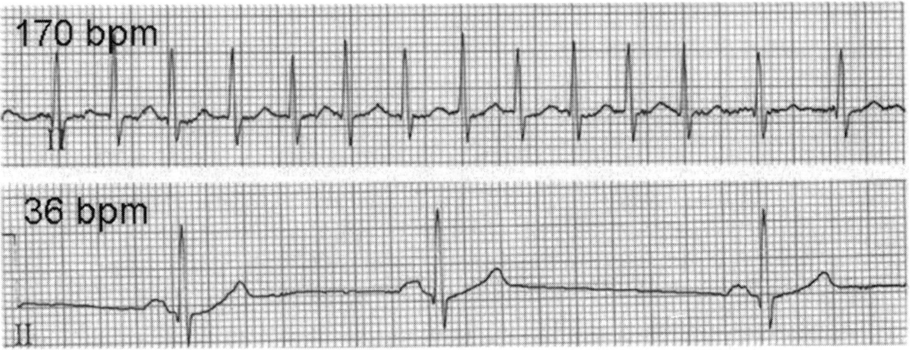

Figure 1.11. Monitor tracings of a patient with alternating atrial fibrillation and sinus bradycardia. The alternation between the rapidly conducted atrial fibrillation at 170 bpm and the sinus bradycardia at 36 bpm is extremely difficult to manage without a permanent pacemaker.

Box 1.2. Commonly Used Medications That May Cause Sinus Node Dysfunction or AV Block

- Digitalis (especially in the setting of hypokalemia)
- Antihypertensive agents (clonidine, methyldopa, guanethidine)
- Beta-adrenergic blockers (Inderal, metoprolol, nadolol, atenolol)
- Calcium channel blockers (verapamil, diltiazem)
- Type 1A antiarrhythmic drugs (quinidine, procainamide, disopyramide)
- Type 1C antiarrhythmic drugs (flecainide, propafenone)
- Type III antiarrhythmic drugs (amiodarone, sotalol)
- Psychotropic medications
  - Tricyclics
  - Phenothiazines
  - Lithium
  - Phenytoin
  - Cholinesterase inhibitors

require comparison of the patient's exercise response with that of age-matched and gender-matched patients using specific exercise protocols.

Although the indications for permanent pacing for sinus node dysfunction are fairly well delineated, there is considerable debate as to which pacing mode is most appropriate. Because of the high incidence of chronotropic incompetence, the need for rate-responsive pacing is generally accepted. However, whether dual-chamber (DDD/DDDR) pacing confers any advantage over the VVIR mode is less well established.[13] Pacing to maintain AV synchrony (AAI/DDD) has been shown to reduce the incidence of atrial fibrillation but does not prevent strokes or prolong survival.[14] Similarly, there is debate about whether patients with intact AV conduction might benefit more from AAI/AAIR than from DDD/DDDR pacing. Single-chamber devices are less complicated and cheaper and allow for normal ventricular activation. These issues are currently being addressed in several large randomized clinical trials and are discussed later in this chapter.

The indications for pacemaker implantation in patients with sinus node dysfunction are listed subsequently.

Class I

1. Sinus node dysfunction with documented symptomatic bradycardia or sinus pauses. Sinus node dysfunction as a result of essential long-term drug therapy of a type and dose, for which there are no acceptable alternatives. (Level of evidence: C.)
2. Symptomatic chronotropic incompetence. (Level of evidence: C.)

Class IIa

1. Sinus node dysfunction occurring spontaneously or as a result of necessary drug therapy, with heart rates less than 40 beats per minute when a clear

association between significant symptoms consistent with bradycardia and the actual presence of bradycardia has not been documented. (Level of evidence: C.)

2. Syncope of unexplained origin when major abnormalities of sinus node function are discovered or provoked in electrophysiologic studies. (Level of evidence: C.)

Class IIb

1. In minimally symptomatic patients, chronic heart rates less than 40 bpm while awake. (Level of evidence: C.)

Class III

1. Sinus node dysfunction in asymptomatic patients, including those in whom substantial sinus bradycardia (heart rate less than 40 beats per minute) is a consequence of long-term drug treatment.
2. Sinus node dysfunction in patients with symptoms suggestive of bradycardia that are clearly documented as not associated with a slow heart rate.
3. Sinus node dysfunction with symptomatic bradycardia due to nonessential drug therapy.

Neurocardiogenic Syncope/Hypersensitive Carotid Sinus Syndrome

Neurally mediated syncope is a form of abnormal autonomic control of the circulation. It may take one of three forms[15]:

I. The cardioinhibitory type is characterized by ventricular asystole of at least 3 seconds due to sinus arrest or (occasionally) complete heart block.
II. The pure vasodepressor response is marked by a decrease in arterial pressure of at least 20 to 30 mm Hg but little or no change in heart rhythm.
III. The mixed type has features of both the cardioinhibitory and vasodepressor types.

Syncope is a common disorder that is estimated to account for approximately 6% of all hospital admissions in the United States annually. Despite extensive evaluation, the cause of syncope may not be found in up to 50% of cases.[16] It is believed that a substantial proportion of these cases may be due to neurally mediated syncope. The exact mechanism of neurally mediated syncope has not been fully elucidated but appears to be initiated by an exaggerated response of the sympathetic nervous system to a variety of stimuli. Although the syncope is most often an isolated event with an obvious precipitating cause such as severe fright or emotional upset, in some individuals these episodes are recurrent and without apparent trigger factors. A variety of other stimuli may give rise to cardioinhibitory or mixed cardioinhibitory responses. These conditions, when recurrent, may also be treated with permanent pacemakers. The conditions include pain, coughing, micturition, swallowing, defecation, and the relatively common vasovagal syndrome. In general, pacemakers may be considered in these patients only when symptoms are recurrent, severe, and cannot be controlled by more conservative measures (e.g., avoidance of stimuli, beta blockers, midodrine hydrochloride [ProAmatine], and/or fludrocortisone acetate [Florinef]). Pacemaker therapy may be successful in patients who predominantly experience the cardioinhibitory type of response. The advent of head-upright tilt testing has had a major impact on the area of neurocardiogenic syncope. Vasodepressor and/or cardioinhibitory responses may be elicited, which appear to correlate only moderately well with the clinical symptoms (Figs. 1.12–1.14). As with the previously mentioned clinical syndromes, permanent pacemakers tend to be effective for patients whose tilt test displays a prominent cardioinhibitory component. The development of permanent pacemakers with the "rate-drop response," which initiates an interval of relatively rapid pacing when the heart rate suddenly drops below a pre-set limit, has stimulated renewed interest in the use of pacing for neurocardiogenic syncope and related disorders. Initial randomized, controlled clinical trials had documented the ability of pacemakers with this feature to reduce syncopal recurrences compared to patients without

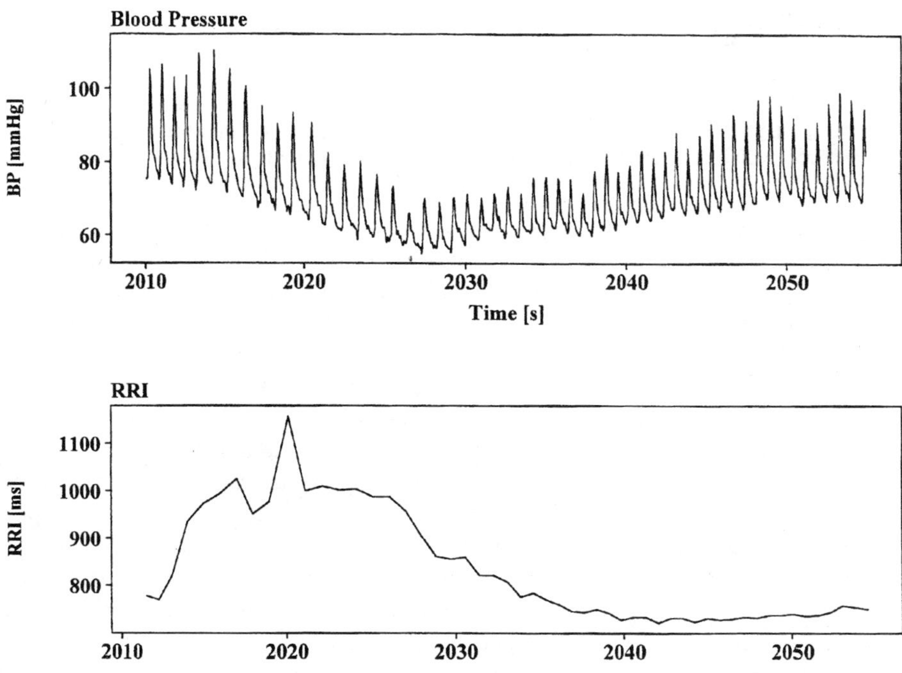

Figure 1.12. An example of a pure vasodepressor response to tilt testing. The upper panel shows blood pressure and the lower panel shows heart rate (R-R intervals, expressed in milliseconds). Note the marked decrease in blood pressure at a time when the heart rate is actually increasing (the R-R interval is shortening). This type of individual is less likely to respond to permanent pacing.

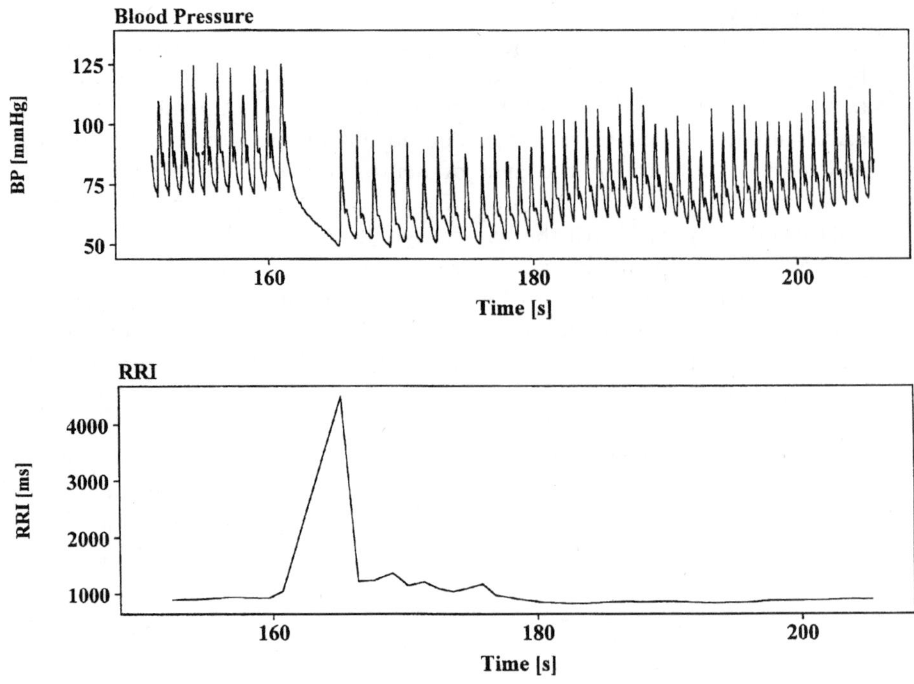

Figure 1.13. Tracings from a tilt test showing a pure cardioinhibitory response. Note the abrupt increase in cardiac cycle length (R-R interval) reflecting marked bradycardia.

pacemakers.[17,18] However, a recent double-blinded, randomized clinical trial (control group received pacemakers, but in ODO mode) showed only a trend toward a reduction in frequency of syncope with active pacing without reaching statistical significance.[19] The final role of pacing in prevention of neurocardiogenic syncope is uncertain; at present, pacing is only used in truly refractory cases in which a significant bradycardic component has been well demonstrated.

One variant of neurally mediated syncope is the hypersensitive carotid sinus syndrome. A mildly abnormal response to vigorous carotid sinus massage may occur in up to 25% of patients, especially if coexisting vascular disease is present. Some patients with an abnormal response to carotid sinus massage may have no symptoms suggestive of carotid sinus syncope. On the other hand, the typical history of syncope—blurred vision and lightheadedness or confusion in the standing or sitting position, especially during movement of the head or neck—should be suggestive of this entity. Classic triggers of carotid sinus syncope are head turning, tight neckwear, shaving, and neck hyperextension. Syncopal episodes usually last only several minutes and are generally reproducible in a given patient. Symptoms associated with this syndrome may wax or wane over several years. Carotid sinus hypersensitivity is most often predominantly cardioinhibitory in nature so that permanent pacing may be very helpful (Fig.

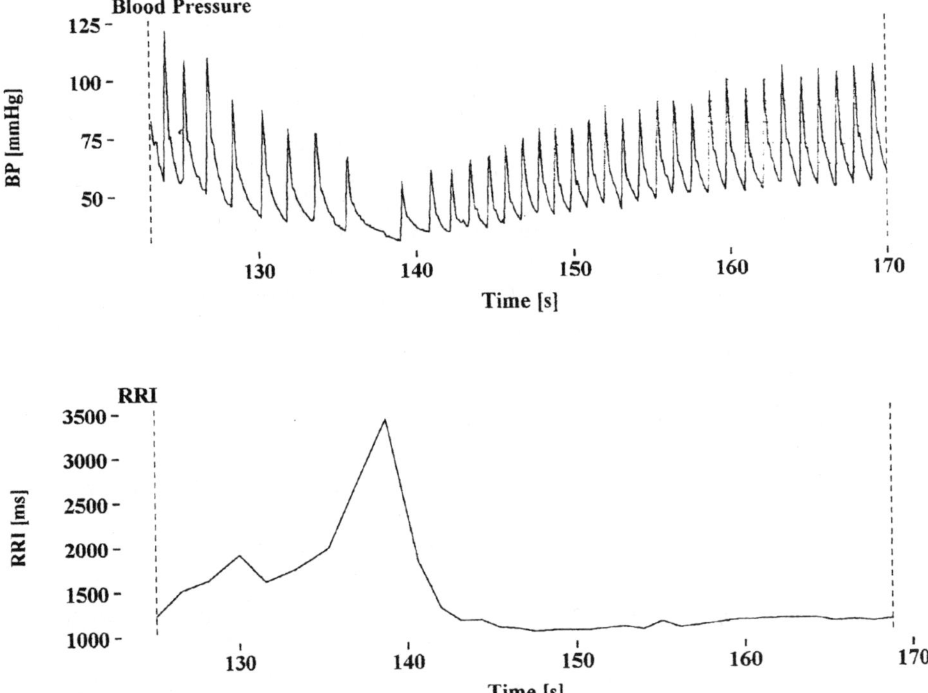

Figure 1.14. An example of a "mixed" cardioinhibitory and vasodepressor response to tilt testing. An initial decrease in blood pressure is followed by a marked increase in cardiac cycle length.

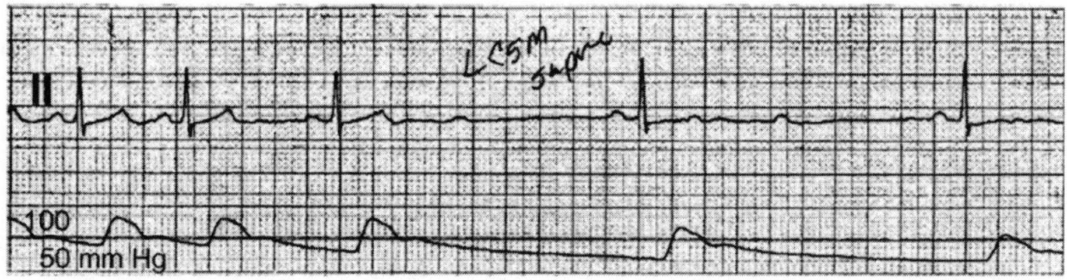

Figure 1.15. A 55-year-old man complained of recurrent presyncopal episodes that occurred when he turned his neck or shaved. Carotid sinus massage produced sinus slowing and 2:1 AV block associated with hypotension as documented by finger plethysmography.

1.15). In contrast, other forms of neurocardiogenic syncope often have a significant vasodepressor component, so that permanent pacing has a more limited role.

The indications for pacemaker implantation in patients with neurally mediated syncope and hypersensitive carotid sinus syndrome are listed subsequently.

Class I

1. Recurrent syncope caused by carotid sinus stimulation; minimal carotid sinus pressure induces ventricular asystole of more than 3-second duration in the absence of any medication that depress the sinus node or AV conduction. (Level of evidence: C.)

Class IIa

1. Recurrent syncope without clear, provocative events and with a hypersensitive cardioinhibitory response. (Level of evidence: C.)
2. Significantly symptomatic and recurrent neurocardiogenic syncope associated with bradycardia documented spontaneously or at the time of tilt-table testing. (Level of evidence: C.)

Class III

1. A hyperactive cardioinhibitory response to carotid sinus stimulation in the absence of symptoms or in the presence of vague symptoms such as dizziness, lightheadedness, or both.
2. Recurrent syncope, lightheadedness, or dizziness in the absence of a hyperactive cardioinhibitory response.
3. Situational vasovagal syncope in which avoidance behavior is effective.

Idiopathic orthostatic hypotension is a related neurocirculatory disorder that may respond to permanent pacing. Several reports have documented a beneficial response to atrial or AV sequential pacing in a small number of patients with idiopathic orthostatic hypotension refractory to salt and steroid therapy.[20] The rationale for pacing in this condition is that by increasing the paced rate (the lower rate in these series varies from 80 to 100 beats per minute), the cardiac output increases and potentially leads to more vasoconstriction. This therapy usually results in some clinical improvement, but it varies considerably from patient to patient. There are currently no class I or class II indications for permanent pacing for idiopathic orthostatic hypotension.

Hypertrophic Cardiomyopathy

Hypertrophic cardiomyopathy is a disorder of the myocardium characterized by excessive myocardial hypertrophy, with a predilection for the interventricular septum. Although there may be obstructive (i.e., a demonstrable gradient across the left ventricular outflow tract) and nonobstructive forms, there might be little difference between them because the gradient is dynamic and affected by preload, afterload, and other factors. Difficulty with diastolic relaxation (and ventricular filling) of the thickened and noncompliant ventricular musculature is present in both forms of this disorder and may be an important determinant of the clinical presentation. Pacing is thought to exert a beneficial effect by inducing paradoxical septal motion and ventricular dyssynchrony and dilatation, thereby improving ventricular filling and reducing the outflow tract gradient.

This is generally achieved with dual-chamber pacing with a short PR interval (i.e., usually 50 to 125 milliseconds) to produce maximal ventricular preexcitation. The acute hemodynamic effects of dual-chamber pacing may be quite dramatic, with a major reduction in left ventricular cavity obliteration and a concomitant decrease in left ventricular outflow tract gradient (Fig. 1.16). More intriguing is the suggestion that the beneficial effects of dual-chamber pacing in this condition do not dissipate immediately once the pacing has been terminated.[21]

The mechanism of the beneficial effects of pacing is incompletely understood and the population who would most reliably benefit has not been fully elucidated. In a recent multicenter trial (the M-PATHY study) using a randomized, double-blind crossover design, Maron and colleagues found that symp-

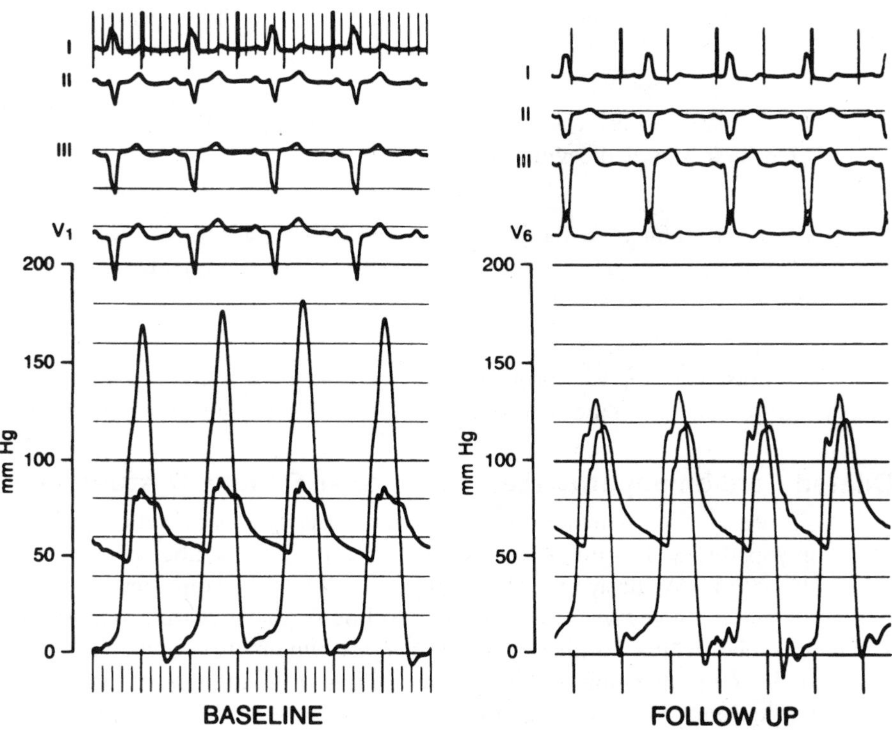

Figure 1.16. Tracings show reduction of left ventricular outflow tract obstruction after chronic dual-chamber pacing. **Left panel**: At baseline, the left ventricular systolic pressure and left ventricular outflow gradient were 180 mm Hg and 90 mm Hg, respectively. **Right panel**: At the follow-up assessment, the left ventricular systolic pressure and left ventricular outflow tract gradient, also measured in sinus rhythm, were reduced to 135 mm Hg and 15 mm Hg, respectively, despite the temporary inhibition of ventricular pacing. This finding suggests remodeling of ventricular function or anatomy by chronic pacing. From top to bottom: I, II, III, V_1 and V_6 are standard ECG leads.

tomatic improvement (quality of life and functional class) was not necessarily accompanied by improvement in objective indices such as treadmill exercise time and peak oxygen consumption.[22] Similarly, in the Pacing in Cardiomyopathy (PIC) study, Linde and colleagues found significant improvement in both the active pacing and inactive pacing (placebo) group, although the improvement was greater in those assigned to active pacing.[23] These two studies suggest that some of the improvement seen in earlier studies may be partly due to placebo effect or the known variability in clinical course of the disorder. Because prolongation of life has not been documented with this therapy, the current role of permanent pacemakers in hypertrophic cardiomyopathy is unclear. Accordingly, it should be remembered that surgical myotomy–myectomy is still considered the gold standard for treatment of this condition.[24] Septal ethanol ablation is an emerging therapy as well. The clinician managing these patients must determine if a device is to be implanted with a dual-chamber pacemaker or if a dual-chamber defibrillator is the most appropriate choice.

The indications for permanent pacing for hypertrophic cardiomyopathy are as follows:

Class I

1. Class I indications for sinus node dysfunction or AV block as previously described. (Level of evidence: C.)

Class IIb

1. Medically refractory, symptomatic hypertrophic cardiomyopathy with significant resting or provoked LV outflow tract obstruction. (Level of evidence: A.)

Class III

1. Patients who are asymptomatic or medically controlled.
2. Symptomatic patients without evidence of LV outflow tract obstruction.

Dilated Cardiomyopathy (Left Ventricular Systolic Dysfunction)

A related area in which permanent pacing may be of benefit is dilated cardiomyopathy. Early studies have suggested that dual-chamber pacing, especially with a short AV delay, may have important hemodynamic benefit in patients with severe congestive heart failure.[25] Although the exact mechanism was not determined, it was postulated that the improvement in hemodynamics may be related to optimization of ventricular filling or reduction of diastolic mitral regurgitation.[26] However, in more recent controlled studies, other groups have failed to confirm these beneficial effects.[27] Studies of right ventricular outflow tract pacing for left ventricular systolic dysfunction have been negative or mixed.[28]

In contrast, there is now considerable evidence that the use of left ventricular or biventricular permanent pacing improves hemodynamics in certain patients with congestive heart failure. Because left ventricular contraction is a key determinant of cardiac output, in theory the properly synchronized contraction of the left ventricle or both ventricles should enhance cardiac performance in patients with intrinsic prolongation of the QRS duration. Randomized, double blinded, controlled clinical trials have clearly established the beneficial role of biventricular pacing therapy in advanced heart failure patients with prolonged QRS duration.[29]

The indications for pacing in patients with heart failure and impaired left ventricular systolic function are:

Class I

1. Class I indications for sinus node dysfunction or AV block as previously described. (Level of evidence: C.)

Class IIa

1. Biventricular pacing in medically refractory, symptomatic NYHA class III or IV patients with idiopathic dilated or ischemic cardiomyopathy, prolonged QRS interval (≥130 milliseconds), LV end-diastolic diameter ≥55 mm and ejection fraction ≤35%. (Level of evidence: A.)

Class III

1. Asymptomatic dilated cardiomyopathy.
2. Symptomatic dilated cardiomyopathy when patients are rendered asymptomatic by drug therapy.
3. Symptomatic ischemic cardiomyopathy when the ischemia is amenable to intervention.

Prevention and Termination of Tachyarrhythmias Including the Prolonged QT Syndrome

Permanent pacing can be used in some situations to prevent or terminate supraventricular (supraventricular tachycardia [SVT]) and ventricular arrhythmias. Individuals with prolongation of the QT or QT-U interval may be prone to a type of polymorphic ventricular tachycardia known as torsades de pointes (Fig. 1.17). Tachycardia is often preceded by a short-long-short series of changes in cycle length. Episodes tend to be paroxysmal, recurrent, and may become life-threatening. Therefore, it is critical that the clinical syndrome be recognized, any offending drugs be stopped, and any electrolyte deficiencies be corrected. A summary of the various conditions associated with torsades de pointes is provided in Box 1.3.

Permanent pacing may also be of help in patients with the long QT syndrome, especially for bradycardic patients who have a history of ventricular arrhythmias or syncope. It provides more uniform repolarization and an increased heart rate, which will shorten the QT interval.[30] Permanent pacing may also permit the use of beta blockers, known to be of benefit in this syndrome, without worsening the resting bradycardia. The potential benefit of an implantable defibrillator should be considered in these patients.

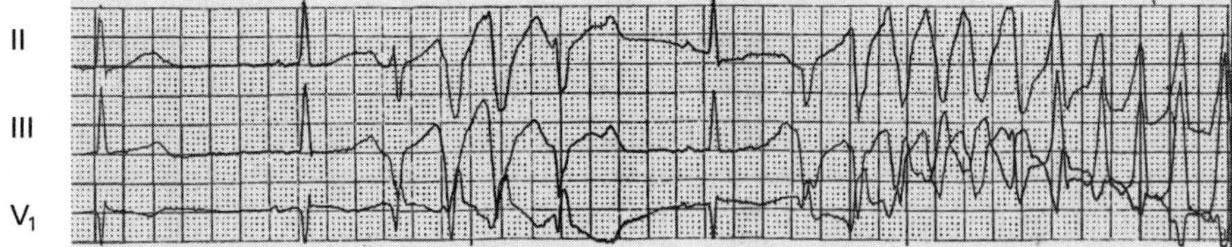

Figure 1.17. A rhythm strip of ECG leads II, III, and V_1 shows paroxysms of polymorphic ventricular tachycardia in an individual with QT interval prolongation and recurrent syncope. Note the short-long-short cycle length sequence that initiates the arrhythmia. In the absence of an identifiable cause, the patient received an implantable cardioverter defibrillator.

Box 1.3. Causes of Torsades de Pointes

- Electrolyte abnormalities
  - Hypokalemia
  - Hypomagnesemia
  - Hypocalcemia
- Antiarrhythmic agents
  - Quinidine
  - Procainamide
  - Disopyramide
  - Amiodarone
  - Sotalol
  - Dofetilide
  - Ibutilide
- Hereditary long QT syndrome(s)
- Bradyarrhythmias
- Liquid protein diets
- Myocardial ischemia/infarction
- Neurologic events
  - Subarachnoid hemorrhage
  - Head trauma
- Noncardiac drugs
  - Antihistamines (astemizole, terfenadine)
  - Tricyclic and tetracyclic antidepressants
  - Phenothiazines
  - Cisapride
  - Erythromycin
  - Trimethoprim sulfamethoxazole
  - Chloroquine
  - Amantadine
  - Pentamidine
- Toxins
  - Organophosphates
  - Arsenic

See www.Torsades.org for updated list.

Because radiofrequency ablation successfully treats most common reentrant SVT arrhythmias, antitachycardia pacing is now rarely used for these arrhythmias. There is, however, growing interest in permanent pacing therapies for atrial fibrillation. In patients with concomitant sinus bradycardia, dual-site atrial pacing combined with drug therapy may reduce the recurrence rates of atrial fibrillation.[31] In addition, preliminary data suggest that antitachycardia pacing may terminate atrial fibrillation and atrial tachycardias in some patients.[32] Ventricular antitachycardia pacing without back-up defibrillation is contraindicated due to the risk of tachycardia acceleration.

The indications for permanent pacing to *prevent or terminate* tachycardias are:

Class I

1. Sustained pause-dependent VT, with or without prolonged QT, in which the efficacy of pacing is thoroughly documented. (Level of evidence: C.)

Class IIa

1. High-risk patients with congenital long-QT syndrome. (Level of evidence: C.)
2. Symptomatic recurrent SVT that is reproducibly terminated by pacing in the unlikely event that catheter ablation and/or drugs fail to control the arrhythmia or produce intolerable side effects. (Level of evidence: C.)

Class IIb

1. Recurrent SVT or atrial flutter that is reproducibly terminated by pacing as an alternative to drug therapy or ablation. (Level of evidence: C.)
2. AV reentrant or AV node-reentrant supraventricular tachycardia not responsive to medical or ablative therapy. (Level of evidence: C.)
3. Prevention of symptomatic, drug-refractory recurrent atrial fibrillation in patients with co-existing sinus node dysfunction. (Level of evidence: B.)

Class III

1. Tachycardias frequently accelerated or converted to fibrillation by pacing.
2. The presence of accessory pathways with the capacity for rapid anterograde conduction whether or not the pathways participate in the mechanism of the tachycardia.
3. Frequent or complex ventricular ectopic activity without sustained VT in the absence of the long-QT syndrome.
4. Torsades de pointes VT due to reversible causes.

Pacing for Children and Adolescents, Including Congenital Heart Block

The general indications for pacing in children and adolescents are similar to those for adults with several additional considerations. The diagnosis of significant bradycardia in children depends on age, presence and type of congenital heart disease, and cardiac physiology. Following surgery for congenital heart disease, patients may have postoperative AV block that if untreated by pacing will worsen their prognosis.[33] Congenital heart disease patients may also have tachycardia-bradycardia syndrome, but the benefits of pacing for this indication are less clear. Congenital heart diseases such as corrected transposition of great arteries, ostium primum atrial septal defects, and ventricular septal defects may be associated with complete heart block.

Congenital complete AV block is a rare anomaly that results from abnormal embryonic development of the AV node and is not associated with structural heart disease in 50% of cases. Congenital complete heart block is also associated with maternal lupus erythematosus. Most of the children with isolated congenital complete AV block have a stable escape rhythm with a narrow complex. Pacing is generally indicated in children with complete heart block if the heart rate in the awake child is less than 50 beats per minute or if associated with left ventricular systolic dysfunction or ventricular arrhythmias. The indications for pacing in congenital complete AV block have been clarified by a prospective study demonstrating improved survival and reduced syncope, myocardial dysfunction, and mitral regurgitation even among asymptomatic patients.[34,35] Exercise testing does not predict future cardiac events in this population.

The indications for permanent pacing in children and adolescents are:

Class I

1. Advanced second- or third-degree AV block associated with symptomatic bradycardia, ventricular dysfunction, or low cardiac output. (Level of evidence: C.)
2. Sinus node dysfunction with correlation of symptoms during age-inappropriate bradycardia. The definition of bradycardia varies with the patient's age and expected heart rate. (Level of evidence: B.)
3. Postoperative advanced second- or third-degree AV block that is not expected to resolve or persists at least 7 days after cardiac surgery. (Levels of evidence: B, C.)
4. Congenital third-degree AV block with a wide QRS escape rhythm, complex ventricular ectopy, or ventricular dysfunction. (Level of evidence: B.)
5. Congenital third-degree AV block in the infant with the ventricular rate less than 50 to 55 beats per minute or with congenital heart disease and a ventricular rate less than 70 beats per minute. (Levels of evidence: B, C.)
6. Sustained pause-dependent VT, with or without prolonged QT, in which the efficacy of pacing is thoroughly documented. (Level of evidence: B.)

Class IIa

1. Bradycardia-tachycardia syndrome with the need for long-term antiarrhythmic treatment other than digitalis. (Level of evidence: C.)
2. Congenital third-degree AV block beyond the first year of life with an average heart rate less than 50 beats per minute, abrupt pauses in ven-

tricular rate that are two or three times the basic cycle length, or associated with symptoms due to chronotropic incompetence. (Level of evidence: B.)
3. Long-QT syndrome with 2:1 AV or third-degree AV block. (Level of evidence: B.)
4. Asymptomatic sinus bradycardia in the child with complex congenital heart disease with resting heart rate less than 40 beats per minute or pauses in ventricular rate more than 3 seconds. (Level of evidence: C.)
5. Patients with congenital heart disease and impaired hemodynamics due to sinus bradycardia or loss of AV synchrony. (Level of evidence: C.)

Class IIb
1. Transient postoperative third-degree AV block that reverts to sinus rhythm with residual bifascicular block. (Level of evidence: C.)
2. Congenital third-degree AV block in the asymptomatic infant, child, adolescent, or young adult with an acceptable rate, narrow QRS complex, and normal ventricular function. (Level of evidence: B.)
3. Asymptomatic sinus bradycardia in the adolescent with congenital heart disease with resting heart rate less than 40 beats per minute or pauses in ventricular rate more than 3 seconds. (Level of evidence: C.)
4. Neuromuscular diseases with any degree of AV block (including first-degree AV block), with or without symptoms, because there may be unpredictable progression of AV conduction disease.

Class III
1. Transient postoperative AV block with return of normal AV conduction. (Level of evidence: B.)
2. Asymptomatic postoperative bifascicular block with or without first-degree AV block. (Level of evidence: C.)
3. Asymptomatic type I second-degree AV block. (Level of evidence: C.)
4. Asymptomatic sinus bradycardia in the adolescent with longest RR interval less than 3 seconds and minimum heart rate more than 40 beats per minute. (Level of evidence: C.)

Orthotopic Cardiac Transplantation

Bradyarrhythmias following orthotopic cardiac transplantation are usually due to sinus node dysfunction, presumably secondary to surgical trauma to the donor sinus node or to interruption of its blood supply. The incidence of sinus node dysfunction in this population is up to 23%, but there is a growing realization that the condition is often benign and reversible within 6 to 12 months after transplant.[36]

The indications for permanent pacing after orthotopic cardiac transplant are:

Class I
1. Symptomatic bradyarrhythmias/chronotropic incompetence not expected to resolve and other class I indications for permanent pacing. (Level of evidence: C.)

Class IIb

1. Symptomatic bradyarrhythmias/chronotropic incompetence that, although transient, may persist for months and require intervention. (Level of evidence: C.)

Class III

1. Asymptomatic bradyarrhythmias.

Permanent Pacing After the Acute Phase of Acute Myocardial Infarction

Bradyarrhythmias and conduction defects are relatively common after acute myocardial infarction. In patients who have these problems, a decision about permanent pacing must be made prior to the patient's discharge from the hospital. It is important to realize that the indications for temporary pacing in the setting of acute myocardial infarction are different from those for permanent pacing following infarction. Unfortunately, there is some uncertainty regarding permanent pacing for these patients because large prospective controlled trials have not been performed. In addition, the criteria for permanent pacing in patients after a myocardial infarction do not necessarily require the presence of symptoms and the need for temporary pacing in the acute stages of infarction is not by itself an indication for permanent pacing.

The prognosis for these patients is strongly influenced by the amount of underlying myocardial damage.[37] In general, sinus node dysfunction tends to be benign and reversible; and permanent pacemakers are rarely required. Similarly, second-degree and even third-degree AV block after inferior wall myocardial infarction is usually reversible and rarely requires permanent pacing. In contrast, conduction defects after an anterior wall myocardial infarction usually warrant permanent pacemaker insertion, although mortality remains extremely high because of pump failure (Fig. 1.18).

The indications for permanent pacing following acute myocardial infarction are:

Class I

1. Persistent second-degree AV block in the His-Purkinje system with bundle branch block or third-degree AV block within or below the His-Purkinje system after acute myocardial infarction. (Level of evidence: B.)
2. Transient advanced (second- or third-degree) infranodal AV block and associated bundle-branch block. If the site of block is uncertain, an electrophysiology study may be necessary. (Level of evidence: B.)
3. Persistent and symptomatic second- or third-degree AV block. (Level of evidence: C.)

Class IIb

1. Persistent second- or third-degree AV block at the AV node level. (Level of evidence: B)

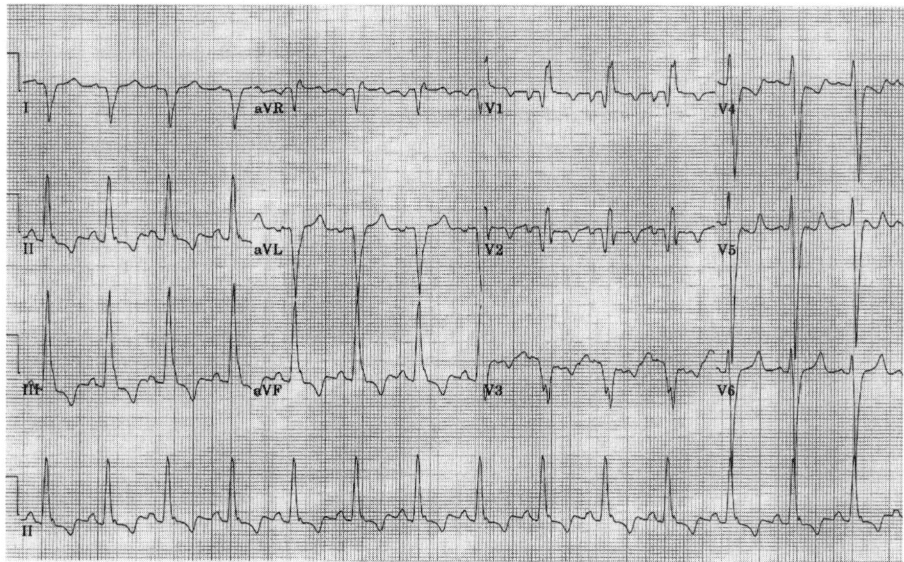

Figure 1.18. A standard 12-lead ECG from an individual with a large anteroseptal myocardial infarction complicated by congestive heart failure and right bundle branch block with right axis deviation, presumably due to left posterior fascicular block. The patient developed transient high-degree AV block 72 hours after admission (a class I indication) and subsequently underwent permanent pacemaker implantation.

Class III

1. Transient AV block in the absence of intraventricular conduction defects. (Level of evidence: B.)
2. Transient AV block in the presence of isolated left anterior fascicular block. (Level of evidence: B.)
3. Acquired left anterior fascicular block in the absence of AV block. (Level of evidence: B.)
4. Persistent first-degree AV block in the presence of bundle-branch block that is old or age indeterminate. (Level of evidence: B.)

Permanent Pacemaker Mode Selection

The selection of a permanent pacing mode for any given patient is largely based on the desire to maintain AV synchrony. Intuitively, the preservation of AV synchrony may seem desirable in all patients. However, the added cost and complexity of dual-chamber systems and the contradictory data concerning the benefits of AV sequential pacing for some patient groups are all a basis for the ongoing evaluation of the true advantages to dual-chamber pacing. It is generally accepted that AV synchrony may benefit patients with left ventricular systolic dysfunction, diastolic dysfunction, or heart failure by preserving the atrial contribution to ventricular filling. In patients with neurally mediated syncope, single-chamber atrial demand inhibited (AAI) or ventricular demand inhibited (VVI) pacing may not relieve symptoms because heart block or pacemaker syndrome, respectively, may occur during pacing. AV sequential pacing is generally accepted in this situation as well. AAI pacing is reserved for patients who have isolated sinus node dysfunction and no known or anticipated AV block. VVI pacing is indicated for patients with chronic atrial arrhythmias that are not expected to return to sinus rhythm. Paroxysmal atrial arrhythmias are no longer a contraindication to universal (DDD)pacing since the advent of mode switching algorithms.

The optimal mode of pacing for sick sinus syndrome, the most common indication for permanent pacing, is less clear. Numerous retrospective uncontrolled studies have suggested that pacing to maintain AV synchrony (AAI/DDD) reduces stroke, atrial fibrillation, heart failure, and mortality when compared to VVI pacing.[38] The current trends are to minimize the use of ventricular pacing even in DDD mode because worsening heart failure and mortality may result. These findings have not been consistently validated in the randomized, controlled studies. The most recent studies to evaluate the benefits of AV sequential versus VVI pacing in this population are listed in Table 1.3.[13,14,39–45] It should be noted that a high incidence of crossover from VVI to DDD pacing in most studies may influence the results. Taken together, the present data suggest that pacing to maintain AV synchrony in sick sinus syndrome does not affect mortality or the incidence of heart failure but does reduce atrial fibrillation and shows a trend toward reduced thromboembolism. Completion of long-term follow-up (mean: 6.4 years) from the Canadian Trial of Physiologic Pacing (CTOPP) trial showed no difference between VVI and DDD pacing with respect to cardiovascular death, stroke, or total mortality, but did show a persistent and significant relative risk reduction of 20% for the development of atrial fibrillation (decreased by physiologic pacing).[40] The high incidence of pacemaker syndrome with VVI pacing also favors the use of DDD/AAI pacing in patients with sick sinus syndrome, this incidence approaching 26% in one study (PASE). General guidelines for pacemaker mode selection are listed in Table 1.4, with the caveat that most recommendations are based on current clinical practice rather than controlled clinical studies.

INDICATIONS FOR TEMPORARY CARDIAC PACING

The following section reviews the clinical settings in which temporary cardiac pacing is indicated. Chapter 4 presents a review of the techniques and complications of temporary cardiac pacing. A summary of the general indications for temporary pacing is given in Box 1.4.

Acute Myocardial Infarction

In the setting of an acute myocardial infarction, several different types of conduction disturbances may become manifest. They include abnormalities of sinus

Table 1.3. Clinical Trials of AV Sequential versus VVI Pacing for Sick Sinus Syndrome and AV Block

Study	Population	No. of Patients	Mean Follow-up Period (mo)	Annualized Mortality	Stroke	Atrial Fibrillation	Crossover
Andersen et al. (39)	SSS without AV block	225	66	6.4% AAI 9.0% VVI	12% AAI 23% VVI★	24% AAI 35% VVI	1.7%
PASE (13)	SSS > 65 yr old	175	18	13.3% DDD 8.0% VVI	20% DDD 31% VVI	19% DDD 28% VVI	28%
CTOPP (40, 41)	Any bradycardia	2568	36	6.3% DDD 6.6% VVI	1.0% DDD 1.1% VVI	5.3% DDD 6.6% VVI★	<5%
Pac-a-Tach (42)	SSS	198	24	3.4% DDD 1.6% VVI	Not reported —	43% DDD 48% VVI	44%
MOST (14)	SSS	2000	30	6% DDD[NC] 7% VVI	1.7% DDD[NC] 2.7% VVI	15% DDD† 21% VVI	37%
Mattioli et al. (43)	SSS or AV block	350	24	Not reported	10% DDD 20% VVI★,‡	8% DDD 21% VVI★,‡	Not reported
STOP-AF (44)	SSS	350	24	Pending	Pending	Pending	—
UK PACE (45)	AV block	2021	54	RR 0.96 (VVI/VVIR vs DDDR)	RR 1.28	Pending	—

★ $P \leq .05$ AV synchronous vs VVI pacing.

† $P = .008$.

‡ Values estimated from graphical representation in original report.

Abbreviations: Crossover = crossover between pacing modes; SSS = sick sinus syndrome; NC = no difference between VVIR and DDDR.

Table 1.4. General Guidelines for Permanent Pacemaker Mode Selection

Mode	Recommended	Not Recommended or Contraindicated	Comment
AAI	• Sinus node dysfunction in absence of known or anticipated AV block	• Heart block known or anticipated • Atrial tachyarrhythmias • Neurally mediated syncope	• Contributions of AV block and vasodepressor response may be variable over time in patients with neurally mediated syncope
VVI	• Chronic atrial tachyarrhythmias	• Heart failure • Left ventricular systolic or diastolic dysfunction • Neurally mediated syncope	• Avoid in patients with structural heart disease when atrial contribution to ventricular filling is important. • Use in SSS may lead to pacemaker syndrome, increased stroke, and AF. • Ventricular pacing associated with CHF and mortality in some patient groups
DDD	• Heart failure • Left ventricular systolic or diastolic dysfunction • Valvular heart disease • Neurally mediated syncope • SSS with AV block	• Chronic atrial tachyarrhythmias	• Recommended in presence of most structural heart disease to preserve AV synchrony. • May reduce stroke and AF in SSS. • Ventricular pacing associated with CHF and mortality in some patient groups
VDD	• Heart block with intact sinus node function and chronotropic competence	• Sinus node dysfunction or chronotropic incompetence • Chronic atrial tachyarrhythmias	• Single pass lead systems simplify implant
Bi V	• Medically refractory class III–IV CHF • Ejection fraction > 35% • QRS ≥ 130 msec	• Class I CHF • Preserved ejection fraction • Absence of ventricular dyssynchrony	• Improves symptoms and possibly survival in some patient groups

Abbreviations: AF = atrial fibrillation; SSS = sick sinus syndrome; Bi V = biventricular; CHF = congestive heart failure; AAI = atrial demand inhibited; DDD = universal; VVI = ventricular demand inhibited; VDD = atrial synchronous ventricular inhibited.

Box 1.4. Indications for Temporary Pacing

In Acute Myocardial Infarction
- Medically refractory symptomatic sinus node dysfunction
- Mobitz II second-degree AV block with acute anterior infarction
- Third-degree AV block with anterior infarction
- New bifascicular block
- Alternating bundle branch block
- Alternating Wenckebach block
- New bundle branch block with anterior infarction
- Bundle branch block of indeterminate age with anterior or indeterminate location infarct
- Medically refractory AV block with bradycardia and symptoms regardless of infarct location

In Absence of Acute Myocardial Infarction
- Medically refractory symptomatic bradycardia
  - sinus node dysfunction
  - second or third degree AV block
- Third-degree AV block with wide QRS escape or ventricular rate <50 bpm

Prophylactic
- Swan-Ganz catheterization or endocardial biopsy in patient with left bundle branch block
- Cardioversion in setting of sick sinus syndrome
- New AV or bundle branch block with acute endocarditis (especially aortic valve endocarditis)
- Perioperatively in patient with bifascicular block and history of syncope
- To allow pharmacologic treatment with drugs that worsen bradycardias

Treatment of Tachyarrhythmias
- Termination of recurrent ventricular or supraventricular tachycardia
- Suppression of bradycardia-dependent ventricular tachyarrhythmias including torsades de pointes

impulse formation or conduction, disorders of atrioventricular conduction, and disorders of intraventricular conduction. In general, any patient with bradyarrhythmias that are associated with symptoms or cause hemodynamic compromise must be treated. The ways of identifying the patient populations at greatest risk for the development of a significant bradyarrhythmia during acute myocardial infarction and in whom temporary pacing should be performed prophylactically are discussed below. It is important to realize that the indications for temporary pacing in the setting of acute myocardial infarction are different from those for permanent pacing following infarction.

Sinus Node Abnormalities: Sinus node dysfunction may include sinus bradycardia, sinus arrest, and/or sinoatrial exit block. The incidence of these electrocardiographic abnormalities is quite variable, ranging from 5% to 30% in different series.[46] Abnormalities of sinus rhythm are more common, with inferoposterior infarction because either the right or left circumflex coronary artery is occluded—these arteries most commonly supply the sinus node. Another potential reason is chemically mediated activation of receptors on the posterior left ventricular wall—these receptors are supplied by vagal afferent fibers. Treatment of sinus bradycardia is not necessary, unless symptoms such as worsening myocardial ischemia, heart failure, or hypotension are documented. Atropine may be administered for vagally mediated bradycardia. If bradycardia is prolonged and severe, or is not responsive to atropine, temporary cardiac pacing is indicated.

Disorders of Atrioventricular Conduction: Atrioventricular block occurs *without* associated intraventricular conduction system abnormalities in 12% to 25% of patients with acute myocardial infarction.[47] The incidence of this finding depends largely on the patient population and the site of infarction. First-degree AV block occurs in 2% to 12% of patients, second-degree AV block in 3% to 10% of patients, and third-degree AV block in 3% to 7% of patients. The majority of patients with abnormalities of atrioventricular conduction without bundle branch block have evidence of an inferoposterior infarction (approximately 70%). The reasons for the increased incidence of AV conduction abnormalities are related to the coronary blood supply to the AV node. The coronary artery supplying the inferoposterior wall of the left ventricle is typically the right or left circumflex coronary, which is occluded during an inferior infarction. In addition, activation of cardiac reflexes with augmentation of parasympathetic tone during inferior ischemia (infarction) may also be responsible. In some cases, AV block may be due to release of adenosine caused by inferior ischemia or during inferior infarction.[48]

The risk of progression from first-degree AV block to high-grade AV block (during inferior infarction) varies from 10% to 30%, and that of second-degree AV block to complete heart block is approximately 35%. As would be expected, the development of high-grade AV block in the setting of acute inferoposterior infarction is usually associated with narrow QRS complex escape rhythms (Figs. 1.19 and 1.20). The junctional escape rhythm usually remains stable at 50 to 60 pulses per minute and can be increased by intravenous atropine, so even complete AV block may not require temporary pacing in this situation.

Type I second-degree AV block with a narrow QRS almost always represents a conduction block in the AV node, and temporary cardiac pacing is rarely required unless the patient has concomitant symptoms. Type I second-degree AV block with a wide QRS complex may represent a conduction block in the AV node or His bundle or contralateral bundle branch block. In these patients, especially in the setting of anterior myocardial infarction, temporary prophylactic pacing must be considered. In patients with type II second-degree AV block and a wide QRS complex in the setting of inferior infarction, or with a wide or narrow QRS complex during an anterior myocardial infarction, a temporary pacemaker should be inserted. Patients with a narrow QRS complex and type II second-degree AV block in the setting of inferior infarction rarely progress to complete heart block.

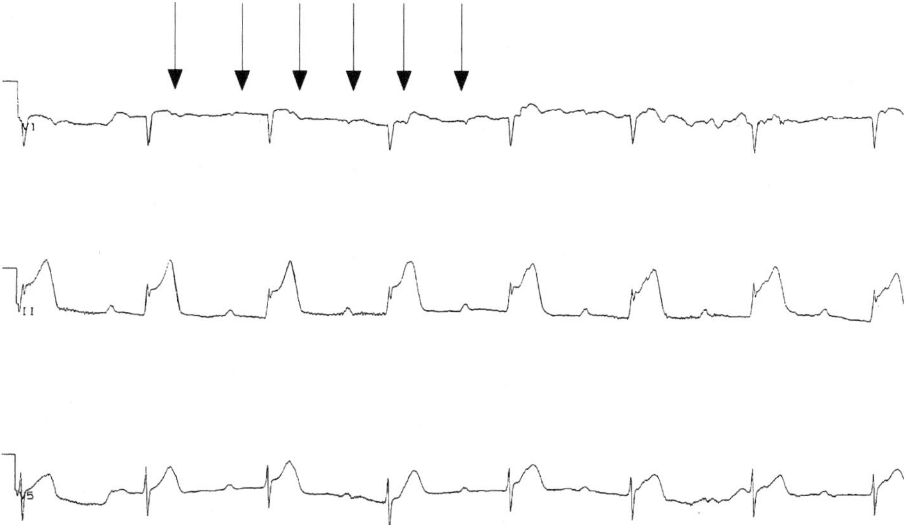

Figure 1.19. A 3-lead (standard leads V_1, II, and V_5) rhythm strip in a 58-year-old man with an acute inferior wall myocardial infarction and complete AV block (the arrows in lead V_1 identify the P waves) with an escape rate of 45 ppm. Despite the slow rate, the patient did not exhibit signs or symptoms of hemodynamic compromise, so no therapy was required. Normal conduction resumed approximately 24 hours later.

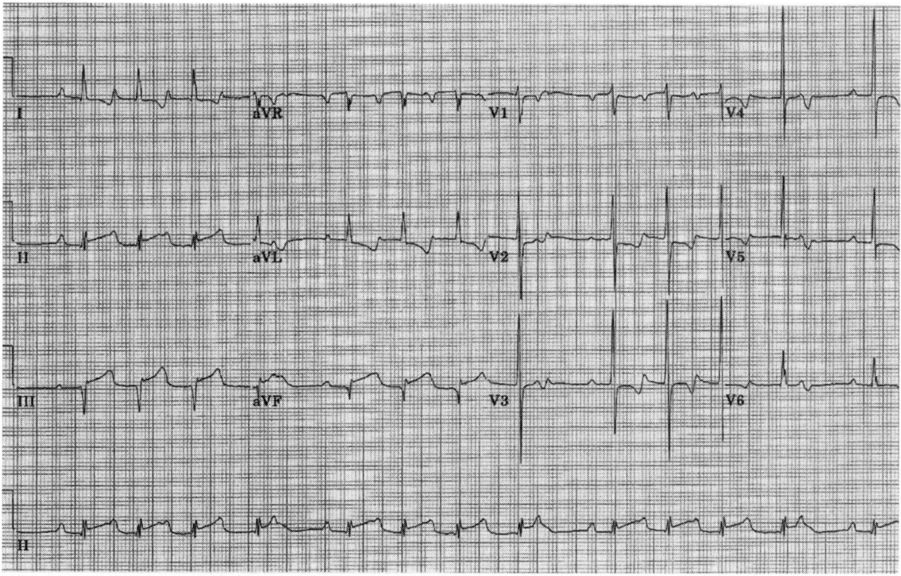

Figure 1.20. A standard 12-lead ECG from a 67-year-old woman with an acute inferior wall myocardial infarction. She received 0.6 mg of atropine intravenously for treatment of sinus bradycardia and developed type I second-degree AV block with a 5:4 Wenckebach sequence. Normal conduction resumed in several hours when the sinus tachycardia due to atropine resolved.

Several special situations are worthy of consideration. Patients with high-grade AV block occurring in the setting of right ventricular infarction tend to be less responsive to intravenous atropine and may demonstrate markedly improved hemodynamics during AV sequential pacing.[49] The mechanism for this hemodynamic improvement is probably a reflection of the restrictive physiology that the infarcted right ventricle demonstrates. Another group of patients who may benefit from prophylactic temporary pacing are those with acute inferior wall infarction with alternating Wenckebach periods. This electrocardiographic finding is rare (2%), but without temporary pacing it frequently leads to hemodynamic embarrassment.

In contrast to inferior wall infarction, high-grade AV block complicating an anterior wall infarction is usually located within the His–Purkinje system. The transition from the first nonconducted P wave to high-grade AV block is often abrupt, and the resulting escape rhythm is typically slow and unreliable. Conducted beats usually have a wide QRS complex. In general, an interruption of the blood supply to the anterior wall and the interventricular septum severe enough to cause AV block usually causes severe left ventricular dysfunction and results in high mortality. Emergency temporary pacing and prophylactic pacing are indicated, although survival may not be significantly improved because of the extent of myocardial damage.[50]

Disorders of Intraventricular Conduction System: A number of studies have examined the incidence of development of new bundle branch block in the setting of acute myocardial infarction and have determined that it varies between 5% and 15%, depending on the site of infarction. New bundle branch block is three times more likely during anterior infarction than during inferior infarction, because the left anterior descending coronary artery provides the major blood supply to the His bundle and the bundle branches. Not surprisingly, there is a high incidence of heart failure in this setting, and the associated high cardiac mortality leads to controversy as to whether temporary or permanent pacing improves the poor prognosis in these patients. As with anterior myocardial infarction and complete heart block, new bundle branch block reflects extensive myocardial damage.

Multiple studies have shown that patients with acute infarction and bundle branch block have a fourfold to fivefold increased risk of progression to high-grade AV block (e.g., an increase from 4% to 18%).[51,52] Both in-hospital and out-of-hospital mortality are higher for patients presenting with bundle branch block during acute infarction. The basis of this increased mortality may be a variety of causes, including heart failure, infarct extension, ventricular tachycardia, and heart block. The mortality of patients with bundle branch block and acute infarction is 30% to 40%, compared with 10% to 15% in patients without bundle branch block. Most of the increase in cardiac mortality appears to be related to the degree of heart failure.

Several small retrospective studies have attempted to identify groups of patients who may be at increased risk of progression to high-grade heart block.[51,52] Unfortunately, many of these studies are limited by their retrospective nature, their small sample size, or their ascertainment bias. On the basis of the results of several studies, patients with conduction system abnormalities who are recommended to have temporary pacemakers inserted prophylactically are listed in Table 1.5.

Patients with a new bundle branch block and first-degree AV block or old bifascicular block and first-degree AV block are at intermediate risk of progression (19% to 29%) to high-grade AV block; they may undergo prophylactic pacing depending on the availability of facilities for emergency placement of a temporary pacemaker. Because the greatest risk of progression to complete heart block occurs in the first 5 days following infarction, these decisions should be made promptly so that temporary pacing may be instituted.

The Multicenter Investigation of the Limitation of Infarct Size (MILIS) study suggested a simpler method of risk stratification.[53] A "risk score" for the development of complete heart block was devised. Patients with any of the following conduction disturbances were given one point: first-degree AV block, type I second-degree AV block, type II second-degree AV block, left anterior fascicular block, left posterior fascicular block, right bundle branch block, and left bundle branch block. The presence of no risk factors was associated with a 1.2% risk of third-degree AV block, one risk factor with a 7.8% risk, two risk factors with a 25% risk, and three risk factors with 36.4% risk of complete heart block. These findings were validated by testing the risk score in over 3000 patients from previously published studies. The risk score appears to be an alternative to risk stratification using combinations of conduction disorders.

The effect of thrombolytic and early interventional therapies on the subsequent development of high-grade AV block in patients presenting with acute infarction and intraventricular conduction system disease has been poorly studied. Although the incidence of complete AV block in acute myocardial

Table 1.5. Risk of High-Grade AV Block during Acute Myocardial Infarction

Patient Group	Risk of High-Grade AV Block
First-degree AV block and new bifascicular BBB	38–43%
First-degree AV block and old bifascicular BBB	20–50%
New bifascicular BBB	15–31%
Alternating BBB	44%
MILIS risk score[a]	
0	1.2%
1	7.8%
2	25%
3	36.4%

[a] 1 point each for first-degree AV block, Mobitz I second-degree AV block, Mobitz II second-degree AV block, left anterior fascicular block, left posterior fascicular block, right bundle branch block, left bundle branch block.

infarctions has decreased following thrombolytic therapy, the mortality still remains high.[54]

The most recent American Heart Association guidelines for temporary transvenous pacing in the setting of acute myocardial infarction are[55]:

Class I

1. Asystole
2. Symptomatic bradycardia (includes sinus bradycardia with hypotension and type I second-degree AV block with hypotension not responsive to atropine)
3. Bilateral bundle branch block (BBB; alternating BBB or right BBB [RBBB] with alternating left anterior fascicular block [LAFB]/left posterior fascicular block [LPFB]) (any age)
4. New or indeterminate age bifascicular block (RBBB with LAFB or LPFB, or LBBB) with first-degree AV block
5. Mobitz type II second-degree AV block

Class IIa

1. RBBB and LAFB or LPFB (new or indeterminate)
2. RBBB with first-degree AV block
3. LBBB, new or indeterminate
4. Incessant ventricular tachycardia, for atrial or ventricular overdrive pacing
5. Recurrent sinus pauses (greater than 3 seconds) not responsive to atropine

Class IIb

1. Bifascicular block of indeterminate age
2. New or age-indeterminate isolated RBBB

Class III

1. First-degree heart block
2. Type I second-degree AV block with normal hemodynamics
3. Accelerated idioventricular rhythm
4. BBB or fascicular block known to exist before acute myocardial infarction

PACING DURING CARDIAC CATHETERIZATION

During catheterization of the right side of the heart, manipulation of the catheter may induce a transient RBBB in up to 10% of patients. This block generally lasts for seconds or minutes but can occasionally last for hours or days. Trauma induced by right ventricular endomyocardial biopsy also may result in temporary, or rarely long-lasting, RBBB. This is a problem only in patients with preexisting LBBB, in whom complete heart block may result. We therefore recommend placement of a temporary transvenous pacing wire in patients who are undergoing right heart catheterization or biopsy in the presence of previously known LBBB. Catheterization of the left side of the heart in patients with known preexisting RBBB only rarely gives rise to complete heart block because of the short length of the left bundle branch. Significant bradycardia and asystole can occur during injection of the right coronary artery. This complication is extremely rare, and the placement of a temporary pacing catheter does not alter the morbidity or mortality of catheterization. The bradycardia usually resolves after several seconds. The same comments apply in general to placement of a temporary pacing wire during angioplasty.

PREOPERATIVE PACING

One of the questions most frequently asked of a consulting cardiologist by both surgeons and anesthesiologists is whether it is necessary to insert a temporary pacing catheter in patients with bifascicular block undergoing general anesthesia. The results of several studies have shown that the incidence of intraoperative and perioperative complete heart block is quite low. There does not appear to be any benefit from preoperative prophylactic pacemaker insertion. Even in patients with first-degree AV block and bifascicular block, there is a very low incidence of perioperative high-grade heart block.

In patients who have bifascicular block and also type II second-degree AV block or a history of unexplained syncope or presyncope; however, the risk of development of high-grade AV block is higher, and a temporary pacemaker should be inserted. The appearance of new bifascicular block in the immediate postoperative period should also lead to insertion of a temporary pacemaker and should raise suspicion of an intraoperative myocardial infarction. The general availability of transcutaneous pacing may make it an acceptable alternative to temporary transvenous pacing in lower risk individuals, although poor patient tolerance is often a limitation.

Open-heart surgery tends to be associated with a somewhat higher incidence of postoperative bradyarrhythmias than does noncardiac surgery, due to the direct trauma to the conduction system and interference with blood supply. Cardiac surgeons generally implant temporary epicardial pacing wires at the time of surgery to facilitate temporary pacing. The major problem then becomes determining how long to wait for resumption of AV conduction and normalization of sinus node function before implanting a permanent pacemaker. Conventionally, a permanent pacemaker is recommended if the problem persists longer than 5 to 7 days after the operation. Although normal conduction may resume after this period of time, in the absence of definitive information about the natural history of these disorders, permanent pacing seems to be a prudent choice.

OTHER TEMPORARY PACING

Temporary pacing is indicated in patients with new AV or BBB in the setting of acute bacterial endocarditis. The development of a new conduction system abnormality generally suggests that there is a perivalvular (ring) abscess that has extended to involve the conduction system near the AV node and/or the His bundle. The endocarditis generally involves the non-coronary cusp of the aortic valve. In one study, high-grade or complete heart block developed in 22% of patients with aortic valve endocarditis and new first-degree AV block.[56] Although these studies are retrospective, the patient with development of new AV block or BBB, especially in the setting of aortic valve endocarditis, should probably undergo temporary pacing while cardiac evaluation continues.

Treatment of tumors of the head and/or neck or around the carotid sinus may in some circumstances give rise to high-grade AV block. Temporary pacing may be required during surgical treatment, radiation therapy, or chemotherapy. If the tumor responds poorly, permanent pacing may be necessary in some cases. The long-term risk for subsequent heart block due to tumor recurrence is difficult to predict in some cases.

Lyme disease, a tickborne spirochete infection, causes a systemic infection with arthritis, skin lesions, myalgias, meningoencephalitis, and cardiac involvement in 5% to 10% of patients.[57] Lyme disease is epidemic in the summer months in the northeastern United States. Carditis typically occurs relatively late in the course of the illness, usually 4 to 8 weeks after the onset of symptoms. AV block is the most common manifestation of carditis and tends to be transient. Block is most common at the level of the AV node and fluctuation between first-degree and higher degrees of AV block is frequent. Temporary cardiac pacing may be required, but the conduction disturbances usually resolve spontaneously, especially with antibiotic treatment, so permanent cardiac pacing rarely is necessary. Similar conduction disturbances can occasionally be seen in patients with viral myocarditis, as well as with other tickborne infections.

A number of medications may produce transient bradycardia that may require temporary pacing until the drug has been stopped (see Box 1.2). These drugs may cause sinus node dysfunction and/or AV block; if used in combination, their effects may become more potent and exacerbate mild or latent conduction system disease. If long-term therapy with these agents is necessary for an underlying disorder and a substitute cannot be found, permanent pacing may be required.

Treatment of Tachycardias with Temporary Pacing

Temporary cardiac pacing has been used for the termination and/or prevention of a variety of arrhythmias. Pacing-termination of ventricular tachycardia is discussed in detail in Chapter 8 on the implantable cardioverter defibrillator and will not be dealt with here. Type I atrial flutter can be successfully pace-terminated approximately 65% of the time in an unselected population and in over 90% of patients in whom atrial flutter develops after surgery.[58] Due to the development of radiofrequency catheter ablation techniques, there is currently less interest in pace-termination of atrial flutter. Similarly, the most common varieties of paroxysmal supraventricular tachycardia are usually pace-terminable but tend to be equally amenable to radiofrequency ablation.

Torsades de pointes is a polymorphic ventricular tachycardia with a sinusoidal electrocardiographic appearance, due to the QRS complex undulating about the baseline. It results from prolongation and dispersion (inequality in different parts of the ventricle) of myocardial repolarization, and is often reflected on the surface ECG by a prolonged QT or QT-U interval. Episodes of tachycardia are often preceded by a short-long-short series of changes in cycle length. Importantly, episodes tend to be recurrent, paroxysmal, and nonsustained initially, but may become sustained later unless the underlying condition is identified and corrected. Therefore, it is critical that the clinical syndrome be recognized, any offending toxins or drugs be stopped, and any electrolyte deficiencies be corrected. (A summary of the causes of torsades de pointes is provided in Table 1.3.) In some patients these treatments will be adequate; in some patients, other forms of therapy must be considered. Overdrive atrial and/or ventricular pacing may be effective in suppressing torsades de pointes because it provides more uniform repolarization and an increased heart rate, which will shorten the QT interval. Intravenous magnesium and also isoproterenol (which also increases heart rate and shortens repolarization) may also be effective in suppressing torsades de pointes, although the latter is associated with troubling side effects. For individuals who have recurrent symptoms refractory to conventional management, implantation of an implantable cardioverter defibrillator should be strongly considered.

REFERENCES

1. Schlant RC, Silverman ME. Anatomy of the heart. In: Hurst JW, ed. The Heart. 6th ed. New York: McGraw-Hill, 1986:16–37.
2. Phibbs B, Friedman HS, Graboys TB, et al. Indications for pacing in the treatment of bradyarrhythmias report of an independent study group. JAMA 1984;252:1307–1311.
3. Gregorators G, Abrams J, Epstein AE. ACC/AHA/NASPE 2002 Guideline update for Implantation of Cardiac Pacemakers and Antiarrhythmia Devices: Summary Article: A Report of the American Heart College of Cardiology/American Heart Association Task Force on Practice Guidelines (ACC/AHA/NASPE Committee to Update the 1998 Pacemaker Guidelines). Circulation 2002;106:2145–2161.
4. Dhingra RC, Denes P, Wu D, et al. Prospective observations in patients with chronic bundle branch block and H-V prolongation. Circulation 1976;53:600–604.
5. McAnulty JH, Rahimtoola SH, Murphy E, et al. Natural history of high risk bundle branch block: final report of a prospective study. N Engl J Med 1982;307: 137–143.
6. McAnulty JH, Rahimtoola SH. Bundle branch block. Prog Cardiovasc Dis 1984;26:333–354.
7. Scheinman MM, Peters RW, Sauve MJ, et al. Value of the H-Q interval in patients with bundle branch block and the role of prophylactic permanent pacing. Am J Cardiol 1982;50:1316–1322.
8. Morady F, Higgins J, Peters RW, et al. Electrophysiological testing in bundle branch; block and unexplained syncope. Am J Cardiol 1984;54:587–591.
9. Salukhe TV, Francis DP, Sutton R. Comparison of medical therapy, pacing and defibrillation in heart failure (COMPANION) trial terminated early; combined biven-

tricular pacemaker-defibrillators reduce all-cause mortality and hospitalization. Int J Cardiol 2003;87:119–120.

10. Barold SS. ACC/AHA guidelines for implantation of cardiac pacemakers: how accurate are the definitions of atrioventricular and intraventricular conduction blocks? Pacing Clin Electrophysiol 1993;16:1221–1226.
11. Sutton R, Kenny R. The natural history of sick syndrome. Pacing Clin Electrophysiol 1986;9:1110–1114.
12. Hilgard J, Ezri MD, Denes PB. Significance of the ventricular pauses of three seconds or more detected on 24-hour Holter recordings. Am J Cardiol 1985;55:1005–1008.
13. Lamas GA, Orav EJ, Stambler BS, et al. Quality of life and clinical outcomes in elderly patients treated with ventricular pacing as compared with dual-chamber pacing. N Engl J Med 1998;338:1097–1104.
14. Lamas GA, Kerry LE, Sweeny MO, et al. Ventricular pacing or dual cahmber pacing for sinus node dysfunction. N Engl J Med 2002;346:1854–1862.
15. Morley CA, Sutton R. Carotid sinus syncope. Int J Cardiol 1984;6:287–293.
16. Manolis AS, Linzer M, Estes NAM. Syncope: current diagnostic evaluation and management. Ann Intern Med 1990;112:850–863.
17. Sheldon R, Koshman ML, Wilson W, Kieser T, Rose S. Effect of dual-chamber pacing with automatic rate-drop sensing on recurrent neurally-mediated syncope. Am J Cardiol 1998;81:158–162.
18. Connolly SJ, Sheldon R, Roberts RS, Gent M. Vasovagal Pacemaker Study Investigators. The North American Vasovagal Pacemaker Study (VPS): a randomized trial of permanent cardiac pacing for the prevention of vasovagal syncope. J Am Coll Cardiol 1999:3316–3320.
19. Connolly SJ, Sheldon R, Thorpe KE, et al. Pacemaker therapy for prevention of syncope in patients with recurrent severe vasovagal syncope: Second Vasovagal Pacemaker Study (VPS II): a randomized trial. JAMA 2003;289:2224–2229.
20. Weissmann P, Chin MT, Moss AJ. Cardiac tachypacing for severe refractory idiopathic orthostatic hypotension. Ann Intern Med 1992;116:650.
21. Fananapazir L, Epstein ND, Curiel RV, et al. Long-term results of dual-chamber (DDD) pacing in hypertrophic cardiomyopathy: evidence for progressive symptomatic and hemodynamic improvement and reduction of left ventricular hypertrophy. Circulation 1994;90:2731–2742.
22. Maron BJ, Nishimura RA, McKenna WJ, et al. For the M-PATHY Study Investigators. Assessment of permanent dual-chamber pacing as a treatment for drug-refractory symptomatic patients with obstructive hypertrophic cardiomyopathy: a randomized double-blind crossover study. Circulation 1999;99:2927–2933.
23. Linde C, Gadler F, Kappenberger L, Ryden L, PIC Study Group. Placebo effect of pacemaker implantation in obstructive hypertrophic cardiomyopathy. Am J Cardiol 1999;83:903–907.
24. Maron BJ. Therapeutic strategies in hypertrophic cardiomyopathy: considerations and critique of new treatment modalities. Heart Failure 1995;February/March:27–32.
25. Hochleitner M, Hortnagel H, Ng CK, et al. Usefulness of physiologic dual-chamber pacing in drug-resistant idiopathic dilated cardiomyopathy. Am J Cardiol 1990;66: 198–202.
26. Nishimura RA, Hayes DL, Holmes DR Jr, Tajik AJ. Mechanism of hemodynamic improvement by dual-chamber pacing for severe left ventricular dysfunction:

an acute Doppler and catheterization study. J Am Coll Cardiol 1995;25:281–288.
27. Gold MR, Feliciano Z, Gottlieb SS, Fisher ML. Dual-chamber pacing with a short atrioventricular delay in congestive heart failure: a randomized study. J Am Coll Cardiol 1995;26:967–973.
28. Stambler BS, Ellenbogen K, Zhang X, et al. Right ventricular outflow versus apical pacing in pacemaker patients with congestive heart failure and atrial fibrillation. J Cardiovasc Electrophysiol 2003;14(11):1180–1186.
29. Abraham WT, Fisher WG, Smith AL, et al. Cardiac resynchronization in chronic heart failure. N Engl J Med 2002;346(24):1845–1853.
30. Moss AJ, Liu JE, Gottlieb SS, et al. Efficacy of permanent pacing in the management of high risk patients with long QT syndrome. Circulation 1991;84:1530.
31. Saksena S, Prakash A, Ziegler P, et al. Improved suppression of recurrent atrial fibrillation with dual-site right atrial pacing and antiarrhythmic drug therapy. J Am Coll Cardiol 2002;40(6):1140–1150.
32. Yung W, Brachmann J, Den Dulk K, et al. Initial clinical experience with a new arrhythmia management device. Circulation 1997;96:1–209.
33. Friedman RA. Congenital AV block. Pace me now or pace me later? Circulation 1995;92:283–285.
34. Michaelsson M, Jonzon A, Riesenfeld T. Isolated congenital complete atrio-ventricular block in adult life. A prospective study. Circulation 1995;92:442–449.
35. Sholler GF, Walsh EP. Congenital complete heart block in patients without anatomic defects. Am Heart J 1989;118:1193–1198.
36. Melton IC, Gilligan DM, Wood MA, Ellenbogen KA. Optimal cardiac pacing after heart transplantation. Pacing Clin Electrophysiol 1999;22:1510–1527.
37. Simons GR, Sgarbosa E, Wagner G, et al. Atrioventricular and intraventricular conduction disorders in acute myocardial infarction: a reappraisal in the thrombolytic era. Pacing Clin Electrophysiol 1998;21:2651–2661.
38. Tang CY, Kerr CR, Connally SJ. Clinical trials of pacing mode selection. Cardiol Clin 2000;18:1–23.
39. Andersen HR, Nielsen JC, Thompsen PE, et al. Long-term follow-up of patients from a randomized trial of atrial versus ventricular pacing for sick-sinus syndrome. Lancet 1997;350:1210–1216.
40. Kerr CR, Connolly SJ, Abdollah H, et al. Canadian Trial of Physiological Pacing. Effects of physiological pacing during long-term follow-up. Circulation 2004;109:357–362.
41. Connolly SJ, Kerr CR, Gent RS, et al. Effects of physiologic pacing versus ventricular pacing on the risk of stroke and death due to cardiovascular cause. N Engl J Med 2000;342:1385–1391.
42. Wharton JM, Sorrentino RA, Campbell P, et al. Effects of pacing modality on atrial tachyarrhythmia recurrence in the tachycardia-bradycardia syndrome: preliminary results of the Pacemaker Atrial Tachycardia Trial. Circulation 1998;98:1–494.
43. Mattioli AV, Castellane ET, Vivoli D, et al. Prevalence of atrial fibrillation and stroke in paced patients without prior atrial fibrillation: a prospective study. Clin Cardiol 1998;21:117–122.
44. Charles RG, McComb JM. Systematic trial of pacing to prevent atrial fibrillation (STOP-AF). Heart 1997;78:224–225.

45. Specialized ECG test may lead to fewer people receiving heart-shocking implants. Available at: http://www.acc.org/media/session_info/late/ACC03/lbct_monday.htm. Accessed September 14, 2004.
46. Parameswaran R, Phe T, Goldberg H. Sinus node dysfunction in acute myocardial infarction. Br Heart J 1976;38:93–96.
47. DeGuzman M, Rahimtoola SH. What is the role of pacemakers in patients with coronary artery disease and conduction abnormalities? Cardiovasc Clin 1983;13: 191–201.
48. Wesley RC, Lerman BB, DiMarco JP, et al. Mechanism of atropine-resistant atrioventricular block during inferior myocardial infarction; possible role of adenosine. J Am Coll Cardiol 1986;8:1232–1234.
49. Topol EJ, Goldschlager N, Ports TA, et al. Hemodynamic benefit of atrial pacing in right ventricular myocardial infarction. Ann Intern Med 1982;96:594–597.
50. Hauer RNW, Lie KI, Liem RL, Durrer D. Long-term prognosis in patients with bundle branch block complicating acute anteroseptal infarction. Am J Cardiol 1982;49:1581–1585.
51. Hindman MC, Wagner GS, JaRo M, et al. The clinical significance of bundle branch block complicating acute myocardial infarction. 1. Clinical characteristics, hospital mortality, and one year follow up. Circulation 1978;58:679–688.
52. Hindman MC, Wagner GS, JaRo M, et al. The clinical significance of bundle branch block complicating acute myocardial infarction. 2. Indications for temporary and permanent pacemaker insertion. Circulation 1978;58:689–699.
53. Lamas GA, Muller JE, Turi ZG, et al. A simplified method to predict occurrence of complete heart block during acute myocardial infarction. Am J Cardiol 1986;57: 1213–1219.
54. Harpaz D, Behar S, Gottileb S, et al. Complete atrioventricular block complicating acute myocardial infarction in the thrombolytic era. J Am Coll Cardiol 1999;34: 1721–1728.
55. Ryan TJ, Antman EM, Brooks NH, et al. ACC/AHA guidelines for the management of patients with acute myocardial infarction: 1999 update: a report of the American College of Cardiology/American Heart Association Task Force on Practice Guidelines (Committee on Management of Acute Myocardial Infarction). J Am Coll Cardiol 1999;34(3):890–911.
56. Roberts NK, Somerville J. Pathological significance of electrocardiographic changes in aortic valve endocarditis. Br Heart J 1969;31:395–396.
57. Cox J, Krajden M. Cardiovascular manifestations of Lyme disease. Am Heart J 1991;122:1449–1455.
58. Peters RW, Weiss DN, Carliner NH, et al. Overdrive pacing for atrial flutter. Am J Cardiol 1994;74:1021–1023.

Basic Concepts of Pacing

G. Neal Kay

2

MYOCARDIAL STIMULATION

An artificial electrical pacing stimulus excites cardiac tissue by the creation of an electrical field at the interface of the stimulating electrode and the underlying myocardium. Although a pacing stimulus can be applied to any portion of the body, a tissue response occurs only in cells that are excitable. For an artificial polarizing pulse to induce a response in excitable tissue, the stimulus must be of sufficient amplitude and duration to initiate a self-regenerating wavefront of action potentials that propagate away from the site of stimulation. Myocardial stimulation depends on an intact source of the electrical pulse (the pulse generator), a conductor between the source of the electrical pulse and the stimulating electrode (the lead conductor), an electrode for delivery of the pulse, and an area of myocardium that is excitable. In this section, the basic properties of myocardial stimulation are reviewed in detail.

BASIC ELECTROPHYSIOLOGY

The property of biologic tissues such as nerve and muscle to respond to a stimulus with a response that is out of proportion to the strength of the stimulus is known as excitability.[1] Excitable tissues are characterized by a separation of charge across the cell membrane that results in a resting transmembrane electrical potential. For cardiac myocytes, the concentration of Na^+ ions outside the cell exceeds the concentration inside the cell. In contrast, the inside of the cell has a 35-fold greater concentration of K^+ ions than the outside of the cell. The resting transmembrane potential is maintained by the high resistance to ion flow, which is an intrinsic property of the lipid bilayer of the cell membrane. Because there is a passive leak of ions through membrane-bound ion channels, the resting potential is further maintained by two active transport mechanisms that exchange Na^+ ions for K^+ and Ca^{2+} ions. The Na^+–K^+ ATPase exchange "pump" extrudes three Na^+ ions for every two K^+ ions that are moved into the cell. The Na^+–Ca^{2+} transport mechanism exchanges three Na^+ ions toward the outside of

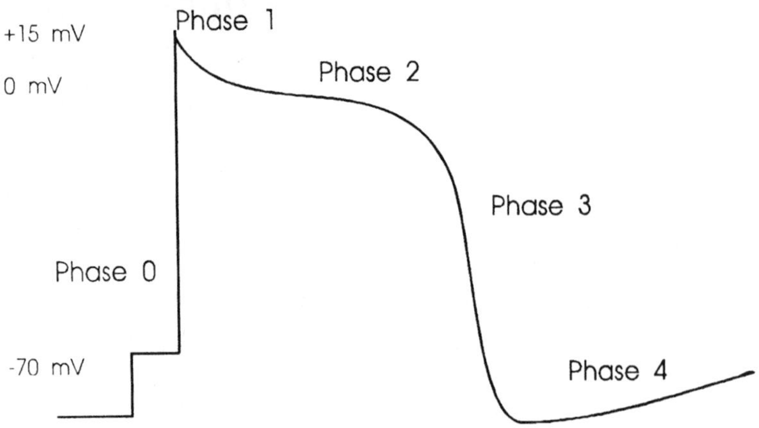

Figure 2.1. The action potential of a Purkinje fiber is illustrated. The resting transmembrane potential is approximately –90 mV. Upon depolarization of the membrane to a threshold potential of –70 to –60 mV, the upstroke of the action potential is triggered (phase 0), carried predominantly by an influx of Na ions into the cell. The transmembrane potential reaches approximately 15 mV (overshoot potential) and is repolarized to approximately 0 mV during phase 1. The plateau phase of the action potential (phase 2) is produced by a complex interaction of inward Ca^{2+} and Na^{+} currents and outward K^{+} currents. Repolarization of the cell occurs during phase 3, during which the cell regains the capability of responding to a polarizing electrical stimulus with another action potential. Phase 4 of the action potential is characterized by a slow upward drift in the transmembrane potential.

the cell for each Ca^{2+} ion that is moved into the cell. Because both these transport mechanisms result in the net movement of three positive charges out of the cell in exchange for two positive charges that are moved in, a net polarization of the cell membrane is produced so that the inside of the cell is maintained electrically negative with respect to the outside. These transport mechanisms depend on the expenditure of energy in the form of high-energy phosphates and are susceptible to disruptions in aerobic cellular metabolism during myocardial ischemia.

Excitable tissues are further characterized by their ability to generate and propagate a transmembrane action potential.[1] The action potential is triggered by depolarization of the membrane from a resting potential of approximately –90 mV to a threshold potential of approximately –70 to –60 mV. Upon reaching the threshold transmembrane potential, specialized membrane-bound protein channels change conformation from an inactive state to an active state, which allows the free movement of Na^{+} ions through the channel.[2] The upstroke of the action potential (phase 0) is a consequence of this sudden influx of Na^{+} into the myocyte and is associated with a change in transmembrane potential from –90 mV to approximately –20 mV (Fig. 2.1).[3,4] It is estimated that the opening of a single Na^{+} channel allows approximately 10^{4} Na^{+} ions to enter the cardiac myocyte. The number of Na^{+} channels is estimated to be on the order of five to 10 channels per square micron of cell membrane.[5,6] In addition to Na^+ channels, specialized proteins are also suspended in the membrane that have differential selectivity for K^+, Ca^{2+}, and Cl^- ions.[7,8] The channels may remain in the open configuration for less than 1 millisecond (characteristic of the Na^+ channel) to hundreds of milliseconds (typical of K^+ channels). The rapid upstroke of the action potential is followed by a short period of hyperpolarization when the transmembrane potential is transiently positively charged. The overshoot potential is quickly abolished (phase 1) by a transient outward K^+ current (I_{to}); and the cell enters the plateau phase (phase 2), during which Ca^{2+} and Na^+ are triggered to enter the cell and outwork K^+ currents are activated.[9,10] The cardiac cell is refractory to further electrical stimulation by a stimulus of any strength during the plateau phase. The net membrane voltage is maintained approximately 0 mV as the inward Na^+ and Ca^{2+} currents are balanced by at least three outward K^+ currents having different time constants (slow, rapid, and ultrarapid, I_{KS}, I_{KR}, and I_{KUR}). These K^+ currents have the property of delayed rectification. After the plateau phase, which lasts several hundred milliseconds, the cardiac cell begins the process of repolarization as the outward currents exceed the inward currents with regeneration of the resting membrane potential and the capability for responding to an electrical stimulus with another action potential (phase 3). The repolarization phase is characterized by the continuation of outward K^+ currents with inactivation of the inward Na^+ and Ca^{2+} currents, which results in a net negative polarization of the inside of the cell. During the repolarization phase an action potential may be induced if the myocyte is challenged by an electrical stimulus of sufficient strength. Following complete repolarization of the membrane, the cell enters a diastolic period during which it is fully excitable (phase 4).[11,12] Tissues demonstrating spontaneous automaticity exhibit a gradual upward drift in transmembrane potential until threshold is reached.

The response of excitable membranes to electrical stimuli is an active process that results in a response exceeding that of simple passive conductance along the membrane. Gap junctions that provide low-resistance intercellular connections conduct the action potential between myocytes.[13,14] The action potential at the site of stimulation results in the depolarization of neighboring areas of the myocyte membrane to threshold voltage, which triggers the Na^+ channels to open and results in regeneration of the action potential. The action potential is not only passively conducted but also actively regenerated at each segment of membrane. However, propagation of the action potential away from the site of electrical stimulation also depends on certain passive cable properties of the myocardium, including the axis of myofiber orientation and the geometry of the connections between fibers.[15] For example, a wavefront of depolarization is conducted with a conduction velocity that is three to five times greater along the longitudinal axis of a myofiber than along the transverse axis.[16,17] These anisotropic conduction properties may be further exaggerated in the presence of myocardial fibrosis in which the intercellular collagen matrix is increased with decreased cell-to-cell communication. Such fibrosis is often present in patients with disorders of the cardiac conduction system. In addition, the safety factor for successful propagation is greater at sites where sheets of myocardium of similar size are joined than where a narrow isthmus of tissue joins a larger mass.[18] Thus, as the structure of cardiac tissue is affected by pathologic conditions such as fibrosis or infarction, the physiologic properties of conduction and excitability may be significantly altered.

STIMULATION THRESHOLD

Cardiac pacing involves the delivery of a polarizing electrical impulse from an electrode in contact with the myocardium with the generation of an electrical field of sufficient intensity to induce a propagating wave of cardiac action potentials.[19] The stimulating pulse may be either anodal or cathodal in polarity, although with somewhat different stimulation characteristics. In addition, the stimulation characteristics are related to the source of the stimulating pulse, with constant-voltage and constant-current generators exhibiting somewhat different stimulation properties. The minimum stimulus intensity and duration necessary to reliably initiate a propagated depolarizing wavefront from an electrode is defined as the stimulation threshold. The stimulation threshold is a fundamental concept that is crucial to programming and troubleshooting permanent pacemakers and pacing leads. In this section, the factors that determine stimulation threshold will be discussed.[20]

Strength–Duration Relation

For a pacing stimulus to produce a self-regenerating wave of depolarization in a cardiac chamber ("capture"), the stimulus must exceed a critical amplitude (measured in volts or milliamperes) and must be applied for a sufficient duration. These factors of stimulus amplitude and duration interact such that the minimal amplitude that is required to capture atrial or ventricular myocardium depends on the duration of the stimulating pulse (pulse duration).[21–24] The stimulus amplitude for endocardial stimulation has an exponential relation to the duration of the pulse, with a rapidly rising strength–duration curve at pulse durations less than 0.25 milliseconds and a relatively flat curve at pulse durations greater than 1.0 milliseconds (Fig. 2.2). As can be appreciated by examining the hyperbolic strength–duration curve, a small change in pulse duration is associated with a significant change in the threshold amplitude at short pulse durations; however, only a small change at longer pulse durations. Because of the exponential relationship between stimulus amplitude and pulse duration, the entire strength–duration curve can be described relatively accurately by two points on the curve, *rheobase* and *chronaxie*.[21] Rheobase of a constant-voltage, strength–duration curve is defined as the least stimulus voltage that will electrically stimulate the myocardium at any pulse duration. For practical purposes, rheobase voltage is usually determined as the threshold stimulus voltage at a pulse duration of 2.0 milliseconds. Pulse durations greater than 2.0 milliseconds provide a negligible lowering of the threshold stimulus voltage. One exception to this rule is with field stimulation, such as with transcutaneous or trans-

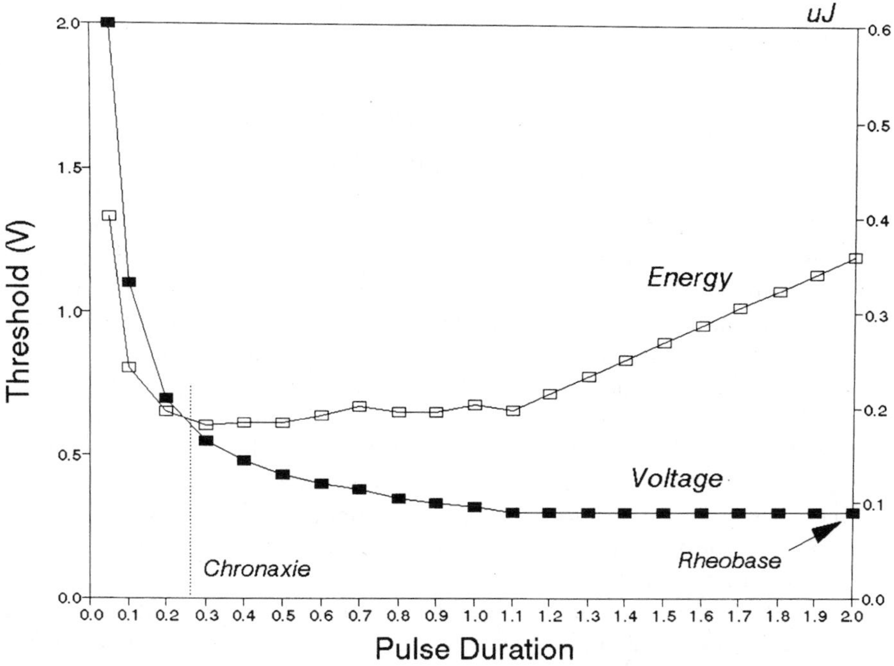

Figure 2.2. Strength-duration curve for constant-voltage stimulation obtained at the time of permanent pacing lead implantation in a patient with complete AV block. The strength-duration relation is characterized by a steeply rising portion at short pulse durations and a relatively flat portion at pulse durations greater than 1 millisecond. The stimulus energy at each point on the strength-duration curve is also demonstrated. The rheobase voltage of a constant-voltage strength-duration curve is defined as the lowest stimulation voltage at any pulse duration. Because the curve is essentially flat at a pulse duration of 2 milliseconds, rheobase can be accurately approximated as the threshold voltage at this point. Chronaxie, the threshold pulse duration at twice rheobase voltage, closely approximates the point of minimum threshold stimulation energy.

esophageal pacing, in which the rheobase voltage is reached at much wider pulse durations (as long as 40 milliseconds for transcutaneous pacing). The chronaxie pulse duration is defined as the threshold pulse duration at a stimulus amplitude that is twice rheobase voltage. Using the rheobase and chronaxie points, Lapicque[21] constructed the following mathematical equation, which can be used to derive the strength–duration curve for constant-current stimulation:

$$I = I_r\left(1 + \frac{t_C}{t}\right) \qquad \text{Eq. 2.1}$$

where I is the threshold current at pulse duration t, I_r is the rheobase current, and t_C is the chronaxie pulse duration.

The relation of stimulus voltage, current, and pulse duration to stimulus energy is provided by the formula:

$$E = \frac{V^2}{Rt} \qquad \text{Eq. 2.2}$$

where E is the stimulus energy, V is the stimulus voltage, R is the total pacing impedance, and t is the pulse duration. The chronaxie pulse duration is important in the clinical application of pacing, as it approximates the point of minimum threshold energy on the strength–duration curve.[25,26] With pulse durations greater than chronaxie, there is relatively little reduction in the threshold voltage. Rather, the wider pulse duration results in the wasting of stimulation energy without providing a substantial increase in safety margin. At pulse durations less than chronaxie there is a steep increase in threshold voltage and stimulation energy. As can be appreciated from Figure 2.2, the chronaxie pulse duration is usually close to the point of minimal stimulation energy. From the energy equation (Eq. 2.2), note that, whereas the energy of a pacing stimulus increases in direct relation to the pulse duration, the energy increases by the square of the voltage. Thus, doubling the stimulus voltage results in a fourfold increase in the stimulus energy.

An appreciation of the threshold strength–duration relation is important for the proper programming of stimulus amplitude and pulse duration. Modern pulse generators offer two major methods for evaluating the stimulation threshold: either automatic decrementation of the stimulus voltage at a constant pulse duration or automatic decrementation of the pulse duration at a constant stimulus voltage. To provide an adequate margin of safety, when the stimulation threshold is determined by decrementing the stimulus amplitude, the stimulus voltage is usually programmed to approximately twice the threshold value. Similarly, for pulse generators that determine threshold by automatically decrementing pulse duration, the pulse duration is usually programmed to at least three times the threshold value. It should be recognized that the hyperbolic shape of the strength–duration curve has important implications for interpreting the results of threshold testing (Fig. 2.3). Although these methods provide comparable margins of safety when the threshold pulse duration is 0.15 milliseconds or less, tripling a threshold pulse duration that is greater than 0.3 milliseconds may not provide an adequate stimulation safety margin.

The threshold strength–duration curve is influenced by several factors, including the method of measurement, the nature of the electrode, the health of the tissue in contact with the electrode, the distance between the electrode and excitable myocardium, and the duration of lead implantation. Stimulation thresholds that are measured by decrementing stimulus voltage until loss of capture are usually 0.1 to 0.2 V lower than when the stimulus intensity is gradually increased from subthreshold until capture is achieved.[27,28] This empiric observation, known as the Wedensky effect, must be considered when accurate measurements of stimulation threshold are required. The Wedensky effect may be greater at narrow pulse durations, potentially reaching clinical significance.

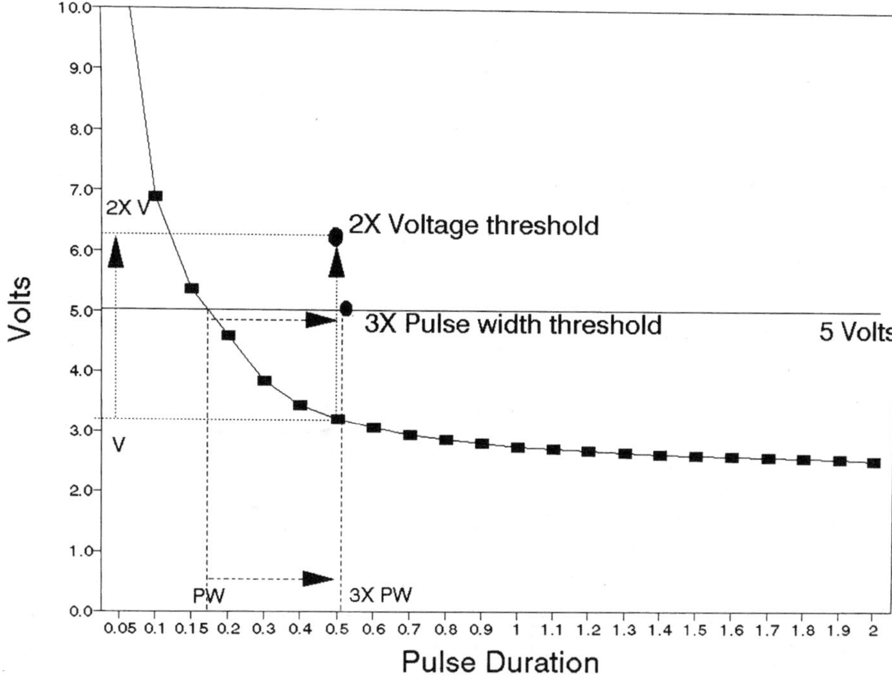

Figure 2.3. The clinical use of the strength–duration relation to determine an adequate margin of safety for stimulation is demonstrated for a patient with a chronically implanted pacing lead. Note that when the stimulation threshold is determined by decrementing pulse duration at a constant voltage (5 V), the strength-duration curve is encountered at the start of the rapidly rising portion of the curve. Tripling of the pulse duration provides an adequate safety margin. When the stimulation threshold is determined by decrementing stimulus voltage at a constant pulse duration (0.5 milliseconds), the strength–duration curve is encountered at a relatively flat portion of the curve. Doubling the stimulation voltage results in a somewhat greater margin of safety than with the alternative method.

When the pacing rate is maintained as a constant during experimental conditions, the Wedensky effect is of marginal significance. This result suggests that this clinical phenomenon is probably explained by the effects of a varying cardiac rate during the gain or loss of capture as the stimulus amplitude is increased or decreased, respectively.

Strength-Duration Curves for Constant-Voltage and Constant-Current Stimulation

There are several differences in the shape of the strength-duration curves for constant-current and constant-voltage stimulation (Fig. 2.4).[25] For example, constant-voltage stimulation usually results in a flat curve at pulse durations greater than 1.5 milliseconds, whereas the constant-current stimulation curve may be slowly downsloping beyond this pulse duration. The strength-duration

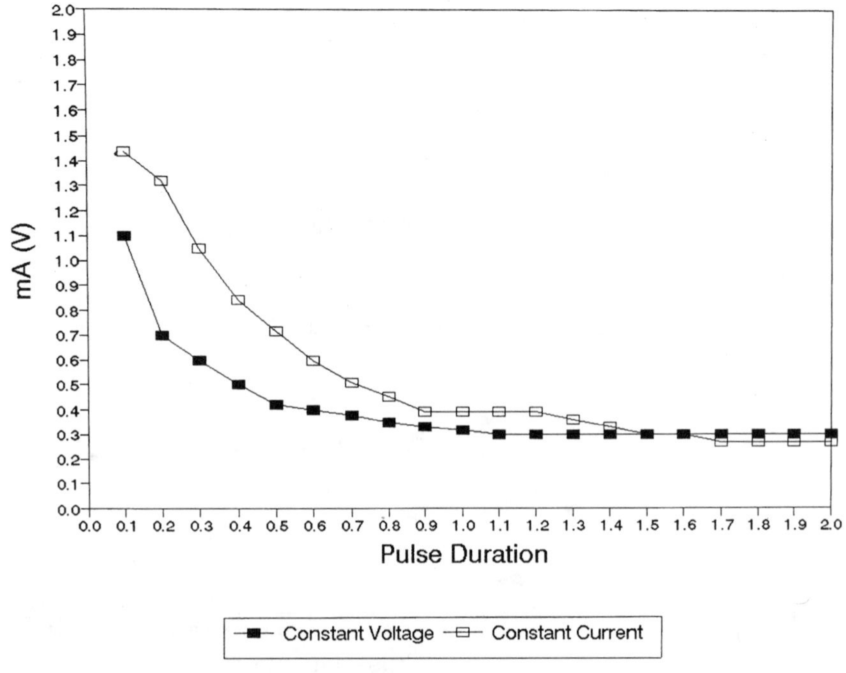

Figure 2.4. Strength-duration curves determined with constant-current and constant-voltage stimulation in a single individual are demonstrated. Note that the constant-current stimulation curve continues to decline gradually at greater pulse durations than that obtained with constant-voltage stimulation.

curve with constant-current stimulation increases more steeply at short pulse durations than it does with constant voltage stimulation. Small changes in pulse duration less than 0.5 milliseconds may result in a significantly greater reduction in stimulation safety margin for constant-current than for constant-voltage pulse generators. Because of this difference in the shape of the strength-duration curves, the chronaxie pulse duration of a constant-current strength-duration relation is significantly greater than that observed with constant-voltage stimulation. Because the most efficient pulse duration for electrical stimulation is at chronaxie (in terms of threshold energy), a constant-voltage pulse generator can be set to deliver a narrower pulse duration than a constant-current generator and yet provide the same safety margin. Virtually all permanent pacemakers presently in use are constant-voltage generators. In contrast, most temporary pacemakers use constant-current generators.

Time-Dependent Changes in Stimulation Threshold

Myocardial stimulation thresholds may change dramatically following positioning of a permanent pacing lead.[29–32] The typical course of events following implantation of an endocardial pacing lead starts with an acute rise in thresh-

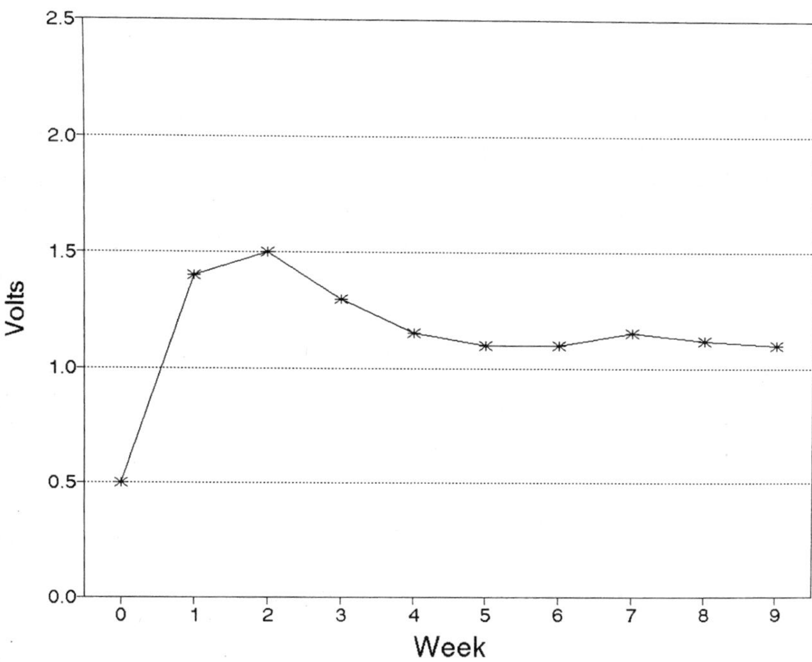

Figure 2.5. Typical evolution of the stimulation threshold over the first 2 months following implantation of a platinum–iridium pacing lead. The stimulation threshold increases from implantation, peaking at 1 to 2 weeks. The chronic stimulation threshold has stabilized by 6 weeks in this individual. Although this curve is typical of those obtained with standard (nonsteroid) permanent pacing leads, there is considerable variability among individuals in the absolute values and slope.

old that begins within the first 24 hours (Fig. 2.5). The threshold usually continues to rise over the next several days, usually peaking at approximately 1 week. The typical stimulation threshold then gradually declines over the next several weeks. By 6 weeks, the myocardial stimulation threshold has usually stabilized at a value that is significantly greater than that measured at implantation of the lead but less than the acute peak. The magnitude of the change in threshold varies widely between individuals and relates to the electrode's size, shape, chemical composition, and surface structure. The stability of the electrode–myocardial interface and the flexibility of the lead also influence the acute-to-chronic change in threshold. In addition to the typical evolution of stimulation threshold following lead implantation, certain leads may exhibit a hyperacute phase of threshold evolution. For example, active fixation electrodes using a screw helix as the active electrode may produce, immediately following implantation, an increased stimulation threshold that gradually decreases over the next 20 to 30 minutes.[33] This transient high threshold is likely related to acute injury at the myocardial–electrode interface and is generally not observed with atraumatic passive fixation leads. Clinically, the hyperacute phase may be manifested by a current of injury in the electrogram. Both the current of injury and the stimulation threshold usually decline rapidly over the first several minutes before pursuing the typical acute-to-chronic threshold evolution, shown in Figure 2.5. Thus, comparisons of changes in stimulation threshold between varying lead designs require an appreciation of the effects of the fixation mechanism. The addition of steroid elution to a pacing electrode (or a steroid-eluting collar around the electrode) markedly attenuates these evolutionary effects, resulting in a much more constant stimulation threshold over time. Several other factors may affect the change in stimulation threshold that occurs with lead maturation such as the mass of lead tip, the stability of the electrode in relation to the myocardial interface, and the force with which the electrode is held in contact with the myocardium. In general, the more stable and the less traumatic the interaction of the electrode and lead with the myocardium, the lower the rise in threshold over time.

Proper programming of the stimulus amplitude of a permanent pacemaker requires an understanding of several factors. First, the strength–duration relation must be appreciated. Second, the safety margin that is chosen for a particular patient must be based on the degree of pacemaker dependency—that is, the likelihood of the patient's developing symptoms should loss of effective pacing occur. For patients judged to be highly pacemaker-dependent, a higher stimulation safety margin may be prudent. As an example, a patient with complete atrioventricular (AV) block with an unreliable ventricular escape rhythm may be more likely to develop symptoms with loss of ventricular capture than is a patient with intermittent sinus node dysfunction. On the other hand, the patient with AV block is likely to be less dependent on atrial than ventricular capture. Thus, a higher safety margin may be needed for the ventricular stimulus than for the atrial stimulus in such an individual. Third, an appreciation of the effect of stimulus amplitude and duration on battery longevity is required. As discussed later in this chapter in the section on output circuits, programming the stimulus intensity greater than 2.8 V results in a marked increase in current drain from the battery. Fourth, the overall metabolic and pharmacologic history of the patient must be considered. For example, patients requiring the addition of an antiarrhythmic drug to their medication regimen may experience a small increase in pacing threshold. Similarly, patients subject to major shifts in potassium concentration or acid–base balance, such as those with renal failure, may have transient increases in pacing threshold. The safety margin that is chosen for these individuals may need to be greater than that for other patients.

Several investigators have reported that pacing threshold varies inversely with the surface area of the stimulating electrode.[34–36] For spherical electrodes, the smaller the surface area of the electrode, the lower the pacing threshold. The explanation for this observation relates to the intensity of the electric field that is generated at the surface of the electrode. For a constant-voltage pulse, the smaller the electrode, the greater the intensity of the electric field and the current density at the surface. The threshold maturation process has been shown to be caused by the growth of an inexcitable capsule of fibrous tissue surrounding the electrode (Fig. 2.6).[37,38] This fibrous capsule effectively increases the surface area of the electrode, thereby decreasing the intensity of the electric field at the junction of the fibrous capsule and the more normal, excitable myocardium.

The cellular events that result in the development of a fibrous capsule have been intensively studied.[39,40] The initial tissue reaction to the implantation of a permanent pacing lead involves acute injury to cell membranes. This damage is rapidly followed by the development of myocardial edema and coating of the electrode by platelets and fibrin. These events are followed by the release of chemotactic factors and the development of a typical cellular inflammatory reaction with the infiltration of polymorphonuclear leukocytes and mononuclear cells. Following the acute polymorphonuclear response, the myocardium at the interface with the stimulating electrode is invaded by macrophages. The extracellular release of proteolytic enzymes and toxic-free oxygen radicals results in an acceleration of tissue injury underlying the electrode. The acute inflammatory response is followed by the accumulation of more macrophages and the influx of fibroblasts into the myocardium. The fibroblasts in the myocardium begin producing collagen, leading to the development of the fibrotic capsule surrounding the electrode.[38]

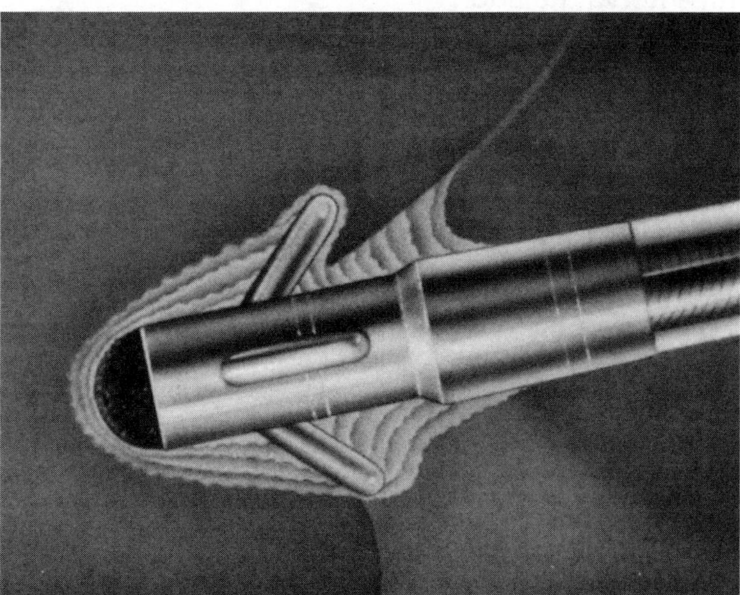

Figure 2.6. Diagram of a fibrous capsule surrounding a chronically implanted pacing electrode. The inexcitable capsule increases the effective radius of the stimulating electrode, reducing the current density at the interface of the capsule and excitable myocardium and increasing the stimulation threshold. (Courtesy of Medtronic, Inc.)

The influences of several pharmacologic agents on the electrode–myocardial maturation process have been studied. Nonsteroidal anti-inflammatory drugs have been shown to have minimal influence on the evolution of pacing thresholds. In contrast, corticosteroids, either systemically or locally administered, may have dramatic effects on the evolution of pacing thresholds.[41] By the use of an infusion pump to deliver dexamethasone sodium phosphate from the center of a ring-shaped electrode, Stokes demonstrated a dramatic decrease in the expected acute-to-chronic rise in pacing threshold with both atrial and ventricular pacing leads in canines. Clinical studies have confirmed these findings and have led to the development of leads that gradually elute dexamethasone from a reservoir beneath the stimulating electrode.[42–45] These corticosteroid-eluting leads have been associated with stable pacing thresholds from the time of implantation and through the follow-up period of several years. Other designs incorporate dexamethasone into a drug-eluting collar that surrounds the stimulating electrode.[46] The application of corticosteroid-eluting collars to active fixation leads has demonstrated that the nature of the electrode remains important to the evolution of pacing thresholds, even in the presence of anti-inflammatory drugs. Nevertheless, steroid elution has been shown to be an effective means of lowering the long-term pacing threshold for leads of virtually all designs, including active and passive fixation endocardial leads as well as epimyocardial screw-in leads.

Strength–Interval Relation

The stimulation threshold is influenced significantly by the coupling interval of electrical stimuli and the frequency of stimulation.[47–50] Figure 2.7 demonstrates a typical ventricular strength–interval curve for both cathodal and anodal stimulation. Note that the stimulus intensity required to capture the ventricle remains quite constant at long extrastimulus coupling intervals, but rises exponentially at shorter intervals. The rise in stimulation threshold at short coupling intervals is related to impingement of the stimulus on the relative refractory period of the ventricular myocardium. As discussed previously, electrical stimuli applied during the repolarization phase of the cardiac action potential may result in a propagated action potential if it is of sufficient intensity.[47] However, during the plateau phase of the action potential, electrical stimuli of any intensity will not be able to generate an action potential as the absolute refractory period is encountered. Figure 2.7 also illustrates the important differences in anodal and cathodal stimulation. Late diastolic stimulation thresholds are lower with cathodal than with anodal stimulation.[47] However, at relatively short extrastimulus coupling intervals, the anodal stimulation threshold may be less than the cathodal threshold.[47] During the relative refractory period, the anodal threshold may actually decline ("dip") before abruptly rising at shorter coupling intervals. With bipolar cardiac pacing, the stimulation threshold is generally determined by the cathode. However, with short extrastimulus coupling intervals, the bipolar stimulation threshold may actually be determined by the anode. If the stimulus intensity exceeds both the cathodal and anodal thresholds, bipolar pacing may

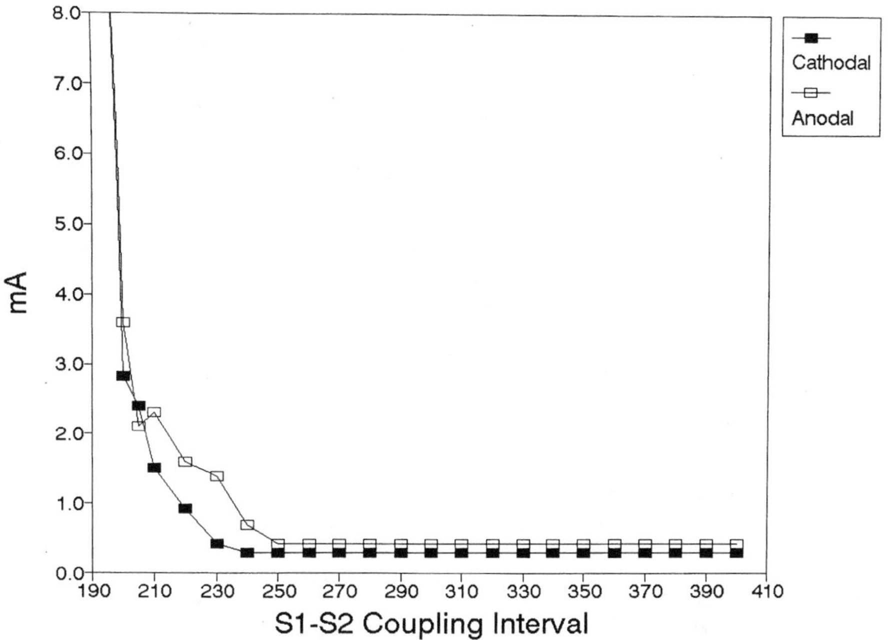

Figure 2.7. The strength-interval relationship for constant current with unipolar anodal and cathodal stimulation is demonstrated in a normal individual. Note that the shape of the curve is relatively flat at long extrastimulus coupling intervals and rises exponentially at short coupling intervals. Also note that cathodal stimulation results in a lower stimulation threshold at long coupling intervals than does anodal stimulation. At short coupling intervals, the anodal stimulation curve may transiently "dip" before rapidly rising.

result in stimulation at both electrode–myocardial interfaces (both anodal and cathodal stimulation).

Effects of Pacing Rate on Myocardial Stimulation

The stimulation frequency may have an important influence on pacing threshold, although increases in threshold have been demonstrated only at very rapid pacing rates.[47,51–53] At shorter stimulation cycle lengths, the action potential of atrial and ventricular myocardium shortens, resulting in a proportional decrease in the relative refractory period. At rapid pacing rates, these factors are manifested by a shift in the strength–interval curve to the left. However, at pacing rates exceeding 250 beats per minute (bpm), pacing stimuli may be delivered during the relative refractory period, resulting in an increase in threshold. The strength–duration curve is shifted upward and to the right at very rapid pacing rates (Fig. 2.8), which may have important implications for antitachycardia pacing.[51] Thus, a stimulation amplitude that provides an adequate safety margin for pacing at slow rates may not be sufficient at rapid pacing rates. Antitachy-

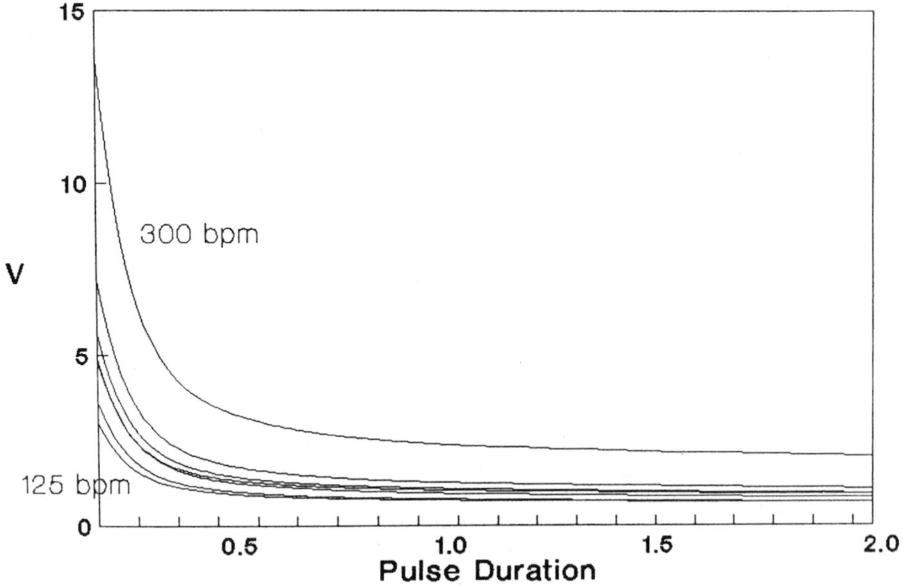

Figure 2.8. The effect of pacing rate on the atrial strength–duration relation for a normal individual is demonstrated. Threshold curves were obtained at pacing rates of 125 to 300 ppm in increments of 25 ppm. Note that the strength-duration curves largely overlap at pacing rates of 125 to 250 ppm. At pacing rates of 275 to 300 ppm, the curve is shifted upward and to the left.

cardia devices provide for this possible increase in stimulation threshold by an automatic increase in the amplitude of pacing stimuli that are delivered at rapid pacing rates. In recognition of the rate-dependence of the pacing threshold, implantable cardioverter-defibrillators typically provide a greater stimulus intensity during antitachycardia pacing than during antibradycardia pacing.

PHARMACOLOGIC AND METABOLIC EFFECTS ON STIMULATION THRESHOLD

The stimulation threshold may demonstrate considerable variability over the normal 24-hour period, generally increasing during sleep and falling during the waking hours.[54,55] The changes in threshold parallel fluctuations in autonomic tone and circulating catecholamines, and consequently there is a decreased threshold during exercise. The stimulation threshold is inversely related to the level of circulating corticosteroids. The stimulation threshold may increase following eating, during hyperglycemia, hypoxemia, hypercarbia, and metabolic acidosis or alkalosis.[56–60] The stimulation threshold may increase dramatically during acute viral illnesses, especially in children. The concentration of serum electrolytes may also influence stimulation threshold. For instance, stimulation threshold typically rises during hyperkalemia.[57–59]

Drugs may also influence stimulation threshold. As mentioned above, catecholamines reduce threshold, and the infusion of isoproterenol may restore capture in some patients with exit block.[55] In contrast, beta-blocking drugs increase the stimulation threshold.[61] Corticosteroids, either orally or parenterally administered, may produce a dramatic decrease in stimulation threshold and are occasionally useful for the management of the acute increase in threshold that may be observed following lead implantation.[41] The list of drugs that raise the stimulation threshold includes the type I antiarrhythmic drugs quinidine,[62] procainamide,[63] flecainide,[64] and encainide. It is not clear whether the type III drug amiodarone has similar effects. Virtually all antiarrhythmic drugs may influence the pacing threshold, although they are usually clinically important only at high serum concentrations.

Occasional patients exhibit a progressive rise in stimulation threshold over time, a clinical syndrome known as exit block. Exit block seems to occur despite optimal lead positioning, as it recurs with the subsequent implantation of new pacing leads. In patients with exit block, the threshold changes in the atrium tend to parallel those in the ventricle. Exit block is best managed by the use of steroid-eluting ventricular leads, which have been associated with low thresholds in patients with this syndrome (Fig. 2.9).[42–45]

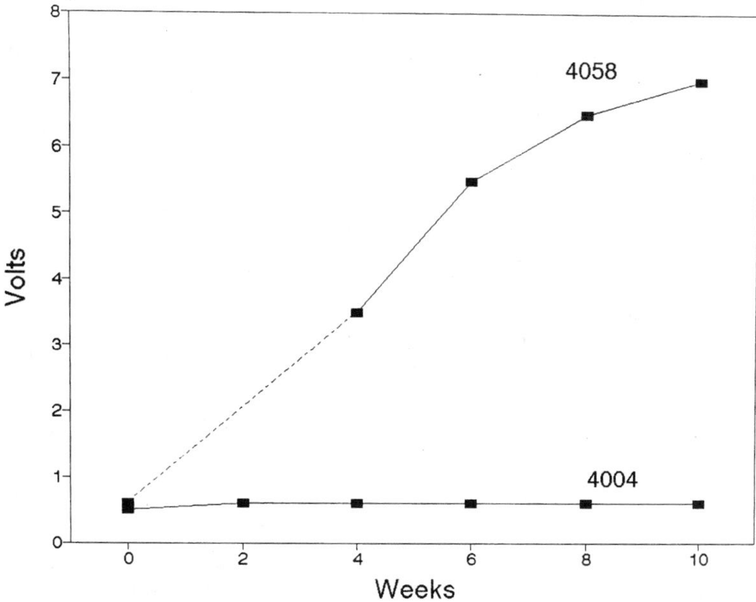

Figure 2.9. The evolution of stimulation threshold voltage (pulse duration 0.5 milliseconds) in the right ventricular apex is demonstrated for an individual with a history of exit block. Note that the stimulation threshold increases progressively from implantation with an active fixation ventricular lead (model 4058). Following implantation of a corticosteroid-eluting electrode (model 4004) in the same patient, the stimulation threshold remains low. Exit block occurs infrequently but usually recurs with standard (nonsteroid) pacing leads.

IMPEDANCE

Impedance is the sum of all factors that oppose the flow of current in an electric circuit. Impedance is not necessarily the same as resistance. The relationship between voltage (V), current (I), and resistance (R) in an electrical circuit is estimated by Ohm's law, $V = IR$. For circuits that follow Ohm's law, impedance and resistance are equal. If voltage is held constant, the current flow is inversely related to the resistance of the circuit ($I = V/R$). The leading-edge voltage of a constant-voltage pulse generator is fixed, and the lower the resistance, the greater the current flow. In contrast, the greater the resistance, the lower the current flow. Because implantable pulse generators are powered by lithium iodine batteries with a fixed amount of charge, pacing impedance is an important determinant of battery longevity.

The total pacing impedance is determined by factors that are related to the lead conductor (resistance), the resistance to current flow from the electrode to the myocardium (electrode resistance), and the accumulation of charges of opposite polarity in the myocardium at the electrode–tissue interface (polarization). Thus, the total pacing impedance (Z_{total}) = Z_c Z_e Z_p, where Z_c is the conductor resistance, Z_e is the electrode resistance, and Z_p is the polarization impedance. The resistance to current flow provided by the lead conductor results in a voltage drop across the lead with a portion of the pacing pulse converted into heat. Thus, this component of the total pacing impedance is an inefficient use of electrical energy and does not contribute to myocardial stimulation. The ideal pacing lead would have a very low conductor resistance (Z_c). In contrast, the ideal pacing lead would also have a relatively high electrode resistance (Z_e) to minimize current flow and maximize battery life.[65] The electrode resistance is largely a function of the electrode radius, with higher resistance provided by a smaller electrode. An electrode with a small radius minimizes current flow in an efficient manner. In addition to providing a greater electrode resistance, pacing electrodes with a small radius provide increased current density and lower stimulation thresholds. Because of these properties, newer pacing and implantable cardioverter-defibrillator (ICD) leads take advantage of smaller electrodes to increase electrode resistance, allowing the total pacing impedance to exceed 1000 ohms. Compared with a standard pacing lead with a total impedance of 500 ohms, a lead with 1000 ohms of impedance would decrease current drain of each pacing pulse by 50%, thereby prolonging the usable battery life of the implantable pulse generator. The routine use of these leads will allow implantable devices to become smaller while maintaining battery longevity. There is a practical lower limit to the size of the electrode, which is related to the likelihood of maintaining stable contact of the electrode with the endocardium throughout the cardiac and respiratory cycles. For example, pacing leads with a very small distal electrode may be associated with a relatively high pacing threshold in a small proportion of patients (<5%), probably as a result of radiographically imperceptible "microdislodgement" of the electrode as it contacts the endocardium.

The third component of pacing impedance, polarization impedance, is an effect of electrical stimulation and is related to the movement of charged ions in the myocardium toward the cathode. When an electrical current is applied to the myocardium, the cathode attracts positively charged ions and repels negatively charged ions in the extracellular space. The cathode rapidly becomes surrounded by a layer of hydrated Na^+ and H_3O^- ions. Farther away from the cathode, a second layer forms of negatively charged ions (Cl^-, HPO_4^{2-}, and OH^-). Thus, the negatively charged cathode induces the accumulation of two layers of oppositely charged ions in the myocardium. Initially, the movement of charged ions results in the flow of current in the myocardium. As the cathode becomes surrounded by an inside layer of positive charges and an outside layer of negative charges, a functional capacitor develops that impedes the further movement of charge. The capacitive effect of polarization increases throughout the application of the pulse, peaking at the trailing edge and decaying exponentially following the pulse as charged layers dissolve into electrical neutrality (Fig. 2.10). Because polarization impedes the movement of charge in the myocardium, it is inefficient and results in an increased voltage requirement for stimulation. Thus, polarization impedance reduces the effectiveness of a pacing stimulus to stimulate the myocardium and wastes current. Polarization impedance is directly related to the duration of the pulse and can be minimized by the use of relatively short pulse durations. Polarization is inversely related to the surface area of the electrode. To minimize the effect of polarization (Z_p) but maximize electrode resistance (Z_e), the surface area of the electrode can be made large but the geometric radius small by the use of a porous coating on the electrode.[66–68] Electrodes constructed with activated carbon,[69,70] or coated with platinum black[71] or iridium oxide, are effective in minimizing the wasteful effects of polarization and in diminishing afterpotentials, which can interfere with sensing.

The evolution of pacing impedance is usually characterized by a fall over the first 1 to 2 weeks following implantation.[32] The chronic pacing impedance then rises to a stable value that is, on average, approximately 15% higher than that at implant. Serial measurements of pacing impedance are extremely valuable for the assessment of lead integrity; low impedance measurements usually reflect a failure of conductor insulation, and high values often suggest conductor fracture or a loose set-screw at the proximal connector. It should be emphasized that the method of measurement greatly influences the impedance value. For example, if the pacing impedance is measured at the leading edge of the pulse, the value reflects Z_c and Z_e but not Z_p. In contrast, measurements near the midpoint of the pulse are a more accurate reflection of total pacing impedance. For clinical purposes, serial assessments of impedance should use a consistent method of measurement.

BIPOLAR VERSUS UNIPOLAR STIMULATION

The term *unipolar pacing* is technically a misnomer, as both bipolar and unipolar configurations require an anode and a cathode to complete the electrical

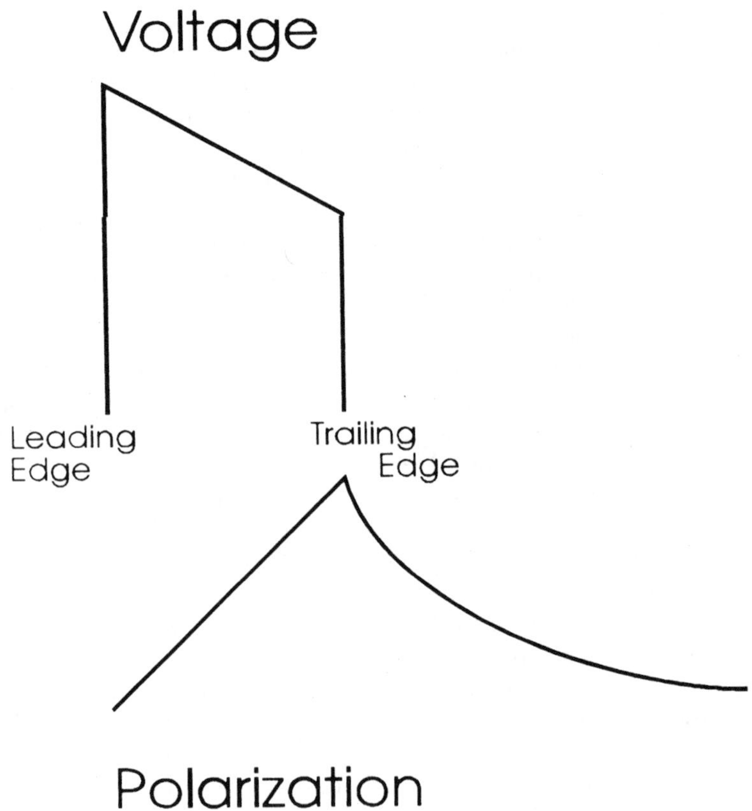

Figure 2.10. The relationship between the voltage waveform of a constant-voltage pulse and the development of polarization effect at the electrode-myocardial interface is illustrated. Note that the polarization effect rises during application of the stimulating pulse and decays exponentially. The trailing edge of the output pulse is less than the leading edge as the output capacitor loses charge during discharge of the pulse.

circuit. Because both unipolar and bipolar pacing use an electrode in contact with the myocardium (usually as the cathode), the difference in these configurations lies in the location of the other electrode (usually the anode). For a unipolar pacing stimulus, the anode is extracardiac in the case of the pulse generator. The anode for bipolar stimulation is located on the pacing lead within the heart, either in contact with the endocardium or lying free within the cardiac chamber. The pacing impedance is slightly higher with bipolar than with unipolar pacing, because two conducting wires are required. However, although the stimulation threshold is slightly lower with unipolar than with bipolar pacing, this is of such a small magnitude that it is rarely of any clinical significance.

The clinically important differences between bipolar and unipolar leads relate to sensing, where the advantages of bipolar leads are substantial, and to the increased diameter and reduced flexibility of bipolar leads. Bipolar pacing is also devoid of the potential for pectoral muscle stimulation, which is sometimes encountered with unipolar stimulation if a high stimulus intensity is required. Bipolar pacing may be especially useful in children when a submuscular pocket is used or in patients with a separate ICD in whom a unipolar stimulus is more likely to be inappropriately sensed by the ICD. However, the increased size of the pacing stimulus on the surface electrocardiogram (ECG) with unipolar pacing may be useful for the assessment of proper pacemaker function, especially with transtelephonic ECG tracings. Bipolar pacing leads also provide for a greater variety of rate adaptive sensors, especially sensors of transthoracic impedance to estimate minute ventilation. Bipolar leads are required of some auto-threshold pacing algorithms that use the ring electrode to determine the presence or absence of capture. Despite these many advantages of bipolar leads, unipolar leads have traditionally had greater reliability than similarly designed bipolar leads.

BIVENTRICULAR PACING

Cardiac resynchronization (CRT) adds another layer of complexity to cardiac stimulation. In its most common configuration, CRT involves electrical stimulation of both the left and right ventricles. At present, unipolar and bipolar leads have been commercially released in the United States for transvenous left ventricular pacing. There are several potential ways in which a unipolar lead in a cardiac vein and either a unipolar or bipolar lead in the right ventricle could be configured for biventricular stimulation.[72,73] The first CRT devices used the tip electrodes of the cardiac venous lead and the right ventricular lead as a split cathode. The anode was usually configured as the ring electrode of a bipolar right ventricular lead (termed the *bipolar split cathodal configuration*)[72] (Fig. 2.11A). In this configuration, the current travels over both tip electrodes in inverse relation to the impedance at the cathodal-tissue interface of the two leads. The return path for current is the shared ring electrode on the right ventricular bipolar lead. Alternatively, when the CRT pulse generator is programmed to the unipolar pacing configuration, the pulse generator casing becomes the anode (termed the *unipolar split cathodal configuration*)[72] (Fig. 2.11B). Both of these split cathodal configurations stimulate the right and left ventricles in parallel. Because the left ventricular (LV) and right ventricular (RV) circuits are stimulated in parallel, the total impedance of the circuit is less than when either the LV or the RV tip electrodes are stimulated alone. However there are several alternative configurations that have been used to achieve CRT, especially when using preexisting leads or pulse generators. One possible configuration uses the tip electrode of the cardiac venous lead as the cathode (or anode) and the tip electrode in the right ventricle as the anode (or cathode). Such a configuration has been used when a preexisting unipolar right ventricular pacing lead has been employed for CRT. This widely split bipolar configuration uses two unipolar leads, each having electrodes with small surface area, thereby increasing the

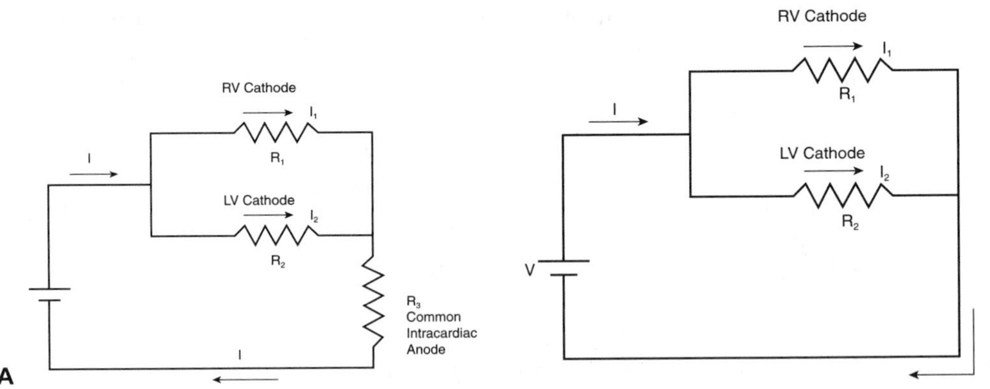

Figure 2.11. (Panel A) Circuit diagram for bipolar split cathodal stimulation in which the tip electrodes of the RV and the LV leads are in parallel with a common anode at the pulse generator housing. **(Panel B)** Circuit diagram for unipolar split cathodal stimulation with the RV and LV tip electrodes in parallel and a common anode at the RV ring electrode. (Reproduced by permission from Barold SS, Levine PA. Significance of stimulation impedance in biventricular pacing. J Intervent Cardiac Electrophysiol 2002;6:67–70.)

overall impedance of the circuit. Alternatively, a Y-adapter can be placed to combine the tip electrodes of two unipolar leads as a split cathode and the pulse generator casing as the anode for unipolar split cathodal stimulation. The split cathodal configurations have several important disadvantages. In studies of these configurations, the apparent left ventricular stimulation threshold approximately doubled with the bipolar split cathodal configuration as compared with the directly measured unipolar LV threshold. The LV stimulation threshold increased from 0.7 ± 0.5 V in the unipolar configuration to 1.0 ± 0.8 V in the unipolar split cathodal configuration ($P = .01$) and from 1.0 ± 0.7 V in the bipolar configuration to 1.3 ± 0.9 V in the bipolar split cathodal configuration ($P < .001$).

The effect of a split cathodal configuration on impedance is complex. In the simplest model of parallel circuits, the total impedance (RT) would be related to the impedances of the RV and LV leads as given by the equation:

$$\frac{1}{R_T} = \frac{1}{R_{RV}} + \frac{1}{R_{LV}} \qquad \text{Eq. 2.3}$$

If the RV and LV lead impedances were equal (500 ohms), then the total impedance would be expected to be 250 ohms. In fact, the observed impedance with a split cathodal configuration is significantly greater than would be predicted by the simple parallel circuit equation. The electrode resistance of a hemispherical electrode is inversely proportional to the square root of the surface area.[74,75] Therefore, to reduce the impedance of an electrode by one-half, it is necessary to quadruple the surface area. Because combining the cathodal electrodes in this study results in an approximate doubling of the electrode surface area, the measured impedance is reduced by a factor of approximately $\sqrt{2}$ (Fig. 2.12). Thus, in practice, the total impedance with the split cathodal configuration of two leads each having an impedance of 500 ohms would be approximated by:

$$R_T = \frac{\left(\frac{R_{LV} + R_{RV}}{2}\right)}{\sqrt{2}} \qquad \text{Eq. 2.4}$$

Thus, the impedance of two 500 ohms leads in a split cathodal configuration would be approximately 350 ohms. This equation gives a value that is much closer to what is observed clinically with a split cathode configuration.

The pacing pulse delivered by the pacing system analyzer is a truncated exponential waveform. The rate of the exponential decay (or droop) of the stimulus waveform is affected by the surface area–dependent values of electrode impedance. The change in the rate of exponential decay that is produced by combining two electrodes as a common cathode can lead to a change in pacing threshold. Because the droop of the waveform contains lower frequencies than the leading edge, it is not only affected by the electrode interface resistance but also by the interface capacitance. Because the capacitance of an electrode is proportional its surface area, the capacitance of two electrodes will approximately double by combining two cathodes. The augmentation of capacitance and decrease in resistance can increase the droop of the stimulus pulse, thereby lowering the voltage before the end of the pulse and increasing the pacing threshold. Another limitation of the split cathodal configuration is that assessment of the electrical integrity of either the LV or the RV lead may be difficult. A complete fracture of the LV lead conductor or the RV tip conductor would have only a small affect on impedance. A fracture of the RV ring conductor would create a dramatic rise in impedance only if the output circuit is programmed bipolar. In addition, a low impedance of one of the leads due to an insulation failure may be difficult to detect because of the already low impedance of the parallel circuit.

More recent generations of US Food and Drug Administration–approved CRT devices use separate output circuits for both the cardiac venous and the right ventricular leads that allow independent programming of stimulation amplitude, pulse duration, and polarity. The use of bipolar leads for both the RV and LV, each with its own output circuit will further simplify CRT, especially sensing.

SENSING

Sensing of the cardiac electrogram is essential to the proper function of permanent pacemakers. In addition to responding to appropriate intrinsic atrial or ventricular electrograms, permanent pacing systems must be able to discriminate these signals from unwanted electrical interference: far-field cardiac events,

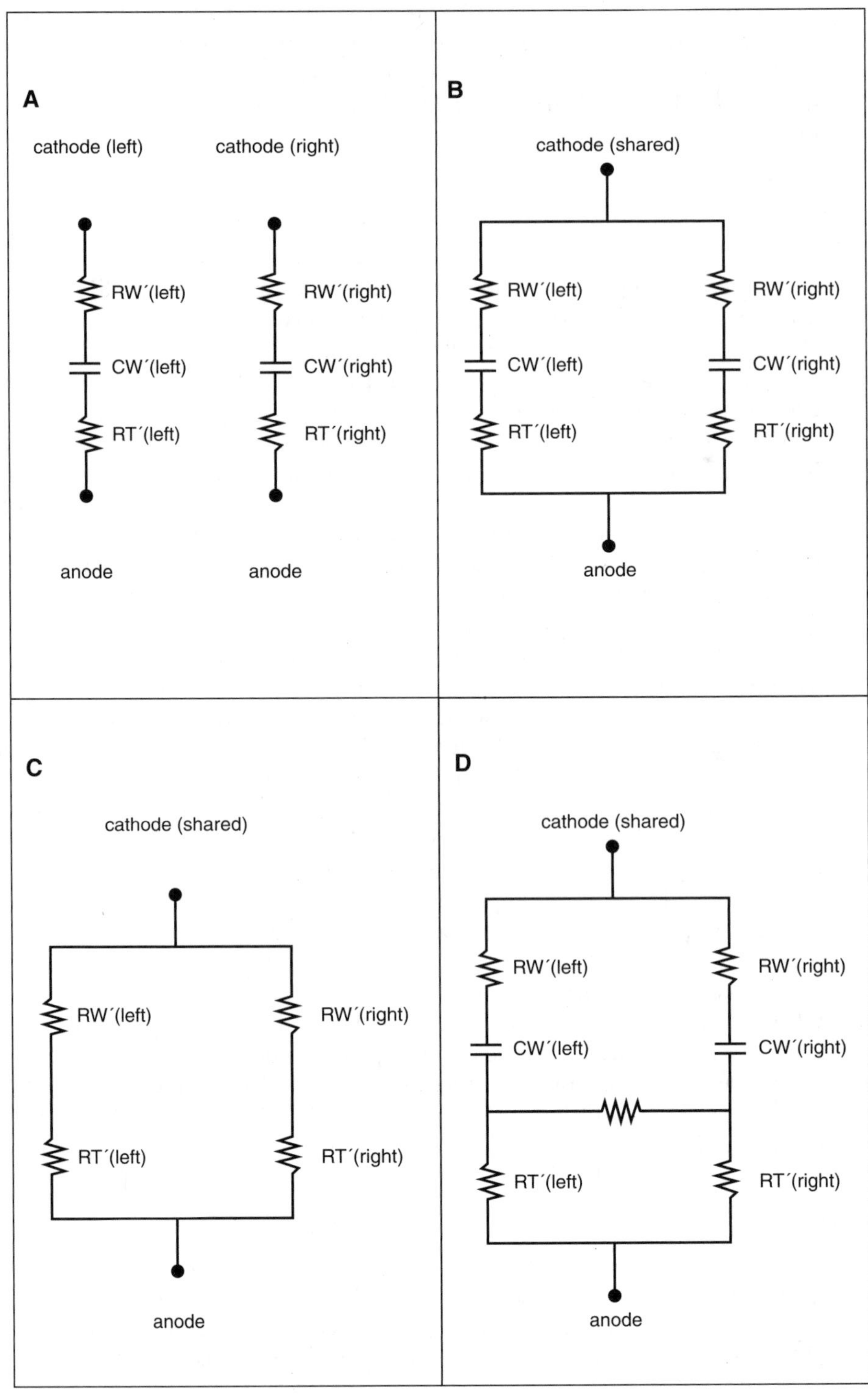
A
cathode (left)
cathode (right)
RW´(left)
CW´(left)
RT´(left)
anode
RW´(right)
CW´(right)
RT´(right)
anode
B
cathode (shared)
RW´(left)
CW´(left)
RT´(left)
RW´(right)
CW´(right)
RT´(right)
anode
C
cathode (shared)
RW´(left)
RT´(left)
RW´(right)
RT´(right)
anode
D
cathode (shared)
RW´(left)
CW´(left)
RT´(left)
RW´(right)
CW´(right)
RT´(right)
anode

diastolic potentials, skeletal muscle signals, and pacing stimuli. In this section, the basic determinants of electrogram sensing will be discussed.

Intracardiac Electrograms

Intracardiac electrical signals are produced by the movement of electrical current through myocardium. An electrode that overlies a region of resting myocardium records from the outside of cardiac myocytes, which are positively charged with respect to the inside of the cell. Despite this, an electrode in one region of resting myocardium will record a charge similar to that recorded by an electrode in another region of resting myocardium (no potential voltage difference between the electrodes). During depolarization, the outside of the cell becomes electrically neutral with respect to the inside. Therefore, as a wavefront of depolarization travels toward an endocardial electrode that records from resting myocardium, the electrode becomes positively charged relative to the depolarized region. This is manifested in the intracardiac electrogram as a positive deflection. As the wavefront of depolarization passes under the recording electrode, the outside of the cell suddenly becomes negatively charged relative to resting myocardium, and a brisk negative deflection is inscribed in the intracardiac electrogram. The peak negative deflection in the intracardiac electrogram, known as the intrinsic deflection (Fig. 2.13), is considered the moment of myocardial activation underlying the recording electrode.[76] The positive and negative deflections that precede and follow the intrinsic deflection represent activation in neighboring regions of myocardium relative to the recording electrode. In clinical practice, the intrinsic deflection in the intracardiac electrogram is usually biphasic, with predominantly negative or positive deflections less frequently observed.[77] Because of the greater mass of myocardium, the normal ventricular electrogram is usually of far greater amplitude than the normal atrial electrogram.

Characteristics of Intracardiac Electrograms: The frequency content of ventricular electrograms has been demonstrated to be similar to that of atrial elec-

Figure 2.12. A common model used to present the electrode to tissue interface based on the Warwick resistor (W) and capacitor (C). The two circuit diagrams are for the left and right sides of the heart before the cathodes were combined. **A:** Faradic resistance is sometimes added in parallel with this circuit to account for behavior with direct current (DC). However, pacing pulses are not considered direct current and, therefore, this resistance was not included for simplification. The anode can be represented by the same series resistor/ capacitor circuit, however, since its values are mostly constant when comparing single and combined cathodes it was not used in the equivalent circuit. **B:** The equivalent circuit for the shared cathode configuration. Notice that the capacitive and resistive values change when the cathodes are combined. **C:** Equivalent circuit for the combined cathodes at the leading edge of the pacing pulse. The interface capacitance is short-circuited at the high frequency leading edge of the pacing pulse. **D:** More complete equivalent circuit in which an additional resistor R is added to account for the possible changes in the current path when the cathodes are combined.

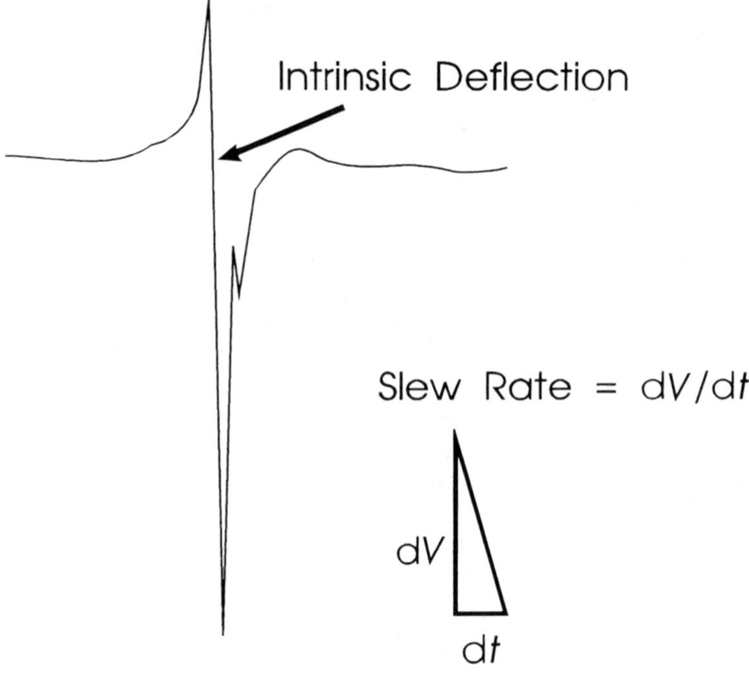

Figure 2.13. A typical bipolar ventricular electrogram in a normal individual. The sharp downward deflection in the electrogram represents the intrinsic deflection and indicates the moment of activation under the recording electrode. The slope of the intrinsic deflection (d*V*/d*t*) is expressed in volts per second and is referred to as the slew rate. For an electrogram to be sensed by a sensing amplifier, the amplitude and slew rate must exceed the sensing threshold.

trograms.[78] By using Fourier transformation, one can express the frequency spectrum of an electrical signal as a series of sine waves of varying frequency and amplitude. Fourier transformation of ventricular electrograms demonstrates that the maximum density of frequencies for R waves is usually found between 10 and 30 Hz.[78] The effects of filtering the atrial electrogram are shown in Figure 2.14. As can be appreciated from the figure, removing frequencies below 10 Hz markedly attenuates the T-wave amplitude without significantly influencing the R wave. The T wave is usually a slower, broader signal that is composed of lower frequencies, generally less than 5 Hz.[78] Similarly, the far-field R wave in the atrial electrogram is composed predominantly of low-frequency signals.[79] Therefore, by high-pass filtering of the intracardiac electrogram, many of the unwanted low-frequency components can be removed. In contrast, the frequency spectrum of skeletal myopotentials ranges from approximately 10 to 200 Hz, with considerable overlap with the intrinsic R and P waves.[78] Although the high-frequency components can be removed with filtering, inappropriate sensing of myopotentials remains a potential problem with the unipolar configuration.

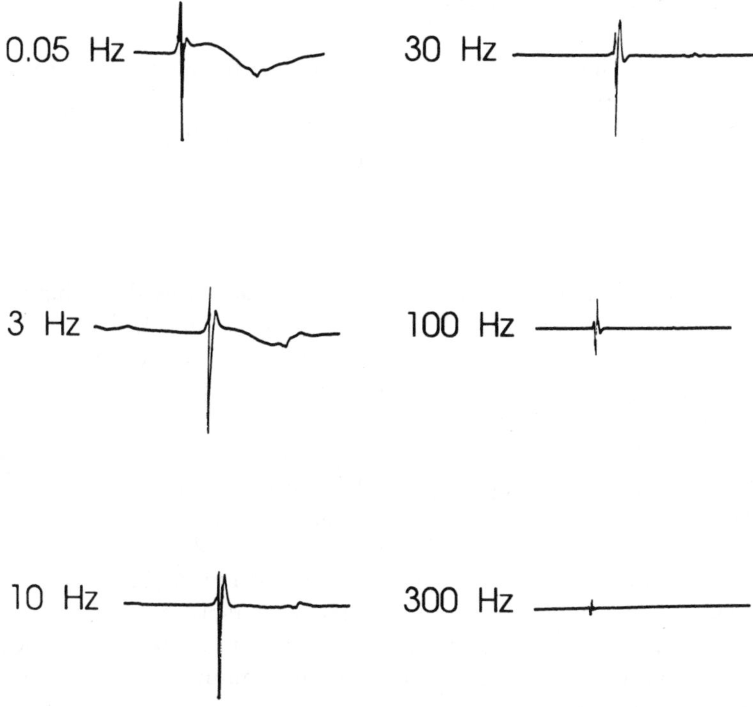

Figure 2.14. The effects of filtering on the bipolar atrial electrogram are demonstrated in an individual. Note that low-pass filtering of the electrogram below 10 Hz has the effect of attenuating the far-field R wave and T wave. Filtering of frequencies greater than 30 Hz results in marked attenuation of the electrogram amplitude. The center frequency of most sensing amplifiers is approximately 30 Hz, consistent with the typical frequency spectra of intra-cardiac electrograms.

For the intracardiac electrogram to be sensed by the sense amplifier of an implantable pulse generator, the signal must be of sufficient amplitude, measured in peak-to-peak voltage. In addition, the intrinsic deflection of the electrogram must have sufficient slope. The peak slope (dV/dt) of the electrogram (also known as the slew rate) is of critical importance to proper sensing (see Fig. 2.13). The sense amplifier of most pulse generators has a center frequency (the frequency for which the amplifier is most sensitive) in the range of 30 to 40 Hz, so frequencies greater than this are attenuated and less likely to be sensed. Components of the electrogram less than the center frequency are also attenuated, with the output of the filter proportional to the slew rate of the waveform. In general, the higher the slew rate of an electrogram, the higher the frequency content. Thus, slow and broad signals with a low slew rate may not be sensed, even if the peak-to-peak amplitude of the electrogram is large. In clinical practice, the slew rate and amplitude of intracardiac electrograms are only modestly proportional. Because of this, both the slew rate and the amplitude of the intracardiac electrogram should be routinely measured.

Unipolar and Bipolar Sensing

Although both unipolar and bipolar sensing configurations detect the difference in electrical potential between two electrodes, the interelectrode distance has a considerable influence on the nature of the electrogram.[80] If a transvenous bipolar lead is used for sensing, both electrodes are located in the heart with an interelectrode distance that is usually less than 3 cm. A unipolar lead uses one electrode in contact with the heart and the other in contact with the pulse generator, often with an interelectrode distance of 30 to 50 cm. Because both electrodes may contribute to the electrical signal that is sensed, the bipolar electrode configuration is minimally influenced by electrical signals that originate outside the heart. In contrast, the unipolar electrode configuration may detect electrical signals that originate near the pulse generator pocket as well as those from inside the heart. These features of unipolar sensing make this electrode configuration much more susceptible to interference by electrical signals originating in skeletal muscle (myopotentials). The myopotentials associated with pectoral muscle contraction may be sensed by unipolar pacemakers, resulting in inappropriate inhibition or triggering of pacing output. Bipolar sensing is relatively immune to myopotentials—a significant clinical advantage. Bipolar sensing is also less likely to be influenced by electromagnetic radiation from the environment than is unipolar sensing. Electrical interference from microwaves, electrocautery, metal detectors, diathermy, or radar is more commonly observed with unipolar than with bipolar sensing.

A bipolar electrogram is actually the instantaneous difference in electrical voltage between the two electrodes. Thus a bipolar electrogram can be constructed by subtracting the absolute unipolar voltage recorded at the cathode (versus ground) from the unipolar voltage recorded at the anode (versus ground). Because the bipolar configuration represents the signal at the cathode minus the signal at the anode, the net electrogram may be considerably different from that of either unipolar electrogram alone. For example, if an advancing wavefront of depolarization is perpendicular to the interelectrode axis of a bipolar lead, each electrode will be activated at exactly the same time. Because the unipolar electrogram at each electrode will be similar and inscribed at the same time, the instantaneous difference in voltage will be minimal. In this situation, the bipolar electrogram will be markedly attenuated. A wavefront of depolarization traveling parallel to the interelectrode axis of a bipolar lead will activate one electrode before the other. The resulting bipolar electrogram may have significantly greater amplitude than either unipolar electrogram alone. From these examples it should be recognized that bipolar sensing is more sensitive to the direction in which the depolarizing wavefront travels than is unipolar sensing. Bipolar electrograms are more likely to be influenced by phasic changes in orientation of the lead with respiration than are unipolar electrograms. Because of these considerations, the electrogram measured at the time of lead implantation should be recorded in the configuration that will be used for sensing by the pulse generator.

Another significant difference between unipolar and bipolar sensing relates to the amplitude of far-field signals. Because of the significantly greater mass of the ventricles, the atrial electrogram often records a far-field R wave (Fig. 2.15). For unipolar atrial leads, the far-field R wave may be equal to or of greater amplitude than the atrial deflection. In contrast, the bipolar atrial electrogram usually records an atrial deflection that is considerably larger than the far-field R wave. The programmable post-ventricular atrial refractory period of dual-chamber pacemakers has effectively reduced inappropriate sensing of far-field R waves in the unipolar atrial electrogram. Despite this, far-field R wave sensing remains an important concern with atrial antitachycardia (AAI) pacemakers and requires the use of long refractory periods in many patients. AAI pacemakers that are designed to interrupt atrial tachycardias require the use of short atrial refractory periods to detect very rapid atrial rates. Because of concerns regarding the inappropriate sensing of far-field R waves and myopotentials with unipolar sensing, antitachycardia pacing systems require the use of bipolar leads.

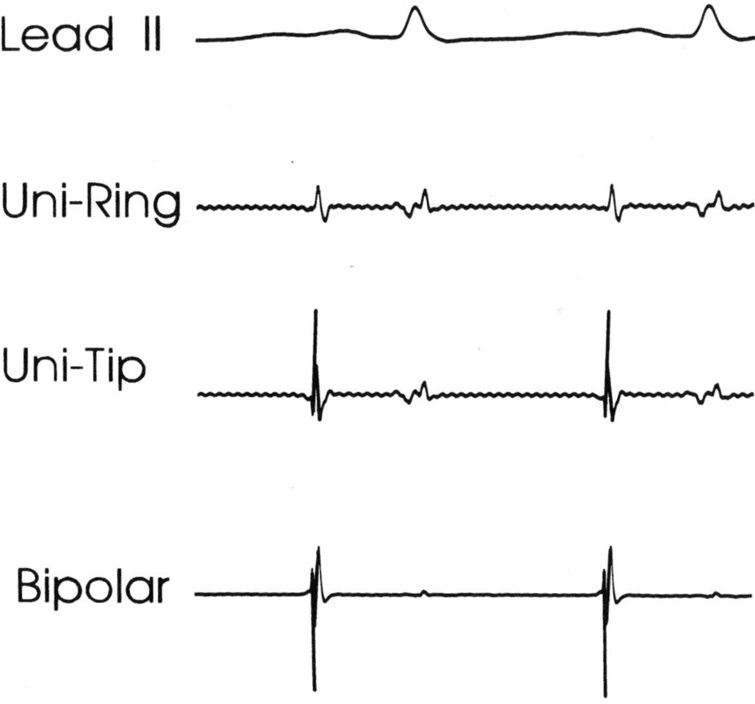

Figure 2.15. Simultaneously recorded unipolar and bipolar atrial electrograms from the ring and tip electrodes of a permanent pacing lead. Note that both of the unipolar electrograms record a far-field R wave. The bipolar electrogram records a sharp atrial deflection and markedly attenuates the far-field R wave. Bipolar sensing is characterized by a relative immunity to far-field electrical events.

The problem of far-field R-wave detection in the atrial electrogram has been addressed by Goldreyer and colleagues by the development of leads incorporating a pair of closely spaced electrodes placed circumferentially around the catheter.[81,82] This concept, known as an orthogonal electrode array, uses electrodes that are separated by 180 degrees around the circumference of the lead body. These electrodes do not contact the atrial myocardium directly but "float" free within the atrial blood pool. The advantage of orthogonal sensing is that both electrodes record ventricular activation nearly simultaneously, with a marked attenuation of the far-field R wave and a greater signal-to-noise ratio. The improved signal-to-noise characteristics of orthogonal electrodes have allowed the use of more sensitive atrial amplifiers and increased reliability of atrial sensing. Orthogonal electrodes have also provided a method for dual-chamber (VDD) pacing that uses a single lead. The single-lead concept uses an electrode at the tip of the catheter, which is placed at the right ventricular apex for ventricular pacing and sensing, and a pair of orthogonally arranged electrodes located more proximally along the catheter in the atrium for atrial sensing.

Sensing in Cardiac Resynchronization Tube Devices

The first generation of CRT devices sensed the electrogram created by combining the left and right ventricular tip electrodes as a single electrode versus the right ventricular ring electrode. The resulting composite electrogram includes both right and left ventricular components (Fig. 2.16). If the width of

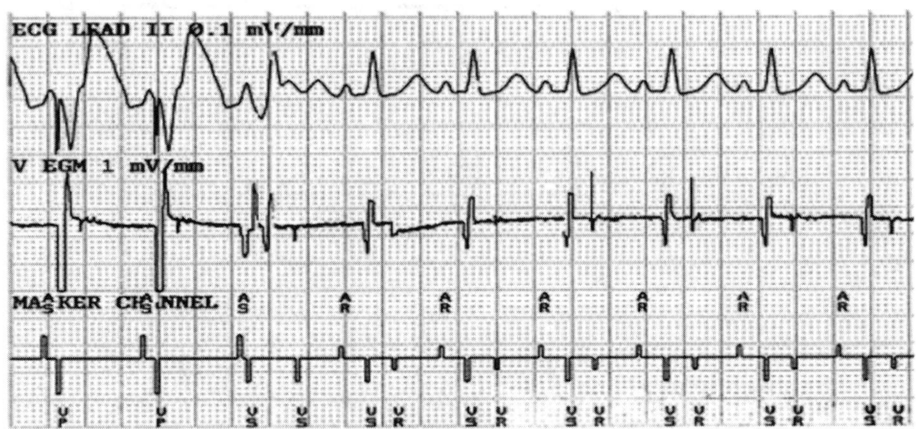

Figure 2.16. An example of loss of atrial tracking by a premature ventricular complex (PVC) that inhibits ventricular pacing for one beat, followed by double counting of the intrinsically conducted ventricular electrogram which represents a composite of RV and LV components. Because of the long intraventricular conduction delay (RV to LV), double counting of the ventricular electrogram resets the ventricular refractory period and the post ventricular atrial refractory period (PVARP) such that the next atrial electrogram occurs during PVARP. As a result, there is perpetuation of intrinsic conduction and failure to maintain consistent cardiac resynchronization therapy.

the combined electrogram exceeds the ventricular blanking period, the potential exists for double counting of the ventricular rate. For pacemakers and ICDs, the most common manifestation is that of increasing the total atrial refractory period (TARP). This is illustrated in Figure 2.17. Remember that the normal post ventricular atrial refractory period begins after a sensed or paced ventricular event. When there is biventricular pacing, both ventricles are paced simultaneously and the post ventricular atrial refractory period begins with the ventricular pacing stimulus. However, when the ventricles are not paced, the sensed biventricular electrogram has two components (right followed by left ventricular components in the case of left bundle branch block). In this situation, the post-ventricular atrial refractory period begins after the second component of the ventricular electrogram. When an atrial event is followed by a biventricular paced event, the total atrial refractory period is equal to the AV delay + PVARP. On the other hand, when an atrial event is followed by a ventricular sensed event, the total atrial refractory period is equal to the AV delay + the RV-LV delay + PVARP. This is illustrated in Figure 2.18, and by the following equations:

$$pTARP = AVD + PVARP$$
(atrial event followed by biventricular pacing) Eq. 2.5

$$iTARP = AVD + IVCD + PVARP$$
(atrial event followed by ventricular sensed event) Eq. 2.6

in which pTARP is the paced total atrial refractory period, iTARP is the intrinsic total atrial refractory period, AVD is the programmed AV delay, and IVCD is the interventricular conduction delay between right and left components of the biventricular sensed electrogram. The consequence of a greater iTARP than pTARP is that ventricular tracking is maintained at faster rates when there is

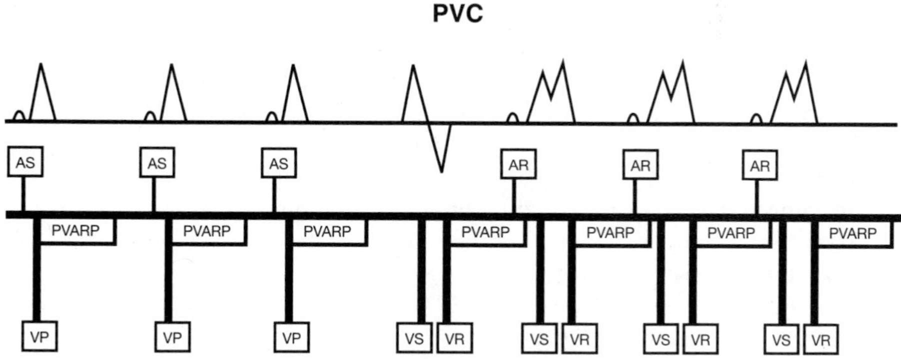

Figure 2.17. Inhibition of atrial tracking by a PVC that extends the PVARP to 400 milliseconds. As a result of post-PVC PVARP extension, the subsequent atrial electrogram falls within PVARP, inhibiting tracking and leading to persistent double counting of the ventricular electrograms during LBBB intrinsic conduction. (Courtesy of Medtronic, Inc.)

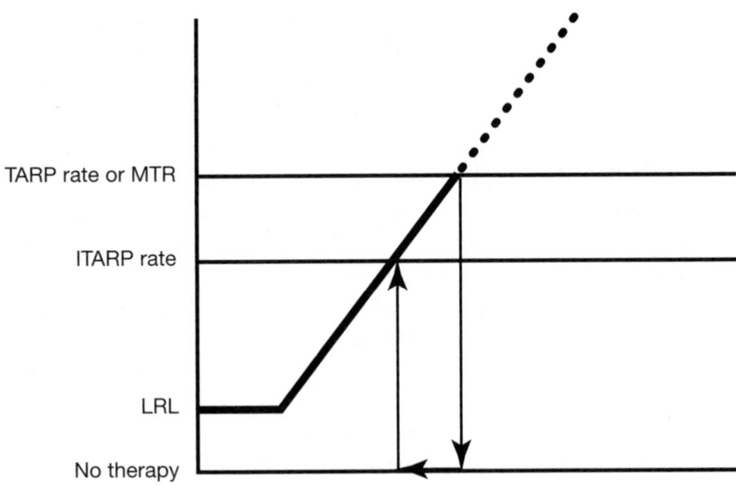

Figure 2.18. Graphical presentation of the maximum tracking rate (MTR) that can be achieved during consistent biventricular pacing (TARP rate) which is determined by adding the AV delay + PVARP. However, during a sensed ventricular rhythm using a composite ventricular electrogram from both the RV and LV, the intrinsic total atrial refractory period (iTARP) is equal to AV delay + IVCD + PVARP. Thus, the atrial rate that will be tracked is equal to the TARP rate during biventricular pacing but the iTARP rate during double sensing of the composite ventricular electrogram. The difference between TARP and iTARP is equal to the IVCD in the ventricular electrogram. (Reproduced by permission from Wang P, Kramer A, Estes M, Hayes DL. Timing cycles for biventricular pacing. PACE 2002;25:62–75.)

consistent biventricular capture than when there is intrinsic conduction (Fig. 2.18). As an example of the practical application of these equations, consider a biventricular pacemaker programmed with a maximum tracking rate of 125 bpm, an AV delay of 150 milliseconds, a PVARP of 300 milliseconds, and an IVCD equal to 200 milliseconds. When there is biventricular pacing, the pTARP equals 450 milliseconds and atrial tracking may occur to the programmed maximum rate of 125 bpm (pTARP equals 450 milliseconds, less than the maximum tracking interval of 480 milliseconds). However, if there is ventricular sensing rather than pacing, the iTARP equals 650 milliseconds and the maximum tracking rate would be limited to 92 bpm. As a result, effective cardiac resynchronization would not be delivered at rates that are considerably slower than the clinician had intended.

Another consequence of double counting of the intrinsic composite biventricular electrogram is the potential for inappropriate detection of ventricular "tachycardias" by an ICD. If there is double counting, the rate identified by the ICD will be double the actual ventricular rate and ICD therapies can be delivered inappropriately. The most common scenario is for sinus tachycardia to be sensed as ventricular tachycardia or ventricular fibrillation. In addition, a relatively slow ventricular tachycardia may be sensed at a rate double that the actual rate so that it falls in the ventricular fibrillation detection zone.

To overcome these limitations of biventricular sensing using a composite ventricular electrogram, the newer generations of ICDs stimulate both the right and left ventricles but only use the right ventricular electrogram to determine ventricular timing. This eliminates the potential for ventricular oversensing and markedly simplifies follow-up of these devices. Nevertheless, if both ventricles are paced but only the right ventricle is sensed, there exists the possibility for left ventricular premature depolarizations to be undersensed. In the worst case scenario, when there is a wide interval between RV and LV pacing, a VPD in the LV could be undersensed and followed by an RV stimulus and then an LV stimulus that falls in the vulnerable period of the LV. To minimize this risk ICD manufacturers have introduced such features as an LV protection period (LVPP) and an interventricular refractory period (IVRP) that allow sensing in the LV to inhibit ventricular pacing after a VPD without altering the basic timing cycle of the device.

Polarization

Following application of a polarizing pulse, an afterpotential of opposite charge is induced in the myocardium at the interface of the stimulating electrode (Fig. 2.19). Immediately after cathodal stimulation, an excess of positive charges surrounds the electrode, which then exponentially decays to electrical neutrality. This positively charged afterpotential can be inappropriately sensed by the sensing circuit of the pulse generator with resulting inhibition of the next pacing pulse.[83] The amplitude of afterdepolarizations is directly related to the amplitude and duration of the pacing stimulus. Thus afterdepolarizations are most likely to be sensed during conditions of maximum stimulus voltage and pulse duration, combined with the maximum sensitivity setting of the pulse genera-

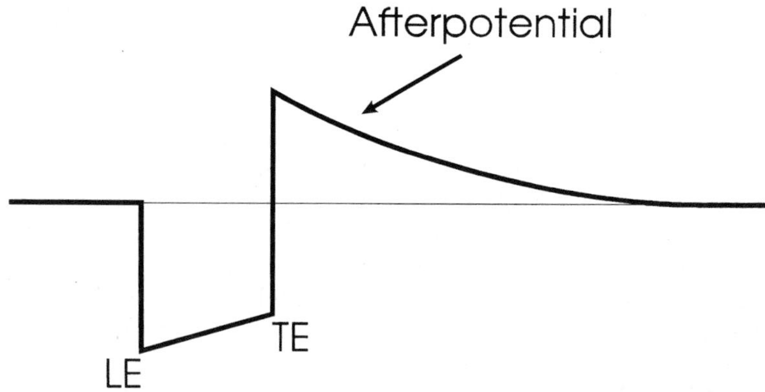

Figure 2.19. Diagram of a constant-voltage output pulse (downward deflection) and a resultant afterpotential of opposite polarity. LE = leading edge, TE = trailing edge.

tor.[84] The inappropriate sensing of near-field afterpotentials has been eliminated by the use of sensing refractory periods that prevent the sensing circuit from responding to electrical signals for a programmable period following the pacing stimulus. However, for dual-chamber pacing systems, afterdepolarizations of sufficient amplitude in one chamber may be sensed by the sensing amplifier in the other chamber. This is most likely to occur with the sensing of atrial afterpotentials in the AV interval by the ventricular sensing circuit, resulting in inappropriate inhibition of ventricular stimulus output (crosstalk). Because of the potential for inhibition of ventricular pacing by the far-field sensing of atrial afterdepolarizations, the ventricular sensing circuit is inactivated for a period (blanking period) following the delivery of an atrial pacing stimulus. Crosstalk is a rare clinical problem with bipolar pacing and sensing, however.

Time-Related Changes in Intracardiac Electrograms

Immediately following implantation of a transvenous lead, the electrogram "ST segment" usually demonstrates a typical injury current. The current of injury is caused by the pressure that is exerted by the distal electrode on myocardial cell membranes. The current of injury is observed with both atrial and ventricular leads and is so typical of the acute electrogram that its absence may reflect malposition of the lead with poor contact of the distal electrode and the endocardium. Lack of an injury current may also reflect placement of the lead in an area of fibrotic myocardium. The injury current is observed with both active and passive fixation electrodes. The injury current usually returns to the isoelectric line over a period ranging from several minutes to several hours.

The amplitude of the intracardiac electrogram typically declines abruptly within several days following implantation, with a gradual increase toward the acute value by 6 to 8 weeks. The chronic R-wave amplitude of passive fixation electrodes has been shown to be approximately 85% of the acute value.[32] The attenuation of the slew rate is considerably greater, with chronic values averaging approximately 50% to 60% of the acute measurement. Corticosteroid-eluting leads have demonstrated minimal deterioration of the electrogram from implantation through regular follow-up assessments.[42–46]

Active fixation leads may be associated with a somewhat different time course than passive fixation leads in the evolution of the intracardiac electrogram, with a markedly attenuated amplitude and slew rate immediately following lead positioning.[33] Over the next 20 to 30 minutes, the electrogram amplitude typically increases. It is likely that the trauma caused by extension of a screw helix into the myocardium is responsible for this hyperacute evolution of the intracardiac electrogram. Recognition of this phenomenon may prevent the unnecessary repositioning of an active fixation lead. In general, active and passive fixation leads are associated with similar chronic electrogram amplitudes.[32–85]

Sensing Impedance

The intracardiac electrogram must be carried by the pacing lead from its source in the myocardium to the sensing amplifier of the pulse generator. The voltage drop that occurs from the origin of the electrical signal in the heart to the proximal portion of the lead depends on the source impedance. The components of source impedance include the resistance between the electrode and the myocardium, the resistance offered by the lead conductor, and the effect of polarization. The electrode resistance is inversely related to the surface area of the electrode.[68] Polarization impedance is also inversely related to electrode surface area. Thus electrodes with large surface area minimize source impedance and contribute to improved sensing.

The electrogram that is sensed by the pulse generator can also be attenuated by a mismatch in impedance between the lead (the source impedance) and the sensing amplifier (input impedance).[86,87] The greater the ratio of input impedance to source impedance, the less the electrogram is attenuated and the more accurately it reflects the true amplitude and morphology of the signal in the myocardium. Thus the drop in electrogram amplitude from the actual voltage in the myocardium to the signal that is sensed by the pulse generator is minimized by a low-source impedance and a high-input impedance. The source impedance of current pacing leads ranges from approximately 400 to 1500 ohms. The sensing amplifiers of currently available pulse generators typically have an input impedance greater than 25,000 ohms. The clinical significance of impedance mismatch (too low a ratio of input impedance to source impedance) is the failure of sensing with insulation failure or conductor fracture. An insulation failure between the conductors of a bipolar lead results in shunting across the amplifier and an effective fall in input impedance. In this situation the electrogram amplitude may be attenuated, with loss of appropriate sensing. A conductor fracture leads to a marked increase in source impedance and a similar impedance mismatch and sensing failure.

Automated Capture Features

To ensure ventricular capture and to allow programming of a low margin of safety, several manufacturers of pacemakers have introduced algorithms that automatically detect ventricular capture and adjust the output of the pacing stimulus. The Autocapture™ feature of St Jude Medical pacemakers allows the pacemaker to automatically adjust the amplitude of the stimulation pulse by detecting capture in the ventricle (Fig. 2.20). These pacemakers require a bipolar ventricular pacing lead that must have low polarization properties for the distal electrode. The presence or absence of ventricular capture is determined by sensing of the evoked response (ER) from the ring electrode. These devices automatically determine the evoked response gain and sensitivity levels by delivering five paired ventricular pulses at 4.5 V and a minimum pulse duration of 0.5 milliseconds or the programmed value. The first of the paired pulses measures the ER while the second pulse is delivered within 100 milliseconds of the first (in the physiologic refractory period of the myocardium) to determine the level of polarization. If the ER amplitude is greater than 2.5 mV, the measured lead polarization is less than 4.0 mV, and the ratio of the ER to the ER sensitivity is greater than 1.8 : 1, the device automatically determines that the safety

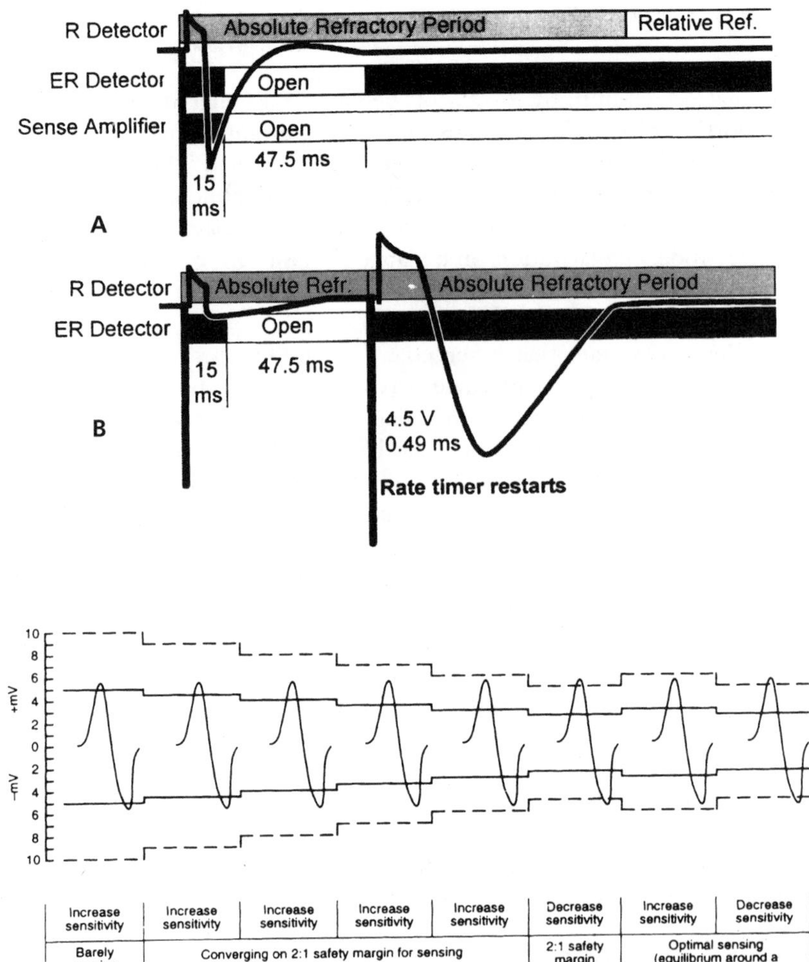

Figure 2.20. Algorithms for automated determination of pacing and sensing thresholds. **Top: (A)** The St. Jude Medical AutoCapture algorithm documents ventricular capture on a beat-to-beat basis by detecting the local evoked electrical response that follows the pacing stimulus. After a 15-millisecond blanking period following the pacing stimulus, the evoked response detection window is open for the next 47.5 milliseconds. If the local evoked electrogram is detected, capture has occurred. **B:** If no evoked response is detected, a high output backup pulse is delivered at the end of the sensing window to provide capture. Two consecutive pulses without capture cause the device to redetermine the capture threshold and adjust the output of the first stimulus to 0.25V above threshold. (Reproduced by permission from Clarke M, Liu B, Schuller H, et al. Automatic adjustment of pacemaker stimulation output correlated with continuously monitored capture thresholds: a multicenter study. European Microny Study Group. Pacing Clin Electrophysiol 1998;21:1567–1575.) **C:** Intermedics automated algorithm to maintain a twofold safety margin for sensing. Inner (*solid line*) and outer (*dotted line*) sensing target levels are monitored. Sensing between the inner and outer target levels drives the sensitivity to more sensitive settings. When the outer target is reached, the sensitivity is moved to less sensitive settings. (Reproduced by permission from Castro A, Liebold A, Vincente J, et al. Evaluation of autosensing as an automatic means of maintaining a 2:1 sensing safety margin in an implanted pacemaker. Autosensing Investigation Team. Pacing Clin Electrophysiol 1996;19:1708–1713.)

margins are acceptable and AutoCapture is recommended. The AutoCapture feature uses unipolar pacing from the tip electrode and determines capture on a beat-to-beat basis. If a ventricular stimulus is not followed by a detectable evoked response, a second test pulse is given at a value equal to 0.25 V above the last threshold measurement (a value known as the automatic pulse amplitude or APA). If a pulse is not followed by detectable capture, a backup pulse is delivered within 80 to 100 milliseconds at an amplitude of 4.5 mV. If two consecutive APA pulses are not followed by an evoked response, the threshold is measured to determine whether the APA needs adjustment. Specifically, the pulse is incremented 0.25 V above the last APA. If capture is not confirmed, the APA is repeated in 0.125-V increments until two consecutive captured events occur. The important point is that all loss of capture pulses are immediately followed by a backup pulse. A potential complicating factor with detection of the evoked response is differentiating fusion from capture. In the DDD(R) pacing mode, precisely timed intrinsic conduction can result in false detection of loss of capture. To differentiate true loss of capture from fusion, the AV delay is incremented by 100 milliseconds after two consecutive loss-of-capture events to search for intrinsic conduction. If intrinsic conduction is indeed present during this extension of the AV delay, the backup pulse is eliminated. On the other hand, if subsequent backup pulses or APA increments are required due to loss of capture, the AV/PV delay is shortened to 50/25 milliseconds. This sequence can introduce confusion into the interpretation of electrocardiographic tracings with irregular AV delays. However, knowledge of the function of the AutoCapture algorithm allows recognition that this is a normal phenomenon.

Other manufacturers offer variants of the automatic capture algorithm that do not deliver backup pulses on a beat-to-beat basis but provide automatic determination of pacing threshold at programmed intervals during the day. These devices determine the pacing threshold and adjust the pacing amplitude to provide a programmed margin of safety. In general, automatic capture algorithms function quite effectively and may reduce the risk of loss of capture due to fluctuations in pacing threshold due to drugs, metabolic derangement, or lead dislodgement. The capability for reducing the programmed margin of safety is effective for prolonging battery life and may reduce the frequency of clinic follow-ups. The Medtronic Ventricular Capture Management™ feature determines a strength duration threshold at a programmable interval (nominal is once per day). The amplitude threshold is determined at a pulse duration of 0.4 milliseconds. Following this, the pulse amplitude is doubled and a pulse duration threshold is measured. The permanent ventricular stimulation amplitude is then automatically reprogrammed using a programmable amplitude safety margin (usually twice threshold) or a programmable minimum amplitude (whichever is higher). The nominal values for ventricular capture management are a safety margin of twice threshold with a pulse duration of 0.4 milliseconds and a minimum ventricular amplitude of 2.5 V. During measurement of pacing threshold, each test pulse is followed by a backup pulse 110 milliseconds later to ensure that a pacing pause does not occur. If the automatically measured ventricular stimulation threshold is greater than 2.5 V at 0.4 milliseconds, the ventricular output is automatically programmed to 5.0 V and 1.0 millisecond.

The Medtronic Atrial Capture Management™ feature is designed to periodically measure the atrial stimulation threshold and adapt the atrial output to a programmable amplitude safety margin. This feature does not use the evoked potential to determine the presence or absence of atrial capture. Rather, the pacemaker searches for evidence that atrial test pulses reset the sinus node (Atrial Chamber Reset Method) or by observing the ventricular response to determine if a captured atrial test pulse is conducted to the ventricles through the AV conduction system. The atrial capture management feature performs an atrial amplitude threshold at 0.4-millisecond pulse duration and after loss of capture is detected (defined as two of three test pulses indicating loss of capture) the amplitude setting is increased until atrial capture is confirmed. Since this feature does not rely on detection of the evoked response, there is no restriction on the type of atrial lead that can be used. This feature will not measure thresholds if the sinus rate is consistently faster than 87 bpm.

Autosensing Functions

Because the most common cause of anomalous pacemaker behavior relates to problems with sensing, several manufacturers have introduced pacemakers that automatically determine the amplitude of P- and R-waves and reprogram the atrial and ventricular sensitivity settings to maintain an acceptable sensing safety margin (see Fig. 2.20). The clinical utility of autosensitivity is highlighted by the observation that programming a 100% sensing safety margin based on a single P-wave measurement provides reliable atrial sensing in only 72% of patients with dual-chamber pacemakers. The Medtronic Sensing Assurance feature measures the amplitude of P- and R-waves and classifies each as *low, high,* or *adequate* based on a non-programmable target-sensing margin. This feature attempts to reprogram the atrial sensitivity value so that the atrial electrogram is maintained within a range that is 4.0 to 5.6 times the programmed sensitivity value. For example, if the atrial sensitivity value is programmed to 0.5 mV, an atrial electrogram amplitude between 0.5 and 2.0 mV the sensing margin is classified as *low* (between 1.0 and 4.0 times sensitivity value); if between 2.0 and 2.8 it is classified as *adequate* (between 4.0 and 5.6 times sensitivity value); and if greater than 2.8 mV, it is classified as *high* (>5.6 times). In the ventricle, the safety margin is maintained between 2.8 and 4.0 times.

LEAD DESIGN

Permanent pacing leads have five major components: 1) the electrode(s); 2) the conductor(s); 3) insulation; 4) the connector pin; and 5) the fixation mechanism. Each of these components has critical design considerations, as well as failure modes. In this section, the factors that are important for design of leads are reviewed.

Electrodes

As discussed previously in this chapter, the stimulation threshold is a function of the current density generated at the electrode.[26,34–36] In general, the smaller the radius of the electrode, the greater the current density. The resistance at the electrode-myocardial interface is higher with smaller electrodes, providing for the efficient use of a constant-voltage pulse and improving battery longevity. Both of these factors favor electrodes with small radius for myocardial stimulation. In contrast, sensing impedance and electrode polarization are decreased with electrodes of larger surface area.[26,68,83,84] Although higher sensing impedance with a small electrode is easily compensated by a higher input impedance of the sensing amplifier, the issue of polarization favors the use of a large electrode to minimize afterpotentials. The ideal pacing lead would have an electrode with a small radius (to increase current density) and a large surface area (to reduce polarization).[68] The solution to these conflicting considerations for optimal stimulation and sensing characteristics has been addressed by the development of electrodes that have a small radius but a complex surface structure that provides a large surface area.[66–70,83]

Electrode Shape: The effect of electrode shape on current density has been studied extensively by Irnich and colleagues. Electrodes with a smooth, hemispherical shape produce a uniform current density. In contrast, electrodes with more complex shapes typically produce an irregular pattern of current density, with "hot spots" at the edges and points of the electrode. Electrodes with an irregular shape enable a high current density to be maintained at these hot spots while presenting a larger overall surface area to the endocardial surface. For example, a ring-tipped electrode resulted in better stimulation thresholds and sensing characteristics than did the older hemispherical electrode designs. Other electrode shapes that were introduced to produce areas of high current density included a grooved hemispherical design and a dish-shaped design with holes bored into the electrode. Leads with helical, screw-shaped electrodes, hooks, and barbs have all been demonstrated to provide areas of increased current density and acceptable stimulation thresholds. Most modern leads have used a small electrode with a complex surface structure to achieve improved stimulation and sensing characteristics.

Surface Structure: Early pacing leads used electrodes with a polished metal surface. The use of electrodes with a textured surface has resulted in a dramatic increase in the surface area of the electrode without an increase in radius.[68–70] The textured surface of modern leads minimizes polarization and improves sensing and stimulation efficiency. The surface of an electrode may be porous, with a structure containing thousands of microscopic pores ranging from 20 to 100 μm. The surface of some leads is coated with sintered microspheres of Elgiloy, platinum, or iridium oxide. In addition, the electrode may be constructed of a woven mesh of microscopic metallic fibers enclosed within a screened basket of wire. The performance of carbon electrodes has been improved by roughening of the surface, a process that is known as *activation*. Each of these porous or roughened surface structures has been shown to minimize polarization greatly; such a structure can lead to the ingrowth of tissue into the electrode.

The ability to differentiate an evoked intracardiac electrogram from afterpotentials is greatly influenced by the polarization characteristics of the electrode. The importance of electrodes with low polarization has greatly increased as pacing systems with the capability to automatically measure the pacing threshold through accurate capture detection have been introduced. In fact, automatic detection of capture may not be possible with some leads having high amplitude afterpotentials. Although sensing is improved by the porous electrode design, the improvement in chronic stimulation thresholds has been mainly accomplished by the use of corticosteroid elution and atraumatic fixation mechanisms.

Chemical Composition: To minimize inflammation and subsequent fibrosis at the tissue interface, electrodes for permanent pacing leads should be biologically inert and resistant to chemical degradation. Certain metals, such as zinc, copper, mercury, nickel, lead, and silver, are associated with toxic reactions in the myocardium and are unsuitable for use in the electrodes of chronically implanted leads.[88] In addition to these materials with direct tissue toxicity, metals that are susceptible to corrosion have been demonstrated to result in increased chronic stimulation thresholds. Stainless steel alloys are variably associated with the potential for corrosion. Titanium and tantalum have been shown to acquire a surface coating of oxides, which may impede charge transfer at the electrode interface. However, titanium that is coated with microscopic particles of platinum or vitreous carbon has been found to have excellent long-term performance as a pacing electrode.[69,70] The polarity of the electrode may also have an important influence on its chemical stability. For example, Elgiloy is a quite acceptable electrode material when used as the cathode. However, when used as the anode, Elgiloy is susceptible to a significant degree of corrosion.

The materials presently in use for the electrodes of permanent pacing leads include platinum-iridium, Elgiloy, platinum coated with platinized titanium, vitreous or pyrolytic carbon coating a titanium or graphite core, platinum, or iridium oxide. The platinized-platinum and iridium-oxide electrodes have been associated with a reduced degree of polarization. Although a small degree of corrosion may occur with any of these materials, the carbon electrodes appear to be less susceptible. The carbon electrodes have been improved by roughening the surface, a process known as activation, which reduces polarization. The chronic thresholds of the activated carbon electrodes compare favorably to those observed with platinum–iridium and Elgiloy.[69]

Steroid-Eluting Electrodes: A major advance in permanent pacing lead technology has been the development of electrodes that elute small amounts of the corticosteroid dexamethasone sodium phosphate.[42–45] The steroid-eluting electrodes incorporate a silicone core that is impregnated with a small quantity of dexamethasone (Fig. 2.21). The core is surrounded by a porous titanium electrode that is coated with platinum. The steroid-eluting leads are characterized by a minimal change in stimulation threshold from implantation to a follow-up period of several years. The acute peak in stimulation threshold is virtually eliminated with these leads. The variation in chronic threshold among individuals is significantly reduced, allowing the confident use of lower pacing amplitudes. It should be emphasized that the corticosteroid eluted from the lead does not affect acute stimulation thresholds. Rather, dexamethasone controls the chronic evolution of the pacing threshold. The design characteristics associated with reduced polarization and chemical stability remain important considerations, even with steroid-eluting leads. Steroid elution may also be accomplished with a drug-impregnated collar that surrounds the tip electrode. Corticosteroid leads are now routinely used for both active and passive fixation designs and have dramatically reduced the risk of exit block (an excessive increase in chronic stimulation threshold) for endocardial pacing and ICD leads as well as for epimyocardial leads.

The studies of Stokes and Bornzin have indicated that the mechanism by which dexamethasone sodium phosphate prevents a rise in chronic stimulation

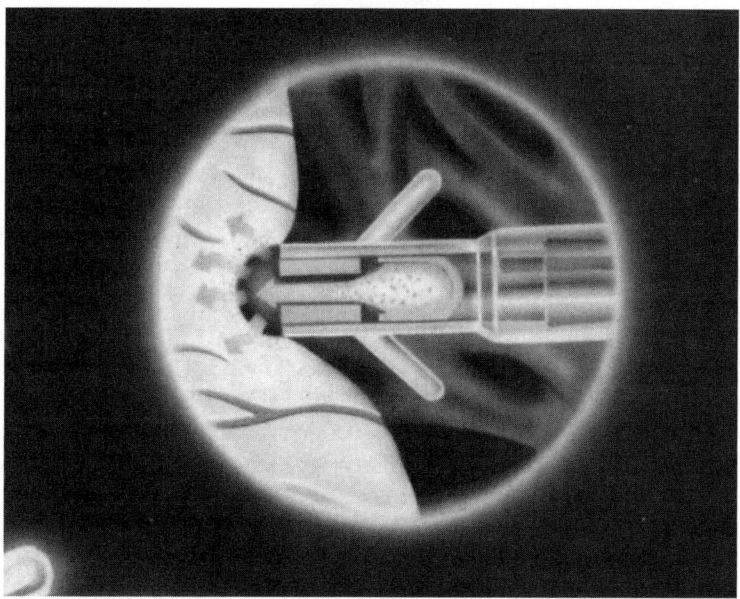

Figure 2.21. Diagram of a steroid-eluting electrode with a reservoir of dexamethasone sodium phosphate that slowly elutes through the electrode into the underlying myocardium. (Courtesy of Medtronic, Inc.)

threshold remains to be fully explained.[46] Although the thickness of the fibrous capsule that surrounds the electrode is reduced, the magnitude is less than would be expected by the evolution in stimulation threshold. This suggests that other mechanisms may be involved. In addition to studies of the steroid-eluting electrodes, clinical studies of pacing leads incorporating a drug-eluting collar surrounding the electrode are ongoing.[46] The duration that drug elution is required for sustained low thresholds remains to be fully defined. Nevertheless, long-term follow-up for over 10 years has indicated that the impressively low chronic thresholds observed with steroid-eluting electrodes appear to be maintained over the usable entire service life of most pacing leads. The routine use of steroid-eluting leads with high electrode resistance has allowed pulse generators to be reduced in size, because of a reduced battery capacity, while maintaining acceptable longevity.

Fixation Mechanism: The chronic performance of permanent pacing leads is critically dependent on stable positioning of the electrode(s). Although early pacing leads were associated with an unacceptably high risk of dislodgment, the development of active and passive fixation mechanisms has dramatically reduced the need for lead repositioning.[89] Previous generations of permanent transvenous pacing leads included several appendages at the distal end that were designed to lodge within the trabeculae of the right atrium or ventricle. However, tines have become the predominant fixation mechanism currently used for passive permanent pacing leads (Fig. 2.22).[90] Passive fixation leads are typically entrapped within the trabeculae of the right heart chambers immediately upon correct positioning of the lead. Effective fixation of the lead can be confirmed at the time of implantation by gentle traction or rotation of the lead. Tines generally add minimal technical difficulty to the implantation procedure, although they may occasionally become entrapped in the tricuspid valve apparatus. The passive fixation devices are rapidly covered by fibrous tissue, making later removal of the lead by simple traction difficult or impossible in as short a time as 6 months. Besides the effectiveness of passive fixation devices to prevent dislodgment, the increased stability that is provided for the distal electrode serves to minimize trauma at the myocardial interface caused by motion. This added stability is likely to result in a smaller fibrous capsule surrounding the electrode and improvement of the chronic stimulation threshold. The passive fixation devices have the relative disadvantage of increasing the maximum external diameter of the lead, requiring the use of a larger venous introducer when the subclavian vein puncture technique is used. Removability of pacing leads is an important consideration. In general, passive fixation leads are more difficult to extract than active fixation leads.

Active Fixation Leads: Although several different fixation methods such as screws, barbs, or hooks have been developed, the present generation of active fixation pacing leads largely relies on a screw helix that is extended into the endocardium (see Fig. 2.22).[91,92] The screw helix may be permanently exposed from the tip

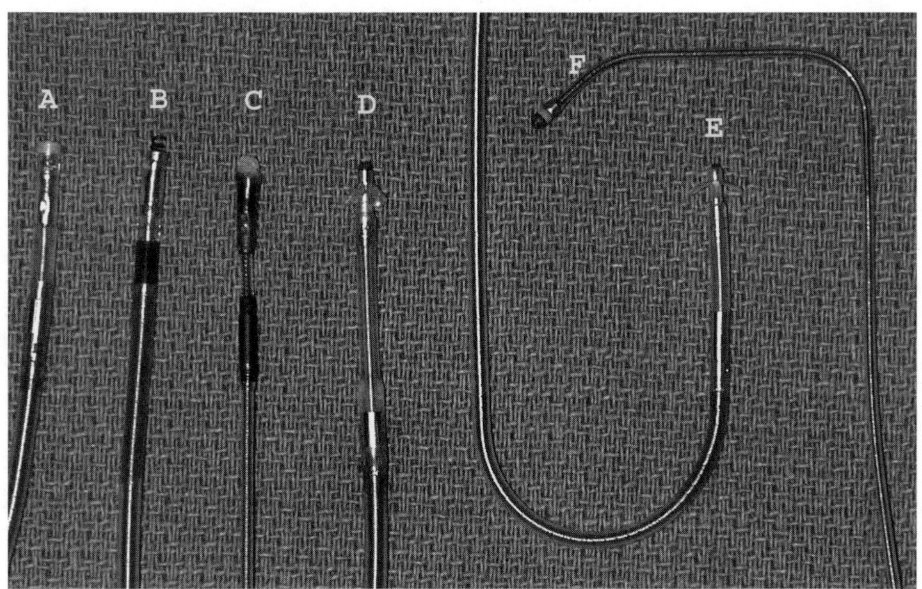

Figure 2.22. Common types of permanent transvenous pacing electrodes. **A:** Active fixation lead with extendable helix (helix retracted). **B:** Active fixation lead with helix extended. **C:** Fixed helix active fixation lead with helix covered by dissolvable mannitol coating. **D:** Straight tined passive fixation lead. **E:** Pre-formed "J" passive fixation tined lead for positioning in the right atrial appendage. This lead has a very small diameter tipo electrode that provides a high pacing lead impedance at the electrode-tissue interface. **F:** Unipolar 4F pre-formed coronary sinus lead for left ventricular pacing. The curved shape helps to hold the lead in position in the coronary veins. All leads except the coronary sinus lead are bipolar but note the differing distances between the ring and tip electrodes.

of the lead (a fixed-screw), requiring the lead to be rotated in a counterclockwise direction during passage through the vasculature. Other leads allow the screw helix to be extended from the tip once the lead has been atraumatically passed through the venous system to the heart (an extendable-retractable screw; Fig. 2.23). The design of Bisping and colleagues incorporates an extendable-retractable helical screw that is well suited for positioning at several sites in the atrium or ventricle at the time of implantation.[91] Active fixation leads may use the screw helix as both the fixation mechanism and the electrically active electrode (see Fig. 2.23). Other designs use a separate electrode at the distal end of the lead for stimulation and sensing with an electrically inactive helix. Although both devices provide similar long-term thresholds, the inactive helix leads are associated with lower acute thresholds. Another approach to active fixation leads uses a cap of mannitol or polyethylene glycol over the screw helix to facilitate introduction of the lead into the vasculature. After approximately 5 minutes in the blood pool, the mannitol or polyethylene glycol dissolves, allowing the screw to engage the endocardium.

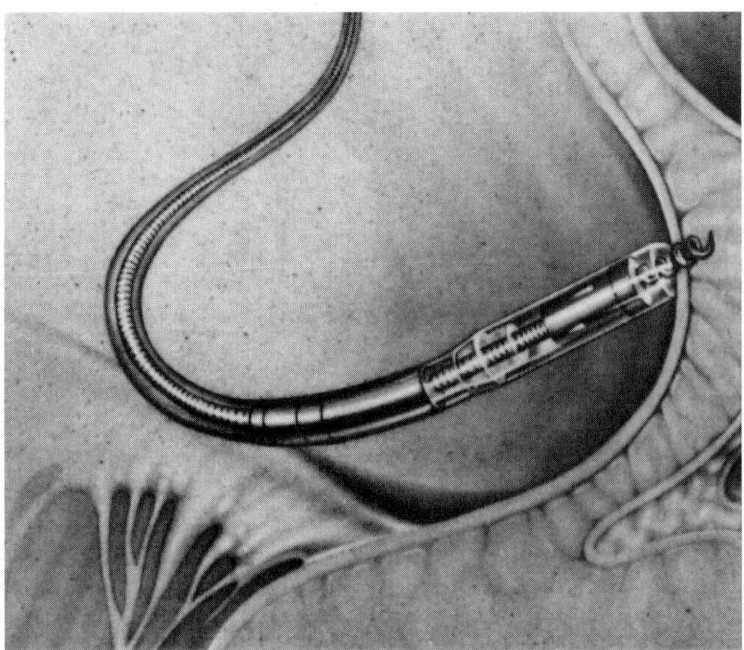

Figure 2.23. A bipolar Bisping-type active fixation that uses the screw helix as the active, distal electrode. The screw helix is extended into the endocardium by rotating the proximal connector of the lead. The screw helix is both extendable and retractable, allowing atraumatic passage through the vasculature. (Courtesy of Medtronic, Inc.)

The extendable-retractable design has become the most widely prescribed active fixation mechanism because of its ease of implantation and because the fixation mechanism can be retracted long after implantation, thereby allowing for an easier extraction procedure.

Active fixation leads offer the implanting physician the capability for stable positioning of the lead at many sites in either the atrium or the ventricle. Although active fixation leads have significantly reduced the risk of atrial lead dislodgment, the chronic pacing thresholds are somewhat higher than those of passive fixation leads. This difference in long-term pacing threshold has become only a minor issue with the routine use of corticosteroid elution in active fixation leads. Active fixation leads may also be used in the ventricle and may have particular usefulness in rheumatic heart disease associated with endocardial scarring. In patients with either congenital or surgically corrected transposition of the great vessels who require transvenous pacing, active fixation leads may be placed in the anatomic left ventricle, which has minimal trabeculae. Although active fixation leads are potentially easier to extract than passive fixation leads, the risk of myocardial perforation during implantation is higher. Because the stimulation thresholds of active fixation leads tend to be similar to those observed with passive fixation leads, with little difference in the rate of lead dislodgment, the choice of active or passive fixation has become largely a matter of preference by the implanting physician.

A special fixation feature of certain discontinued lead models must be mentioned: the J-retention wire. Manufactured by Cordis Corporation and later by Telectronics, the Accufix leads incorporated a thin, flexible, J-shaped metal ribbon that was welded to the proximal electrode and positioned between the outer polyurethane insulation and the outer conductor coil. This retention wire provided the lead with a permanent "J" shape. When combined with a unique method of extending and retracting the electrically inactive helix (accomplished by rotating a stylet), these leads were very easy to implant and became popular. Unfortunately, with continued flexing during cardiac motion, the J-retention wire developed metal fatigue and commonly fractured. The retention wire could then protrude through the outer polyurethane insulation and produce myocardial perforation, occasionally with pericardial tamponade. After an extensive program of fluoroscopic screening of these leads for J-retention wire fracture and perforation with selective extraction, it has become clear that a conservative approach to management of these leads is indicated for most patients as the risks of lead extraction usually exceed the risk of spontaneous injury.[93] Nevertheless, patients with an Accufix lead should be carefully followed for signs or symptoms related to J-retention wire protrusion and injury.

The Telectronics Encor leads use a similar J-retention wire in a tined, passive-fixation design. In contrast to the Accufix leads, the J-retention wire was placed within the inner conductor coil of the Encor leads. These leads have been demonstrated to have a much lower risk of J-retention wire fracture and protrusion. The risk of spontaneous injury appears to be far lower than the risk of lead extraction for Encor leads and a conservative management strategy is indicated for patients implanted with these leads.

Conductors

The conducting wire that connects the stimulating and sensing electrode(s) to the proximal connector pin of the lead is a critical determinant of the useable service life of permanent pacing leads. At a minimum pacing rate of 70 ppm (pulses per minute) the heart contracts and relaxes at least 36 million times a year, producing substantial mechanical stress on a permanent pacing lead.

If one considers that the lead must flex with each heartbeat in a complex manner having longitudinal, transverse, and rotational components, one can appreciate the potential for metal fatigue and fracture of the conductor. The most common site for lead fracture is at the fulcrum of a freely moving conductor with a stationary point. Thus the junction of the subclavian vein and the first rib is a common site of conductor failure. In addition, leads may fail at the site of mechanical injury, such as with excessively tight fixation sutures, especially when an anchoring sleeve is not used. Although early pacing leads were made of a single conductor wire and were associated with a high rate of fracture, modern leads use multiple wires that are coiled (Fig. 2.24). The use of mul-

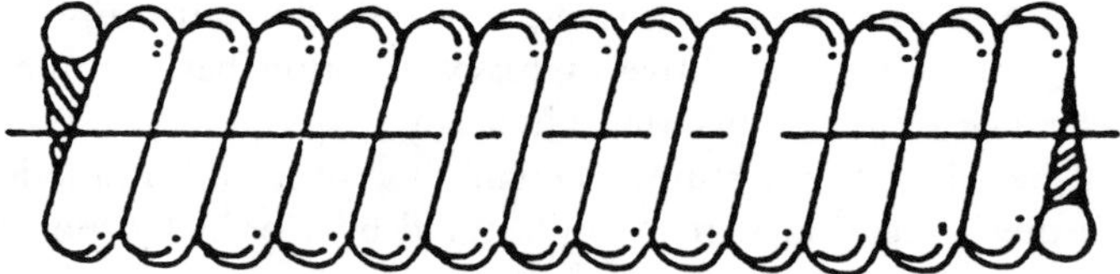

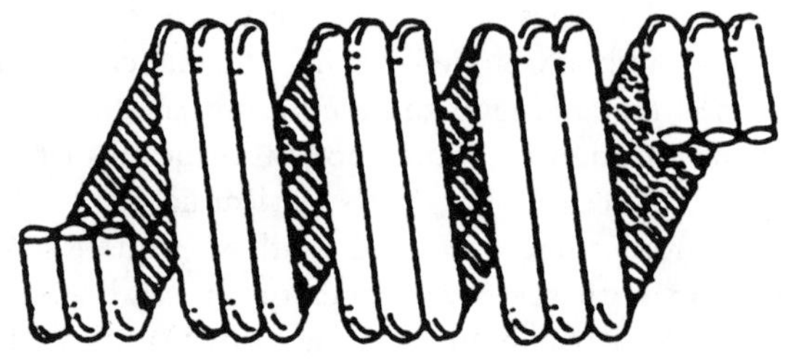

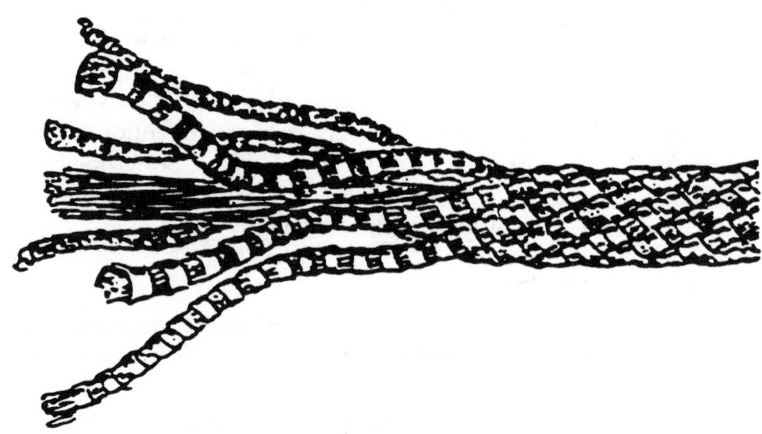

Figure 2.24. **Top:** A unifilar conducting coil that consists of a single wire wound around a central axis. (Courtesy of Medtronic, Inc.) **Center:** A trifilar conducting coil constructed with three wires wound in parallel around a central axis. **Bottom:** A braided (tinsel-type) lead conductor constructed of multiple wires woven around a central conductor wire.

tiple conducting coils has dramatically improved the conductor's resistance to metal fatigue and tensile strength.

Stainless steel was used for the conducting coils of early multifilar leads. Stainless steel eventually was abandoned because of the potential for corrosion, and was replaced by Elgiloy or MP35N, an alloy of nickel. More recently, conductors manufactured with the drawn-brazed-strand (DBS) technique have been introduced. The DBS conductor is made of six nickel alloy wires that are drawn together with heated silver. The silver forms the matrix of the conductor, occupying the central core and the spaces between the nickel alloy wires. Silver also forms a thin outer layer that coats the conductor. DBS conductors are characterized by excellent resistance to flexion-related fracture. This conductor also has a very low ohmic resistance, allowing more efficient delivery of the stimulating pulse to the electrode and reduced sensing impedance. The Medtronic 6972 polyurethane-insulated lead was found to be associated with insulation failures that were related to internal oxidation of the polyurethane by silver chloride from the DBS conductor. Because of the potential for oxidation of polyurethane by silver complexes, DBS conductors are no longer used with polyurethane-insulated leads.

Bipolar leads are usually constructed of the coaxial design, with the conductor coil to the distal electrode within the outer conductor coil, which ends at the proximal electrode (Fig. 2.25). Older bipolar leads incorporate two conductor coils wound side by side within the insulating sleeve (see Fig. 2.25A). The coaxial design also requires that insulation be placed around both conductors, making the overall external diameter rather large (see Fig. 2.25B). Coaxial bipolar leads are also less flexible than unipolar leads (see Fig. 2.25B). These characteristics have inhibited some physicians from using bipolar pacing leads routinely. A newer generation of bipolar pacing leads uses two conductors that are coiled in parallel, allowing the external diameter of a bipolar lead to be no larger than with a standard unipolar design (see Fig. 2.25A, bottom). These "Fine-Line" leads have been proven to provide excellent durability with a very thin lead body.

Insulation

The materials used for the insulation of permanent pacing leads are of two varieties, silicone rubber and polyurethane (Table 2.1). Silicone rubber has proven to be a reliable insulating material in over four decades of clinical experience. Silicone is a relatively fragile material, however, with a low tear strength. Because the insulation of permanent pacing leads may be subjected to trauma during or after implantation, the silicone layer must be thicker than it would be if it were stronger. Although the size of silicone-insulated unipolar leads has been clinically acceptable, coaxial bipolar leads constructed of this material have been of relatively large external diameter (often 10-F or greater). In addition, silicone rubber exposed to blood has a high coefficient of friction, making the manipulation of two leads in a single vein difficult. These disadvantages have been addressed by the introduction of platinum-cured silicone rubber, which is characterized by improved mechanical strength. The coefficient of friction has been greatly reduced by the development of a lubricious, "fast-pass" coating. These improved silicone leads are of smaller external diameter and are far easier to manipulate when in contact with another lead.

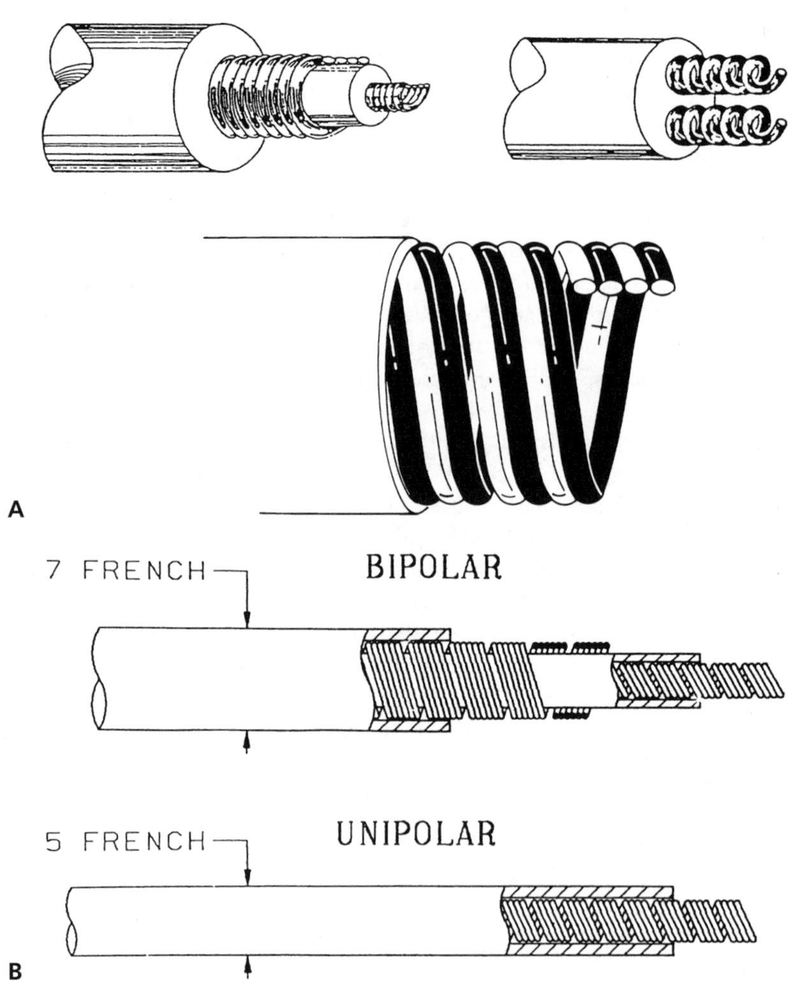

Figure 2.25. A (Top left): A bipolar lead with two conductor coils that are wound coaxially. The inner coil connects to the tip electrode, and the outer coil connects to the ring electrode. A sleeve of insulation separates the coils. **Top right:** A bipolar lead conductor using two unifilar coils placed in parallel (side by side) with surrounding insulation. (Courtesy of Medtronic, Inc.) **Bottom:** A schematic representation of a multiconductor lead with two Teflon-insulated conducting wires wound in parallel and encased within a polyurethane insulating sleeve. This construction provides a smaller diameter to the lead body than does the standard coaxial design. (Courtesy of St. Jude Medical, Inc.) **B (Top):** A schematic of a standard bipolar coaxial lead with inner and outer conductor coils and inner and outer insulation sleeves. **Bottom:** A schematic of a unipolar lead with a quadrafilar conducting coil surrounded by a sleeve of insulation. (Courtesy of St. Jude Medical, Inc.)

Table 2.1. Pacemaker Lead Insulation

	Advantages	Disadvantages
Silicone rubber	• 30-year proven history • Repairable • Low process sensitivity • Easy fabrication/molding • Very flexible	• Tears easily (nicks, ligatures) • Cuts easily • Low abrasion resistance • High friction in blood • Requires thicker walls (large diameter) • More thrombogenic and fibrotic • Subject to cold flow failure • Absorbs lipids (calcification)
Polyurethane	• 10-year proven history (55D) • High tear strength • High cut resistance • Low friction in blood • High abrasion resistance • Thinner walls possible (small diameter) • Relatively nonthrombogenic	• Relatively stiff (especially 55D) • Not repairable • Manufacturing process sensitive • Environmental stress cracking (ESC) • Metal ion oxidation (MIO) • History of clinical failures (80A)

Polyurethane was introduced as an insulation material because of its superior tear strength and low coefficient of friction. These properties allow polyurethane leads to be constructed with smaller external diameter than those made with conventional silicone rubber. The smaller polyurethane leads have contributed to the increased acceptance of bipolar pacing and have allowed two leads to be placed in a single vein, also contributing to the ease of dual-chamber pacemaker implantation.

Two major forms of polyurethane, known as P80A and P55D, have been used to insulate permanent pacing leads. The P80A polymer, which is less stiff than the P55D variety, was used in the first polyurethane-insulated cardiac pacing leads. The P55D polymer, which has greater tensile and tear strength, has been used as the insulating material for the pacing leads of several manufacturers. The P55D polymer is now the predominant form of polyurethane used for pacing leads.

Within 4 years of the first human implant, polyurethane insulation failures became clinically apparent. The model 6991U unipolar atrial lead with a preformed J shape demonstrated a pattern of insulation failure in the J-region in a minority of cases.[94] The model 6972 bipolar ventricular lead was found to have surface cracks in the P80A polyurethane insulation and clinical evidence of insulation failure (Fig. 2.26). The initial polyurethane-insulated leads have shown a high incidence of microscopic cracks in the outer surface of the insulation material. Extensive investigations by Stokes have shown that the surface cracks are likely related to environmental stresses rather than to biologic degra-

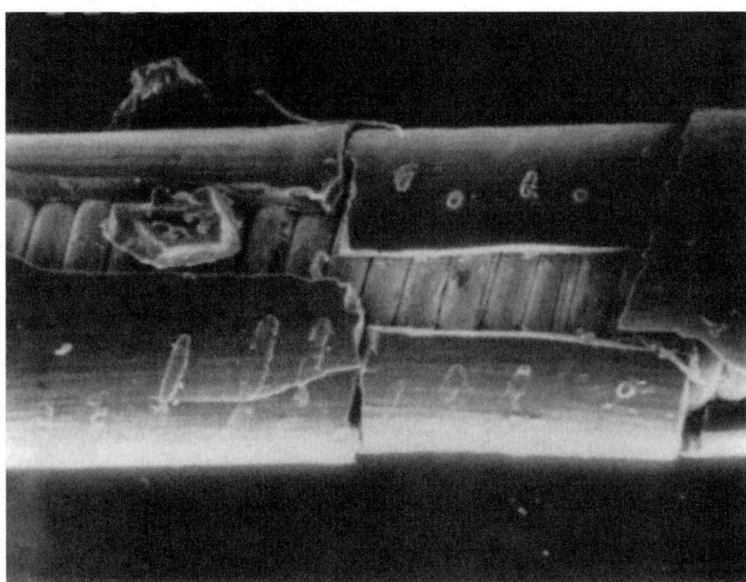

Figure 2.26. Cracking of polyurethane insulation (P80A) covering a bipolar permanent pacing lead 2 years after implantation. (Courtesy of St. Jude Medical, Inc.)

dation.[95] The surface cracks in the polyurethane develop in the manufacturing process as the heated polyurethane cools more rapidly than the inner core, leading to opposing stresses within the insulation. Although microscopic cracks in the outer surface of the polyurethane are usually clinically unimportant, these cracks may predispose the insulation to further degradation by trauma during or after lead implantation. At sites of additional mechanical stress, such as at the anchoring suture or during stylet insertion, the surface cracks may propagate deeper into the polyurethane, leading to insulation failure. Polyurethane may also be oxidized by silver chloride. Thus, degradation of polyurethane from the inside of the lead from silver contained in DBS conductors may occur.[96]

The mechanisms of polyurethane failure have been addressed by changes in the manufacturing process (slower cooling of the heated polyurethane and the elimination of solvents) and by the recognition that conductors made with silver should not be used with leads insulated with this material. Nevertheless, the P80A polymer has an unacceptable risk of insulation failure when used for permanent pacing leads, at least as it is manufactured by some companies. The poor performance of the Medtronic models 6972, 4012, and 4004 bipolar polyurethane leads has led to a shift to the P55D polymer. At this point, either polyurethane P55D or silicone rubber are acceptable insulating materials. The relatively low incidence of unipolar leads to develop clinically detectable insulation failure is a declining clinical advantage.

Epimyocardial Leads

Permanent pacing leads that are sutured to the epicardium or screwed into the myocardium of either the atrium or ventricle are presently used in clinical situations involving abnormalities of the tricuspid valve, congenital heart disease, or when permanent pacing leads are implanted during intrathoracic surgical procedures (Fig. 2.27). Epimyocardial electrodes use a fishhook shape that is stabbed into the atrial myocardium, a screw helix that is rotated into the ventricle, or loops that are placed within epicardial stab wounds in the ventricle. The chronic stimulation thresholds with myocardial leads tend to be higher than with modern endocardial electrodes, although there is considerable overlap. The use of three turns on an epicardial screw has been demonstrated to decrease the risk of exit block when compared to a two-turn screw. The incorporation of corticosteroid-eluting electrodes into the design of myocardial leads has significantly improved the long-term performance of epicardial pacing, especially in children with congenital heart disease, a group of patients with a very high risk of exit block with older lead designs. Epicardial leads now incorporate bipolar electrodes with steroid elution that can be sutured onto the epicardial surface without the requirement for a traumatic screw. These leads have greatly improved the outcome of epicardial pacing for selected patients. The introduction of CRT devices has provided for a resurgence in the clinical use of epicardial leads for left ventricular stimulation.

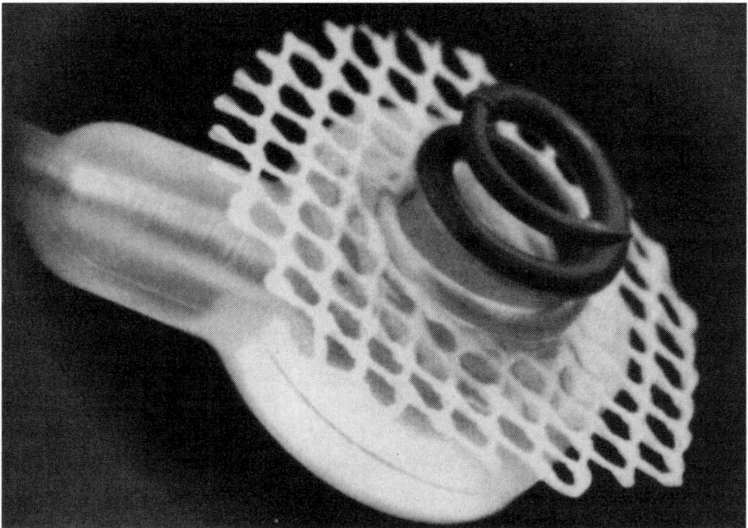

Figure 2.27. Unipolar epicardial screw-in electrode with a screw helix that is rotated into the myocardium. (Courtesy of St. Jude Medical, Inc.)

Connectors

Over the first three decades of pacing, a major problem for pacemaker and lead manufacturers as well as for implanting physicians was incompatibility of lead connectors and pulse generator headers that resulted from the lack of a consistent standard. Permanent pacing leads have evolved from a standard 5- to 6-mm connector pin for unipolar and bifurcated bipolar models to an "in-line" bipolar connector with a 3.2-mm diameter (Fig. 2.28). The considerable variability in the design of the in-line bipolar connector led to considerable confusion among physicians as to whether a particular lead of one manufacturer would match the pulse generator of another. Much of this confusion was related to the location of sealing rings; some manufacturers preferred to place the sealing rings in the header of the pulse generator, and others preferred the sealing rings to be on the connector of the lead. Because of this chaotic situation (Fig. 2.29), an international meeting of manufacturers agreed on a voluntary standard for leads and connectors incorporating the sealing rings on a 3.2-mm lead connector (VS-1). After continued problems with universal acceptance of the VS-1 connector, the incompatibility problem has been largely resolved with an industry-wide standard configuration known as IS-1 (Fig. 2.30).

Despite this vast improvement in standardization, implanting physicians encountering previously implanted leads must be aware that not all pulse generators will accept the connector pin of all 3.2-mm leads. For example, the IS-1 pulse generator will not accept an older Medtronic or Telectronics 3.2-mm or a Cordis 3.2-mm connector pin. The IS-1B connector will accept any of the VS-1, IS-1, Medtronic 3.2-mm, or Cordis 3.2-mm lead connectors. Although these incompatibility problems have been eliminated with new implants, the physician must be aware of these potential problems when planning to replace a pulse generator with an older model of lead. The introduction of cardiac

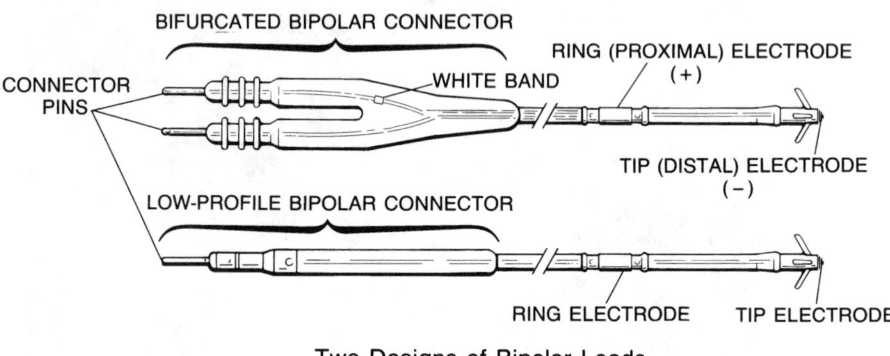

Figure 2.28. A white band marks the conductor leading to the distal electrode on a standard bifurcated bipolar lead connector with two connector pins. On a low-profile "Medtronic" type bipolar connector that has a single pin, the distal electrode connects to the pin.

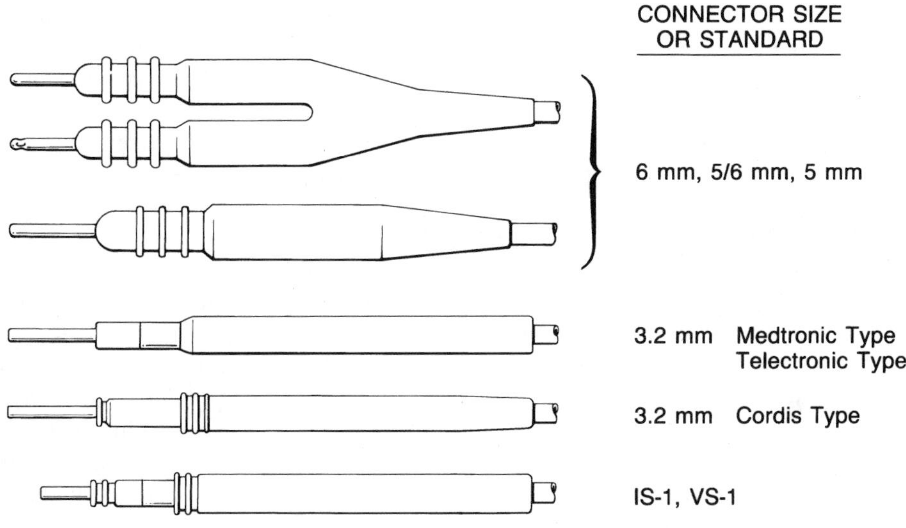

Figure 2.29. Five common varieties of lead connectors. 1) The upper connector is a bifurcated bipolar design with two connector pins, each 5 to 6 mm in diameter with sealing rings on the lead. 2) The second connector is a standard unipolar design of 5- or 6-mm diameter incorporating sealing rings. 3) The Medtronic-type, low-profile connector has a 3.2-mm diameter and no sealing rings. 4) The 3.2-mm Cordis-type connector is similar and incorporates sealing rings on the proximal portion of the lead. 5) The IS-1 and VS-1 connectors are incompatible with the other designs and include sealing rings on the proximal portion of the lead.

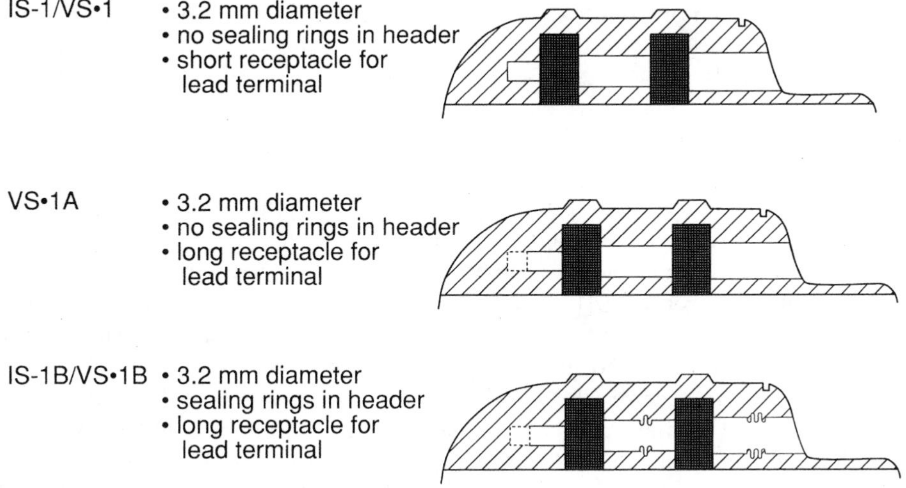

Figure 2.30. Three varieties of in-line bipolar pulse generator headers.

venous pacing leads for cardiac resynchronization has led to another potential conflict between the lead connector and pulse generators. Whereas the other manufacturers offer cardiac venous leads with an IS-1 connector, Guidant manufacturers leads with an LV-1 connector that will only connect to a specialized LV-1 pulse generator (manufactured only by Guidant). This presents a potential difficulty at the time of pulse generator replacement.

Specialized Coatings to Prevent Tissue Ingrowth

Because pacing and ICD leads may need to be extracted, newer leads are being designed so that the trauma of lead extraction can be minimized. The first consideration is to make the lead isodiametric so that there are no ridges or areas of increased diameter along the lead that would increase the risk of removal. A novel advance is the introduction of ePTFE (expanded polytetrafluoroethylene) coating over the ICD coils of the Guidant Reliance G leads. This coating prevents the ingrowth of tissue into the coil electrodes while having no significant effect on the conduction of electrical energy. Such coatings are likely to minimize the risks of later lead extraction.

PULSE GENERATORS

All pulse generators presently used in permanent pacing systems have several basic functional elements that are critical to the operation of the device. These include a power source, an output circuit, a sensing circuit, and a timing circuit. Pulse generators also contain a telemetry coil for sending and receiving programming instructions and diagnostic information. In addition to these basic elements, almost all new pulse generators contain circuits for sensing the output of an artificial, rate-adaptive sensor. The integrated circuit of most pulse generators also contains the capability of storing information in memory—either read-only memory (ROM) or random access memory (RAM)—which can be used to process diagnostic data or alter the feature set of the device following its implantation. In this section, the important aspects of each of these basic elements of pulse generators are reviewed.

Power Source

The power source of all pulse generators presently in use is a chemical battery. Modern pulse generators almost exclusively use lithium as the anodal element and iodine as the cathodal element (Fig. 2.31). The energy provided by a chemical battery is generated by the transfer of electrons from the anodal element to the cathodal element of the battery. In the case of lithium batteries, lithium is the anodal element and provides the supply of electrons. The cathodal element of the battery receives the electrons. In a lithium–iodine cell, iodine serves as the cathodal element and accepts electrons from lithium. Poly-2-vinyl pyridine is combined with the cathodal element to assist in the transfer of electrons to iodine. At the battery terminals, the anode gives up electrons and is negatively charged, and the cathode accepts electrons and is positively charged. Internally,

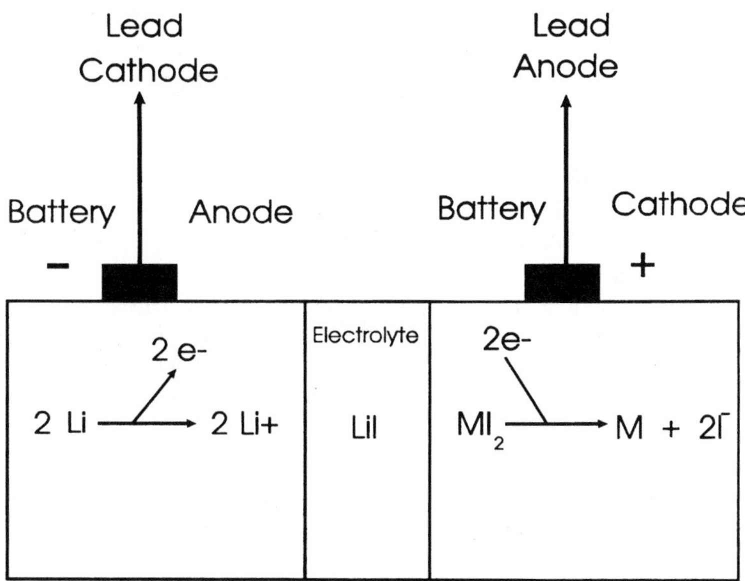

Figure 2.31. Schematic of a lithium-iodine battery. The anodal terminal of the battery is negatively charged as lithium releases electrons to the lead. The battery anode leads to the cathode of the pacing lead (which is also negatively charged). The anodal portion of the battery itself becomes positively charged with the reaction 2Li $\rightarrow$ $2Li^+$ + $2e^-$. The cathodal terminal of the battery is positively charged and connects to the anode of the lead. The cathodal reaction is $MI2 + 2e^- \rightarrow M + 2I^-$, where *M* represents poly-2-vinyl pyridine.

the anodal reaction proceeds as 2Li $\rightarrow$ $2Li^+ + 2e^-$ with the cathodal reaction being $2I + 2e^- \rightarrow 2I^-$. Thus, within the battery, the anode is positively charged and the cathode is negatively charged; the overall chemical reaction is 2Li + 2I $\rightarrow$ 2LiI. The electrons are carried from the anodal terminal of the battery to the cathodal terminal when the circuit is completed through the external load. For a stimulating pulse, the output circuit of the pulse generator, the pacing lead, and the myocardium provide the external load.

The battery also contains an electrolyte, the material separating the anodal and cathodal elements; this material serves as a conductor of ionic movement but is a barrier to the transfer of electrons. The electrolyte for a lithium-iodine battery is composed of a semisolid layer of lithium iodide that gradually increases in thickness over the life of the cell. As the LiI layer grows, the internal impedance of the battery increases. A major advantage of the lithium–iodine battery is the solid nature of the material, allowing the cell to be hermetically sealed and relatively resistant to corrosion. In contrast to the solid electrolyte of lithium-iodine batteries, the lithium–cupric-sulfide battery previously manufactured by Cordis used a liquid electrolyte. Although this electrochemical cell was associated with a low impedance over 90% of its useable life, it also has been associated with corrosion of the terminal feed-through and early failure. The zinc-mercury battery used in early pulse generators contained sodium hydroxide as the electrolyte, a material that was corrosive and associated with the potential for sudden failure. Zinc-mercury batteries were also characterized by the production of hydrogen gas as a by-product of the battery reaction. The requirement for the venting of hydrogen gas from the battery prevented hermetic sealing of the pulse generator and permitted the influx of tissue fluid, further increasing the risk of sudden failure.

The battery voltage depends on the chemistry of the cell. For example, the lithium-iodine cell generates approximately 2.8 V at the beginning of its life. The lithium–silver-chromate cell generates 3.2 V and the lithium–thionyl-chloride cell produces 3.6 V at beginning of life, whereas the lithium–lead-iodide cell has a voltage of only 1.9 V. Because the voltage of each of these cells is less than what may be required for chronic myocardial stimulation, a voltage multiplier in the output circuit must be used to allow output pulses of greater amplitude than the cell voltage. If the lithium-iodine battery potential is 2.8 V, how is it possible for a pacemaker to deliver an amplitude of 5 V? There are two potential methods for delivering a stimulus with an amplitude that is greater than that generated by the chemical reaction of the battery.

First, the pacemaker could use two batteries placed in series. Using cells in series increases the output voltage of the battery but does not increase battery capacity. Electrochemical cells may also be connected in parallel to increase capacity. However, cells in parallel do not generate an increased voltage. The alternative method is to use the battery charge of two capacitors in parallel and then to discharge the two capacitors to the lead in series. In this way a single battery with a potential of 2.8 V could generate 5.6 V with two capacitors, or 8.4 V with three capacitors. The total capacitance (C_T) of two capacitors (C_1 and C_2) charged in parallel is equal to $C_T = C_1 + C_2$. Because the total charge (Q) is related to the voltage (V) and capacitance (C) of the capacitor by the equation $Q = CV$, a double amount of charge is drawn from the battery. However, when these two capacitors are then discharged in series onto the lead, the capacitance is given by the equation.

$$\frac{1}{CT} = \frac{1}{C_1} + \frac{1}{C_2}$$

Thus, the discharge of these two capacitors in series results in a capacitance that is equal to one-half that for a single capacitor. Because an equal amount of charge must flow from each capacitor in series, the remaining voltage on the capacitor after discharge is $V_f/2$, where V_f is the final voltage. The net result is that by programming the pacemaker to a voltage that is double the battery voltage, the charge taken from the battery is equal to twice that delivered to the lead and the total amount of charge drained from the battery increases fourfold.

The longevity of a battery is determined by several factors, including the chemical elements of the battery, the size of the battery, the amount of internal discharge, and the voltage decay characteristics of the cell. To maximize battery life, the ideal electrochemical cell would have no internal discharge. However, batteries used for permanent pacemakers have been associated with internal discharge of variable degrees. For example, the initial zinc-mercury cells were associated with an internal rate of self-discharge of over 15% per year. The lithium-iodine cell is associated with a low rate of self-discharge following the initial reaction of lithium and iodine in the cell, generally less than 1% per year in chronic use.

For a battery to be suitable for use in permanent pacemakers, the decay characteristics of the cell should be predictable (Fig. 2.32). The ideal battery should have a predictable fall in voltage near the end of life, yet provide sufficient service life after the initial voltage decay to allow time for the elective replacement indicator to be detected and for replacement to be performed. The early zinc-mercury batteries were associated with a nearly constant cell voltage until end of life, when the voltage declined abruptly. These characteristics were generally unacceptable because of the difficulty of anticipating battery depletion. Lithium cells are associated with a more predictable behavior at end of life. The lithium–silver-chromate cell is characterized by two distinct plateau phases of voltage, the first phase (3.2 V) representing approximately 70% of the service life and a second phase of approximately 2.5 V. This two-phase decay characteristic is an attractive feature of this cell and allows a wide period in which to detect the elective replacement indicator.

Another battery that has been used for permanent pacemakers is the lithium–thionyl-chloride cell. This battery was associated with instances of an abrupt fall in battery voltage related to a sudden rise in cell impedance and

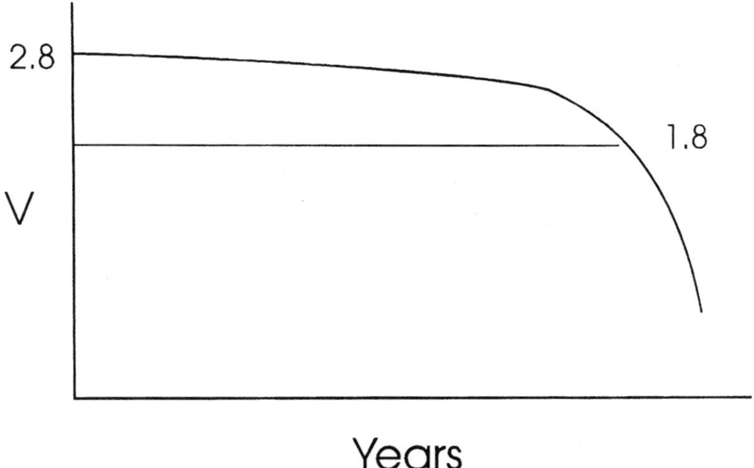

Figure 2.32. Typical voltage decay characteristics of a lithium-iodine battery. At beginning of life, the lithium-iodine cell generates 2.8 V. At end of useable life (90% depletion), the battery voltage decreases to approximately 1.8 V.

unexpected end-of-life behavior. The voltage produced by a lithium-iodine cell is inversely related to the internal battery impedance. The internal impedance of the battery increases with the thickness of the lithium-iodide electrolyte layer, from less than 1 kohm at the beginning of life to over 15 kohm at the extreme end of life. The voltage generated by the cell declines almost linearly from the initial value of 2.8 V to 2.4 V at approximately 90% of the useable battery life. Following this, the voltage declines exponentially to 1.8 V at the end of life. The magnet-related pacing rate of the pulse generator is related to the cell voltage, usually declining once the voltage falls below 2.4 V. The end-of-life indicator of pulse generators is usually signaled by a decrease in the magnet-related pacing rate to a fixed percentage of the beginning-of-life rate. Unfortunately, the end-of-life magnet rate is variable between manufacturers and between models. Some manufacturers signal the end of life by a two-step process, with an initial decrease in the magnet rate to an intermediate value followed by a stepwise decrease in rate to a second, lower value in association with a change in pacing mode, such as from DDD to VVI. In addition to a decrease in the magnet rate, the cell impedance of many pulse generators can be directly telemetered from the device, allowing a more accurate estimation of the useable service life. Some manufacturers also include an automatic increase in the pulse duration of the output circuit so that the total energy of the pulse delivered remains constant. Although the output energy may remain constant by the stretching of the pulse duration, loss of capture will occur if the stimulus voltage falls below rheobase.

The useable service life of a pulse generator not only depends on the characteristics of the battery, but is greatly influenced by the current drain of the integrated circuit, the amplitude and duration of the output pulse, the frequency of stimulation, the total impedance of the pacing lead, and the additional energy required to monitor and generate the output of a rate-adaptive sensor. Advances in the design of integrated circuits have greatly minimized the static current drain required to operate the circuit to less than 2 μA. The major source of current drain for the present generation of pulse generators is the output pulse. Thus, the amplitude, duration, and frequency of stimulating pulses are major contributors to the life of the power source. The pacing impedance is another critical influence on the current drain of the output pulse. Advances in pacing leads that have improved pulse generator longevity while providing an adequate safety margin include the use of electrodes with steroid elution, high electrode-tissue impedance, and low polarization. With the introduction of these high-performance leads, the nominal output energy has been significantly reduced. The addition of automatic threshold tracking and capture verification also holds the potential to increase pulse generator longevity by optimizing the energy of the stimulating pulse for each patient.

Output Circuits

The output pulse of the pulse generator is generated from the discharge of a capacitor to the anode and cathode of the pacing leads. The output capacitor is charged from the battery at a relatively slow rate to the programmed output voltage. Because the battery voltage of lithium–iodine cells is approximately 2.8 V, delivery of a stimulus of amplitude greater than this requires the use of a voltage multiplier. The voltage multiplier involves charging more than one capacitor from the battery. For example, if a stimulus voltage of 5.6 V is programmed, two capacitors must be charged from the battery in parallel and discharged in series. The cost of doubling the output voltage is a fourfold increase in current drain from the battery. If the stimulus amplitude is programmed to 8.4 V (three times the voltage of a lithium-iodide cell), three capacitors must be charged. In this case, a threefold increase in stimulus voltage results in a ninefold increase in current drain from the battery, markedly shortening battery life.

Output Pulse Waveforms: Most pulse generators used for permanent cardiac pacing deliver a capacitively coupled, constant-voltage pulse of programmable duration. When the fully charged capacitor is discharged, the resulting voltage at the leading edge of the pulse is independent of the pacing impedance. However, the trailing edge of the pulse is less than that of the leading edge, with the magnitude of the voltage drop being a function of the pacing impedance (Fig. 2.33). Because the capacitor stores a charge of fixed quantity, the greater the current flow, the smaller the charge (and voltage) remaining on the capacitor at the end of the pulse. Therefore, the lower the impedance, the greater the current delivered and the greater the drop in voltage from leading edge to trailing edge during the pulse. Thus, even though the term *constant voltage* is used to describe the stimulus waveform of permanent pacemakers, in reality the output voltage of the pulse is not constant from beginning to end.

Constant-current generators are no longer being implanted for permanent pacing, though a few pulse generators manufactured by Cordis are still in service. However, constant-current pulse generators are typical of many external pacing systems. The constant-current pulse is typically flat, with little or no change in current from leading edge to trailing edge. However, as the polarization impedance rises during the pulse, the resulting voltage must also rise proportionally to maintain the current at a constant level. Although either constant-current or constant-voltage pulse generators are capable of providing reliable pacing in the vast majority of clinical circumstances, at extremely high lead impedances the voltage required to maintain a constant-current pulse may exceed the capabilities of the battery.

The output waveform of the pulse generator is followed by a low-amplitude, long-duration wave of opposite polarity known as the afterpotential. The afterpotential is caused by polarization at the electrode–tissue interface and is dependent on the stimulus amplitude and duration. The afterpotential is also influenced by the polarization characteristics of the electrode. Afterpotentials may be inappropriately sensed by the sensing circuit if the stimulus amplitude and pulse duration are great and the sensing threshold is low. To reduce the afterpotential, the output circuit of some manufacturers incorporates a fast recharge pulse, during which the electrode polarity is reversed for a short period

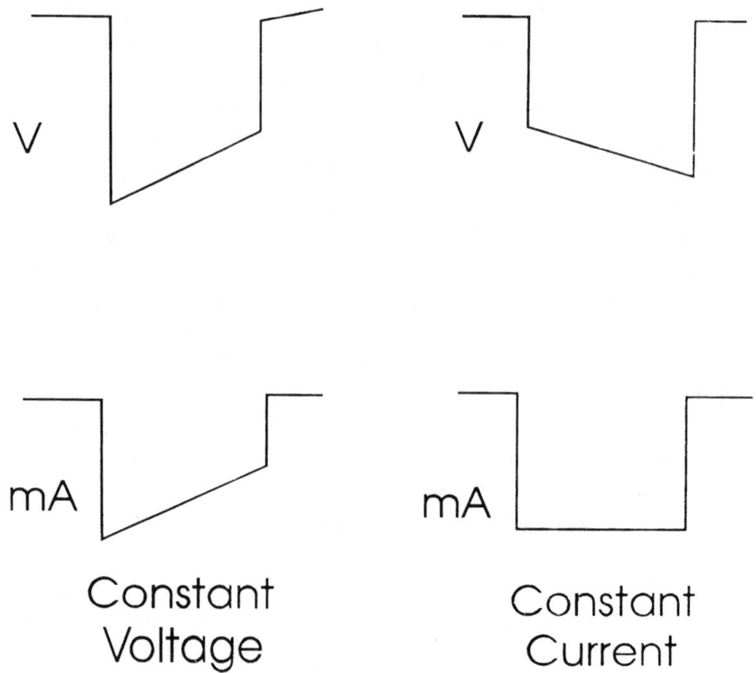

Figure 2.33. Output voltage and current waveforms for constant-voltage **(left)** and constant-current **(right)** stimulation. With a constant-voltage pulse, the leading-edge voltage is independent of load. The trailing-edge voltage depends on the total pacing impedance. The delivered current also declines from leading edge to trailing edge. With constant-current stimulation, the current remains constant throughout the pulse (provided that the cell can generate the required voltage). The delivered voltage increases with rising impedance during the pulse.

following the output pulse. This diminishes the polarization at the electrode-tissue interface, although it does not eliminate the need for low-polarization electrodes. As mentioned previously, the major clinical impact of afterpotentials relates to the ability of the pulse generator to automatically determine myocardial capture.

Sensing Circuits

The intracardiac electrogram is conducted from the electrodes to the sensing circuit of the pulse generator, where it is amplified and filtered. As discussed previously in this chapter, to minimize attenuation of the signal the sensing amplifier must have an input impedance greatly in excess of the sensing impedance. The greater the input impedance, the less the electrogram is attenuated by the amplifier. The input impedances of the sense amplifiers used in permanent pacing systems are greater than 25,000 ohms. The intracardiac electrogram is filtered to remove unwanted frequencies, a process that markedly affects the amplitude of the processed signal. A bandpass filter attenuates components of the electrogram on either side of the center frequency (the frequency with least attenuation) (Fig. 2.34). The bandpass filters of different manufacturers vary significantly with regard to center frequency (from approximately 20 to 40 Hz), so intracardiac electrograms measured with a pacing system analyzer of one manufacturer may produce considerably different electrogram amplitudes than will the pulse generator sensing amplifier of another manufacturer. It is also somewhat difficult to compare the sense amplifiers of different manufacturers because the shape of the test waveform has an important influence on the amplitude of the filtered electrogram, such that square-wave and sinusoidal test pulses may produce frequency attenuation spectra that differ from those of intracardiac electrograms. Following filtering of the intracardiac signal, the processed signal is compared with a reference voltage to determine if the signal exceeds a threshold detection level. Signals with amplitude greater than the sensitivity threshold level are sensed as intracardiac events, whereas signals of lower amplitude are discarded as noise. Signals that exceed the threshold level are marked by an output voltage pulse that is sent to the timing circuit.

Permanent pacemakers also contain noise reversion circuits that change the pulse generator to an asynchronous pacing mode when the sensing threshold level is exceeded at a rate faster than the noise reversion rate. The noise reversion mode prevents inhibition of pacing in the presence of electromagnetic

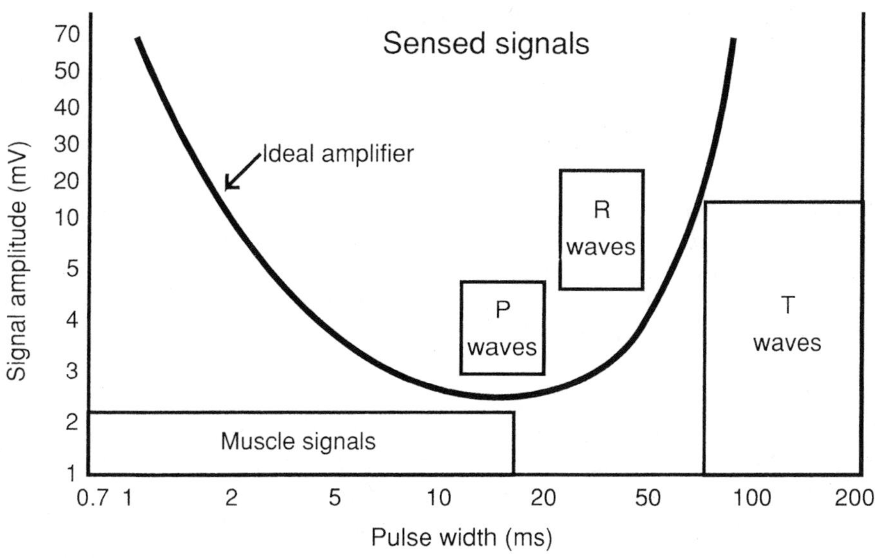

Figure 2.34. Signal processing with bandpass filtering of a sine-squared test waveform by a ventricular sensing amplifier. The curve denotes the signal amplitude required to be detected by the sensing amplifier with a threshold sensitivity value of 2.5 mV. Note that the amplitude of the signal that is needed for appropriate sensing is markedly increased at frequencies below and above the center frequency.

interference. The electronic circuitry of the pulse generator must also be protected from damage caused by overwhelming electrical energy generated in the clinical environment. The input voltage to the sensing amplifier is limited by a Zener diode that is designed to protect the integrated circuit from high external voltages such as may occur during defibrillation shocks or electrocautery. When the input voltage carried by the pacing leads exceeds the Zener voltage, the excess energy is shunted back to the myocardium through the leads. In addition to these features, which are designed to manage external electromagnetic interference, the sensing amplifier must prevent the detection of unwanted intracardiac signals such as far-field R waves in the atrial electrogram, afterpotentials, T waves, and retrogradely conducted P waves.

The potential for inappropriate inhibition of the ventricular output of a dual chamber pacemaker by far-field ventricular sensing of the atrial pacing stimulus or its afterpotential can be effectively reduced by the use of a ventricular blanking period. During the ventricular blanking period, the ventricular sensing amplifier is turned off immediately following the atrial pacing pulse. Although the blanking period has been quite effective in decreasing the frequency of ventricular crosstalk (inappropriate inhibition of ventricular pacing by far-field atrial pacing stimuli), several manufacturers also provide a nonphysiologic AV delay with delivery of a ventricular pacing pulse on sensing a ventricular event early in the AV interval. The inappropriate detection of intracardiac signals is also managed by the use of sensing refractory periods, during which the sense amplifier is not responsive to events such as T waves or retrogradely conducted P waves. The initial portion of the refractory period is a blanking period during which the sense amplifier is totally insensitive to electrical signals.

The remainder of the refractory period is typically a noise-sampling period. Events in this portion of the refractory period do not reset the timing circuit but initiate a new blanking period. Although sensing refractory periods are extremely effective for the management of unwanted signals, there are relative disadvantages to this approach, such as the inability of a DDD pacing system to track rapid atrial rates when a prolonged atrial refractory period is required to manage retrograde ventriculoatrial conduction. Newer pacing systems that incorporate variable refractory periods that change in proportion to the output of a metabolic sensor are likely to reduce the importance of these disadvantages.

Timing Circuits

The pacing cycle length, sensing refractory and alert periods, pulse duration, and AV interval are precisely regulated by the timing circuit of the pulse generator. The timing circuit of a pulse generator is a crystal oscillator that generates a very accurate signal with a frequency in the kHz range. The output of the crystal oscillator is sent to a digital timing and logic control circuit that operates internally generated clocks at divisions of the oscillator frequency. The output of the logic control circuit is a logic pulse that triggers the output pacing pulse, the blanking and refractory intervals, and the AV delay. The timing circuit also receives input from the sense amplifier to reset the escape intervals of an inhibited pacing system or trigger initiation of an AV delay for triggered pacing modes. The pulse generator also contains a rate-limiting circuit that prevents the pacing rate from exceeding an upper limit in the case of a random component failure. This runaway protection rate is typically in the range of 180 to 200 ppm.

Telemetry Circuits

Programmable pulse generators have the capability of responding to radiofrequency signals emitted from the programmer as well as sending information in the reverse direction, from the pulse generator to the programmer. The pulse generator is capable of both transmitting information from a radiofrequency antenna and receiving information with a radiofrequency decoder. Telemetry information may be sent as radiofrequency signals or as a pulsed magnetic field. Information that is sent from an external programmer to the pulse generator is sent in coded programming sequences with a preset frequency spectrum. Most pulse generators require the radiofrequency signal to be pulsed with a specific frequency in a sequence that is typically 16 pulses in duration. Thus the radiofrequency signal is quite precise, decreasing the likelihood of inappropriate alteration of the program by environmental sources of radiofrequency energy or magnetic fields. This characteristic also prevents the programmers of one manufacturer from programming the pulse generator of another. The detected telemetry bursts from the programmer are sent as digital information from the radiofrequency demodulator to the telemetry control logic circuit of the pulse generator. This logic circuit also provides for properly timed pulses to be sent from the antenna of the pulse generator to the programmer. *Real-time telemetry* is the term used to describe the capability of a pulse generator to transmit information to the programmer regarding measurements of pulse amplitude and duration, lead impedance, battery impedance, and delivered current, charge, and energy. These measurements may provide useful information for troubleshooting pacing systems. The pulse generator may also allow telemetry of intracardiac electrograms and timing circuit markers that can be extremely valuable for the evaluation of sensing (see Chapters 7 and 10).

Microprocessors

Microprocessors have become the standard control circuits of implantable pacemakers and ICDs. Microprocessors have several advantages over older integrated circuits, including a far greater circuit density and greatly reduced current drain. Microprocessors also allow very sophisticated algorithms, requiring multiple calculations to be incorporated into implantable devices, and have vastly increased data storage. The microprocessor can respond to changes in programming instructions that allow functions to be added or changed after implantation. The integrated circuit of pulse generators may contain both ROM and RAM.

ROM (typically 1 to 2 kilobytes of 8 to 32 bits) is used to guide the sensing and output circuits. Devices with 8- or 16-bit processors usually require several clock cycles to decode an instruction from memory. The processors operating with larger instruction words (such as 32 bits) may load and execute an instruction in a single clock cycle, improving the efficiency of the repetitive tasks that are required for pacing and sensing.

In addition, RAM is used to store diagnostic information regarding pacing rate, intrinsic heart rates, and sensor output. The amount of RAM that is included in the pulse generator varies between models and manufacturers. The amount of RAM in modern pulse generators is rapidly increasing and will increase the amount of diagnostic information that can be stored in the pulse generator. Such data include histograms of paced and intrinsic heart rate, sensor function, trends of heart rate and sensor function over time, storage of intracardiac electrograms from episodes of high atrial or ventricular rates, and mode-switching events. The rapidly expanding diagnostic capabilities of pacemakers will allow improved assessment of the physiologic condition of the patient. Thus, information may be stored that relates to heart rate variability, respiration, intracardiac pressure, patient activity, lung water, and arrhythmias.

Almost all manufacturers offer fully RAM-based pulse generators. There are several important advantages to microprocessor-based pacemakers, including decreased production costs for an entire product line, increased flexibility to upgrade features in subsequent pacemaker models, and the capability for downloading new features into previously implanted pacemakers by telemetry. It is important to emphasize that the microprocessors used in permanent pacemakers must be custom designed to minimize current drain and operate with a lithium-iodine battery. Thus, a microprocessor that is used in a microcomputer and has access to a virtually unlimited power supply (AC current operating at 110 V) would not be feasible for inclusion in a permanent pacemaker.

RATE-ADAPTIVE SENSORS

Widespread appreciation of the importance of rate modulation in the augmentation of cardiac output with exercise has led to the development of a variety of physiologic sensors. Although the normal sinus node may be an ideal rate-adaptive sensor for many patients who require pacemakers, the frequent occurrence of sinus node dysfunction and atrial fibrillation in clinical practice limits the applicability of atrial sensing for reliably modulating pacing rate in many individuals. Thus, artificial sensors that correlate with the level of metabolic demand either directly or indirectly have assumed increased importance in the design and application of permanent pacing systems. In this section, the design considerations of these sensors are discussed. For practical concerns, two major rate-adaptive sensors have come to dominate the pacing market: accelerometers and minute ventilation. Although there have been a host of other potential sensors, including the continued use of the QT interval and intracardiac impedance, only accelerometers and minute ventilation sensors have achieved widespread acceptance for standard pacemakers.

The ideal rate-adaptive pacing system should provide pacing rates that are proportional to the level of metabolic needs. The speed of change in the pacing rate should be similar to that of the sinus node. The ideal sensor demonstrates sensitivity and specificity. It should demonstrate sensitivity to both exercise- and non-exercise-related changes, such as mental stress. Specificity is demonstrated by the failure of the sensor to be affected by stimuli that should not cause an increase in pacing rate.

Multiple technical considerations are important in the implementation of the sensor. These include the stability of the sensor and the size of the sensor, as well as its biocompatibility and the ease of its programming. Excessive energy consumption by a sensor will limit the life span of the pulse generator. Sensors that are large or require the placement of additional electrodes or a new type of electrode may present a technical problem. The response of the sensor is determined by its intrinsic properties in response to stimuli, by the algorithm used to relate changes in the sensed parameter to changes in paced heart rate, and by the ease and way it is programmed.

Activity Sensors and Accelerometers

Rate-adaptive pacing systems that detect mechanical vibration are based on the clinical association of increasing body motion with increasing levels of exercise. These devices are designed to detect low-frequency vibrations in the range of the resonant frequency of the human body (approximately 4 Hz). A piezoelectric ceramic crystal functioning as a strain gauge is bonded to the inside of the pulse generator case or to the circuit board (Fig. 2.35). As the ceramic crystal flexes and deforms in response to mechanical vibration or pressure, an electric current is generated. The magnitude of the electric current from the crystal is related to the frequency and amplitude of vibrations. The output of the sensor is processed electronically and used to modulate changes in pacing rate.

Early motion-sensitive pacing systems simply counted the occurrence of sensor output exceeding a programmable threshold level (Fig. 2.36, top).[97,98]

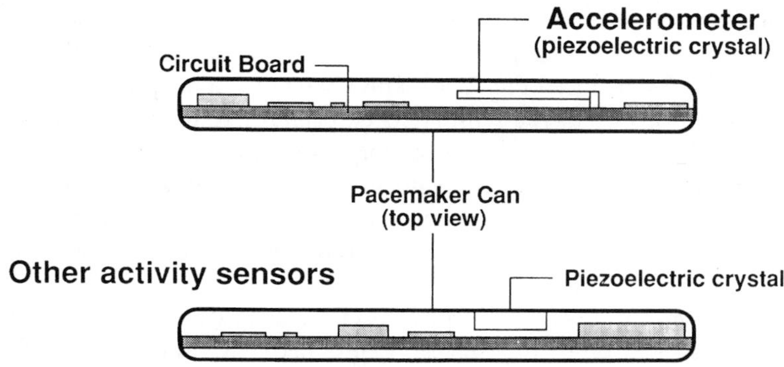

Figure 2.35. Schematic of two motion-sensing, rate-adaptive pacing systems. **Top:** An accelerometer (piezoelectric crystal) is mounted on the circuit board of the pulse generator. **Bottom:** The alternative sensor location, with the piezoelectric crystal mounted on the inside of the pulse generator case. (Courtesy of Intermedics, Inc.)

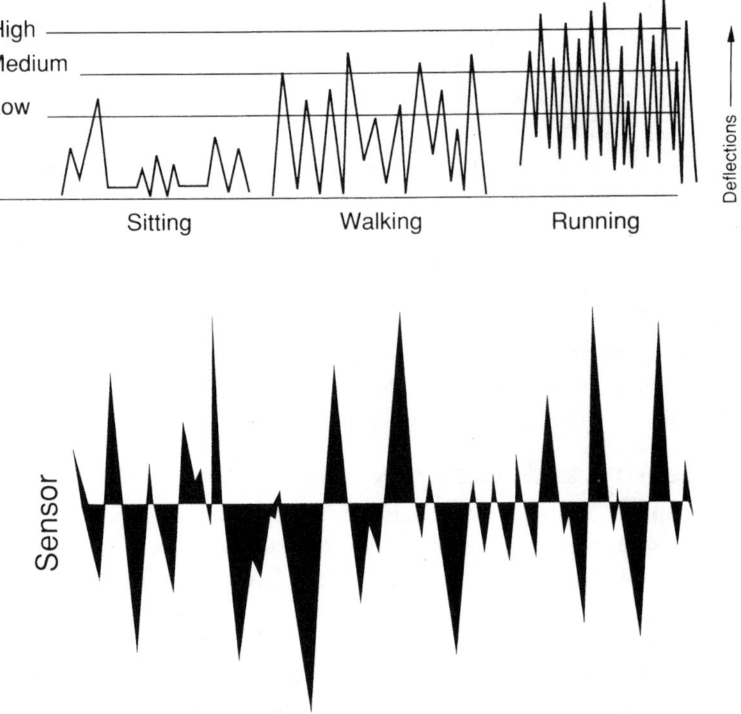

Figure 2.36. **Top:** Processing of the activity sensor signal by simple counting of the frequency of deflections above a threshold amplitude (high, medium, or low). **Bottom:** Processing of the activity signal by integration of the amplitude and frequency of sensor deflections above a threshold value.

Because vibrations that greatly exceeded the threshold registered the same as those that exceeded this level only slightly, the function of these devices was frequently an all-or-none increase in pacing rate. Newer devices integrate the output of the sensor, responding to both the frequency and the amplitude of the electrical signal (see Fig. 2.36). This change in signal processing has improved the proportionality of the sensor-related pacing rate to the level of exercise. The threshold level for the detection of vibrations is programmable from low to high, allowing the device to be individualized to the resonant characteristics of the individual. The slope of the relationship between sensor output and pacing rate is also programmable. Newer devices also allow separate programming of rate onset and rate offset.

Motion-sensitive, rate-adaptive pacing systems are characterized by a rapid response to the onset of exercise. Combined with simplicity of function and compatibility with any standard pacing lead, these devices have become the most widely prescribed rate-adaptive pacing systems presently in use. There are important limitations to these sensors, however, as they are related only indirectly to metabolic demand. For example, exercise that generates significant mechanical vibration (such as walking or arm motion) leads to a greater rate increase than exercise that produces less motion (such as bicycling). Similarly, the pacing rate produced by descending stairs is typically greater than that produced by climbing stairs.[99] In addition, these sensors are susceptible to environmental noise from vibrations produced by transportation or direct pressure over the pulse generator. Finally, these sensors respond poorly to some types of exercise (e.g., swimming, isometric exercise).

Because of these limitations of activity sensors, body motion is now detected by the use of accelerometers. Acceleration sensors use either piezoelectric or piezoresistive materials.[100] The piezoelectric accelerometer is mounted on the hybrid circuitry in the pulse generator rather than bonded to the pulse generator case and has become the standard method for detection of body motion. This allows the accelerometer to be mechanically insulated from the case, preventing increases in pacing rate as a result of simple pressure on the pulse generator. As the patient moves in the anterior-posterior axis, the mass of the accelerometer deflects in proportion to the change in velocity (acceleration $= dV/dt$). Accelerometers that are piezoelectric generate an electrical potential as a result of deformation of the piezoceramic material. In contrast, piezoresistive accelerometers measure changes in electrical resistance that occur with mechanical deformation of the sensor and require a somewhat greater current drain to power the sensor.

Although motion of the body during walking or bicycling occurs in both the anterior-posterior and vertical axes, exercise workload is more proportional in the anterior-posterior axis than in the vertical axis. Because accelerometers tend to detect acceleration in the anterior–posterior axis to a greater extent than in the vertical axis, these sensors offer the potential for greater proportionality of response than do activity sensors. Accelerometers have been shown to be somewhat less susceptible to excessive rate increases during descending stairs than activity sensors. Accelerometers have also been demonstrated to produce a rate response that is closer to the expected behavior of the sinus node during bicycle exercise than has been observed with activity sensors. In general, accelerometers offer rate modulation that is somewhat more proportional to exercise workload than is usual with activity sensors. As a result, accelerometers have largely replaced activity sensors for rate-adaptive pacing.

Because accelerometers have a constant coupling mass of the sensor that is independent of the body, these devices offer a more predictable range of responses during exercise than do activity sensors. In fact, the acceleration signals that are recorded with accelerometers are remarkably consistent among individuals who vary in body weight, age, or physiologic condition. These devices also have improved resolution (ability to detect small changes in motion) as compared with activity sensors. The raw accelerometer signal is rectified and integrated to produce a value that represents the energy content of the signal. Because the frequency range of the accelerometer signal associated with exercise is known to have a maximal amplitude less than 4 Hz, the signal can be filtered to remove external noise, which typically has maximal amplitude in the range of frequencies between 10 and 50 Hz. The typical accelerometer is designed to respond to frequencies between 0.5 and 10 Hz. This ability to filter unwanted signals is an advantage of accelerometers as compared with activity sensors, which are less able to discriminate body motion from external noise.

The most characteristic attribute of accelerometers is their ability to respond rapidly to the onset of exercise. The interval from the onset of exercise to an increase in sensor energy is often instantaneous. For the accelerometer to modulate the pacing rate, the sensor energy must be converted to a *desired* pacing rate. For any given sensor energy, the desired pacing rate must be calculated from the lower pacing rate, the upper sensor rate, the upper tracking rate, the rate adaptive slope, and any rate-smoothing or mode-switching constraints. In addition, reaction and decay constants, which may or may not be programmable, translate the time required to change the *actual* pacing rate to the *desired* pacing rate. The sensor slope parameter determines the rate of change in pacing rate that will occur for a given change in the accelerometer signal energy. For a given change in sensor energy the greater the programmed slope, the greater the pacing rate that will be calculated. However, the effect of the upper sensor rate on the pacing rate that will be achieved at any given level of exercise and slope setting should be emphasized. For example, programming the maximum sensor rate from 120 bpm to 160 bpm will have a marked influence on the rate adaptive function of the pacemaker that is at least as important as the slope value that is programmed.

Accelerometers have been demonstrated to provide a more physiologic rate adaptation than activity sensors can provide during treadmill or bicycle exercise testing.[101,102] The response to walking downstairs has been far more physiologic with accelerometers than with activity sensors.[102] Newer pacemakers offer automatic adjustment of the rate adaptive slope of the accelerometer by comparing the rate-adaptive histograms observed over time to a set of expected responses. If the accelerometer provides pacing rates that exceed the target rates more frequently than expected, the slope parameter is reduced. If the pacing rate does not reach the target rate the slope value is gradually increased until an expected target rate is achieved. Although the ability of these algorithms to achieve a physiologic rate modulation during exercise may not be ideal in all patients, these algorithms tend to prevent extremes of overpacing or underpacing in the population of pacemaker patients.

The major advantage of accelerometers over activity sensors is that they can be applied to any pacing lead, regardless of the polarity or electrical integrity. They have a proven ability to provide a rapid heart rate response to the onset of exercise, and there is now widespread clinical experience with these devices. For these reasons accelerometers are the most commonly prescribed rate-adaptive sensors implanted.

Minute Ventilation Sensors

Respiratory rate (RR), tidal volume (TV), and minute ventilation (the product of these two parameters) increase in proportion to changes in carbon dioxide production (VCO_2). At exercise workloads less than anaerobic threshold, the minute ventilation is closely associated with oxygen consumption (VO_2).

Minute-ventilation–sensing, rate-adaptive pacing systems have been demonstrated to provide rate modulation that is closely correlated with VO_2 in most patients implanted with these devices.[103–106] Minute ventilation is estimated by frequent measurements of transthoracic impedance between an intracardiac lead and the pulse generator case using a tripolar system. A low-energy pulse of known current amplitude (1 mA with pulse duration 15 microseconds) is delivered from the ring electrode of a standard bipolar pacing lead (Fig. 2.37). The resultant voltage between the tip electrode and the pulse generator case is measured and the impedance calculated. The impedance pulses are subthreshold and are delivered every 50 milliseconds. Transthoracic impedance increases with inspiration and decreases with expiration. By measuring the frequency of respiration-related fluctuations in impedance (correlated with respiratory rate) and the amplitude of those excursions (correlated with tidal volume), the estimated minute ventilation can be calculated.

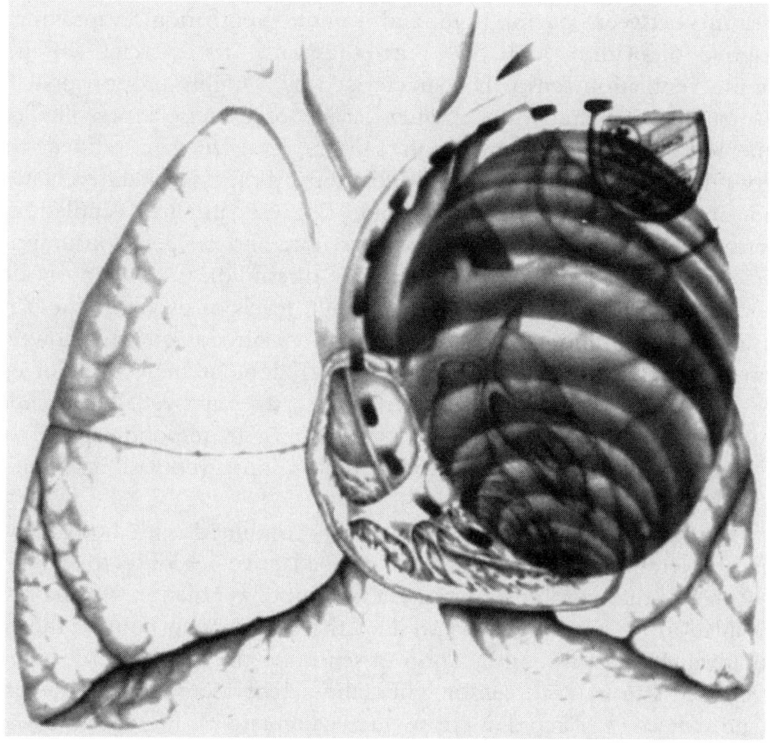

Figure 2.37. Diagram of a tripolar transthoracic impedance (minute-ventilation) sensing rate-adaptive pacing system. A low-energy pulse is emitted from the ring electrode every 50 milliseconds with measurement of the resultant voltage between the tip electrode and the pulse generator case. (Courtesy of St. Jude Medical, Inc.)

The transthoracic impedance signal is a complex parameter that is influenced by several factors. However, the transthoracic impedance is most closely related to the volume and resistivity of blood in the right heart chambers and systemic venous system. The impedance signal fluctuates in response to both respiration and cardiac motion (right ventricular ejection). The impedance signal may also change with thoracic motion due to arm movements. To minimize the cardiac-related component of the impedance signal, low-pass filtering of frequencies greater than 48 to 60 Hz is performed. A potential problem of this approach is that respiratory rates greater than 48 to 60 breaths per minute, which may be observed in children, may be inappropriately sensed.

The impedance signal is processed by comparing the average impedance values accumulated over two periods (1 minute and 1 hour). When the short-term average (1 minute) exceeds the long-term average (1 hour), the pacing rate is increased. The slope of the relationship between changes in minute ventilation and pacing rate is a programmable parameter. Because the initial minute-ventilation pacing systems decreased the paced cycle length linearly with respect to the minute-ventilation signal, the sensor was characterized by a relatively slow onset of rate modulation. Newer generations of devices offered a linear relationship between pacing rate and minute ventilation, improving the rate-adaptive algorithm and the initial response to exercise. In general, the minute-ventilation sensor is characterized by a highly proportional relationship to metabolic demand over a wide variety of exercise types. The most recent generation of minute-ventilation sensors have further refined the relation between heart rate and minute ventilation by the use of different slopes below and above the anaerobic threshold. Because minute ventilation normally increases out of proportion to the heart rate and oxygen consumption at high exercise workloads (above the anaerobic threshold), newer sensors decrease the heart rate/minute-ventilation slope at high levels of exercise. These refinements have made the minute-ventilation sensor very physiologic. By allowing a steeper slope at low levels of exercise and a flatter slope at high levels of exercise, the rate adaptation that can be achieved is greatly improved. The steeper slope at low minute-ventilation levels allows the sensor to respond rapidly to the onset of exercise. By reducing the slope at high minute-ventilation levels, overpacing is prevented.

Minute-ventilation sensing has been combined with both activity sensors and accelerometers to improve the rate adaptive response to exercise.[107] Early pacemakers that combined activity and minute-ventilation sensors provided rate modulation by allowing the fastest of these sensors to control the pacing rate. An advantage of this combination of sensors is the ability to separately program the upper rate of each sensor. Thus, the activity sensor could be programmed to provide a very rapid increase in pacing rate at the onset of exercise, yet prevent excessive increases in rate by limiting the maximum activity rate. After minute ventilation increases during more sustained exercise, the rate response can be controlled by the minute-ventilation sensor. The clinical utility of this sensor combination has been demonstrated in a multicenter trial.

Minute-ventilation pacemakers generally require the use of a bipolar pacing lead to measure transthoracic impedance, limiting the use of this sensor in patients with previously implanted pacing leads. However, DDDR pacing systems manufactured by ELA Medical (Talent II) use the atrial lead to sense the minute-ventilation signal. Although a bipolar atrial lead is required for this device, a unipolar ventricular lead may be used. This device offers continuous self-modulation of the rate-adaptive slope based on a rolling trend of minute-ventilation signals. The ELA Talent II pacemaker allows minute ventilation to be determined with a unipolar lead. The Guidant Pulsar Max and Medtronic Kappa 400 series pacemakers have combined minute-ventilation and accelerometer sensors with blending of the sensor output to modulate pacing rate. Although providing quite different rate adaptive algorithms, both of these devices emphasize the accelerometer at low levels of exercise and the minute-ventilation sensor at high levels of exercise. Both devices also incorporate a cross-checking feature of the sensors such that overpacing in response to false-positive sensor activation. These devices also automatically adjust the rate adaptive slope of the sensors by comparing the pacing rate achieved to an expected sensor target rate or histogram profile.

QT Interval

The intracardiac QT interval has been demonstrated to shorten with exercise or sympathetic tone and to lengthen at rest. The QT interval also shortens with increasing pacing rate and lengthens at slow heart rates. The QT interval is measured from the onset of the pacing stimulus to the apex of the T wave in the intracardiac ventricular electrogram. Although the QT interval varies widely among individuals, it is quite consistent in an individual at rest. The QT interval can be markedly influenced by medications or electrolyte concentrations, however. Initial QT-sensing pacing systems suffered from a high incidence of T wave undersensing and degradation of the ventricular electrogram over time. In addition, electrodes with high polarization properties were associated with large afterpotentials that interfered with accurate measurement of the QT interval. These problems were significantly improved by the addition of a fast-recharge pulse that minimized afterpotentials and by changes in the T wave filter.

The QT-pacing system includes an absolute refractory period of 250 milliseconds, which is followed by a programmable T wave sensing window (250 to 450 milliseconds). A subthreshold marker pulse that is visible on the surface electrocardiogram is useful for confirming appropriate T wave sensing. Further improvements in this sensor have involved the use of a curvilinear slope that improves the initial rate response to the onset of exercise. Automation of the slope measurement has also improved the function of this sensor and reduced the time required for calibration of the pacemaker. Disadvantages of the QT sensor involve the requirement for a low-polarization electrode, potentially complex programming, and the fact that the T wave can be reliably sensed only with paced beats. The potential advantages of this sensor are its responsiveness to emotional factors and the lack of a specialized lead. It is also clear that the function of the sensor underwent continuous and significant refinement in the rate-adaptive algorithm. The disadvantages of the QT sensor have been largely overcome by combining this sensor with an activity sensor (Vitatron Diamond). This dual-sensor pacing system allows a programmable blending of sensor response to modulate pacing rate. Although this sensor has been reliable and effective, its market share has been relatively small.

Other Sensors

Other sensors that have been demonstrated to provide clinically acceptable rate modulation include central venous temperature, mixed venous oxygen saturation, right ventricular dP/dt, peak endocardial acceleration, and intracardiac impedance. Each of these sensors has been demonstrated to have highly physiologic rate response characteristics. Nevertheless, the requirement for a specialized pacing lead has hindered the widespread acceptance of most of these products.

REFERENCES

1. Hodgkin AL, Huxley AF. A quantitative description of membrane current and its application to conduction and excitation in nerves. J Physiol (Lond) 1952;117: 500–544.
2. Grant AO. Evolving concepts of cardiac sodium channel function. J Cardiovasc Electrophysiol 1990;1:53–67.
3. Cohen CJ, Bean BP, Tsien RW. Maximal upstroke velocity (Vmax) as an index of available sodium conductance: comparison of Vmax and voltage clamp measurements of INa in rabbit Purkinje fibers. Circ Res 1984;54:636–651.
4. Bodewei R, Hering S, Lemke B, et al. Characterization of the fast sodium current in isolated rat myocardial cells: simulation of the clamped membrane potential. J Physiol (Lond) 1982 Apr; 325:301–315.
5. Angelides KJ, Nutter TJ. Mapping the molecular structure of the voltage-dependent sodium channel. J Biol Chem 1983;258:11958–11967.
6. Noda M, Ikeda T, Suzuki H, et al. Expression of functional sodium channels from cloned cDNA. Nature 1986;322:826–828.
7. Tsien RW. Calcium channels in excitable cell membranes. Ann Rev Physiol 1983;45:341–358.
8. Tsien RW, Hess P, McCleskey EW, et al. Calcium channels: mechanisms of selectivity permeation and block. Ann Rev Biophys Biochem 1987;16:265–290.
9. Hume JR, Giles W. Ionic currents in single isolated bullfrog atrial cells. J Gen Physiol 1983;81:153–194.
10. Hume JR, Giles W, Robinson K, et al. A time and voltage dependent K current in single cardiac cells from bullfrog atrium. J Gen Physiol 1986;88:777–798.
11. Brown HF, DiFrancesco D, Noble SJ. How does adrenalin accelerate the heart? Nature 1979;280:235–236.
12. DiFrancesco D, Ferroni A, Mozzanti M, et al. Properties of the hyperpolarizing activated current (if) in cells isolated from the rabbit sinoatrial node. J Physiol 1986;377:61–88.

13. DeMello WC. Intracellular communication in cardiac muscle. Circ Res 1982;51: 1–9.
14. Barr L, Dewey MM, Berger W. Propagation of action potentials and the structure of the nexus in cardiac muscle. J Gen Physiol 1965;48:797–823.
15. Walton MK, Fozzard HA. Experimental study of the conducted action potential in cardiac Purkinje strands. Biophys J 1983;44:1–8.
16. Spach MS, Miller WT III, Geselowitz DB, et al. The discontinuous nature of propagation in normal canine cardiac muscle. Evidence for recurrent discontinuities of intracellular resistance that affect the membrane currents. Circ Res 1981;48:39–54.
17. Spach MS, Dolber PC, Heidlage JR, et al. Propagating depolarization in anisotropic human and canine cardiac muscle: apparent directional differences in membrane capacitance. A simplified model for selective directional effects of modifying the sodium conductance on Vmax, tau foot, and the propagation safety factor. Circ Res 1987;60:206–219.
18. Inoue H, Zipes DP. Conduction over an isthmus of atrial myocardium in vivo: a possible model of Wolff-Parkinson-White syndrome. Circulation 1987;76:637–647.
19. Winfree AT. The electrical thresholds of ventricular myocardium. J Cardiovasc Electrophysiol 1990;1:393–410.
20. Irnich W. The fundamental law of electrostimulation and its application to defibrillation. Pacing Clin Electrophysiol 1990;13:1433–1477.
21. Lapicque L. Définition expérimentale de l'excitabilité. Soc Biol 1909;77:280–283.
22. Hoorweg L. Über die elektrische nerve merregung. Pflugers Arch Physiol 1892;52:87–99.
23. Weiss G. Sur la possibilité de rendre comparable entre eux les apparels servant a l'excitation électrique. Arch Ital Biol 1901;35:413–446.
24. Blair HA. On the intensity–time relations for stimulation by electric currents. J Gen Physiol 1932;15:709–729.
25. Irnich W. The chronaxie time and its practical importance. Pacing Clin Electrophysiol 1980;3:292.
26. Ripart A, Mugica J. Electrode–heart interface: definition of the ideal electrode. Pacing Clin Electrophysiol 1983;6:410.
27. Sylven JC, Hellerstedt M, Levander-Lingren M. Pacing threshold interval with decreasing and increasing output. Pacing Clin Electrophysiol 1982;5:646.
28. Timmis GC, Westveer DC, Holland J, et al. Precision of pacemaker thresholds: the Wedensky effect. Pacing Clin Electrophysiol 1983;6:A-60.
29. Luceri RM, Furman S, Hurzeler P, et al. Threshold behavior of electrodes in long-term ventricular pacing. Am J Cardiol 1977;40:184.
30. Kertes P, Mond H, Sloman G, et al. Comparison of lead complications with polyurethane tined, silicone rubber tined and wedge tip leads: clinical experience with 822 ventricular endocardial leads. Pacing Clin Electrophysiol 1983;6:957.
31. Williams WG, Hesslein PS, Kormos R. Exit block in children with pacemakers. Clin Prog Electrophysiol Pacing 1983;4:478–489.
32. Platia EV, Brinker JA. Time course of transvenous pacemaker stimulation impedance, capture threshold, and electrogram amplitude. Pacing Clin Electrophysiol 1986;9:620–625.
33. de Buitleir M, Kou WH, Schmaltz S, Morady F. Acute changes in pacing threshold and R- or P-wave amplitude during permanent pacemaker implantation. Am J Cardiol 1990;65:999–1003.

34. Furman S, Parker B, Escher D. Decreasing electrode size and increasing efficiency of cardiac stimulation. J Surg Res 1971;11:105.
35. Smyth NPD, Tarjan PP, Chernoff E, et al. The significance of electrode surface area and stimulation thresholds in permanent cardiac pacing. J Thorac Cardiovasc Surg 1976;71:559.
36. Irnich W. The electrode myocardial interface. Clin Prog Electrophysiol Pacing 1985;3:338–348.
37. Parsonnet V, Zucker IR, Kannerstein ML. The fate of permanent intracardiac electrodes. J Surg Res 1966;6:285.
38. Beyersdorf F, Schneider M, Kreuzer J, et al. Studies of the tissue reaction induced by transvenous pacemaker electrodes. I. Microscopic examination of the extent of connective tissue around the electrode tip in the human right ventricle. Pacing Clin Electrophysiol 1988;11:1753–1759.
39. Guarda F, Galloni M, Ossone F, et al. Histological reactions of porous tip endocardial electrodes implanted in sheep. Int J Artif Organs 1982;5:267.
40. Szabo Z, Solti F. The significance of the tissue reaction around the electrode on the late myocardial threshold. In: Schaldach M, Furman S, eds. Advances in pacemaker technology. New York: Springer-Verlag, 1975:273.
41. Nagatomo Y, Ogawa T, Kumagae H, et al. Pacing failure due to markedly increased stimulation threshold two years after implantation: successful management with oral prednisolone: a case report. Pacing Clin Electrophysiol 1989;12:1034–1037.
42. Mond H, Stokes K, Helland J, et al. The porous titanium steroid eluting electrode: a double blind study assessing the stimulation threshold effects of steroid. Pacing Clin Electrophysiol 1988;11:214–219.
43. Kruse IM, Terpstra B. Acute and long-term atrial and ventricular stimulation thresholds with a steroid eluting electrode. Pacing Clin Electrophysiol 1985;8:45.
44. King DH, Gillette PC, Shannon C, et al. Steroid-eluting endocardial lead for treatment of exit block. Am Heart J 1983;106:1438.
45. Pirzada FA, Moschitto LJ, Diorio D. Clinical experience with steroid-eluting unipolar electrodes. Pacing Clin Electrophysiol 1988;11:1739–1744.
46. Brewer G, Mathivanar R, Skolsky M, Anderson N. Composite electrode tips containing externally placed drug-releasing collars. Pacing Clin Electrophysiol 1988;11: 1760–1769.
47. Brooks CMcC, Hoffman BF, Suckling EE, Orias O. Excitability of the heart. New York: Grune & Stratton, 1955:196–197.
48. Orias O, Brooks CM, Suckling EE, et al. Excitability of the mammalian ventricle throughout the cardiac cycle. Am J Physiol 1950;163:272–279.
49. Buxton AE, Marchlinski FE, Miller JM, et al. The human atrial strength–interval relation. Influence of cycle length and procainamide. Circulation 1989;79:271–280.
50. Boyett MR, Jewell BR. A study of the factors responsible for rate-dependent shortening of the action potential in mammalian ventricular muscle. J Physiol 1978; 285:359–380.
51. Kay GN, Mulholland DH, Epstein AE, Plumb VJ. Effect of pacing rate on the human–strength duration curve. J Am Coll Cardiol 1990;15:1618–1623.
52. Plumb VJ, Karp RB, James TN, Waldo AL. Atrial excitability and conduction during rapid atrial pacing. Circulation 1981;63:1140–1149.
53. Johnson EA, McKinnon MG. The differential effect of quinidine and pyrilamine on the myocardial action potential at various rates of stimulation. J Pharmacol Exp Ther 1957;120:460–468.

54. Preston TA, Fletcher RD, Lucchesi BR, Judge RD. Changes in myocardial threshold. Physiologic and pharmacologic factors in patients with implanted pacemakers. Am Heart 1967;74:235.
55. Levick CE, Mizgala HF, Kerr CR. Failure to pace following high dose antiarrhythmic therapy-reversal with isoproterenol. Pacing Clin Electrophysiol 1984;7:252.
56. Sowton E, Barr I. Physiological changes in threshold. Ann NY Acad Sci 1969;167:679.
57. O'Reilly MV, Murnaghan DP, Williams MB. Transvenous pacemaker failure induced by hyperkalemia. JAMA 1974;228:336.
58. Gettes LS, Shabetai R, Downs TA, Surawiez B. Effect of changes in potassium and calcium concentrations on diastolic threshold and strength–interval relationships of the human heart. Ann NY Acad Sci 1969;167:693.
59. Lee D, Greenspan R, Edmands RE, Fisch C. The effect of electrolyte alteration on stimulus requirement of cardiac pacemakers. Circulation 1968;38(suppl 6):124.
60. Hughes HC, Tyers GFO, Forman HA. Effects of acid–base imbalance on myocardial pacing thresholds. J Thorac Cardiovasc Surg 1975;69:743.
61. Kubler W, Sowton E. Influence of beta-blockade on myocardial threshold in patients with pacemakers. Lancet 1970;2:67.
62. Wallace AG, Cline RE, Sealy WC, et al. Electrophysiologic effects of quinidine. Circ Res 1966;19:960–969.
63. Gay RJ, Brown DF. Pacemaker failure due to procainamide toxicity. Am J Cardiol 1974;34:728.
64. Hellestrand KF, Burnett PJ, Milne JR, et al. Effect of the antiarrhythmic agent flecainide acetate on acute and chronic pacing thresholds. Pacing Clin Electrophysiol 1983;6:892.
65. Irnich W, Gebhardt U. The pacemaker–electrode combination and its relationship to service life. In: Thalen HJT, ed. To pace or not to pace, controversial subjects in cardiac pacing. The Hague: Martinus Nyhoff, 1978:209.
66. Amundson D, McArthur W, MacCarter D, et al. Porous electrode–tissue interface. Pacing Clin Electrophysiol 1979;2:40–50.
67. MacGregor DC, Wilson GJ, Lixfeld W, et al. The porous-surfaced electrode. A new concept in pacemaker lead design. J Thorac Cardiovasc Surg 1979;78:281.
68. Sinnaeve A, Willems R, Backers J, et al. Pacing and sensing: how can one electrode fulfill both requirements? Pacing Clin Electrophysiol 1987;10:546–559.
69. Elmqvist H, Schuller H, Richter G. The carbon tip electrode. Pacing Clin Electrophysiol 1983;6:436.
70. Garberoglio B, Inguaggiato B, Chinaglia B, et al. Initial results with an activated pyrolytic carbon tip electrode. Pacing Clin Electrophysiol 1983;6:440–447.
71. Walton C, Gergely S, Economides AP. Platinum pacemaker electrodes. Origins and effects of the electrode–tissue interface impedance. Pacing Clin Electrophysiol 1987;10:87–99.
72. Mayhew MW, Johnson PL, Slabaugh JE, Bubien RS, Kay GN. Electrical characteristics of a split cathodal pacing configuration. PACE 2003;26:2264–2271.
73. Barold SS, Levine PA. Significance of stimulation impedance in biventricular pacing. J Interventional Card Electrophysiol 2002;6:67–70.
74. Ripart A, Mugica J. Electrode-heart interface: Definition of the ideal electrode. PACE 1983;6:410–421.

75. Irnich W. Paradigm shift in lead design. PACE 1999;22:1321–1332.
76. Lewis T. The mechanism and graphic registration of the heartbeat. London: Shaw and Sons, 1925.
77. Furman S, Hurzeler P, DeCaprio V. The ventricular endocardial electrogram and pacemaker sensing. J Thorac Cardiovasc Surg 1977;73:258.
78. Kleinert M, Elmqvist H, Strandberg H. Spectral properties of atrial and ventricular signals. Pacing Clin Electrophysiol 1979;2:11.
79. Parsonnet V, Myers GH, Kresh YM. Characteristics of intracardiac electrogram II. Atrial endocardial electrograms. Pacing Clin Electrophysiol 1980;3:406.
80. DeCaprio V, Hurzeler P, Furman S. Comparison of unipolar and bipolar electrograms for cardiac pacemaker sensing. Circulation 1977;56:750.
81. Goldreyer BN, Knudson M, Cannom DS, Wyman MG. Orthogonal electrogram sensing. Pacing Clin Electrophysiol 1983;6:464.
82. Aubert AE, Ector H, Denys BG, DeGeest H. Sensing characteristics of unipolar and bipolar orthogonal floating atrial electrodes: morphology and spectral analysis. Pacing Clin Electrophysiol 1986;9:343–359.
83. Thull R, Schaldach M. Electrochemistry or after-pacing potentials on electrodes. Pacing Clin Electrophysiol 1986;9:1191–1196.
84. Hauser RG, Susmano A. After potential oversensing by a programmable pulse generator. Pacing Clin Electrophysiol 1981;4:391.
85. Shandling AH, Castellanet M, Rylaarsdam A, et al. Screw versus nonscrew transvenous atrial leads: acute and chronic P-wave amplitudes (abstract). Pacing Clin Electrophysiol 1989;12:689.
86. Greatbatch W, Piersma B, Shannon FD, et al. Polarization phenomena relating to physiological electrodes. Ann NY Acad Sci 1969;167:722.
87. Raber MB, Cuddy TE, Israel DA. Pacemaker electrodes act as high-pass filter on the electrogram. In: Watanabe Y, ed. Cardiac pacing. Amsterdam and Oxford: Excerpta Medica, 1977:506.
88. Brummer SB, Robblee LS, Hambrecht FT. Criteria for selecting electrodes for electrical stimulation: theoretical and practical considerations. Ann NY Acad Sci 1983;405:159–171.
89. Holmes DR, Nissen RG, Maloney JD, et al. Transvenous tined electrode systems: an approach to acute dislodgement. Mayo Clin Proc 1979;54:219–222.
90. Furman S, Pannizzo F, Campo I. Comparison of active and passive adhering leads for endocardial pacing. Pacing Clin Electrophysiol 1979;2:417–427.
91. Bisping HJ, Kreuzer J, Birkenheir H. Three-year clinical experience with a new endocardial screw-in lead with introduction protection for use in the atrium and ventricle. Pacing Clin Electrophysiol 1980;3:424–435.
92. Pehrsson SK, Bergdahl L, Svane B. Early and late efficacy of three types of transvenous atrial leads. Pacing Clin Electrophysiol 1984;7:195–202.
93. Kay GN, Brinker JA, Kawanishi DT, et al. Risks of spontaneous injury and extraction of an active fixation pacemaker lead: report of the Accufix Multicenter Clinical Study and Worldwide Registry. Circulation 1999;100:2344–2352.
94. Byrd CL, McArthur W, Stokes K, et al. Implant experience with unipolar polyurethane pacing leads. Pacing Clin Electrophysiol 1983;6:868–882.
95. Stokes KB, Frazer WA, Christopherson RA. Environmental stress cracking in implanted polyurethanes. In: Proceedings of the Second World Congress on Biomaterials, tenth annual meeting of the Society of Biomaterials. Washington, DC: Society of Biomaterials, 1984:254.

96. Phillips RE, Thoma RJ. Metal ion complexation of polyurethane. A proposed mechanism of calcification. In: Plank H, et al., eds. Polyurethanes in biomedical engineering II: Proceedings of the Second International Conference on Polyurethanes in Biomedical Engineering. Amsterdam: Elsevier, 1987:91–108.
97. Humen DP, Kostuk WJ, Klein GJ. Activity-sensing rate responsive pacing: improvement in myocardial performance with exercise. Pacing Clin Electrophysiol 1985;8:52.
98. Benditt DG, Mianulli M, Fetter J, et al. Single chamber cardiac pacing with activity-initiated chronotropic response. Evaluation by cardiopulmonary exercise testing. Circulation 1987;75:184.
99. Lau CP, Butrous G, Ward DE, Camm AJ. Comparison of exercise performance of six rate-adaptive right ventricular cardiac pacemakers. Am J Cardiol 1989;63: 833–838.
100. Matula M, Alt E, Fotuhi P, et al. Influence of varied types of exercise on the rate adaptation of activity pacemakers. Pacing Clin Electrophysiol 1992;15:578.
101. Matula M, Alt E, Fotuhi P, et al. Influence of varied types of exercise to the rate modulation of activity pacemakers. Pacing Clin Electrophysiol 1992;15:1578.
102. Bacharach DW, Hilden RS, Millerhagen JO, et al. Activity-based pacing: comparison of a device using an accelerometer versus a piezo-electric crystal. Pacing Clin Electrophysiol 1992;15:188.
103. Kay GN, Bubien RS, Epstein AE, Plumb VJ. Rate-modulated cardiac pacing based on transthoracic impedance measurements of minute ventilation: correlation with exercise gas exchange. J Am Coll Cardiol 1989;14:1283–1289.
104. Alt E, Heinz M, Hirgsletter C, et al. Control of pacemaker rate by impedance-based respiratory minute ventilation. Chest 1987;92:247.
105. Lau CP, Antoniou A, Ward DE, Camm AJ. Initial clinical experience with a minute ventilation sensing rate modulated pacemaker: improvements in exercise capacity and symptomatology. Pacing Clin Electrophysiol 1988;11:1815–1822.
106. Val F, Bonnet JL, Ritter PH, Pioger G. Relationship between heart rate and minute ventilation, tidal volume and respiratory rate during brief and low level exercise. Pacing Clin Electrophysiol 1988;11:1860–1865.
107. Alt E, Theres H, Heinz M, et al. A new rate-modulated pacemaker system optimized by combination of two sensors. Pacing Clin Electrophysiol 1988;11:1119.

Hemodynamics of Cardiac Pacing

Richard C. Wu and Dwight W. Reynolds

3

Knowledge as well as interest in hemodynamics has evolved substantially since 1960, essentially pari passu with the technology of cardiac pacing. Although general knowledge of this subject has played an important role in the evolution of sophisticated pacing capabilities, the technology itself has facilitated the expansion of knowledge of cardiovascular hemodynamics generally and as it relates to pacing.

The vogue in pacing since 1980 has been the accomplishment of "physiologic" pacing. Our concepts of physiologic pacing have evolved in concert with our understanding of pacing-related cardiovascular hemodynamics, as well as with technologic sophistication. In 2004, we speak of "minimal right ventricular pacing" to avoid prolonging the QRS, optimizing and providing for rate-varied atrioventricular (AV) intervals, using alternative right ventricular pacing sites for improved hemodynamic performance, and selecting patients with heart failure for cardiac resynchronization therapy. The key concepts of physiologic pacing, considered most broadly, include *the proper sequencing of atrial and ventricular contraction and physiologic rate modulation*. These topics are discussed in this chapter along with consideration of special applications as a practical guide for selection of a pacing mode as it relates to these physiologic and hemodynamic issues.

ATRIOVENTRICULAR SYNCHRONY

The hemodynamics of AV synchrony have been addressed both qualitatively and quantitatively for centuries.[1] Elegant work was published in the past century.[2,3] The topic has been more extensively examined since 1960, during which time pacemakers have been developed that are capable of providing AV synchrony. The hemodynamics of AV synchrony are discussed in the context of advantages that might accrue from maintaining AV synchrony. The physiologic basis of these hemodynamic benefits result from the ability of AV synchrony to: 1) maximize ventricular pre-load and therefore contractility; 2) close AV valves before ventricular systole, limiting AV valvular regurgitation; 3) maintain low mean atrial pressures, thus facilitation venous return; and 4) regulate autonomic and neurohumoral reflexes involving atrial pressure and volume.

Advantages of Atrioventricular Synchrony

Blood Pressure: Systemic blood pressure and cardiac output have been the subjects of much of the discussion regarding the importance of maintaining AV synchrony. For grouped patient data, AV synchrony generally provides similar or slightly greater systolic and mean blood pressures than ventricular pacing.[4] A typical example of the blood pressure comparison among atrial, AV, and ventricular pacing is shown in Figure 3.1. In this case, essentially no differences exist between the blood pressures when comparing atrial to AV pacing. The blood pressure during ventricular pacing is slightly lower than during either atrial or AV pacing. A heterogeneous group of pacemaker patients studied at the

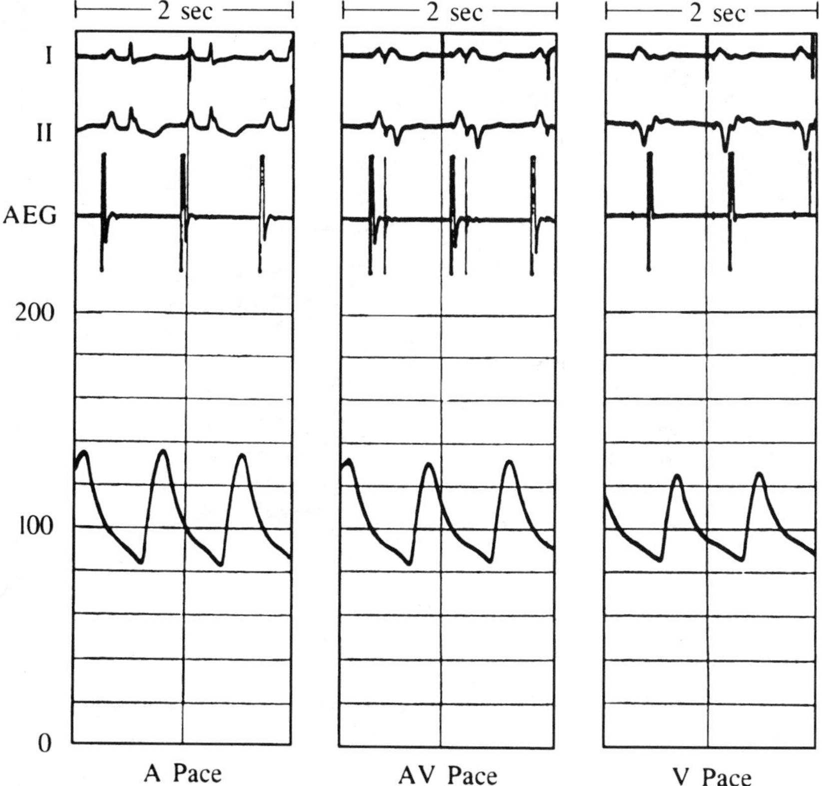

Figure 3.1. Femoral artery pressure recordings from one patient. **Left:** During atrial pacing (A Pace). **Center:** During AV sequential pacing (AV Pace). **Right:** During ventricular pacing (V Pace). All tracings are at 80 ppm with AV interval of 150 milliseconds during AV pacing. Scale in mmHg. I, II, III = standard ECG leads; AEG = atrial electrogram.

University of Oklahoma[4] showed statistically significant differences in their femoral artery systolic pressure (Fig. 3.2) but not in their diastolic and mean pressures (Table 3.1). The measurements in this study were performed with supine patients, which may have masked potentially more dramatic differences if evaluations had been done with the patients in an upright posture.

It has, however, been observed that some individuals have marked decreases in blood pressure when ventricular pacing is instituted.[5,6] Although this is not the typical response to ventricular pacing, some individuals do have dramatic and symptomatic decreases in systemic blood pressure (Fig. 3.3). Several mechanisms may be responsible for this phenomenon. Loss of left ventricular preload volume from mistimed atrial contraction (loss of atrial "kick") and loss of inhibitory cardiac reflexes (due also to inappropriately timed atrial contraction)

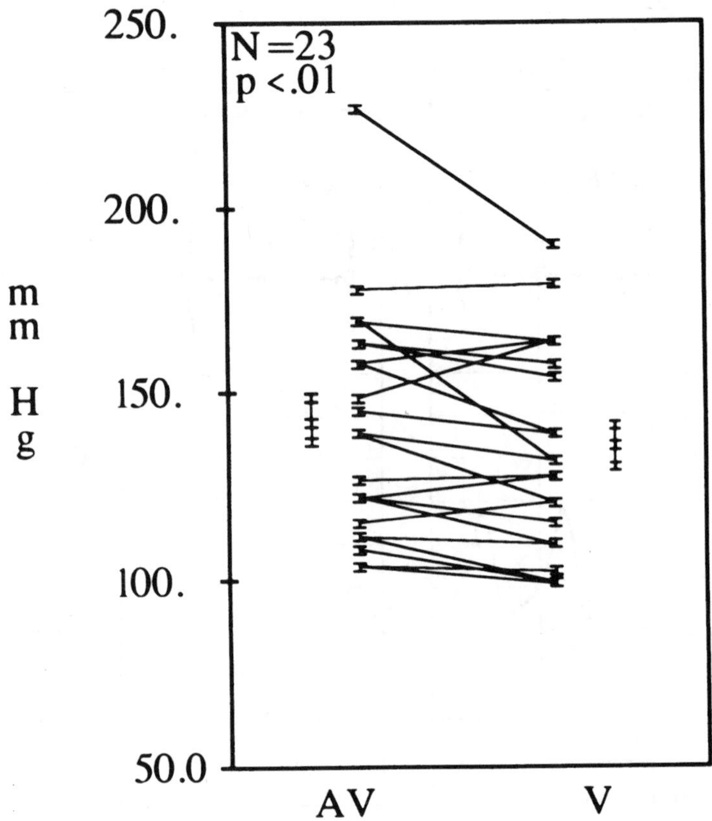

Figure 3.2. A comparison of femoral artery systolic pressures in a group of 23 pacemaker patients. **Left:** During AV sequential pacing. **Right:** During ventricular pacing. Both are at 80 ppm with AV interval during AV pacing equal to 150 milliseconds. Individual comparisons are inside and connected by solid lines. Group comparison ±SEM is outside. Paired *t* tests were used for statistical comparison.

Table 3.1. Hemodynamic Evaluation of Atrioventricular and Ventricular Pacing

Parameter	Av*	V*	N	$P^{\dagger}$
RA mean (mm Hg)	6.0 ± 0.6	8.1 ± 0.6	22	<.001
PA systolic (mm Hg)	24.5 ± 1.6	28.3 ± 1.7	23	<.001
PA diastolic (mm Hg)	12.6 ± 1.0	14.3 ± 1.1	23	<.02
PA mean (mm Hg)	17.1 ± 1.1	20.6 ± 1.2	23	<.001
PCW mean (mm Hg)	7.7 ± 1.0	13.4 ± 1.2	22	<.001
LV systolic (mm Hg)	141.3 ± 5.2	132.0 ± 5.1	23	<.01
LV end-diastolic (mm Hg)	9.8 ± 1.4	10.1 ± 0.8	22	NS
FA systolic (mm Hg)	141.4 ± 5.1	133.4 ± 5.1	23	<.01
FA diastolic (mm Hg)	80.3 ± 2.0	80.9 ± 2.4	23	NS
FA mean (mm Hg)	105.6 ± 2.8	103.1 ± 3.4	23	NS
CI.TD (L/min/m^2)	2.575 ± 0.148	2.073 ± 0.126	23	<.001
CT.Angio (L/min/m^2)	3.337 ± 0.210	2.878 ± 0.157	19	<.001
LV.EDVI (mL/m^2)	85.7 ± 7.4	76.6 ± 6.8	19	<.001
LV.ESVI (mL/m^2)	46.2 ± 5.9	42.2 ± 5.4	19	<.05
LV.SVI (mL/m^2)	39.7 ± 2.6	34.3 ± 2.0	19	<.001
LV.EF (%)	48.9 ± 2.8	47.6 ± 2.8	19	NS
SVR (dyne · sec · cm^{-5})	1856.1 ± 160.3	2178.0 ± 180.6	23	<.001
PVR (dyne · sec · cm^{-5})	169.0 ± 16.3	152.1 ± 15.0	22	NS

* Mean ± SEM.

† Paired *t* test.

Angio = angiography; CI = cardiac index; EDVI = end-diastolic volume index; EF = ejection fraction; ESVI = end-systolic volume index; FA = femoral artery; LV = left ventricle; NS = not statistically significant; PA = pulmonary artery; PCW = pulmonary capillary wedge; PVR = pulmonary vascular resistance; RA = right atrium; SVI = stroke volume index; SVR = systemic vascular resistance; TD = thermodilution.

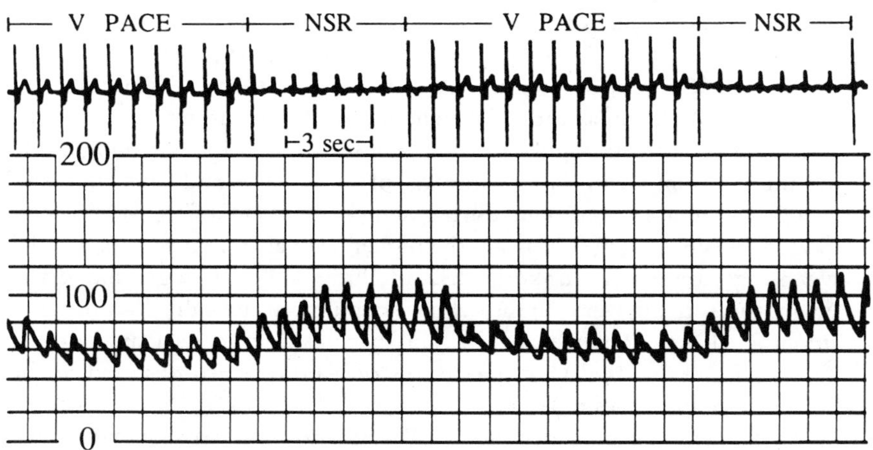

Figure 3.3. Radial artery pressure recording from a patient during right ventricular pacing (V PACE) at 80 ppm and normal sinus rhythm (NSR) (scale in mm Hg). This patient's blood pressure, measured by radial artery line, drops from approximately 110/70 mm Hg during sinus rhythm to approximately 75/55 mm Hg during ventricular pacing.

have been the mechanisms most commonly implicated. This marked hypotension can produce dramatic symptoms, including syncope. In a clinical setting, if this problem is suspected but hypotension with symptoms cannot be reproduced in a supine position, an upright or semiupright posture may unmask the problem, especially if it is related to a left ventricular preload deficiency caused by loss of atrial contribution to ventricular filling. An important consideration in the hemodynamic response to ventricular pacing is ventriculoatrial (VA) conduction. VA conduction, the ability to conduct electrical impulses retrograde from the ventricles through the AV junction to the atria, can lead to atrial contraction during ventricular systole or in cases of long VA conduction, early diastole. This can cause loss of the atrial contribution to ventricular filling as well as other hemodynamic problems, as discussed below. VA conduction has been found in as many as 90% of patients with sick sinus syndrome and in 15% to 35% of individuals with a variety of degrees of AV block.[7–9] This has been a major issue in the use of hysteresis, a feature commonly included in ventricular pacemakers since 1980.[10] During ventricular pacing, even when VA conduction is not intact, if the ventricular pacing rate is unequal to the atrial rate, there will be periods of time when atrial contraction occurs during ventricular systole with the resulting disadvantageous hemodynamics.

Cardiac Output: Cardiac output, more than any other hemodynamic feature, has been the focus of discussions and investigations relating to AV synchrony.[11–13] Properly timed atrial contraction provides a significant increase in ventricular end-diastolic volume and is responsible for the so-called atrial kick. Studies have shown a wide range in the actual importance of the atrial contribution to ventricular filling depending on the patient populations and study conditions. By increasing the end-diastolic volumes (right and left ventricles), the cardiac output is, in turn, increased. The average increase in cardiac output in a broad-based pacing population, if AV synchrony is maintained, appears to be between 15% and 25% in comparison to non–AV-synchronized ventricular pacing.

In the Oklahoma study, the benefits of AV synchrony were confirmed in a broad-based pacing population (Fig. 3.4; see Table 3.1). AV pacing at 80 pulses per minute (ppm) with an AV interval of 150 milliseconds was compared with ventricular pacing at 80 ppm during which VA conduction was intact or was created by VA pacing. Consistently higher cardiac outputs maintained by AV synchrony were seen in both thermodilution and angiographic evaluations. Again, the patients were supine when examined; an upright posture might have amplified these differences, because in that position ventricular diastolic filling depends more on atrial kick due to loss of venous return of blood to the heart (lower extremity pooling).[14]

The hemodynamic benefits of AV-synchronized versus ventricular pacing have also been demonstrated for patients after myocardial infarction[15] and cardiac surgery.[16,17] Patients with reduced cardiac output—especially if such reduced function is due to relative volume depletion or only mild to moderately depressed left ventricular function—frequently benefit significantly from main-

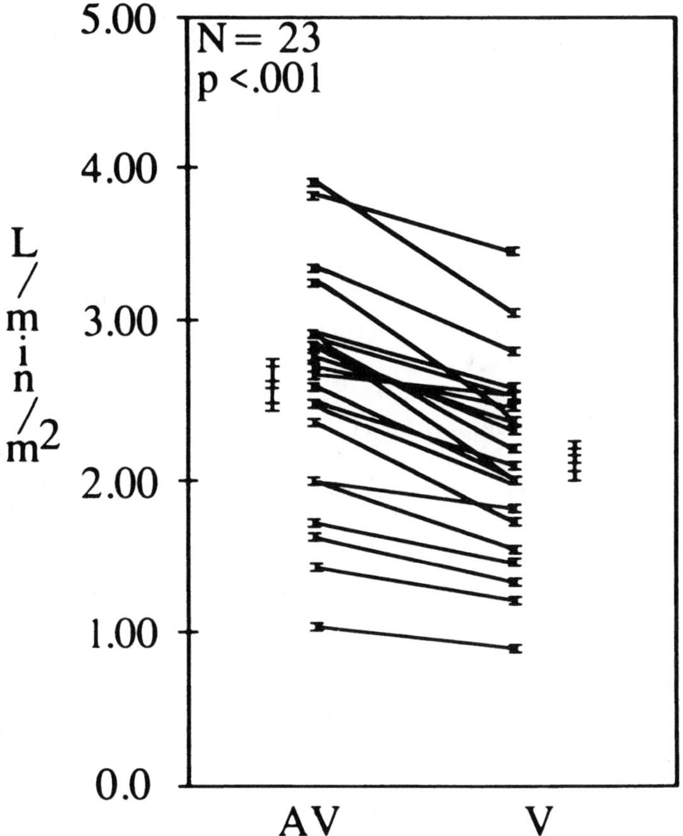

Figure 3.4. A comparison of the cardiac index, measured by thermodilution technique, in 23 pacemaker patients. **Left:** During AV sequential pacing. **Right:** During ventricular pacing. Both are at 80 ppm with AV interval during AV pacing = 150 milliseconds. Individual comparisons are inside and connected by solid lines. Group comparison ±SEM is outside. Paired *t* tests are used for statistical comparison.

tenance of AV synchrony; this should be kept in mind when dealing with patients in these and other situations.

There has been a general perception that patients with abnormal cardiac function benefit most from maintenance of AV synchrony. This may be true, but the reasons are frequently not due to better cardiac output.[12,18] In fact, if cardiac output were the only consideration hemodynamically (and obviously it is not), it is patients with very poor ventricular function (markedly increased end-diastolic volume and depressed ejection fraction) that benefit least from AV synchrony. This can be best understood by using the concept of ventricular function curves that compare stroke volume or cardiac output to left ventricular (LV) end-diastolic volume or preload.

Figure 3.5 shows hypothetical ventricular function curves for a patient with normal ventricular function (curve 1), one with moderate LV dysfunction (curve 2), one with very poor LV function and a markedly dilated ventricle (curve 3), and a patient with hypertrophic cardiomyopathy (curve 4). These curves describe the performance of the left ventricle in generating stroke volume (or cardiac output) in relationship to the end-diastolic volume (or preload). In patients with normal LV function (curve 1), as end-diastolic volume increases, stroke volume (and cardiac output) increases until the flat or descending portion of the curve is reached. In patients with depressed LV function (curves 2 and 3) there is a lesser increase in stroke volume that depends on end-diastolic volume to the point that in patients with poor LV function (curve 3) there is negligible improvement in stroke volume with further increases in end-diastolic volume. On the other hand, patients with hypertrophic cardiomyopathies tend to have small ventricles that are normal (i.e., normal systolic function) or hyperdynamic in function (curve 4). Small increases in end-diastolic volume can significantly increase stroke volume in this situation. As has been discussed, AV synchrony provides the atrial kick that increases end-diastolic volume. Point A on these curves represents the hypothetical stroke volume and end-diastolic volume during AV pacing. Point B represents stroke volume and end-diastolic volume during ventricular pacing (with associated loss of atrial kick). In the normal situation (curve 1), although end-diastolic volume is greater and hence stroke volume is greater during AV-synchronized pacing, the loss of AV synchrony during ventricular pacing does not drop the end-diastolic volume and the stroke volume significantly. This, however, might not be the case if filling volume were otherwise reduced by volume depletion due to blood loss, diuresis, and so on. In these situations, even with normal LV function, the higher end-diastolic volumes and stroke volumes provided by properly timed atrial contraction might

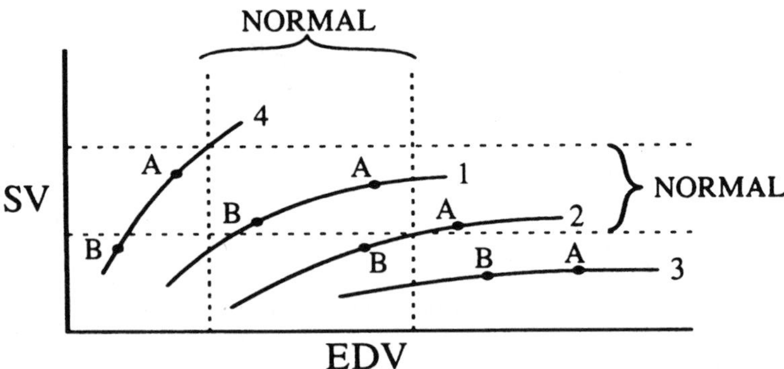

Figure 3.5. Hypothetical ventricular function curves comparing **(1)** stroke volume (SV) and left ventricular end-diastolic volume (EDV) in patients with normal ventricular function; **(2)** moderately depressed ventricular function; **(3)** severely depressed ventricular function; and **(4)** hyperdynamic ventricular function. Point **A** = with normal AV sequence; and Point **B** = without normal AV sequence.

be important. With depressed LV function of a moderate degree (curve 2), although maintenance of AV synchrony provides for a greater end-diastolic volume, the stroke volume advantage is diminished. It is possible that, due to overall reduction in stroke volume (and cardiac output), even this modest increment in stroke volume would be of important benefit. In patients with more severely depressed LV function and extremely flat LV function curves (curve 3), end-diastolic volume can be augmented with maintenance of AV synchrony, but there is little advantage in stroke volume. With regard to patients with hypertrophic cardiomyopathies or highly non-compliant ventricles (curve 4) maintenance of AV synchrony may be very important in enhancing stroke volume and cardiac output because of the relatively small end-diastolic volumes. This is because small increments in end-diastolic volume may substantially increase the stroke volume due to the steep slope of the curve. This relatively steep-sloped ventricular function curve is also characteristic of patients with ventricular diastolic dysfunction, a group for whom maintenance of AV synchrony is also very important. Figure 3.6 displays this concept in a relatively small number of patients studied using quantitative nuclear techniques.[18] Although only data from the supine position at 80 ppm are shown (AV interval 150 milliseconds during AV-synchronized pacing), the same situation hemodynamically was found to be present at a faster pacing rate (100 ppm) and in an upright posture.

Movement along single ventricular function curves is probably simplistic in that such variables as afterload, which could be modulated by a number of factors, might cause shifting from one curve to another as well as movement along a given curve. However, for practical understanding, this conceptual approach is useful.

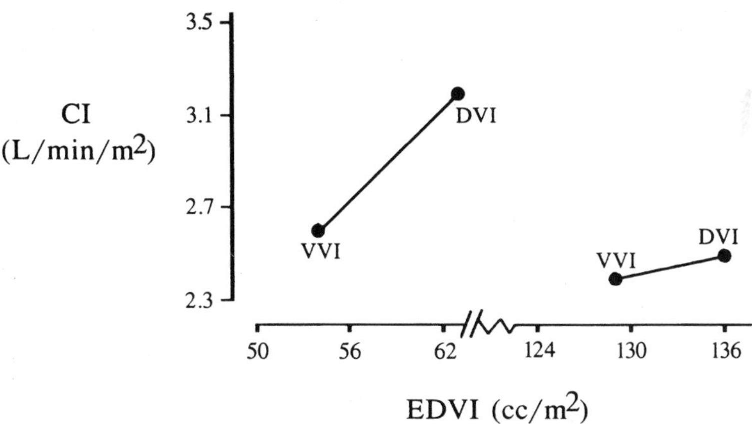

Figure 3.6. Ventricular function curves comparing cardiac index (CI) and left ventricular end-diastolic volume index (EDVI) from **(left)** a group of nine patients with relatively normal ventricular function and **(right)** a group of four patients with markedly depressed ventricular function. The patients were studied in supine position at pacing rate = 80 ppm; AV interval during DVI pacing = 150 milliseconds. Points are group mean. VVI = ventricular pacing (no AV synchrony); DVI = AV sequential pacing (AV synchrony).

Atrial Pressures: Cardiac output and blood pressure have been the primary foci of most discussions about the importance of AV synchrony, and the most extreme cases of intolerance to ventricular pacing relate to these factors. It is likely, however, that an increase in atrial pressures during ventricular pacing is the most common mechanism by which symptoms are produced when AV synchrony is not maintained. During AV synchrony, atrial contraction augments ventricular end-diastolic filling pressure while maintaining a low mean atrial pressure throughout diastole. In the absence of AV synchrony, a higher mean atrial pressure is required to achieve the same degree of ventricular filling. By this mechanism, AV synchrony is associated with lower venous and left atrial pressures (Fig. 3.7).

In Figure 3.7, the left panel shows recordings of pulmonary capillary wedge pressure in one patient during AV-synchronous pacing (80 ppm/AV interval 150 milliseconds). The right panel shows pulmonary capillary wedge pressure during ventricular pacing (80 ppm) with intact ventriculoatrial conduction. A relatively normal pulmonary capillary wedge pressure tracing is produced during AV pacing with mean pressures between 4 and 8 mm Hg and without significant phasic aberration. In contrast, during ventricular pacing, one can see that the mean pressures are elevated to between 8 and 12 mm Hg with large A waves (or VA waves) that, at times, exceed 16 mm Hg. This elevation in atrial pressures, and specifically the production of giant or "cannon" A waves, occurs because of left atrial contraction against a closed mitral valve; the increased pressure wave is present not only in the left atrium but also in the pulmonary veins and pulmonary capillary wedge position. The same phenomenon occurs on the right side of the heart. Figures 3.8 to 3.10 display simultaneous pulmonary capillary wedge and right atrial recordings during ventricular pacing (80 ppm) in which

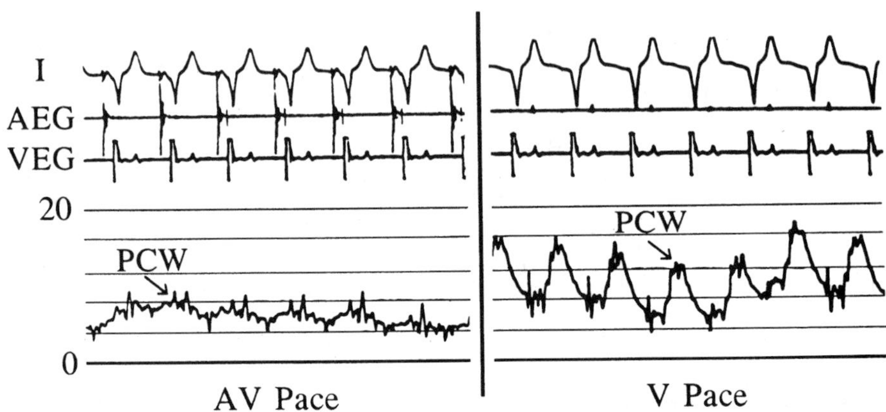

Figure 3.7. Pulmonary capillary wedge (PCW) pressure recordings from a single patient during **(left)** AV pacing (AV Pace) and **(right)** ventricular pacing (V Pace) at 80 ppm with AV interval = 150 milliseconds. (Scale = mm Hg; I = ECG lead I; AEG = atrial electrogram; VEG = ventricular electrogram.)

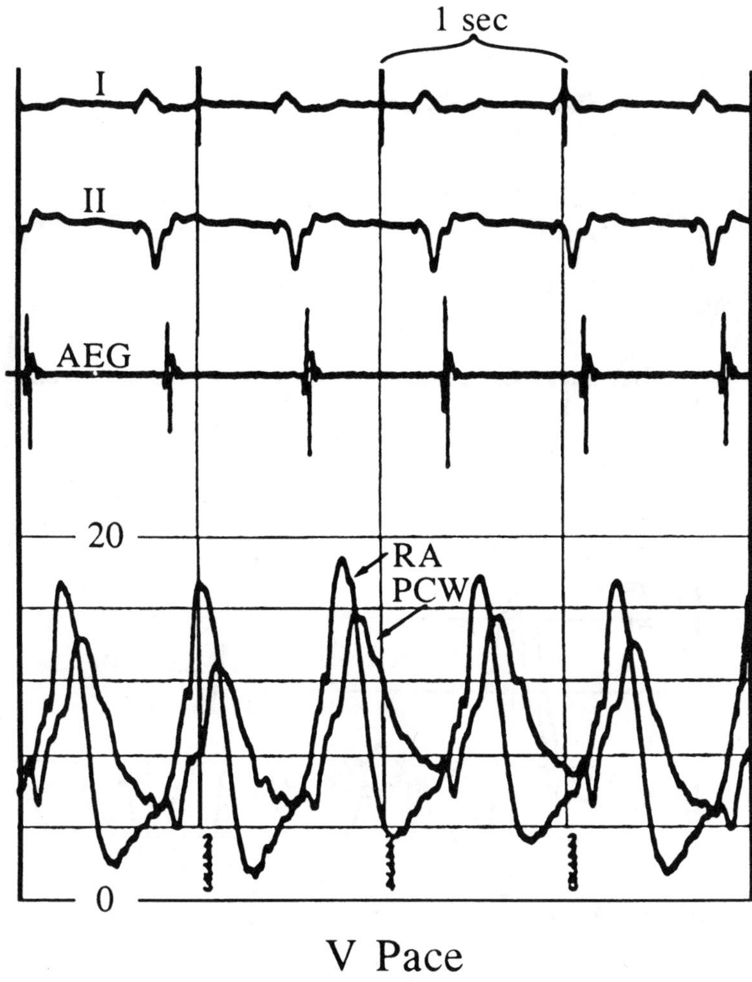

Figure 3.8. Right atrial (RA) and pulmonary capillary wedge (PCW) pressure recordings during ventricular pacing (V Pace) at 80 ppm with 1 : 1 VA conduction. (Scale = mm Hg; I, II standard ECG leads; AEG = atrial electrogram.)

VA conduction is intact. Intact VA conduction produces consistent elevations in pressure in the left atrium and right atrium due to the contraction of the atria against closed AV valves. Even when VA conduction is not intact, because of unequal atrial and ventricular rates there will be frequent periods when atrial contraction occurs during ventricular systole, during which the AV valves are closed; hence the problems of elevated pressures in the atria and pulmonary veins occur. It has been our experience that some patients are actually more symptomatic when VA conduction is not intact, due to the intermittency of these elevated pressures, thus preventing patients from establishing tolerance for this phenomenon.

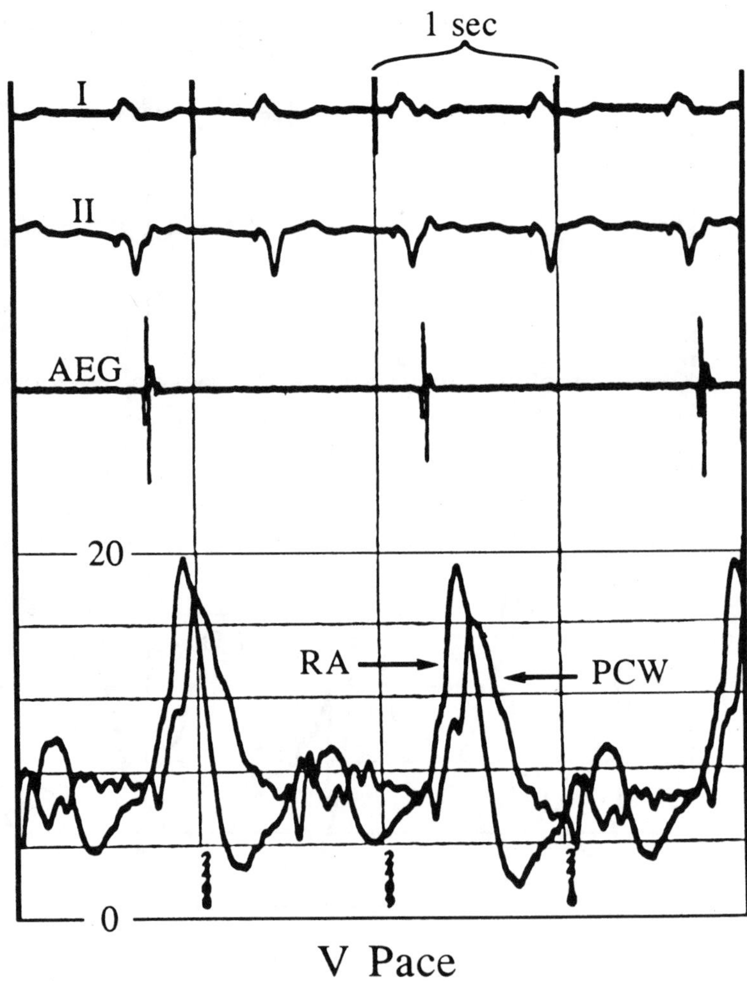

Figure 3.9. Right atrial (RA) and pulmonary capillary wedge (PCW) pressure recordings during ventricular pacing (V Pace) at 80 ppm with 2:1 VA conduction. Scale = mmHg; I, II standard ECG leads; AEG = atrial electrogram.

The relationship of the phasic changes in the pulmonary capillary wedge (and left atrial) pressures to LV pressures can be seen in Figures 3.11, 3.12, and 3.13. Figure 3.11 is a display of normal LV and pulmonary capillary wedge pressure recordings during AV pacing (80 ppm/AV interval of 150 milliseconds). The appropriately timed A wave can be seen in both the LV and pulmonary capillary wedge pressure recordings. In contrast, as Figure 3.12 shows, during ventricular pacing (80 ppm) with a consistent 1:1 VA relationship, the loss of the A wave contribution to the upstroke of the LV pressure recording and the giant A wave, late in ventricular systole, can be seen consistently in the pulmonary

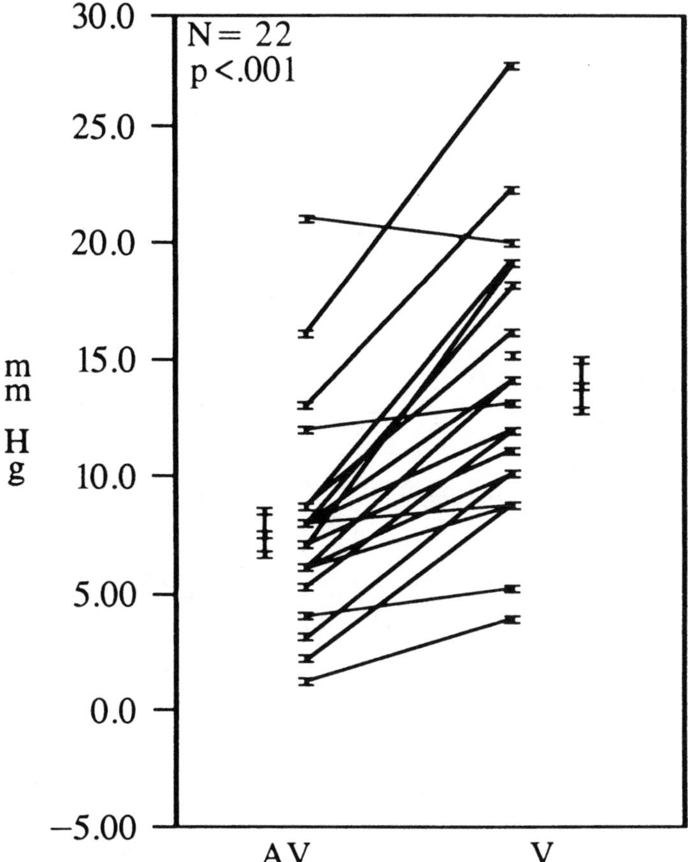

Figure 3.10. A comparison of pulmonary capillary wedge pressures in a group of 22 pacemaker patients during **(left)** AV sequential pacing and **(right)** ventricular pacing, both at 80 ppm with AV interval during AV pacing = 150 milliseconds. Individual comparisons are inside and connected by solid lines. Group comparison ±SEM is outside. Paired *t* tests used for statistical comparison.

capillary wedge pressure recording. Figure 3.13 displays this relationship when the atrial contraction is random in relationship to ventricular contraction.

Although it is relatively clear that the mechanism for the giant A waves is the contraction of the atria against closed AV valves, some have speculated that AV valvular regurgitation is responsible for much of the increase in phasic pressure in the atria[19,20]; however, worsening of AV regurgitation appears to play a lesser role in elevating atrial pressure. In the University of Oklahoma study, pacemaker patients underwent LV cineangiography for assessment of mitral regurgitation during both AV and V pacing.[21] Of the 16 patients who underwent paired LV cineangiograms, five (approximately 30%) had slight worsening in the

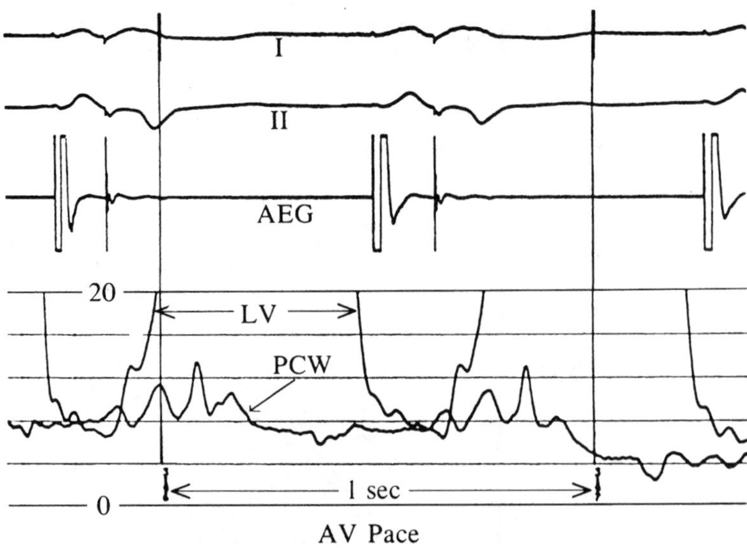

Figure 3.11. Left ventricular (LV) and pulmonary capillary wedge (PCW) pressure recordings during AV pacing at 80 ppm with AV interval = 150 milliseconds. Scale = mm Hg; I, II = standard ECG leads; AEG = atrial electrogram.

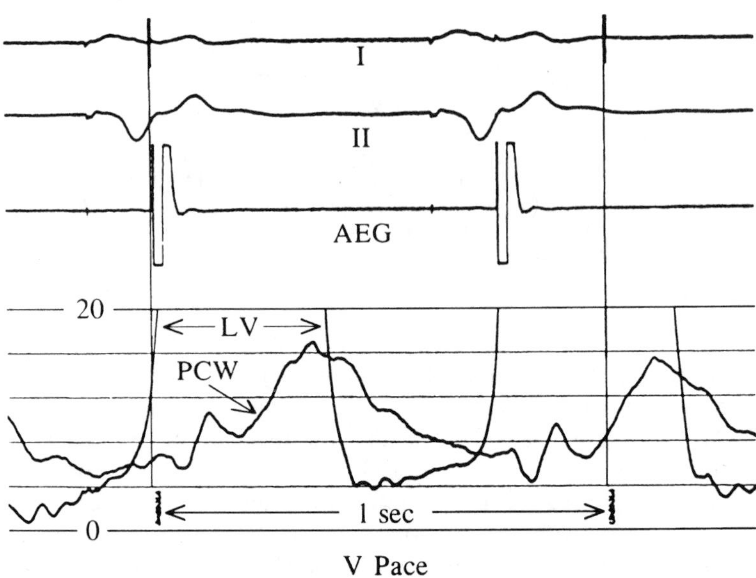

Figure 3.12. Left ventricular (LV) and pulmonary capillary wedge (PCW) pressure recordings during ventricular pacing at 80 ppm with AV interval = 150 milliseconds. Scale = mm Hg; I, II = standard ECG leads; AEG = atrial electrogram.

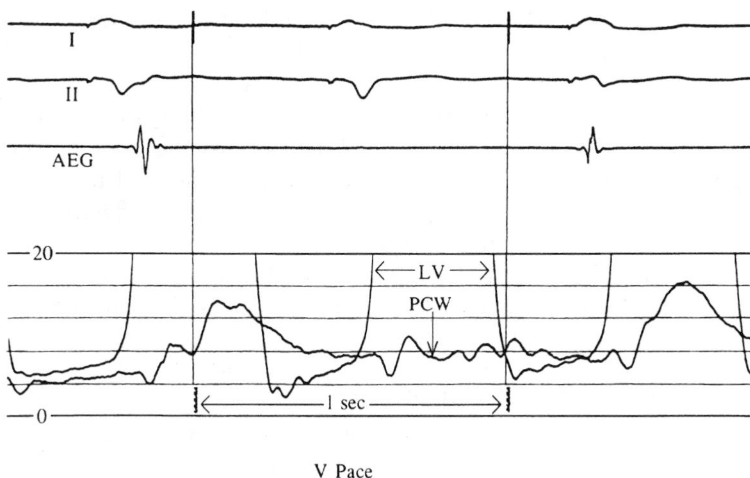

Figure 3.13. Left ventricular (LV) and pulmonary capillary wedge (PCW) pressure recordings during ventricular pacing at 80 ppm with AV interval = 150 milliseconds with VA dissociation. Scale = mm Hg; I, II = standard ECG leads; AEG = atrial electrogram.

degree of mitral regurgitation during ventricular pacing compared with AV pacing. It is possible that an occasional patient will have substantial worsening or production of mitral and tricuspid regurgitation during ventricular pacing, but it is unlikely that in a majority of patients this contributes significantly to the problem of atrial pressure elevation and giant A waves seen consistently during ventricular pacing. To reiterate, it appears that the primary mechanism of these increases in atrial pressure is related to the contraction of the atria against the closed AV valves during ventricular systole with worsening of AV valvular regurgitation occurring less frequently.

Other Advantages: Pulmonary vascular resistance was not significantly different between AV and V paced patients. Systemic vascular resistance may be significantly higher during ventricular pacing. Mechanistically, it is likely that this increase in systemic vascular resistance is related to neural reflexes supportive of blood pressure when cardiac output is diminished.[5,6] A hemodynamic variable that is usually not significantly affected in most individuals (AV versus V pacing) is ejection fraction (see Table 3.1). Although the components of ejection fraction—both end-diastolic volume and stroke volume—are significantly lower during ventricular pacing, ejection fraction is unaffected because both the numerator (stroke volume) and the denominator (end-diastolic volume) of the ejection fraction vary in the same proportion. Ejection fraction is a crude measurement of contractile performance, so it is not surprising that presence or absence of AV synchrony, which primarily affects preload and cardiac output, has no effect on ejection fraction.

It appears that pacing modalities have little effect on most hormonal levels, but atrial natriuretic peptide (ANP), an atrially produced hormone, does appear to be increased during ventricular pacing. This increase is probably related to release of the hormone in response to the stress of higher atrial pressures.[22] The importance of the increase is unclear. Ventricular pacing does, however, increase peripheral sympathetic nerve tone and circulating catecholamine levels.[23]

While non-randomized studies have reported differences in survival between patients undergoing AV synchronous and ventricular pacing, the results of controlled randomized trials have dispelled these findings.[24–27] It is now believed that AV synchronous pacing provides no survival benefit over ventricular pacing alone.

Effects of Atrioventricular Interval

The mere presence of a consistent AV relationship does not assure optimal hemodynamics and as described, some relationships are detrimental as with 1:1 VA conduction. Similarly, inappropriately short or long AV delays can be detrimental. An excessively long AV delay may inadequately fill the ventricle by causing early mitral valve closure and truncating diastolic filling time. In addition, diastolic AV valvular regurgitation may occur with re-opening of the valve before ventricular systole. An excessively short AV delay may limit active filling of the ventricle and promote systolic AV valvular regurgitation as ventricular contraction begins while the AV valves are still open. It appears that, at rest, 125 to 200 milliseconds is generally the optimal range if the right atrium and ventricle are paced.[28,29] On the other hand, more precise optimization may be possible, although it may vary from patient to patient and from time to time in a specific patient. In addition, with conventional right heart pacing systems, the activation sequence of the left-sided chambers may be quite different from the programmed values due to marked interatrial and interventricular conduction delays. Doppler echocardiography is commonly used to optimize the AV interval by assessing the pattern of early and late diastolic mitral valve flow and the aortic flow velocity integral (Figs. 3.14 and 3.15). While AV interval can be optimized at rest, assessing the adequacy of this parameter upright and during exercise presents greater technical difficulties.

There is some predictability in certain aspects of AV interval optimization. It is consistent that optimal hemodynamics at higher heart rates require shorter AV delays than are optimal at lower rates. With exercise, there is a relatively linear decrease in the normal PR interval as exercise increases from the resting state to near maximal exertion.[30] The total reduction in spontaneous PR interval in normal individuals appears to be about 20 to 50 milliseconds or approximately 4 milliseconds for each 10-beat increment in heart rate. Sophisticated pacing systems have already been developed that incorporate this concept. It appears that cardiac output can be more effectively increased and pulmonary capillary wedge pressures (and presumably atrial pressures) can be effectively maintained at lower levels using rate-variable AV intervals rather than fixed AV intervals.

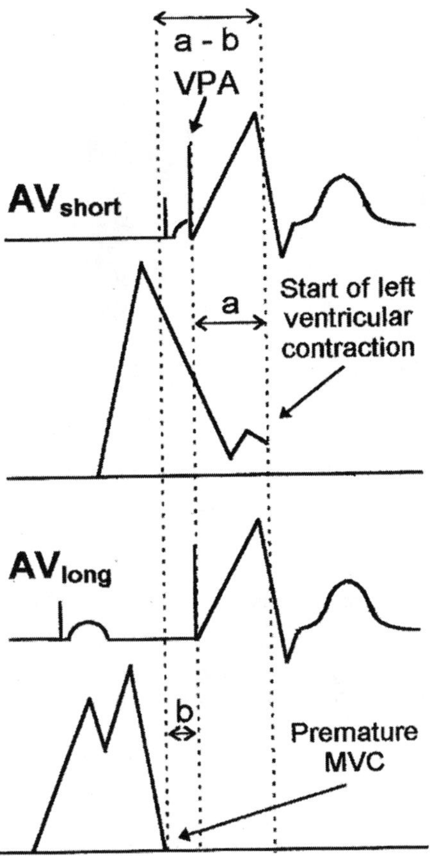

Figure 3.14. One Doppler technique for optimizing the AV interval. The surace ECG and Doppler mitral inflow pattern in depicted schematically for a very short AV interval (eg. 50 milliseconds) in the top of the figure and a very long AV interval (eg. 250 milliseconds) in the bottom of the tracing. Interval "a" represents the longest time between ventricular pacing artifact (VPA) and the mitral valve closure (MVC) for the short AV interval. Interval "b" represents the time between ventricular pacing and mitral valve closure during the long AV interval and may be a negative value due to diastolic regurgitation. The optimal AV delay is calculated as the long AV delay minus the difference between intervals a and b. (Adapted from Kinderman M, et al. Optimizing the AV delay in DDD pacemaker patients with high degree AV block: mitral valve Doppler versus impedance cardiography. PACE 1997;20:2453–2462.)

Atrial Sensed versus Atrial Paced Atrioventricular Intervals: Another issue relating to hemodynamics involves the difference in the appropriate AV intervals, depending on whether the atrium is sensed or paced. If atrial activity is sensed, this marks the initiation of the pacemaker AV interval. Because some atrial activation has already occurred at this time, the AV interval based on sensed atrial activity should be shorter than when the atrium is paced to begin both the AV interval and atrial electrical activation (Fig. 3.16). The appropriate dif-

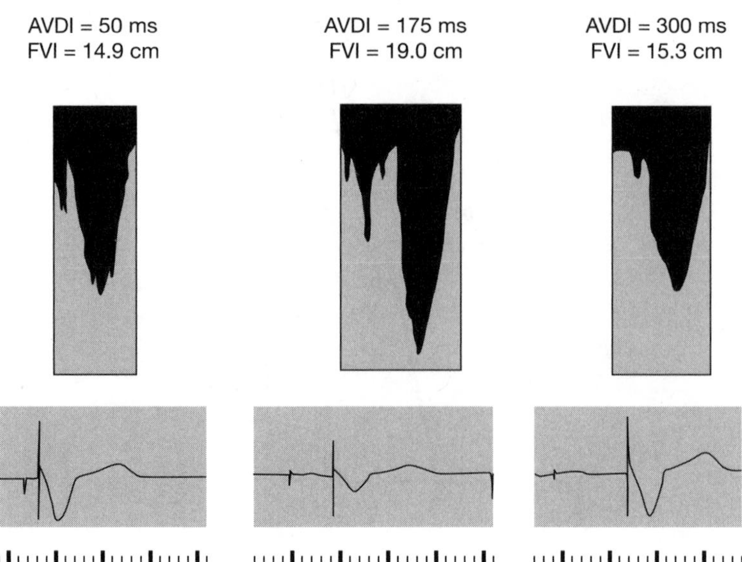

Figure 3.15. Doppler aortic flow velocity integrals (FVI) recorded from the same patient at varying AV pacing intervals. Note the maximal aortic flow velocity at AV interval (AVI) of 175 milliseconds. (Reproduced by permission from Janosik DL, Pearson AC, Buckingham TA, et al. The hemodynamic benefit of differential atrioventricular delay intervals for sensed and paced atrial events during physiologic pacing. J Am Coll Cardiol 1989;14:499–507.)

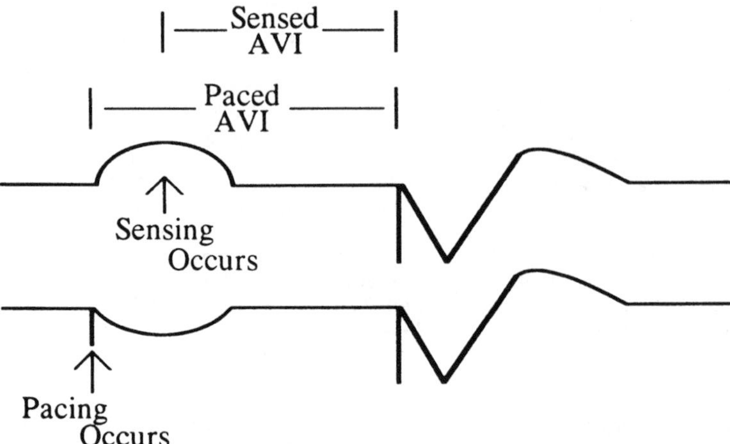

Figure 3.16. Hypothetical relationship of appropriate AV intervals (AVI) during atrial sensing versus atrial pacing at initiation of the AVI.

ference in the atrial sensed AV interval setting and the atrial paced AV interval setting is probably variable in different patients; the most appropriate values for these parameters are somewhat empirically determined.[31] Generally, an atrial sensed AV interval 20 to 50 milliseconds less than the atrial paced AV interval has been used at our institution.

Atrial versus Atrioventricular Pacing

Both atrial and AV pacing have the advantage of providing AV synchrony. The choice of atrial versus AV pacing is usually made on the basis of considerations other than hemodynamics. We compared the hemodynamics of atrial and AV pacing in a group of pacemaker patients who were not selected for hemodynamic status.[32] The results of the comparison are shown in Table 3.2. The pacing rate in this study was 80 ppm, and the AV interval during AV pacing was 150 milliseconds. The study was done with patients in the supine position. Except for pulmonary artery and pulmonary capillary wedge pressures, there were no statistically significant differences found when comparing atrial to AV pacing. For example, the cardiac index for the group as a whole showed no significant difference between atrial and AV pacing, although small differences were seen in some patients. It is likely that the small but statistically significant differences in pulmonary artery and pulmonary capillary wedge pressures are related to a suboptimal AV interval during AV pacing. Other studies have shown improved cardiac output, ejection fraction and pulmonary capillary wedge pressure with AAI compared to DDD pacing.[33,34]

Table 3.2. Hemodynamic Evaluation of Atrial and Atrioventricular Pacing

Parameter	A*	Av*	N	P†
RA mean (mm Hg)	5.8 ± 0.7	6.7 ± 0.6	19	NS
PA systolic (mm Hg)	24.1 ± 1.5	25.4 ± 1.7	20	.05
PA diastolic (mm Hg)	12.1 ± 0.9	13.4 ± 1.0	20	.01
PA mean (mm Hg)	16.5 ± 1.0	18.0 ± 1.2	20	.02
PCW mean (mm Hg)	6.7 ± 0.9	8.3 ± 1.0	20	.01
LV systolic (mm Hg)	143.8 ± 7.1	145.7 ± 7.2	20	NS
LV end-diastolic (mm Hg)	8.8 ± 0.9	10.7 ± 1.4	20	NS
AO systolic (mm Hg)	145.0 ± 7.0	146.2 ± 7.1	20	NS
AO diastolic (mm Hg)	81.8 ± 2.0	82.1 ± 2.4	20	NS
AO mean (mm Hg)	107.2 ± 3.2	108.1 ± 3.5	20	NS
CI (L/min/m^2)	2.66 ± 0.15	2.62 ± 0.15	20	NS
PVR (dyne · sec · cm^{-5})	168 ± 17	174 ± 20	20	NS
SVR (dyne · sec · cm^{-5})	1769 ± 148	1816 ± 166	20	NS

* Mean ± SEM.

† Paired *t* test.

AO = aortic; CI = cardiac index; LV = left ventricle; NS = not statistically significant; PA = pulmonary artery; PCW = pulmonary capillary wedge; PVR = pulmonary vascular resistance; RA = right atrium; SVR = systemic vascular resistance.

Besides differing AV intervals, another difference between atrial and AV sequential pacing is the ectopic ventricular activation with the dual-chamber mode. In detailed human studies, ventricular pacing compared to intrinsic ventricular activation can produce measurable increases in left ventricular filling pressures and end-systolic volume as well as reductions in regional septal ejection fraction, ventricular d*P*/d*t*, stroke volume, and indices of diastolic function.[34] As a result there is growing concern over the long-term consequences of right ventricular pacing and pacemaker algorithms that allow for maintenance of AV synchrony and minimize unnecessary ventricular pacing evolving.

Pacemaker Syndrome

Pacemaker syndrome is a term proposed in 1974 to describe a condition comprising a variety of symptoms and signs produced by ventricular pacing.[23,35,36] Pacemaker syndrome has been defined differently by different investigators, but the broadest definition is probably most appropriate. It is best thought of as any combination of the variety of symptoms and signs occurring with ventricular pacing that are relieved by restoration of AV synchrony. Although it is most often the result of VVI pacing, pacemaker syndrome can result from any pacing mode that results in AV dyssynchrony, even AAI pacing with long PR intervals.

Two difficulties in ascribing symptoms and signs specifically to pacemaker syndrome are commonly encountered. First, patients who have pacemakers implanted are frequently patients with other cardiovascular problems that produce the symptoms and signs described. Second, unfortunately, many pacemaker patients have the belief that having the pacemaker, de facto, forces them to accept a less than normal sense of well-being. An extreme symptom frequently associated with pacemaker syndrome is syncope. Syncope is very uncommon and is most likely related to profound hypotension—and, in some, a decrease in cardiac output—associated with loss of AV synchrony. Additional symptoms related to blood pressure and cardiac output include malaise, easy fatigability, a sense of weakness, lightheadedness, and dizziness. Symptoms related to higher atrial and venous pressures include dyspnea (frequently at rest), orthopnea, paroxysmal nocturnal dyspnea, a sensation of fullness and/or pulsations in the neck and chest, as well as palpitations, chest pain, nausea, and peripheral edema. Experience has shown that careful questioning is frequently necessary to elucidate these symptoms. It is not uncommon for patients who have had a pacemaker implanted for some time to deny symptoms, but on specific questioning, to admit to having experienced symptoms that can be directly related to ventricular pacing with loss of AV synchrony.

Careful examination is necessary to find physical signs related to ventricular pacing. Some of these signs include relative or absolute hypotension that can be continuous or fluctuating, neck vein distension with prominent "cannon" A waves, pulmonary rales, and rarely peripheral edema.

Pacemaker syndrome is most severe when intact retrograde VA conduction is present. Besides the reduced stroke volume and cardiac output from the loss of atrial kick, the elevated venous pressures resulting from atrial contraction against closed AV valves activate atrial and pulmonary vagal afferent nerves. This in turn produces peripheral vasodilation and hypotension. Patients with pacemaker syndrome have a failure to increase systemic vascular resistance in response to VVI pacing despite elevated peripheral sympathetic nerve traffic and circulating catecholamines. These findings suggest offsetting parasympathetic activation or failure of end-organ responsiveness.

Pacemaker syndrome can often be prevented by simple hemodynamic evaluation at the time of pacer implant. Pacemaker syndrome is likely to result from VVI pacing if the blood pressure drops by more than 20 mmHg during ventricular pacing. Retrograde conduction is not uncommon even in patients with complete heart block. If hypotension develops, implantation of a dual-chamber pacing system is requisite. Because retrograde conduction may be intermittent, absence of hypotension at implant does not preclude pacemaker syndrome. The management of patients with VVI-pacemaker syndrome after VVI-pacemaker implantation include upgrading to a DDD system, reducing the lower pacing rate to encourage conduction of sinus rhythm, use of hysteresis, or withdrawal of medications that impair sinus node function. For the rare patients with pacemaker syndrome and dual-chamber systems, programming to ensure atrial capture, avoidance of atrial non-pacing modes (VDD) or atrial non-tracking modes (DDI or DVI) may be useful. Fortunately, in the United States, there has been a dramatic reduction in the use of VVI/VVIR pacing of the past 20 years and this has in turn dramatically reduced the prevalence of pacemaker syndrome.

Hemodynamics of Alternative Site Right Ventricular Pacing

Pacing from the right ventricular outflow tract (RVOT) offers the theoretical advantages of a more normal electrocardiographic vector of ventricular activation due to basilar to apical conduction and earlier activation of the bundle of His. One study has demonstrated the feasibility of permanent para-Hisian pacing to produce a narrow paced QRS complex identical to that in sinus rhythm.[37] Despite these theoretical advantages, the clinical benefits of RVOT pacing have been difficult to demonstrate. Some studies have found significant acute hemodynamic advantages; however, several randomized controlled chronic studies have demonstrated either modest or negligible benefit to RVOT or multisite right ventricular pacing compared to right ventricular apical (RVA) pacing.[38–42] These studies did not fully examine the role of patient selection for such factors as presence of atrial fibrillation, type and degree of heart failure, interventricular conduction delay, degree of mitral regurgitation and diastolic dysfunction, which may influence the response to pacing.

A large, multicenter, prospective, randomized cross-over trial was designed to examine differences between single site RVA pacing and alternative site RVOT pacing, as well as dual-site (RVA and RVOT) pacing. In the Right Ventricular Outflow Versus Apical Pacing (ROVA) study, all patients (103 enrolled) had indications for VVIR pacing, a history of heart failure (NYHA class II or III), LV dysfunction (LV ejection fraction [LVEF] $\leq$ 40%), and chronic atrial fibrillation (AF > 7 days).[43] The primary endpoint was health-related quality of life after 3 months. Secondary endpoints were NYHA functional class, LVEF, severity of mitral regurgitation by echocardiography, exercise capacity, and lead-related complications. At 3 months follow-up, the main finding was that no significant benefit was observed in RVOT or dual-site RV pacing compared to RVA pacing. Although QRS duration significantly shortened during RVOT (149 ± 19 milliseconds) and dual-site RV pacing (164 ± 18 milliseconds, respectively) compared with RVA pacing (180 ± 23 milliseconds), surprisingly, at 9 months of follow-up, LVEF was higher in those assigned to RVA pacing (47.3 ± 17.6%) than during RVOT pacing (34.3 ± 13.4%).

Right ventricular septal (RVS) pacing has also been examined in small clinical studies. Several studies have suggested acute hemodynamic benefits during RVS pacing in patients with reduced left ventricular function, presumably due to a shorter activation time between the septum and left ventricle (shorter QRS) during RVS pacing compared to other right ventricular sites.[38–40] However, long-term clinical benefit has not been demonstrated.[40,43,44] One study (14 patients) tested whether RVS pacing functionally correlated with a shorter QRS duration and higher ejection fraction when compared to RVA pacing.[45] The QRS duration was generally shorter with RVS pacing in most patients (64%), but sometimes longer (29%) or unchanged compared to RVA pacing. Overall, the QRS duration was not significantly different between RVS and RVA pacing (156 ± 10 milliseconds vs 166 ± 18 milliseconds, respectively). The study found that a shorter QRS duration positively correlated with a higher left ventricular ejection fraction, but that RVS pacing site did not necessarily produce the shortest QRS or consistently result in improved left ventricular function.

Detrimental Effects of Continuous Right Ventricular Pacing

Continuous right ventricular pacing may have detrimental effects on myocardial function and result in progression of heart failure in patients with left ventricular dysfunction. Right ventricular pacing produces an asynchronous pattern of activation, contraction, and relaxation between the left and right ventricles.[41,46,47] Experimental studies have shown that chronic right ventricular pacing induces abnormal histologic changes, left ventricular hypertrophy or thinning, and subsequent impairment of left ventricular function.[41] In patients with complete AV block and normal ventricular function at the time of permanent lead implantation, chronic right ventricular pacing may induce regional myocardial perfusion defects, wall motion abnormalities, and impaired left ventricular systolic and diastolic function.[46,47]

In a recent study of patients with sinus node dysfunction, continuous right ventricular apical pacing was associated with an increased risk of heart failure and atrial fibrillation, even among patients with preserved AV synchrony and normal baseline QRS duration.[46] The study was a subgroup analysis of patients (n = 1339) enrolled in the MOde Selection Trial (MOST), a large, multicenter, randomized trial comparing single-chamber rate-modulated pacing (VVIR) pacing versus dual-chamber rate-modulated pacing (DDDR). The main finding was that ventricular desynchronization imposed by RVA pacing in the DDDR mode greater than 40% of the time conferred a 2.6-fold increased risk of heart failure hospitalization compared with lesser pacing among similar patients with a normal baseline QRS duration. Ventricular pacing in the VVIR mode greater than 80% of the time was also associated with increased heart failure risk. In absolute terms, the average risk of heart failure in those receiving RVA pacing was approximately 10%; however, the risk was approximately 2% if RVA pacing was minimal (<10% of the time). The risk of atrial fibrillation increased linearly with cumulative RVA pacing in both groups. The investigators concluded that both heart failure progression and atrial fibrillation may be reduced by implementing strategies that minimize ventricular pacing and preserve normal ventricular activation.

The use of implantable cardioverter defibrillator (ICD) therapy with backup ventricular pacing has become standard treatment for patients with cardiomyopathies at increased risk for life-threatening ventricular arrhythmia. Because bradycardia (sinus node dysfunction) is also prevalent in the ICD patient population, cardiologists have implanted more dual-chamber devices to treat both bradyarrhythmias and tachyarrhythmias. Studies also suggest that synchronous dual-chamber pacing may improve hemodynamics or suppress arrhythmias.[48] However, heart failure is a common comorbidity in patients with indications for ICDs. MADIT II, the first ICD clinical trial which included patients with dual-chamber ICDs in their study, reported a significant association between heart failure hospitalization with the presence of an ICD.[49] The study implicates continuous right ventricular pacing as a potential risk factor for heart failure progression.

The Dual Chamber and VVI Implantable Defibrillator (DAVID) trial tested the hypothesis that dual-chamber pacing for rate support would be more efficacious than backup pacing in patients receiving ICDs. The trial was a multicenter, randomized, blinded, parallel study of 506 patients with standard indications for ICD implantation (VT/VF, LVEF $\leq$ 40%) but without indications for antibradycardia pacing.[50] All patients had a dual-chamber, rate-responsive pacing ICD implanted and were randomized to ventricular backup pacing (VVI 40) or dual chamber rate-responsive pacing (DDDR 70, average AV delay 180 milliseconds). The primary end point was freedom from death and absence of hospitalization for heart failure. The study was prematurely discontinued by the data and safety monitoring board because of increased mortality and hospitalization for patients treated with dual-chamber pacing (73.3% 1-year survival and 22.6% requiring hospitalization) compared to backup pacing (83.9% survival and 13.3% hospitalization).

At the University of Oklahoma, adult patients with a primary indication for bradycardia pacing generally undergo right ventricular lead placement at the apex (RVA). Lead placement in the RVA usually offers easier technical positioning, a lower incidence of lead complications, and increased long-term stability (see Chapter on Techniques of Pacemaker Implantation). Additionally, in patients with ventricular arrhythmias undergoing ICD implant, placement of an integrated pacing and defibrillation lead at the RVA favorably lowers the defi-

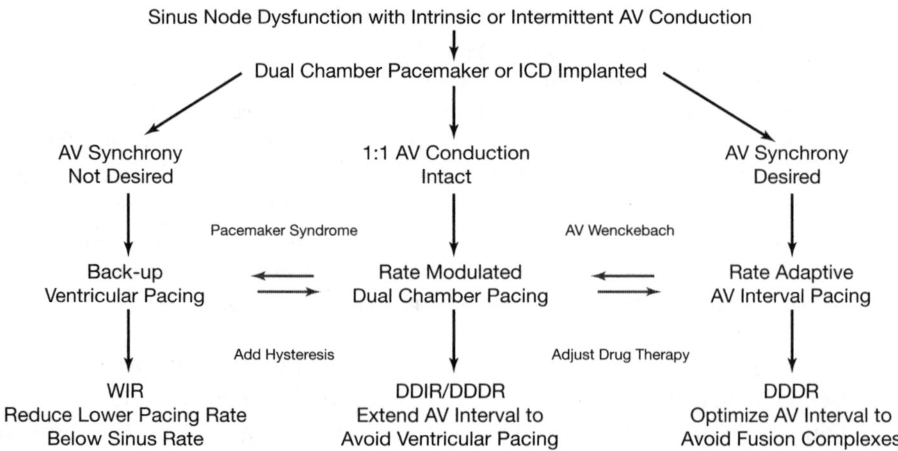

Figure 3.17. Minimal ventricular pacing strategy to promote intrinsic AV conduction after implant of a dual chamber pacemaker or ICD for treatment of sinus node dysfunction with impaired AV conduction (present or anticipated). **Left:** Back-up VVIR pacing is used if AV synchrony is not required. The lower pacing rate is programmed below sinus rate and rest hysteresis is added when appropriate. Change to dual-chamber pacing if pacemaker syndrome (due to retrograde VA conduction) develops. **Middle:** Rate modulated dual chamber pacing is preferred for patients with intrinsic AV conduction. The programmed AV interval is extended to promote normal ventricular activation in patients capable of maintaining 1:1 AV conduction. Discontinue or adjust drugs that affect AV conduction when appropriate. Add rate adaptive pacing if patient is symptomatic with extended AV delays. **Right:** Rate varied AV interval pacing is used for patients requiring physiologic AV intervals. During programming, sensed and paced AV intervals should be optimized to avoid ventricular fusion complexes.

brillation threshold (see chapter on the implantable cardioverter defibrillator). Backup RVA pacing is preferable in patients with preserved AV conduction and normal left ventricular function. Based on the findings of adverse events occurring in patients receiving frequent cumulative right ventricular pacing, all attempts are made to minimize ventricular pacing when intrinsic AV conduction is present (Fig. 3.17). At times, in patients with symptomatic bradycardia and heart failure, we pace from the right ventricular septum or outflow tract. However, for patients meeting criteria for cardiac resynchronization therapy, implantation of a biventricular device is our standard practice (see chapter on cardiac resynchronization therapy).

HEMODYNAMICS OF PACING IN HYPERTROPHIC OBSTRUCTIVE CARDIOMYOPATHY

Hypertrophic obstructive cardiomyopathy (HOCM) represents a special situation for which pacing may have a role in some patients. These patients have obstruction to LV outflow caused by hypertrophy of the interventricular septum, typically in the subaortic valve area, combined with systolic anterior motion of the mitral valve. A number of studies documented that, by producing dyssynchrony of LV contraction, dual-chamber pacing reduces the degree of outflow obstruction and symptoms in many patients.[51–54] Objective as well as subjective improvement in such parameters as oxygen consumption at peak exercise has been documented.[55] An example of modest improvement in left ventricular outflow gradient is shown in Figure 3.18.

A full understanding of the mechanisms responsible for improvement is lacking, and the possible role of pacing in improving diastolic function and mitral regurgitation is debated. Despite the theoretical and acute hemodynamic effects of ventricular pacing, the results of controlled, randomized trials of pacing for HOCM have been disappointing. The placebo effect of pacing system implantation appears to play an important role in overall subjective improvement.[53] In these patients, pacing has not been shown to reduce mortality in this condition and that the long-term benefits from this therapy are less than what were suggested by early reports. Data from a recent multicenter review document a very high incidence of sudden cardiac death in this condition.[56] Whether AV pacing incorporated into implantable defibrillators will play an important role in the treatment of these patients in the future must be determined.

Hemodynamics of Left Ventricular Pacing

Although the inefficacy of simple right ventricular pacing for dilated cardiomyopathy has been recognized,[51–55] there is growing enthusiasm for biventricular pacing therapy in treating patients who have baseline QRS prolongation and severely depressed left ventricular systolic function. A more complete discussion of left ventricular pacing is given in the chapter on cardiac resynchronization therapy. This therapy seeks to optimize left ventricular contraction by normalizing the dysfunctional activation patterns associated with ventricular conduction delays. The biventricular devices pace the right atrium, the right ventricle, and the left ventricle, accessed via the coronary sinus transvenously or from the epicardium surgically. There is evidence that, in some patients, pacing the right atrium and just the left ventricle is hemodynamically beneficial.[57] The studies to date have primarily focused on patients with severely reduced left ventricular systolic function, refractory heart failure, markedly prolonged QRS durations (usually due to left bundle branch block), and no bradycardiac indication for pacing.

Numerous acute studies have shown that pacing both ventricles simultaneously is of hemodynamic benefit in patients with QRS prolongation and depressed ejection fraction. Much uncertainty remains about the mechanisms by which hemodynamic improvement occurs, but several factors are likely. The first is improvement of atrial/left ventricular synchrony to optimize end-diastolic filling and reduce diastolic mitral regurgitation.[57–59] Second, is a lengthening of diastolic filling times due to a shorted QRS duration. The third and probably most important factor is "resynchronization" of the severely uncoordinated and dysfunctional patterns of ventricular contraction in patients with prolonged native QRS complexes (Fig. 3.19).[60,61] With marked *intra*ventricular conduction

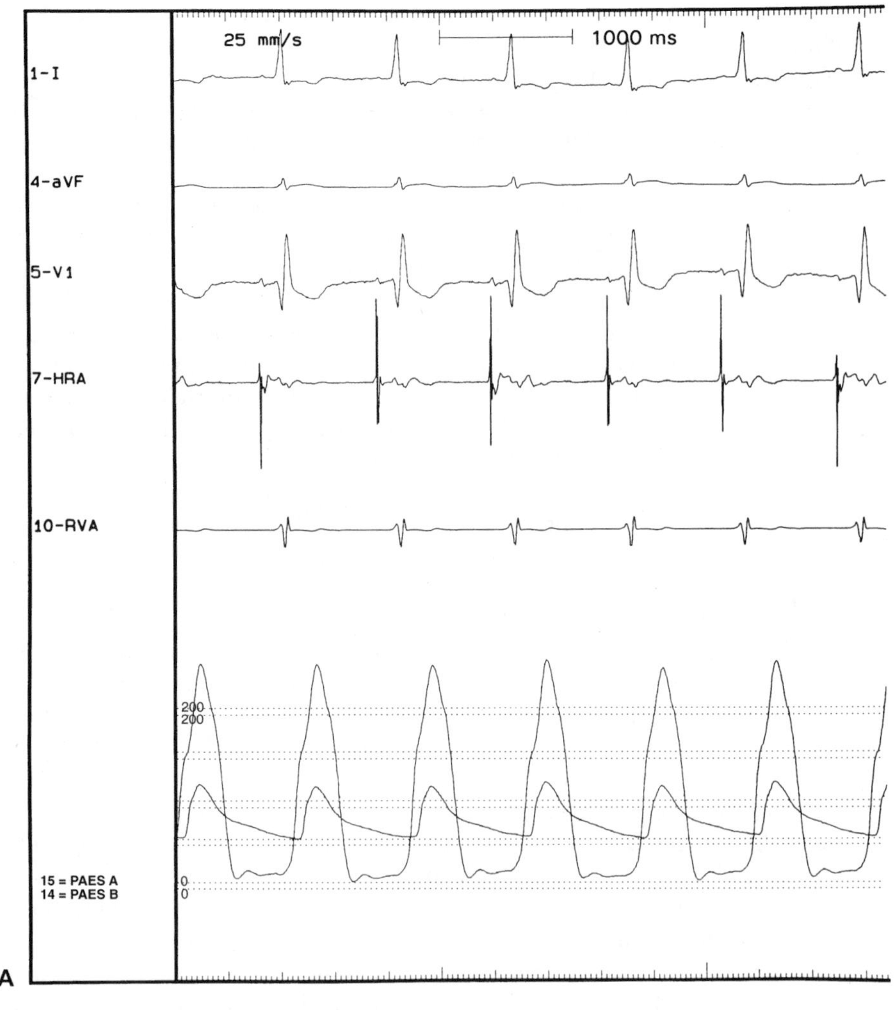

Figure 3.18. Tracings showing the impact of AV sequential pacing on left ventricular and femoral arterial pressure in selected patient with hypertrophic obstructive cardiomyopathy. **A:** The presence of a nearly 150 mm Hg pressure gradient at baseline during sinus rhythm. **B:** With AV sequential pacing at an AV interval of 75 milliseconds, the pressure gradient decreases to 50 to 90 mmg. The beat-to-beat variability of the measurement of this gradient is highlighted by the bottom tracing. **Top to bottom:** I, aVf, V_1 = surface ECG leads; RA, right atrial intracardiac recording; RV, right ventricular intracardiac recording and femoral and left ventricular pressure tracings (in mm Hg) superimposed on each other. (Reproduced by permission from Sweeney MO, Ellenbogen KA. Implantable devices for the electrical management of heart disease: overview of indications for therapy and selected recent advances. In: Antman EM, ed. Cardiovascular Therapeutics. 2nd ed. Philadelphia: WB Saunders, 2002.) The left ventricular to femoral artery peak systolic gradient is approximately 150 mm Hg during sinus rhythm, whereas during AV pacing with an AV interval of 75 milliseconds the pressure gradient decreases to between 50 and 90 mm Hg.

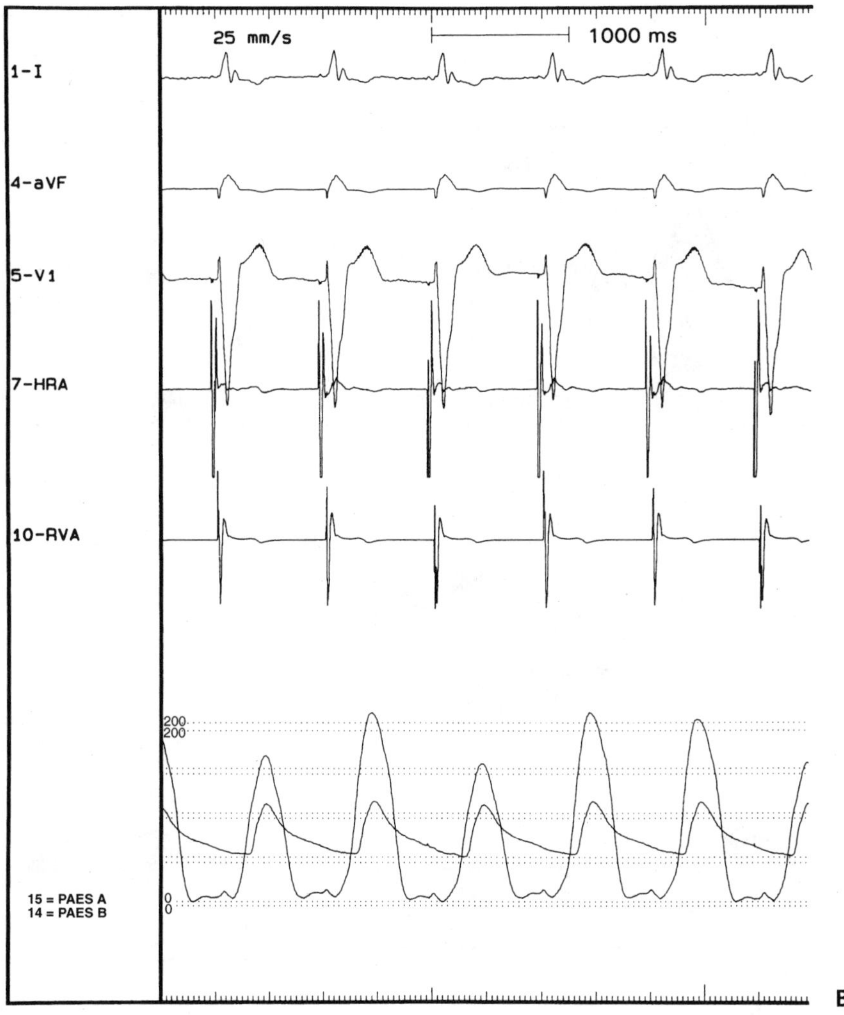

Figure 3.18. *Continued*

delays, regions of the ventricle may still be actively contracting while other regions are relaxing and filling in diastole (see Fig. 3.19). The result is that part of the contractile effort does not contribute to cardiac ejection. In addition, *inter*ventricular conduction delays may impair the synergy provided by simultaneous right and left ventricular contraction.

In acute studies, there is improvement in systolic blood pressure, wedge pressure, cardiac output, and reduced V wave amplitude with biventricular pacing compared to intrinsic conduction or right ventricular pacing.[57–61] Several large multicenter, randomized trials have been completed to definitively evaluate long-

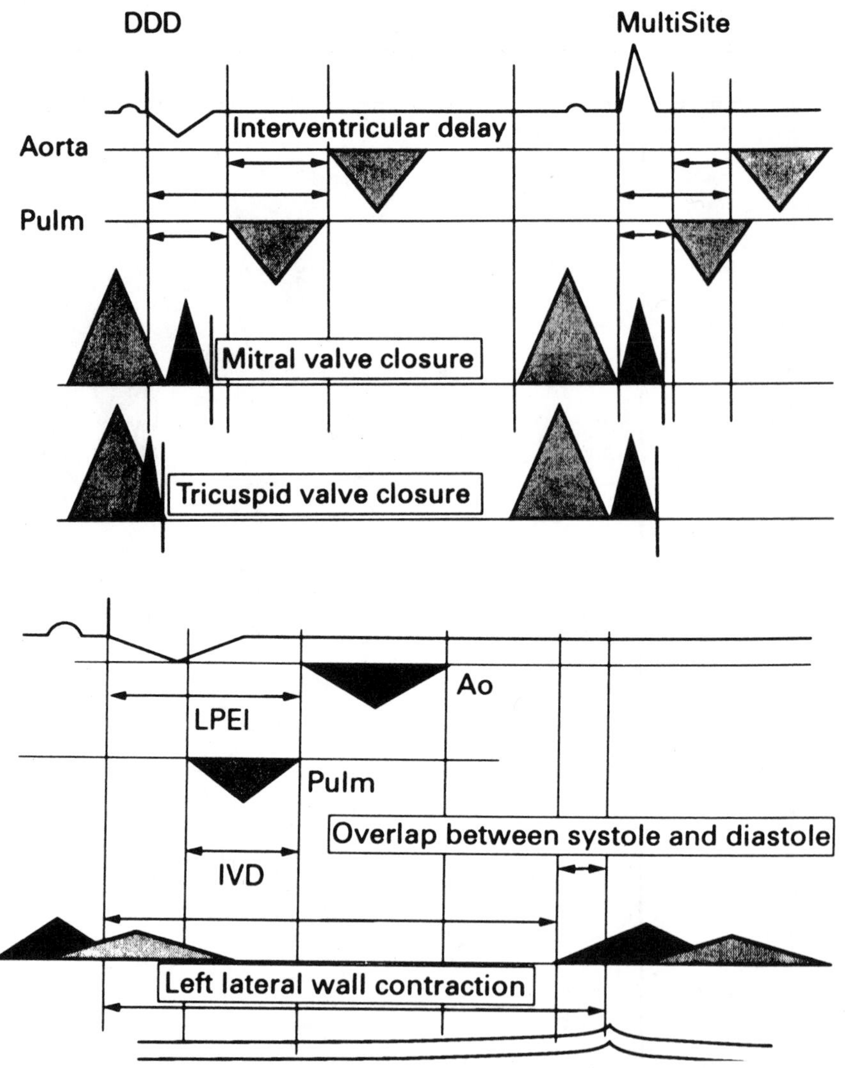

Figure 3.19. Effects of biventricular pacing on ventricular hemodynamics. The schematic represents Doppler flow patterns as seen by the four-chamber apical view. **Top panel:** Surface ECG is top tracing. When comparing ventricular activation with DDD right ventricular (RV) and biventricular (multisite) pacing, left ventricular activation occurs earlier in systole during biventricular pacing. Aortic and pulmonary ejection flow velocities are represented by the downward triangles. Left ventricular (LV) and RV filling are shown by the upright triangles representing E and A waves. The AV delay no longer needs to be set at very short values to lengthen the ventricular filling times. The total duration of systole is shortened rather than lengthened. **Bottom panel:** Surface ECG is top tracing. Aortic and pulmonary ejection are indicated as in top panel. LV filling E and A waves are illustrated in the lower tracing. With marked delay of activation of the lateral wall, active contraction of this segment is still ongoing during the initial phase of ventricular filling. An overlap of systole and diastole between different wall segments results in negation of part of the contractile effort. The successful elimination of late lateral wall contraction often decreases the severity of mitral regurgitation. (Reproduced by permission from Cazeau S, Gras D, Lazarus A, et al. Multisite stimulation for correction of cardiac asynchrony. Heart 2000;84:579–581.)

term outcomes. These trials are described in the chapter on cardiac resynchronization therapy.

Because biventricular pacing avoids the detrimental effects of right ventricular pacing alone, the demonstration of long-term benefits from biventricular pacing would serve a growing population of patients who have heart failure and potentially a broad scope of patients who have left ventricular dysfunction and require anti-bradycardia ventricular pacing. Biventricular pacing will likely expand in use for patients with chronic atrial fibrillation, particularly those who require atrioventricular junction ablation for either heart rate control or treatment of symptoms. A small study demonstrated that CRT in patients with congestive heart failure and previous AV junction ablation with RV pacing for chronic atrial fibrillation had improvement of symptoms and LV systolic function following upgrade to biventricular pacing.[62] Preliminary result for the Post AV Nodal Ablation Evaluation (PAVE) Trial support the use of biventricular pacing. The prospective, randomized study compared biventricular pacing with RV pacing in 252 patients (NYHA class I to III) who underwent AV junction ablation. The exercise capacity (primary endpoint, 6-minute walk test) was significantly better in patients receiving biventricular pacing (mean distance 25.55 m further) compared to those receiving RV pacing. Functional capacity (peak VO_2) and LV ejection fraction (44.9% vs 40.7%) were also greater in the group with biventricular pacing, although there was no significant difference in survival.

RATE MODULATION

As with AV synchrony, terminology here can be confusing. The earliest term used to describe the physiologic property of pacing systems was *rate responsive*. Significant objection to this term (for grammatical reasons) has led to the more acceptable use of the terms *rate adaptive* and *rate modulating*. All these terms are used to describe the capacity of a pacing system to respond to physiologic need by increasing and decreasing pacing rate. The capability of a pacing system depends on the presence of one of a variety of physiologic sensors that monitor need or indication for rate variability.

The predominant need for rate modulation derives from physical activity or exertion. There are other physiologic situations in which normally there are modulations of heart rate—for example, with fever and emotional stress. These, however, are substantially less important, especially in the context of pacing systems. The technology of physiologic sensors is discussed in Chapter 2. A comprehensive discussion of exercise physiology is beyond the scope of this book, but the more important and relevant concepts will be addressed.

Exercise Physiology

The importance of rate modulation in pacing systems is related directly and specifically to the importance of matching cardiac output with body need. A brief discussion of exercise physiology is warranted.

During exercise—or "work," as it is frequently referred to by physiologists—the body tissues increase their demand for oxygen.[14] In addition, there is increased need for removal of metabolic by-products, such as CO_2, from the tissues. The body has a number of mechanisms in place to provide for these increased needs during exercise. Redistribution of blood flow to working tissues, increased ability of working tissues to extract oxygen from the blood, and, most important, increased cardiac output are these mechanisms. Here, we focus on the last of these—the body's ability to increase cardiac output with exercise—as this is what rate modulation provides.

The importance of cardiac output during work must be appreciated. A direct, relatively linear relationship exists between the amount of work accomplished and oxygen consumption. Maximal work capacity, therefore, is specifically related to maximum oxygen consumption. Further, consistent with the Fick principle,

$$\text{Cardiac output} = O_2 \text{ consumption}/\text{AV } O_2 \text{ difference}$$

where AV means arterial–venous. Also,

$$\text{Cardiac output} = \text{Stroke volume} \times \text{Heart rate}$$

By substitution in these equations,

$$O_2 \text{ consumption} = \text{Stroke volume} \times \text{Heart rate} \times \text{AV } O_2 \text{ difference}$$

Because oxygen consumption is directly, linearly proportional to work (Fig. 3.20),

$$\text{Work} \approx \text{Stroke volume} \times \text{Heart rate} \times \text{AV } O_2 \text{ difference}$$

Increasing any of these variables will support an increased ability to do work, but the increase in heart rate is the most important. Maximum work, in

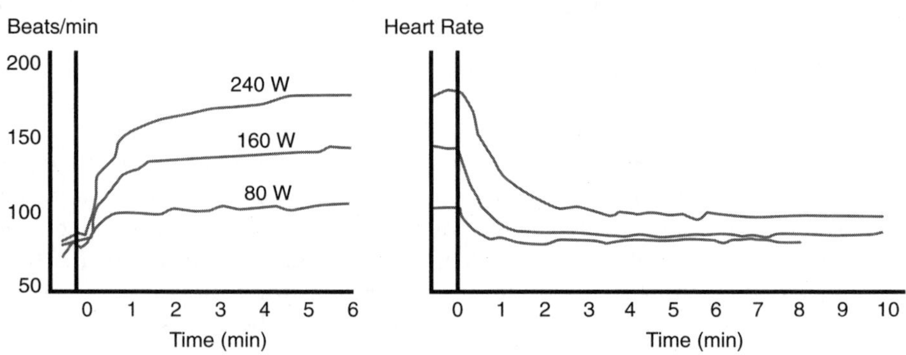

Figure 3.20. Heart rate response at onset and termination of exercise in 8 healthy young men at different work loads. W = watts. At onset of exercise, the majority of the total increment in heart rate occurs in the first minute of effort. (Reproduced by permission from Linnarsson D. Dynamics of pulmonary gas exchange and heart rate changes at start and end of exercise. Acta Physiol Scand 1974;415:1–68.)

normal individuals, is accomplished by an increase in stroke volume to approximately 150% of the resting value, an increase in heart rate to approximately 300% of the resting value, and an increase in AV O_2 difference by approximately 250% of the resting value. These changes allow an increase in work to over ten times resting levels. In normal individuals, peak cardiac output can be increased to 300% of resting values simply by an increase in heart rate. During peak exercise, the stroke volume is increased to approximately 150% of the resting value. This increase in stroke volume, as depicted in Figure 3.19, is not linear and is achieved at approximately the halfway point between the rest and maximal exercise levels. The increased stroke volume is accomplished by an increase in venous return, ventricular filling, and contractility. Loss of AV synchrony can compromise stroke volume, even with exercise, although it appears that AV synchrony is usually less important during exercise in providing ventricular filling than it is at rest. It is ideal, however, to optimize stroke volume because this is a more energy-efficient way of accomplishing cardiac output (milliliters of cardiac output/milliliters of O_2 consumption) than by an increase in heart rate.

Clearly, the most important mechanism by which cardiac output is increased during exercise is by increasing heart rate. The normal heart rate response to exercise follows a triphasic response (Fig. 3.20).[63] Heart rate increases most rapidly within the first 10 to 15 seconds of exercise and reaches 70% of the total heart rate increased in this phase. A slower exponential rise in heart rate follows during the next 60 to 90 seconds. Finally, a slow linear increase or plateau phase finally results from sustained activity. Heart rate deceleration with cessation of exercise is generally slower than the rate acceleration and also follows a biphasic or triphasic response.

Advantage of Rate Modulation

As is obvious by the foregoing discussion of exercise physiology, the ability of patients to increase heart rate with exercise is the primary means of meeting this and other metabolic demands. Exertional intolerance, manifested by a number of clinical symptoms, can be very limiting, but it is almost obligatory if heart rate cannot be increased.

In pacemaker patients, compromised ability to increase heart rate due to the underlying cardiac electrical problem and/or superimposed drug therapy is common. The inability to increase and maintain heart rate appropriately with exercise has been called chronotropic incompetence.[64] Some patients are ultimately able to achieve the appropriate heart rate for the level of exercise but do so more slowly than is normal. Patients with any of these forms of chronotropic incompetence are candidates for pacing systems with rate-modulation capabilities. The diagnosis of chronotropic incompetence is relatively easy to make at times. Patients with third degree, and frequently lesser degrees, of AV block are typically chronotropically incompetent. The diagnosis of chronotropic incompetence in patients with sinus node dysfunction is frequently more difficult. A number of different criteria have been proposed, including the inability to increase heart rate with exercise to at least 70% to 85% of the maximum predicted heart rate (maximum predicted heart rate = 220 − age in years). This is a useful criterion for diagnosing chronotropic incompetence, but it cannot be used in many individuals due to limitations on their exercise function unrelated to cardiopulmonary status. Further, there are patients with delayed chronotropic responses who could benefit from rate-modulating pacing systems but might be missed by this criterion.

More complicated formulas have been developed to allow determination of the presence of chronotropic incompetence by exercise testing with assessments made by stage.[65] The Wilkoff chronotropic assessment exercise protocol (CAEP) is an easily performed treadmill test that has become widely used for chronotropic competency evaluation (Table 3.3). It uses gradual increases in both elevation and speed, and can be used for the evaluation of devices with a variety of sensor types.

Quantification of the improvement in work capacity in pacemaker populations comparing non–rate-modulating with rate-modulating modes has consistently shown the advantages of the rate-modulating systems. Rate-modulating pacing systems have been shown not only to improve the heart-rate response with exercise but also to increase work. Compared to VVI pacing, VVIR mode improves exercise duration and cardiac index in patients undergoing paired stress testing.[66,67] These improvements are independent of patient age and ejection fraction. Even greater improvements in exercise hemodynamics are documented with DDDR pacing compared to either VVIR or DDD modes.[68] Compared to VVIR, DDDR pacing has demonstrated to improve exercise capacity, cardiac output, and cardiac metabolic indices, suggesting more efficient cardiac work.[69] In patients with sick sinus syndrome, DDDR pacing provides greater maximal heart rates, exercise times, higher maximal oxygen uptake, and higher oxygen

Table 3.3. Chronotropic Assessment Exercise Protocol

Stage		Speed (mph)	Grade (%)	Time (min)	Cumulative Time	METs
Warmup	0	1.0	0	—	—	1.5
	1	1.0	2	2.0	2.0	2.0
	2	1.5	3	2.0	4.0	2.8
	3	2.0	4	2.0	6.0	3.6
	4	2.5	5	2.0	8.0	4.6
	5	3.0	6	2.0	10.0	5.8
	6	3.5	8	2.0	12.0	7.5
	7	4.0	10	2.0	14.0	9.6
	8	5.0	10	2.0	16.0	12.1
	9	6.0	10	2.0	18.0	14.3
	10	7.0	10	2.0	20.0	16.5
	11	7.0	15	2.0	22.0	19.0

METs = metabolic equivalents.

uptake at anaerobic threshold than DDD pacing (Fig. 3.21).[70] These benefits have been attributed largely to the increased heart rate in the rate-responsive mode.

The importance of AV synchrony diminishes at higher heart rates as the early and late diastolic filling phases converge. Nordlander and colleagues, in review of studies addressing work capacity in rate-modulating versus non–rate-modulating systems, noted that for every 40% increase in paced rate during rate-modulated pacing compared with non–rate-modulated pacing, there is a 10% increase in work capacity.[44] Despite acute hemodynamic benefits during formal exercise testing, improvements in quality of life and symptoms have not been clearly established.

Exercise testing and assessment of improvement in maximal work capacity represent quantifiable parameters for assessing improvement in patients with pacemakers; but most pacemaker patients, like most normal individuals, function at submaximal levels of exertion most of the time. Optimization of heart rate at these submaximal levels of exertion by providing rate modulation is the principal gain of enfranchising this physiologic concept. Protocols such as CAEP can be helpful.

In Figures 3.22 and 3.23, the relative hemodynamic benefits of rate modulation and stroke volume and rate modulation and AV synchrony scaled from rest to maximum exertion can be seen for a general population. At rest, AV synchrony is of preeminent benefit, whereas this benefit is diminished as one

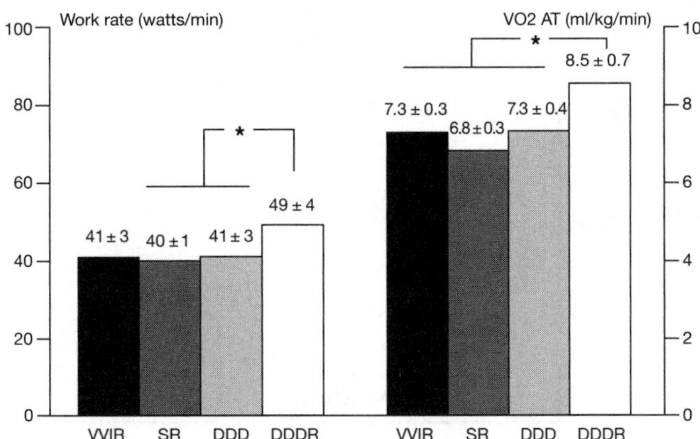

Figure 3.21. Work rate versus oxygen uptake at anaerobic threshold in 9 patients with sinus node dysfunction. Each patient underwent testing in sinus rhythm (SR), VVIR, DDD and DDDR pacing modes using a respiratory sensor pacemaker. Oxygen uptake was greater in DDDR mode compared to all others at anaerobic threshold. (Reproduced by permission from Lemke B, et al. Aerobic capacity in rate modulated pacing. PACE 1992;15:1914–1918.)

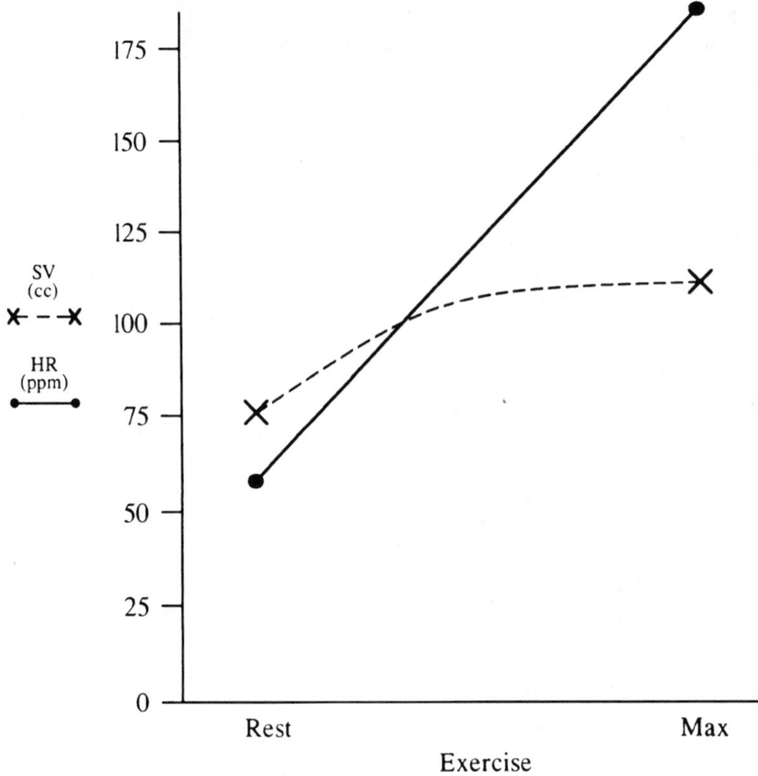

Figure 3.22. Normal stroke volume (SV) and heart-rate (HR) response to exercise.

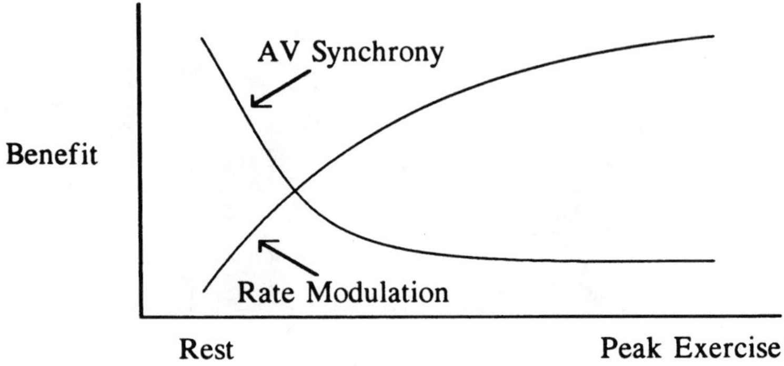

Figure 3.23. Hypothetical, general relationship between AV synchrony and rate modulation with respect to hemodynamic benefit, both at rest and during exercise.

approaches maximal exercise, especially in relationship to rate modulation. Rate modulation is of very little value at rest, but it becomes quite important early in exercise and increases in relative benefit approaching maximal exercise. Rate modulation and AV synchrony are complementary, not competitive, physiologic concepts.

MODE SELECTION AND STRATEGIES TO MINIMIZE VENTRICULAR PACING

Selection of the appropriate bradyarrhythmia pacing mode to fit the patient's electrical and hemodynamic status is usually not difficult. Striving to provide both AV synchrony and rate modulation, when clinical evidence supports a benefit, assists in this decision-making process.[44,48] Mode-selection decisions related to electrical considerations take into account three principal issues: atrial rhythm status, status of AV conduction, and presence of chronotropic competence. An expanding indication for chronotropic support includes heart failure patients who meet criteria for cardiac resynchronization therapy. A mode selection flow chart is shown in Figure 3.24.

Difficulties may arise in the assessment of atrial rhythm status; however, the availability of mode switching functions in most devices has rendered the presence of atrial arrhythmias relatively inconsequential in all but cases of chronic

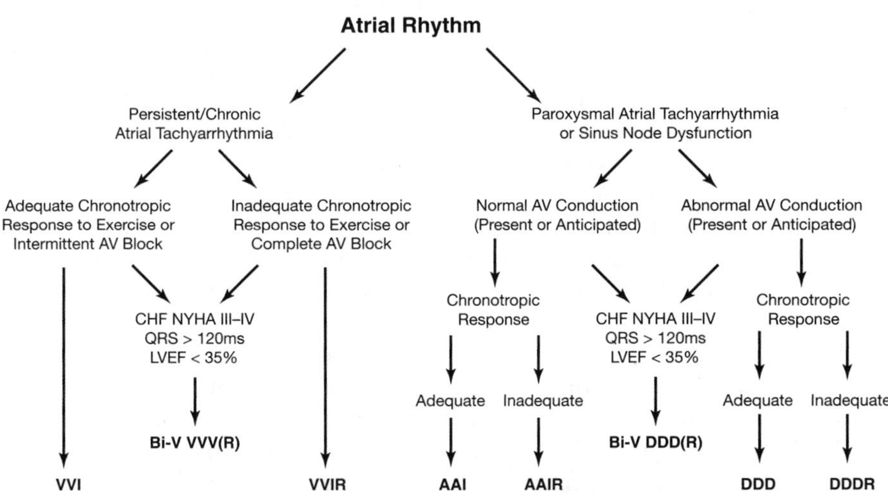

Figure 3.24. Mode-choice algorithm based on the presence and persistence of atrial tachyarrhythmias, status of AV conduction, and adequacy of chronotropic response to exercise. VVI = ventricular demand pacing, VVIR = rate-modulated ventricular demand pacing, DDD = AV universal pacing, DDDR = rate-modulated AV universal pacing, AAI = atrial demand pacing, AAIR = rate-modulated atrial demand pacing, Bi-V = biventricular, (R) with or without rate-modulation. (Pacemaker codes are discussed in detail in Chapter 6.)

arrhythmias. At present, at the University of Oklahoma, preservation of AV synchrony using dual chamber pacemakers is typically chosen if there are any periods of significant sinus rhythm. This practice is supported by randomized clinical trials that show an improved quality of life, a reduction of atrial fibrillation, and avoidance of pacemaker syndrome (VVIR to DDDR crossover up to 26%) with dual-chamber pacing compared to single-chamber right ventricular pacing.[27,44]

Another difficulty in mode selection is related to the determination of AV conduction status. Careful evaluation of AV conduction status dramatically reduces the likelihood that subsequent AV conduction problems will develop, but a small risk remains of approximately 2% to 6% in 5 years.[71] For this reason, although we may program an atrial pacing mode for patients with sinus node dysfunction and normal AV conduction, a dual-chamber pacing system is usually implanted.

Although the maintenance of physiologic AV intervals has hemodynamic benefits, recent clinical studies have shown that frequent or unnecessary right ventricular apical pacing, particularly dual-chamber pacing, increases the risk of atrial fibrillation, progression of heart failure, or death.[45,50] Of note, the majority of patients that received dual-chamber (DDDR) pacing in these trials utilized "physiologic AV delays" in the range of 120 to 200 milliseconds, resulting in a high percentage of ventricular pacing. The risks of frequent or continuous right ventricular stimulation may be reduced by using "minimal ventricular pacing" strategies that use backup ventricular pacing (VVI or VVIR) when AV synchrony is not required, or extended AV intervals during dual chamber pacing, to allow for intrinsic ventricular activation (see Fig. 3.24). Rate-adaptive AV interval pacing is reserved for patients that are symptomatic with long AV delays or high-grade AV block. As mentioned previously, simple measures include lengthening the AV delay to avoid ventricular fusion complexes, programming a lower pacing rate below the resting sinus rate, adding hysteresis for periods of inactivity, and adjusting drugs that affect AV nodal conduction. Newer dual chamber bradyarrhythmia devices use algorithms that essentially provide AAIR pacing with ventricular monitoring and backup DDDR pacing as needed during AV block, and can extend AV delays up to 350 milliseconds, without causing symptoms.[72]

The mode of pacing selected in the last 100 pacemaker and 100 ICD implants performed at the University of Oklahoma is shown in Figure 3.25. For a historical comparison, in the current pacemaker series there are almost no AAIR implants (1% vs 9% 8 years earlier) and more DDDR implants (67% vs 49% 3 years earlier). This reflects a better capacity to avoid ventricular pacing with intact AV conduction with the DDDR mode with and without mode switching than was the case with the early mode-switching devices. The number of VVI and VVIR implants for ICDs (38%) compared to pacemakers (18%) reflects the different pacing indications. (ICD patients receive VVI mode for backup bradyarrhythmia pacing in the absence of a true bradycardia indication for pacing and pacemaker patients virtually all receive VVIR mode for

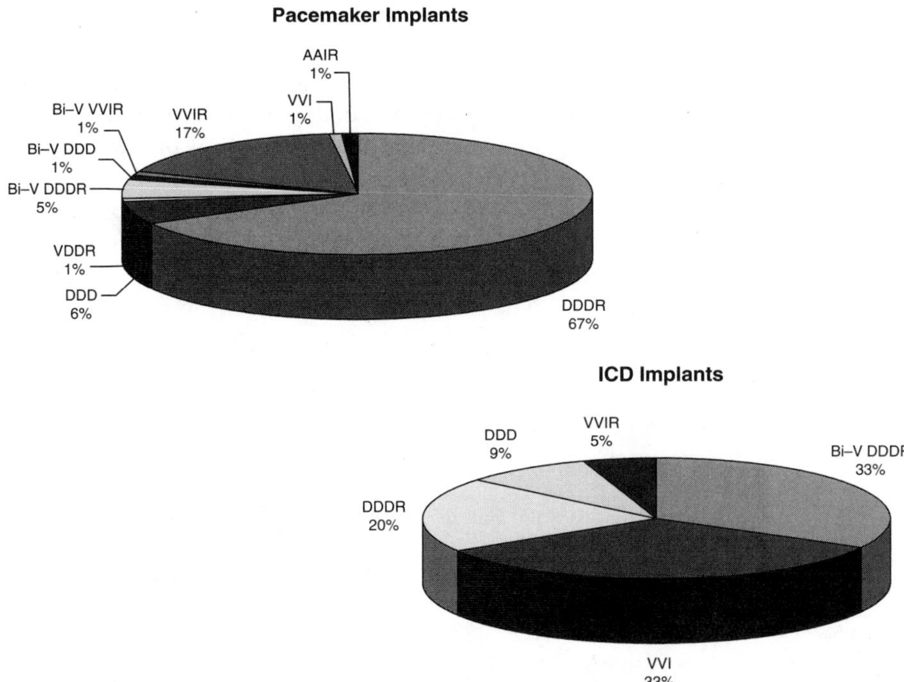

Figure 3.25. **A:** Mode selected at pacemaker implant in a recent series of 100 consecutive patients at the University of Oklahoma. **B:** Mode selected at Implantable Cardioverter Defibrillator (ICD) implant in a series of 100 consecutive patients. The modes are the same as those in Figure 3.24.

chronotropic response with chronic atrial fibrillation.) Finally, the past 3 years has marked the advent of cardiac resynchronization therapy and the growth of biventricular device implants. Although clinical trials of CRT excluded patients with a history of sinus node dysfunction and utilized an atrial sensed-biventricular stimulation mode (Bi-VDD) to establish the independent benefit of biventricular resynchronization, atrial arrhythmias and chronotropic incompetence are common in heart failure patients and rate response is added when appropriate. This is reflected in our confidence of the mode-switching and rate response capabilities of our biventricular ICD implant population (33% received Bi-V DDDR).

In summary, current pacemaker guidelines for mode-selection are to preserve AV synchrony with atrial or, most commonly, AV pacing in all but the most extenuating circumstances. Evidence-based practice now supports the following conclusions about atrial based compared to ventricular pacing: 1) atrial-based pacing reduces the incidence of atrial fibrillation, 2) atrial-based pacing has an inconsistent effect on heart failure, and 3) atrial-based pacing does not reduce mortality of strokes compared to ventricular pacing.[44] Based on recent evidence, there is growing concern that continuous right ventricular pacing increases the risk of heart failure progression; therefore, all attempts to avoid unnecessary right ventricular pacing by implementing strategies to preserve normal ventricular activation are recommended. It is quite possible that studies currently in progress will lead to a more widespread use of biventricular pacing whenever significant ventricular stimulation is anticipated. Further, we judge the patient's chronotropic response capabilities; and when symptoms or heart failure are exacerbated by a blunted or absent rate response, we treat using devices with simple, automatic but appropriate physiologic sensors.

REFERENCES

1. Harvey W. Exercitatio anatomica de motu cordis et sanguinis in animalibus (1628). R Willis, translator. England: Barnes Survey, 1874.
2. Lewis T. Fibrillation of the auricles: its effects upon the circulation. J Exp Med 1912;16:395–398.
3. Gesel RA. Auricular systole and its relation to ventricular output. Am J Physiol 1911;29:32–63.
4. Reynolds DW, Olson EG, Burow RD, et al. Hemodynamic evaluation of atrioventricular and ventriculoatrial pacing. Pacing Clin Electrophysiol 1984;7:463.
5. Erlebacher JA, Danner RL, Stelzer PE. Hypotension with ventricular pacing: an atrial vasodepressor reflex in human beings. J Am Coll Cardiol 1984;4:550–555.
6. Alicandri C, Fouad FM, Tarazi RC, et al. Three cases of hypotension and syncope with ventricular pacing: possible role of atrial reflexes. Am J Cardiol 1978;42: 137–142.
7. Goldreyer B, Bigger T. Ventriculoatrial conduction in man. Circulation 1970;41: 935–946.
8. Klementowicz P, Ausubel K, Furman S. The dynamic nature of ventriculoatrial conduction. Pacing Clin Electrophysiol 1986;9:1050–1054.
9. Levy S, Corbelli JL, Labrunie P. Retrograde (ventriculoatrial) conduction. Pacing Clin Electrophysiol 1983;6:364–371.
10. Petersen MEV, Chamberlain-Webber R, Fitzpatrick AP, et al. Permanent pacing for cardioinhibitory malignant vasovagal syndrome. Br Heart J 1994;71:274–281.
11. Karloff I. Hemodynamic effect of atrial triggered vs. fixed rate pacing at rest and during exercise in complete heart block. Acta Med Scand 1975;197:195–210.
12. Greenberg B, Chatterjee K, Parmley WW, et al. The influence of left ventricular filling pressure on atrial contribution to cardiac output. Am Heart J 1979;98: 742–751.
13. Kruse I, Arnman K, Conradson TB, Ryden L. A comparison of the acute and long-term hemodynamic effects of ventricular inhibited and atrial synchronous ventricular inhibited pacing. Circulation 1982;675:846–855.
14. Astrand PO, Rodahl K. Textbook of work physiology. 2nd ed. New York: McGraw-Hill, 1977.
15. Topol E, Goldschlager N, Ports TA, et al. Hemodynamic benefit of atrial pacing in right ventricular myocardial infarction. Ann Intern Med 1982;96:594–597.
16. Hartzler GO, Maloney JD, Curtis JJ, Barnhorst DA. Hemodynamic benefits of atrioventricular sequential pacing after surgery. Am J Cardiol 1977;40:232–236.

17. Chamberlain DA, Leinbach RC, Vassaux CE, et al. Sequential atrioventricular pacing in heart block complicating acute myocardial infarction. N Engl J Med 1970;282: 577–582.
18. Reynolds DW, Wilson MF, Burow RD, et al. Hemodynamic evaluation of atrioventricular sequential vs. ventricular pacing in patients with normal and poor ventricular function at variable heart rates and posture. J Am Coll Cardiol 1983;1:636.
19. Ogawa S, Dreifus LS, Shenoy PN, et al. Hemodynamic consequences of atrioventricular and ventriculoatrial pacing. Pacing Clin Electrophysiol 1978;1:8–15.
20. Morgan DE, Norman R, West RO, Burggraf G. Echocardiographic assessment of tricuspid regurgitation during ventricular demand pacing. Am J Cardiol 1986;58: 1025–1029.
21. Reynolds DW, Olson EG, Burrow RD, et al. Mitral regurgitation during atrioventricular and ventriculoatrial pacing. Pacing Clin Electrophysiol 1984;7:476.
22. Nakaoka H, Kitahara Y, Imataka K, et al. Atrial natriuretic peptide with artificial pacemakers. Am J Cardiol 1987;60:384–385.
23. Ellenbogen KA, Wood MA, Stambler BS. Pacemaker syndrome: clinical, hemodynamic and neurohumoral features. In: Barold SS, Mugica J, eds. New perspectives in cardiac pacing 3. Armonk, NY: Futura Publishing, 1993:85–112.
24. Alpert M, Curtis J, Sanfelippo J, et al. Comparative survival after permanent ventricular and dual-chamber pacing for patients with chronic high degree atrioventricular block with and without preexistent congestive heart failure. J Am Coll Cardiol 1986;7:925–932.
25. Rosenqvist M, Brandt J, Schuller H. Long-term pacing in sinus node disease: effects of stimulation mode on cardiovascular morbidity and mortality. Am Heart J 1988;116:16–22.
26. Connolly SJ, Kerr CR, Gent M, et al. Effects of physiologic pacing versus ventricular pacing on the risk of stroke and death due to cardiovascular causes. Candadian Trial of Physiologic Pacing Investigators. N Engl J Med 2000;342: 1385–1391.
27. Lamas GA, Lee KL, Sweeney MO, et al. Ventricular pacing or dual-chamber pacing for sinus-node dysfunction. N Engl J Med 2002;346:1854–1862.
28. Haskell RJ, French WJ. Optimum AV interval in dual-chamber pacemakers. Pacing Clin Electrophysiol 1986;9:670–675.
29. Janosik DL, Pearson AC, Buckingham TA, et al. The hemodynamic benefit of differential atrioventricular delay intervals for sensed and paced atrial events during physiologic pacing. J Am Coll Cardiol 1989;14:499–507.
30. Luceri RM, Brownstein SL, Vardeman L, Goldstein S. PR interval behavior during exercise: implications for physiological pacemakers. Pacing Clin Electrophysiol 1990;13:1719–1723.
31. Alt E, von Bibra H, Blomer H. Different beneficial AV intervals with DDD pacing after sensed or paced atrial events. J Electrophysiol 1987;1:250–256.
32. Reynolds DW, Olson EG, Burow RD, et al. Atrial vs. atrioventricular pacing: a hemodynamic comparison. Pacing Clin Electrophysiol 1985;8:148.
33. Leclercq C, Gras D, Le Helloco A, et al. Hemodynamic importance of preserving the normal sequence of ventricular activation in permanent pacing. Am Heart J 1995;129:1133.
34. Santomauro M, Fazio S, Ferraro S, et al. Fourier analysis in patients with different pacing modes. PACE 1991;14:1351.

35. Hass JM, Strait GB. Pacemaker induced cardiovascular failure: hemodynamic and angiographic observations. Am J Cardiol 1974;33:295–299.
36. Ausubel K, Boal BH, Furman S. Pacemaker syndrome: definition and evaluation. Clin Cardiol 1985;3:587–594.
37. Deshmukh P, Casavant DA, Romanyshyn M, Anderson K. Permanent direct His-bundle pacing: a novel approach to cardiac pacing in patients with normal His-Purkinje activation. Circulation 2000;101:869–877.
38. Gold MR, Brockman R, Peters RW, et al. Acute hemodynamic effects of right ventricular pacing site and pacing mode in patients with congestive heart failure secondary to either ischemic or idiopathic dilated cardiomyopathy. Am J Cardiol 2000;85:1106–1109.
39. Gold MR, Shorofsky SR, Metcalf MD, et al. The acute hemodynamic effects of right ventricular septal pacing in patients with congestive heart failure secondary to ischemic or idiopathic dilated cardiomyopathy. Am J Cardiol 1997;79:679–681.
40. Bourke JP, Hawkins T, Keavey P, et al. Evolution of ventricular function during permanent pacing from either right ventricular apex or outflow tract following AV-junctional ablation for atrial fibrillation. Europace 2002;4:219–28.
41. Tse HF, Yu C, Wong KK, et al. Functional abnormalities in patients with permanent right ventricular pacing: the effect of sites of electrical stimulation. J Am Coll Cardiol 2002;40:1451–1458.
42. Giudici MC, Thornburg GA, Buck DL, et al. Comparison of right ventricular outflow tract and apical lead permanent pacing on cardiac output. Am J Cardiol 1997;79:209–212.
43. Stambler BS, Ellenbogen K, Zhang X, et al. Right ventricular outflow versus apical pacing in pacemaker patients with congestive heart failure and atrial fibrillation. J Cardiovasc Electrophysiol 2003;14:1180–1186.
44. Lamas GA, Ellenbogen KA, Hennekens CH, Montanez A. Evidence base for pacemaker mode selection from physiology and randomized trials. Circulation 2004;109:443–451.
45. Schwaab B, Frohlig G, Alexander C, et al. Influence of right ventricular stimulation site on left ventricular function in atrial synchronous ventricular pacing. J Am Coll Cardiol 1999;33:317–323.
46. Sweeney MO, Hellkamp AS, Ellenbogen KA, et al. Adverse effect of ventricular pacing on heart failure and atrial fibrillation among patients with normal baseline QRS duration in a clinical trial of pacemaker therapy for sinus node dysfunction. Circulation 2003;107:2932–2937.
47. Tantengco MV, Thomas RL, Karpawich PP. Left ventricular dysfunction after long-term right ventricular apical pacing in the young. J Am Coll Cardiol 2001;37: 2093–2100.
48. Gregoratos G, Abrams J, Epstein AE, et al. ACC/AHA/NASPE 2002 guideline update for implantation of cardiac pacemakers and antiarrhythmia devices: summary article: a report of the American College of Cardiology/American Heart Association Task Force on Practice Guidelines (ACC/AHA/NASPE Committee to Update the 1998 Pacemaker Guidelines). Circulation 2002;106:2145–2161.
49. Moss A, Zareba W, Hall W, et al. for the Multicenter Automatic Defibrillator Implantation Trial II Investigators. Prophylactic implantation of a defibrillator in patients with myocardial infarction and reduced ejection fraction. N Engl J Med 2002;346:877–883.

50. Wilkoff BL, Cook JR, Epstein AE, et al. Dual-chamber pacing or ventricular backup pacing in patients with an implantable defibrillator: the Dual Chamber and VVI Implantable Defibrillator (DAVID) Trial. JAMA 2002;288:3115–3123.
51. Jeanrenaud X, Goy JJ, Kappenberger L. Effects of dual-chamber pacing in hypertrophic cardiomyopathy. Lancet 1992;339:1318–1323.
52. Fananapazir L, Cannon RO, Tripodi D, Panza JA. Impact of dual-chamber permanent pacing in patients with obstructive hypertrophic cardiomyopathy with symptoms refractory to verapamil and β-adrenergic blocker therapy. Circulation 1992;85:2149–2161.
53. Fananapazir L, Epstein ND, Curiel RV, et al. Long-term results of dual-chamber (DDD) pacing in obstructive hypertrophic cardiomyopathy. Evidence for progressive symptomatic and hemodynamic improvement and reduction of left ventricular hypertrophy. Circulation 1994;90:2731–2742.
54. Nishimura RA, Trusty JM, Hayes DL, et al. Dual-chamber pacing for hypertrophic cardiomyopathy: a randomized, double-blind, crossover trial. J Am Coll Cardiol 1997;29:435–441.
55. Simantirakis EN, Kanoupakis EM, Kochiadakis GE, et al. The effect of DDD pacing on ergospirometric parameters and neurohormonal activity in patients with hypertrophic obstructive cardiomyopathy. Pacing Clin Electrophysiol 1998;21:2269–2272.
56. Maron BJ, Olivotto I, Spirito P, et al. Epidemiology of hypertrophic cardiomyopathy related death: revisited in a large non-referral-based patient population. Circulation 2000;102:858–864.
57. Auricchio A, Stellbrink C, Block M, et al. Effect of pacing chamber and atrioventricular delay on acute systolic function of paced patients with congestive heart failure. The pacing therapies for congestive heart failure study group. Circulation 1999;99:2993–3001.
58. Kass DA, Chen CH, Curry C, et al. Improved left ventricular mechanics from acute VDD pacing in patients with dilated cardiomyopathy and ventricular conduction delay. Circulation 1999;99:1567–1573.
59. Saxon LA, Kerwin WF, DeMarco T, et al. Acute effects of AV synchronous biventricular pacing on left atrial to left ventricular activation/contraction sequence in dilated cardiomyopathy. J Cardiac Failure 1998;4:138.
60. Kerwin WF, Botvinick EH, O'Connell JW, et al. Ventricular contraction abnormalities in dilated cardiomyopathy: effect of biventricular pacing to correct interventricular dyssynchrony. J Am Coll Cardiol 2000;35:1121–1227.
61. Cazeau S, Gras D, Lazarus A, et al. Multisite stimulation for correction of cardiac asynchrony. Heart 2000;84:579–581.
62. Leon AR, Greenberg JM, Kanuru N, et al. Cardiac resynchronization in patients with congestive heart failure and chronic atrial fibrillation: effect of upgrading to biventricular pacing after chronic right ventricular pacing. J Am Coll Cardiol 2002;39:1258–1263.
63. Linnarsson D. Dynamics of pulmnary gas exchange and heart rate changes at start and end of exercise. Acta Physiol Scand 1974;415:1–68.
64. Ellestad MH, Wan MKC. Predictive implications of stress testing: follow-up of 2700 subjects after maximum treadmill testing. Circulation 1975;51:363–369.
65. Wilkoff BL, Corey J, Blackburn G. A mathematical model of the cardiac chronotropic response to exercise. J Electrophysiol 1989;3:176–180.

66. Buckingham TA, Woodruff RC, Pennington DG, et al. Effect of ventricular function on the exercise hemodynamics of variable rate pacing. J Am Coll Cardiol 1988;11:1269.
67. Lau CP, Camm J. Role of left ventricular function and Doppler derived variables in predicting hemodynamic benefits of rate-responsive pacing. Am J Cardiol 1988;62:174.
68. Proctor EE, Leman RB, Mann DL, et al. Single-versus dual-chamber sensor-driven pacing: Comparison of cardiac outputs. Am Heart J 1991;122:728.
69. Jutzy RV, Florio J, Isaeff DM, et al. Limitations of testing methods for evaluation of dual-chamber versus single-chamber adaptive rate pacing. Am J Cardiol 1991;61:1715.
70. Cappuci A, Boriani G, Speechia S, et al. Evaluation by cardiopulmonary exercise testing of DDDR versus DDD pacing. PACE 1992;15:1908.
71. Santini M, Aexidou G, Ansalone G, et al. Relation of prognosis in sick sinus syndrome to age, conduction defects, and modes of permanent cardiac pacing. Am J Cardiol 1990;65:729–735.
72. Sweeney MO, Shea JV, Fox V, et al. Randomized trial of a new minimal ventricular pacing mode in patients with dual chamber ICDs. PACE 2003;26:973.

Temporary Cardiac Pacing

Mark A. Wood and Kenneth A. Ellenbogen

4

Temporary cardiac pacing serves as the definitive therapy for the acute management of medically refractory bradyarrhythmias. The applications of temporary pacing also include management of certain tachyarrhythmias and use in provocative diagnostic cardiac procedures. It is essential for cardiologists, intensivists, and emergency room personnel to be familiar with temporary pacing. The indications for temporary pacing are given in Chapter 1. The purpose of this chapter is to describe the salient clinical aspects of the temporary pacing techniques currently in use.

TRANSCUTANEOUS CARDIAC PACING

Transcutaneous cardiac pacing has emerged as the preeminent initial mode of cardiac pacing for bradyasystolic arrest situations and prophylactic pacing applications. The technique can be quickly and safely initiated by minimally trained personnel. A variable incidence of cardiac capture and poor patient tolerance represent the disadvantages to transcutaneous pacing.

Transcutaneous cardiac pacing produces depolarization of myocardial tissue by pulsed electrical current conducted through the chest between electrodes adherent to the skin. The self-adhesive surface patch electrodes are large—typically 8 cm in diameter—nonmetallic, and impregnated with a high-impedance conductive gel. Transcutaneous pacing generators are usually incorporated into external defibrillator units (Fig. 4.1). These units provide up to 200 mA of current and use a rectangular or truncated exponential pulse waveform of 20 to 40 milliseconds duration. The long pulse widths permit the lowest pacing thresholds while minimizing the stimulation of skeletal muscle and cutaneous nerves.

To initiate transcutaneous pacing, the patch electrodes are secured anteriorly and posteriorly to the chest wall. Several electrode configurations have been recommended and appear to be equally effective in healthy subjects.[1] For effective capture, it is essential that the anterior chest electrode be of *negative* polarity. Thresholds may be unobtainable or intolerably painful if the negative

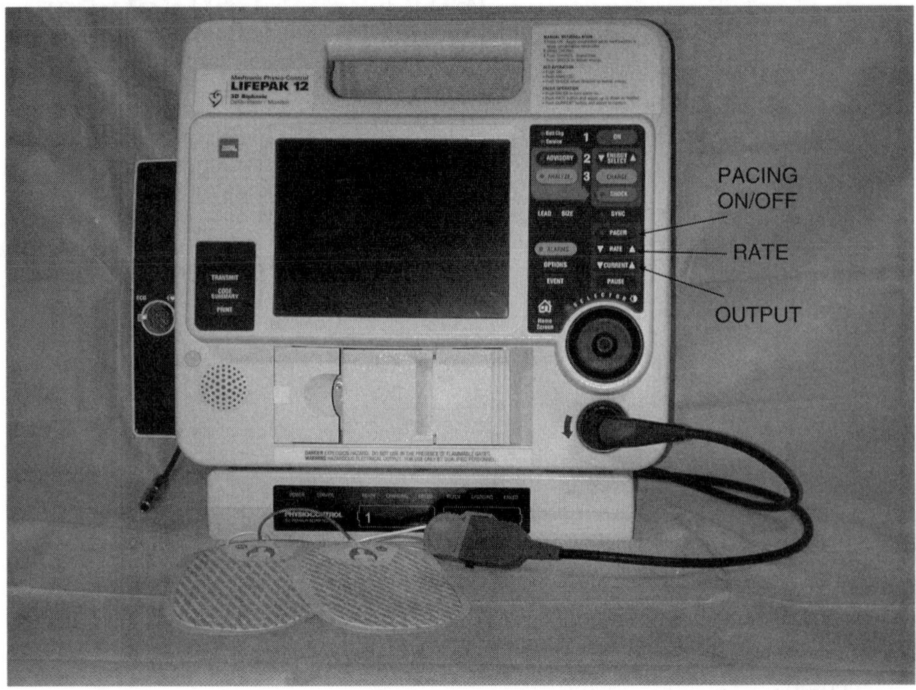

Figure 4.1. Transcutaneous cardiac pacing generator/defibrillator and surface patch electrodes. The controls for transcutaneous pacing are indicated. (Courtesy of Medtronic, Inc.)

electrode is placed posteriorly. The anterior (negative) electrode can be centered over the palpable cardiac apex, or over the chest lead V_3 position along the left sternal border (Fig. 4.2). The posterior (positive) electrode is centered at the level of the inferior aspect of the scapula between the spine and either the right or left scapula, but it is equally effective when positioned on the anterior right chest in healthy subjects.[2] Placement directly over the scapula or spine may increase the pacing threshold. Before electrode placement, the skin should be thoroughly cleaned with alcohol to remove salt deposits and skin debris, which contribute to patient discomfort and/or elevate pacing thresholds. Excessive body hair beneath the electrode interface raises transthoracic and impedance. Shaving beneath the patches can reduce the impedance by up to 13.8% and is further reduced by pressure applied to the patches.[2] Abrading the skin by shaving may worsen discomfort, however.

In emergency bradyasystolic situations, transcutaneous pacing should be initiated at maximal current output to ensure ventricular capture. Chest compressions may be performed directly over the electrodes without disruption of pacing or danger to medical personnel. The large pacing stimulus artifact obscures ancillary electrocardiography (ECG) monitors; thus, the electronically filtered display on the generator itself must be followed. Cardiac capture is suggested by the appearance of depolarization artifacts following the pacing

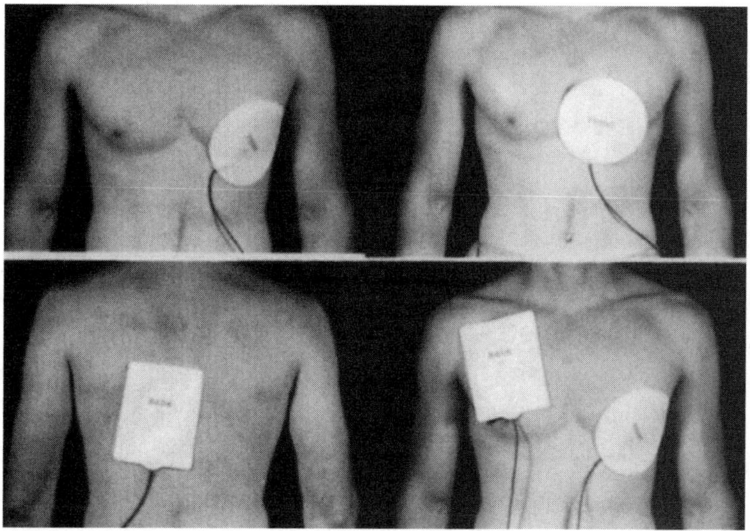

Figure 4.2. Transcutaneous pacing electrode positions. **Upper left:** Anterior cathodal patch placement over cardiac apex. **Upper right:** Alternate anterior cathodal patch position over position of electrocardiographic chest lead V_3. **Lower left:** Posterior anodal patch centered between lower aspect of the left scapula and the spine. **Lower right:** Placement of anterior anodal patch on the right chest. Note that cathodal (negative) electrode must be positioned anteriorly.

stimuli, but capture *must* be confirmed by palpation of a pulse or by Doppler auscultation (Fig. 4.3). Once capture is documented, the current may be decreased gradually until loss of capture defines the pacing current threshold.

In conscious patients, transcutaneous pacing is begun at rates slightly faster than the native rhythm and at minimal current output. The current is gradually increased until cardiac capture is documented or until intolerable discomfort develops. The final current output is left at or slightly (5 to 10 mA) above threshold.

Transcutaneous pacing thresholds tend to be lowest in healthy subjects and in patients with minimal hemodynamic compromise. In these settings, thresholds generally range from 40 to 80 mA.[3–6] In clinical use, thresholds of 20 to 140 mA are encountered.[5] The current output that produces intolerable pain is highly variable among individuals; however, the majority of patients can be paced at manageable levels of discomfort.[4,5] The pain results from stimulation of cutaneous afferent nerves and intense pacing-induced skeletal muscle contraction. No correlation has been defined between transcutaneous pacing threshold and age, body weight, body surface area, chest diameter, cardiac drug therapy, or etiology of underlying heart disease.[4,5,7] However, thresholds are elevated for 24 hours following intrathoracic surgery, possibly due to entrapped pericardial and mediastinal air, or transient myocardial ischemia.[7] Elevated thresholds may also occur in the presence of emphysema, pericardial effusion, positive-pressure

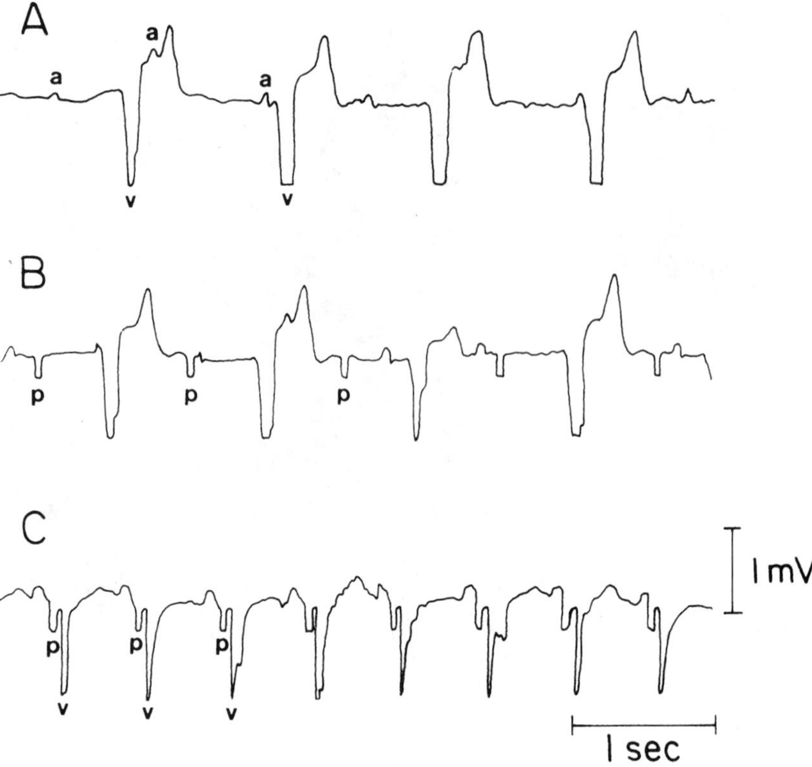

Figure 4.3. Successful transcutaneous cardiac pacing during complete heart block. **A:** Complete heart block with wide complex ventricular escape rhythm (a = atrial depolarization; v = ventricular depolarization). **B:** Subthreshold transcutaneous pacing stimuli (p) at 20 mA fail to capture the ventricle. **C:** A 1:1 ventricular capture achieved with increased generator current output to 60 mA. Ventricular capture was confirmed by palpation of femoral pulses.

ventilation, and when used to pace terminate ventricular tachycardias.[5,8,9] As with other forms of cardiac pacing, thresholds tend to be higher and incidence of capture lower during prolonged or delayed resuscitation efforts. Thresholds may decrease after adequate myocardial perfusion is restored, however.

Electrophysiologically, transcutaneous pacing affects ventricular pacing in humans.[9,10] Retrograde activation of the atria may occur. Intracardiac, electrocardiographic, and pressure monitoring during transcutaneous pacing have shown the right ventricle to be the site of earliest myocardial activation.[9,10] Theoretically, this follows from the proximity of the right ventricle to the anterior (negative) electrode and from the fact that the stimulating current density declines proportionally to the square of distance from the electrode. Despite initial right ventricular activation, echocardiographic studies in healthy subjects undergoing transcutaneous pacing have shown normal synchronous left ventricular contraction without alterations in ventricular end-diastolic dimension or fractional shortening when compared to sinus rhythm.[3] This pattern suggests near-simultaneous activation of the entire left ventricle. When measured at or near the transcutaneous pacing threshold, ventricular effective refractory periods may be significantly longer than values obtained during right ventricular endocardial stimulation.[4]

Modest reductions in left ventricular systolic pressure and stroke index may occur during transcutaneous pacing when compared to sinus rhythm or atrioventricular (AV) sequential pacing as a result of AV dyssynchrony.[11] The alterations in systemic pressures are similar to those induced by endocardial ventricular demand inhibited pacing. Right heart pressures may increase due to loss of AV synchrony. Compared with atrial or ventricular endocardial pacing, transcutaneous pacing reportedly provides greater cardiac output and systolic indices.[10] This phenomenon has been associated with an increased O_2 consumption during transcutaneous pacing and is believed to result from enhanced skeletal muscle metabolism secondary to electrical stimulation. Systemic vascular resistance appears to be unaltered, however. Alternatively, the enhanced cardiac output from transcutaneous pacing may result from chest, diaphragmatic, and abdominal muscle contractions simulating cough-induced resuscitation synchronized to cardiac activation.[12]

The incidence of ventricular capture with transcutaneous pacing is greatly influenced by the setting in which it is used. In healthy subjects, the ability to capture and tolerate transcutaneous pacing is high, ranging from 50% to 100%.[4,9,13] Clinically, success rates appear to be highest when transcutaneous pacing is used prophylactically or early (within 5 minutes) in the course of bradycardic arrests.[5] In these situations, success rates may exceed 90%.[5] In emergency situations, the success of transcutaneous pacing is lower, but ranges from 10% to 93%.[1,5,14] In the largest study, Zoll and co-workers report ventricular capture in 105 of 134 patients (78%) in diverse clinical situations.[5] Electrical capture was obtained in only 58% of cardiac arrests but in 95% of cases of prophylactic use. Transcutaneous pacing has been used continuously in humans for up to 108 hours and intermittently for 17 days without complications.[5,15] This pacing mode has been used to terminate both ventricular and supraventricular tachycardia.[14,16]

A variety of causes may contribute to failure of transcutaneous pacing. These are outlined with possible solutions in Table 4.1. The causes of excessively painful pacing and their corrections are listed in Table 4.2.

In more than 40 years of experience, complications related to transcutaneous pacing have been extraordinarily rare. Although limited areas of focal myofibrillar coagulation necrosis and perivascular microinfarcts have been demonstrated in dogs undergoing transcutaneous pacing, no such lesions have been described in humans.[9] Transcutaneous pacing produces no measurable release of myoglobin, myocardial creatine kinase, or myocardial lactate dehydrogenase in normal individuals.[3] There are no reports of damage to skeletal muscle, lungs, myocardium, or skin (other than mild erythema and irritation) associated with transcutaneous pacing in humans. Caution has been suggested in using

Table 4.1. Failure to Capture during Transcutaneous Pacing

Cause	Solution
Suboptimal lead position	Reposition leads avoiding scapula, sternum, and spine
Negative electrode placed posteriorly	Place negative electrode anteriorly over apex or V_3
Poor skin-electrode contact	Clean skin of sweat and debris; shave body hair
Faulty electrical contacts	Check electrical connections
Generator battery depletion	Charge battery or plug-in generator
Increased intrathoracic air	Reduce positive pressure ventilation; relieve pneumothorax
Pericardial effusion	Drain
Myocardial ischemia/metabolic	CPR, ventilation, correct acidosis/hypoxia/electrolyte derangements abnormalities
High threshold	Shave hair beneath electrodes, apply pressure to patches, apply patches with fresh gel

Table 4.2. Painful Transcutaneous Pacing

Cause	Solution
Conductive foreign body beneath electrode	Remove foreign body
Electrode over skin abrasions	Reposition; use care in shaving beneath electrodes
Apprehension or low pain tolerance	Administer narcotics or benzodiazepines
Sweat or salt deposits on skin	Clean skin, remove foreign material (increased local current density)
High threshold	Apply pressure to patches, apply patches with fresh gel

this technique within 3 days of sternotomy; however, actual wound dehiscence from pacing-induced muscle contractions appears to be more a theoretical concern than a practical one. Coughing and discomfort from cutaneous nerve and skeletal muscle stimulation are the most frequent problems. When properly used the technique poses no electrical danger to personnel attending the patient. Transcutaneous pacing appears remarkably free from arrhythmic complications despite its use in acute myocardial infarction, digitalis toxicity, during anesthesia, and in cases of endocardial pacing-induced ventricular arrhythmias.[5] There is only one reported case of ventricular tachycardia induced by therapeutic transcutaneous pacing.[17] In dogs, ventricular fibrillation thresholds during the ventricular vulnerable period average 12.6 times the pacing threshold and exceed the current capacity of clinically available generators.[18] The ability to prolong ventricular refractoriness may contribute to its low arrhythmogenic potential.

TRANSVENOUS PACING

Transvenous pacing provides the most consistent and reliable means of temporary cardiac pacing in clinical practice. The technique permits reliable atrial and/or ventricular pacing, a feature unique to this modality. Once initiated, pacing is generally stable and extremely well tolerated. Considerable knowledge and technical skills are required to implement transvenous pacing safely and effectively, however.[19] Even so, a variety of complications may attend its use. The procedure also requires significant time to implement, making it less than ideal for emergency situations.

Transvenous cardiac pacing uses intravenous catheter electrodes to stimulate atrial or ventricular myocardial tissue directly with electrical current pulses provided by an external generator. Stimulation may be accomplished by bipolar electrode configurations—in which both anode and cathode are intracardiac in location; or by unipolar pacing—in which one pole, preferably the anode, is extracardiac in location. The bipolar configuration is most commonly used for temporary pacing, and a variety of pacing leads are available (Fig. 4.4). These catheters are typically 3 to 6F in diameter, use platinum-coated electrodes, and are constructed of flexible plastic. These catheters may be flaccid and flow-directed (floating) by means of an inflatable balloon between the electrodes, or they may be semirigid (semifloating) without balloons for more responsive manipulation. Semirigid catheters may be straight or possess preformed distal curvatures (J configurations) to facilitate manipulation and stable atrial positioning. Temporary screw-in pacing leads have been introduced to enhance lead stability.[20,21] These leads have been used for prolonged pacing up to 32 days and permit ambulatory temporary pacing (see Fig. 4.4B).[20–22] Alternatively, screw-in permanent pacing electrodes may be introduced percutaneously for prolonged pacing.

Other specialized electrode designs include single-pass dual-chamber pacing leads and pulmonary artery catheters with proximal atrial and/or distal ventricular electrodes (Figs. 4.4 and 4.5). Lead stability may be problematic with pacing pulmonary artery catheters, however.

Temporary pacing generators are typically constant-current output devices (Fig. 4.6). These generators are designed to function against loads of 300 to 1000 ohms. The stimulus pulse width is usually 1 to 2 milliseconds. Temporary pacing generators typically feature adjustable rates (30 to 180 pulses per minute [ppm]), sensitivity (0.1 mV-asynchronous), and current output (0.1 to 20 mA). Temporary universal (DDD) generators provide a variety of programmability and are capable of most common single- and dual-chamber pacing modes as well as high-rate pacing for arrhythmia termination.

Decisions regarding the site of venous access for pacing should take into consideration the urgency to initiate pacing, desired lead stability, need to avoid specific complications, and anticipated duration of pacing. Proper catheter position is most easily and rapidly obtained from the right internal jugular approach.[23] This site and the left subclavian route are the sites of choice during

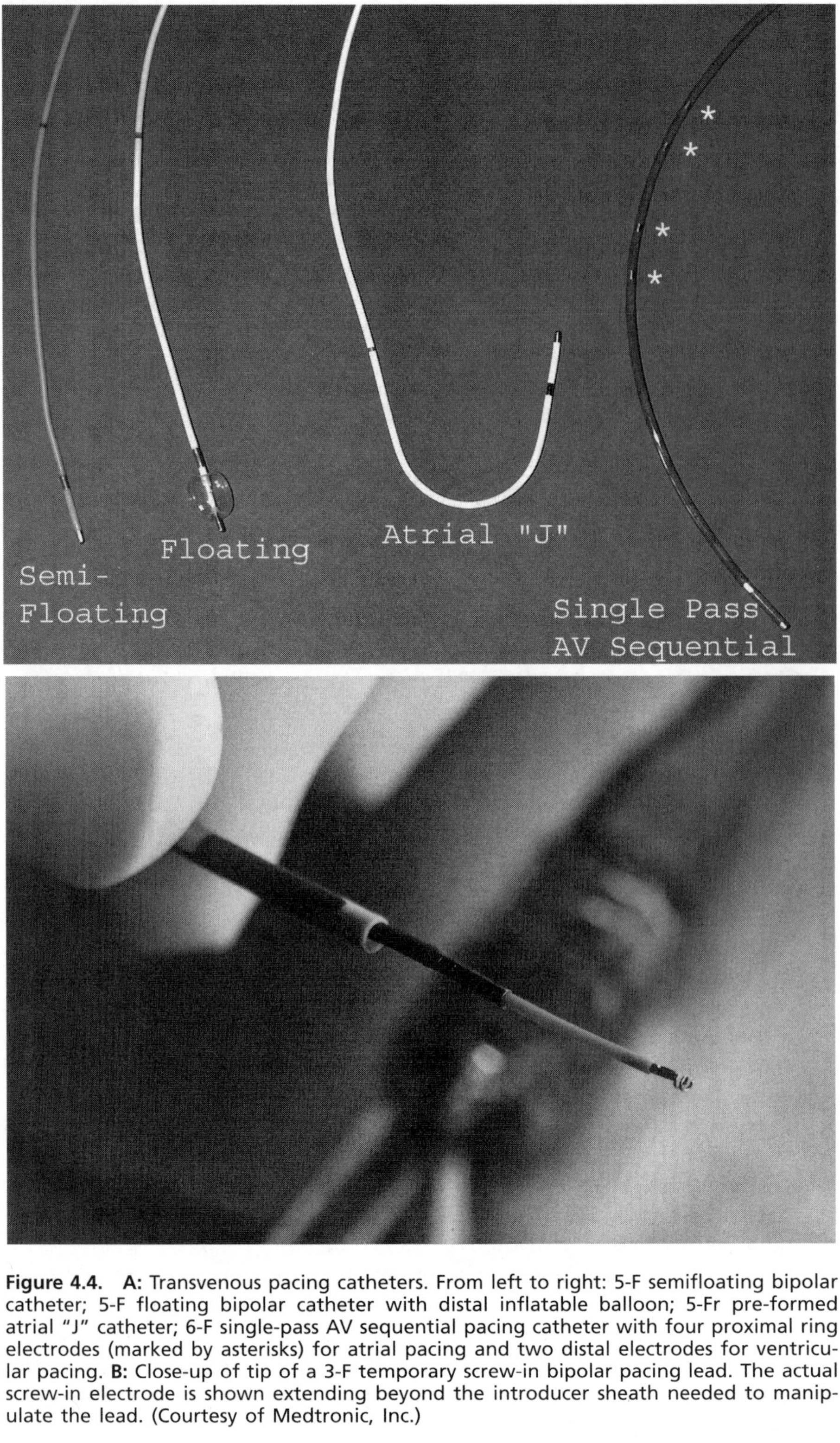

Semi-
Floating
Floating
Atrial "J"
Single Pass
AV Sequential

A

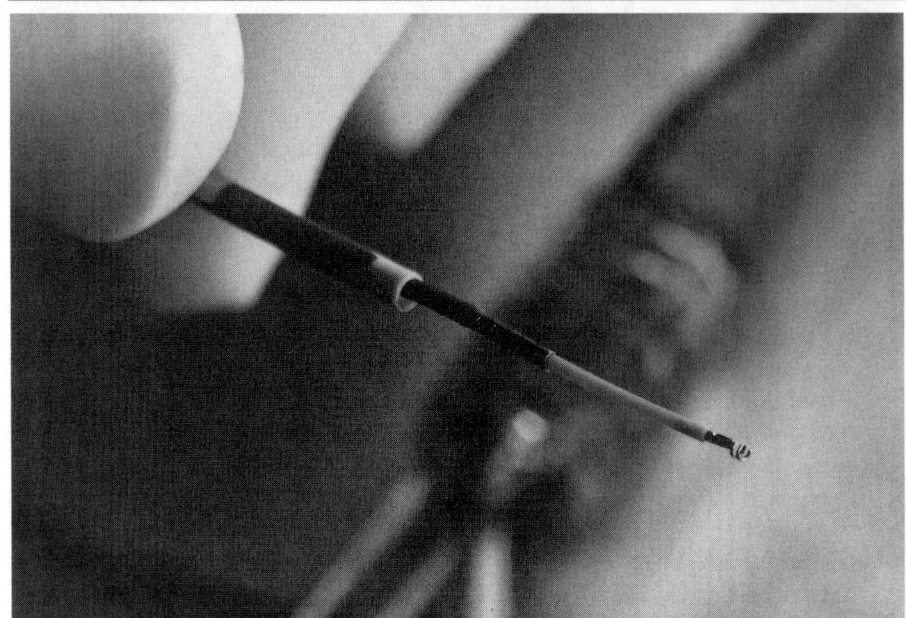

B

Figure 4.4. A: Transvenous pacing catheters. From left to right: 5-F semifloating bipolar catheter; 5-F floating bipolar catheter with distal inflatable balloon; 5-Fr pre-formed atrial "J" catheter; 6-F single-pass AV sequential pacing catheter with four proximal ring electrodes (marked by asterisks) for atrial pacing and two distal electrodes for ventricular pacing. **B:** Close-up of tip of a 3-F temporary screw-in bipolar pacing lead. The actual screw-in electrode is shown extending beyond the introducer sheath needed to manipulate the lead. (Courtesy of Medtronic, Inc.)

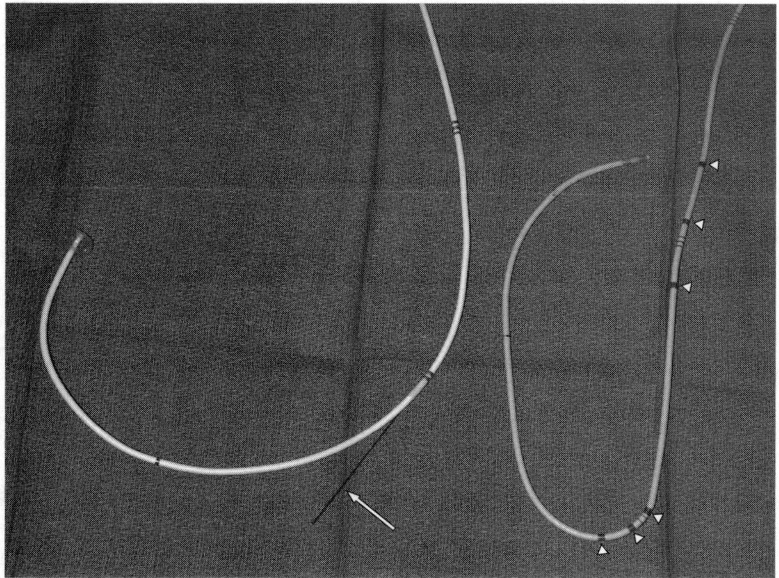

Figure 4.5. Pacing pulmonary artery pressure monitoring catheters. **Left:** Ventricular pacing pulmonary artery catheter using a 3-F wire electrode (*arrow*) deployed into the right ventricle through a port in the body of the catheter. **Right:** AV sequential pacing pulmonary artery catheter with three proximal atrial ring electrodes and two distal ventricular ring electrodes. The electrodes are highlighted by the *arrowheads*.

emergency situations. The external jugular and brachial routes are too circuitous to negotiate without fluoroscopy. The cephalic vein is frequently impassable even with fluoroscopy due to its acute junction with the axillary vein. Catheter stability is maximized by use of the internal jugular or subclavian routes; it is most problematic with peripheral sites, especially brachial, because of movement of the extremities. The peripheral routes do, however, permit greatest control of bleeding complications and avoid pneumothorax and inadvertent puncture of the carotid or subclavian arteries. Femoral venous pacing carries the greatest risks of thrombosis, phlebitis, and infection, thus necessitating site changes every 24 hours. Temporary pacing for extended periods is best tolerated and least complicated by using the internal jugular or subclavian routes; however, subclavian access may preclude immediate use of this vein for permanent pacing if it is needed.

Once venous access is obtained, the catheter may be directed to the desired intracardiac position by electrocardiographic, echocardiographic, or, ideally, fluoroscopic guidance. Optimal pacing thresholds and lead stability are usually achieved in the right ventricular apex and right atrial appendage. An external defibrillator should *always* be present during catheter manipulation. For placement in the right ventricular apex, non-floating catheters usually require formation and rotation of a loop in the atrium under fluoroscopy but may advance

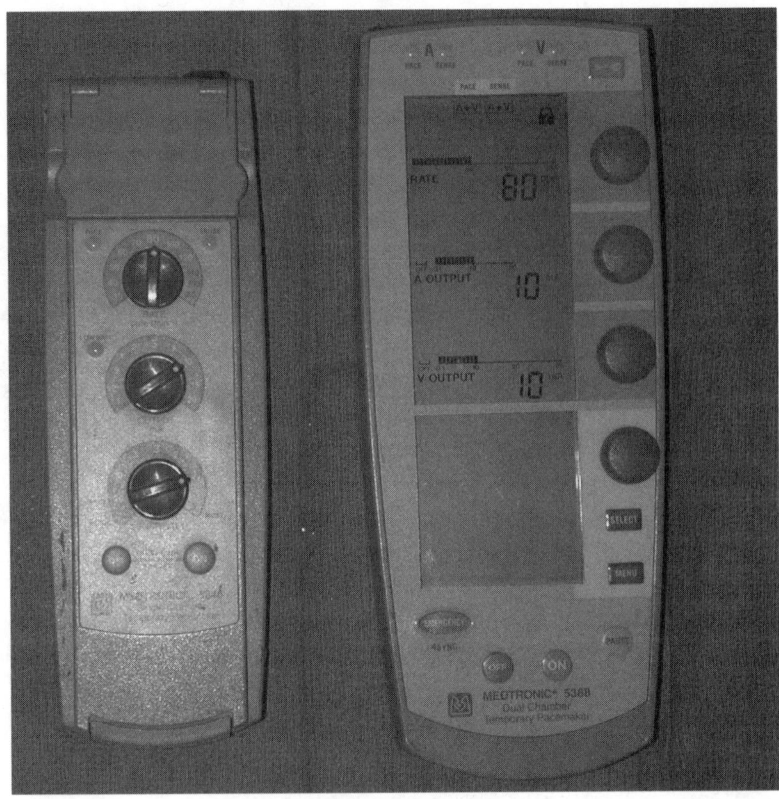

Figure 4.6. Temporary external transvenous pacing generators. **Left:** Single chamber generator with adjustable rate, output, and sensitivity. This device is capable of single chamber demand and asynchronous pacing modes. **Right:** Temporary DDD generator. This highly programmable unit is capable of most common single-chamber and dual-chamber modes as well as high-rate pacing. (Courtesy of Medtronic, Inc.)

directly across the tricuspid valve by deflecting off the tricuspid annulus (Figs. 4.7 and 4.8).

Once in the ventricle, catheters coursing the superior vena cava tend to orient superiorly and require counter-clockwise torque and gentle advancement to reach the right ventricular apex (see Fig. 4.7). The inferior vena caval approach may orient the catheter tip inferiorly toward the ventricular apex but still requires clockwise torque during advancement to reach the apex (see Fig. 4.8). Under fluoroscopy, the atrial appendage is accessed from the superior vena cava by orienting preformed J catheters anteriorly and slightly medially in the low right atrium. The catheter is withdrawn slowly until the tip demonstrates the typical to and fro "wagging" motion of the atrial appendage. Following cardiac surgery, the atrial appendage may be deformed or absent, requiring approximation of curved atrial catheters against the atrial wall or interatrial septum (see Figs. 4.7 and 4.8).

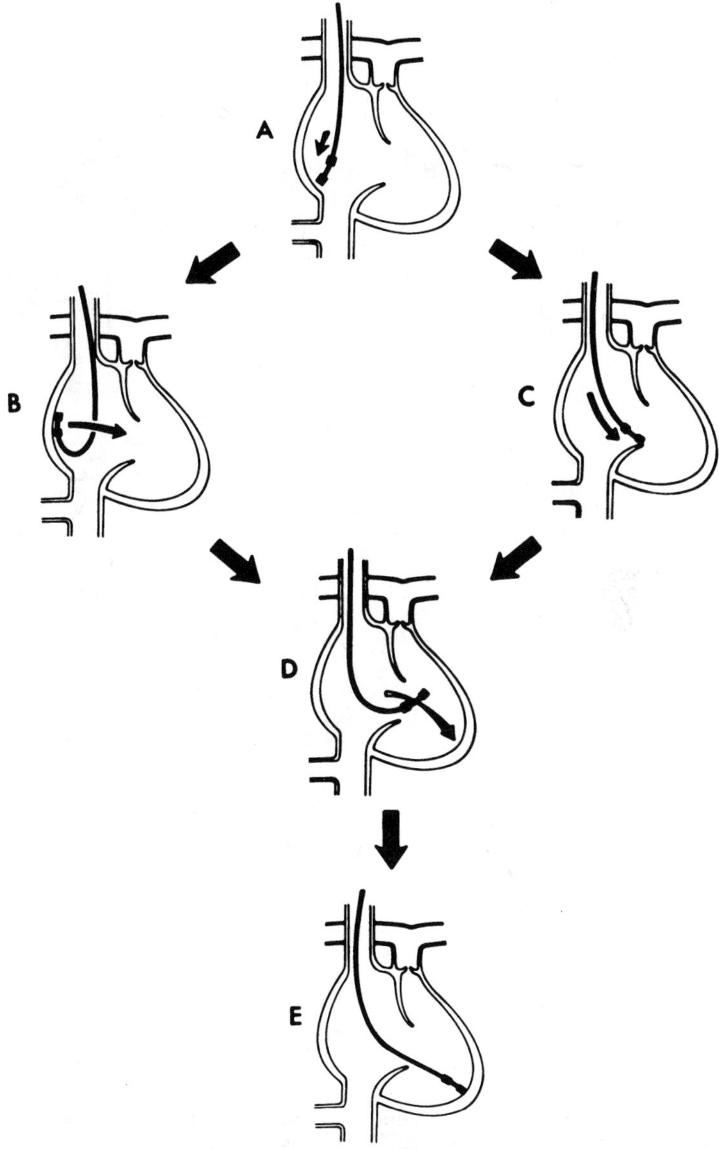

Figure 4.7. Techniques for right ventricular catheter placement from the superior vena cava under fluoroscopic guidance. **A:** Catheter advanced to the low right atrium. **B:** Further advancement produces a loop or bend in the distal catheter, which is then rotated medially. **C:** Alternatively, catheter in low right atrium deflects off tricuspid annulus directly into the right ventricle. **D:** Superior orientation of the catheter tip in the ventricle requires counterclockwise torque during advancement to reach the apex. **E:** Final catheter position in the right ventricular apex. Catheter position in **(B)** may be suitable for atrial pacing.

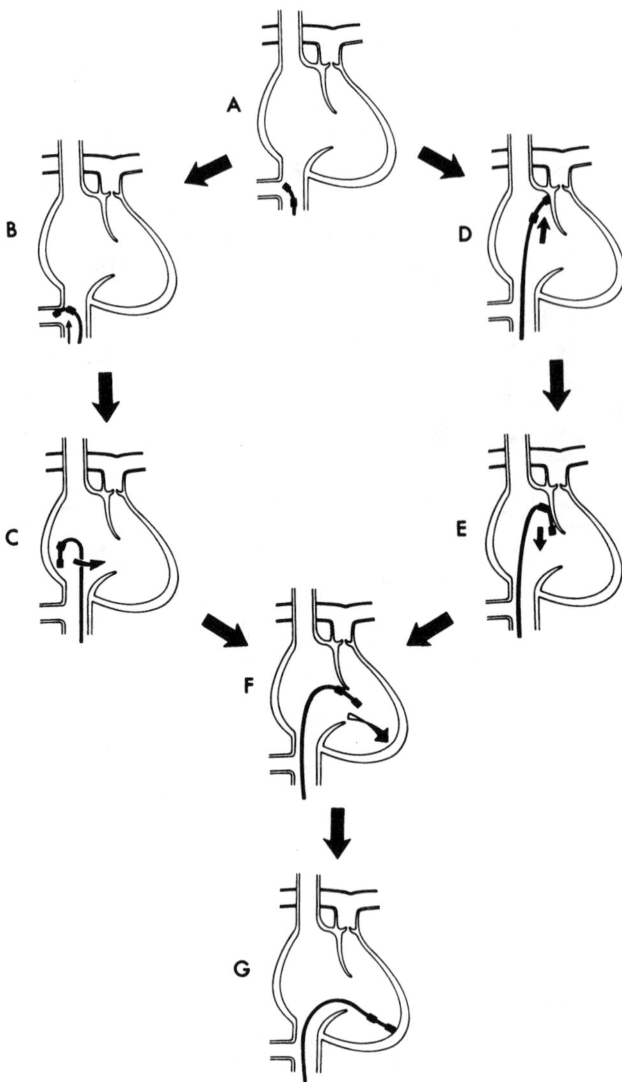

Figure 4.8. Techniques for right ventricular catheter placement from the inferior vena cava under fluoroscopic guidance. **A:** Catheter is advanced to the hepatic vein. **B:** Catheter tip engages proximal hepatic vein and is advanced further, forming a bend in the catheter. **C:** The bend in the distal catheter is then rotated medially. **D:** Alternatively, the catheter is advanced to the high medial right atrium. **E:** With advancement, a bend is formed in the catheter, which is then quickly withdrawn or "snapped" back to the level of the tricuspid orifice. **F:** After crossing the tricuspid valve, the catheter is advanced with gentle clockwise torque to reach the apex. **G:** Final catheter position in the right ventricular apex. Catheter positions in **(C)** and **(D)** can be used for atrial pacing.

When fluoroscopy is unavailable or impractical, electrocardiographic guidance is possible using flow-directed balloon-tipped catheters or semirigid catheters. While advancing these leads, the distal electrode is connected to lead V_1 of a standard ECG recorder. Balloon-tipped catheters are inflated in the central circulation. The catheter location is known from the characteristic unipolar electrograms recorded in each chamber (Fig. 4.9). Balloon-tipped catheters are deflated upon entry into the ventricle to avoid displacement into the pulmonary artery. Large ventricular electrograms (≥6 mV) with ST segment elevation (injury pattern) signal contact with ventricular endocardium. There appears to be no correlation between the magnitude of ST (or PR) segment elevation and pacing threshold, however.[24] Echocardiographic guidance of catheter position is possible by filling the balloon of flow-directed catheters with echogenic fluid.[25] In asystole, a semi-floating catheter is advanced during asynchronous pacing at maximal output until ventricular capture is documented by ECG monitoring or palpation of a pulse. Flow-directed catheters provide the shortest insertion times.[26]

Once positioned, the electrodes are connected to the pacing generator; for bipolar pacing, the distal pole serves as the cathode (negative pole), and the proximal pole serves as the anode (positive pole). During unipolar pacing, *cathodal* intracardiac stimulation reduces thresholds and pacing-related arrhythmic complications.[27] The anodal (positive) pole of the generator is secured to a subcutaneous wire electrode or surface patch electrode with surface area ≥50 mm² to reduce thresholds. During emergency situations, pacing is initiated asynchronously, at maximal outputs. Following capture, current output is reduced until loss of capture defines the pacing threshold. During non-emergency situations, pacing is begun at low outputs in the demand mode at rates slightly above (10 ppm) the intrinsic heart rate. Current is increased until capture is achieved. Optimal ventricular and atrial pacing thresholds are less than 1.0 mA. Pacemaker output is maintained at three to five times threshold to compensate for subsequent threshold elevations due to inflammation and edema at the electrode-tissue interface, physiologic alterations, or pharmacologic interventions.

Sensing threshold in the demand mode is determined by setting the pacemaker rate below the intrinsic heart rate, then reducing sensitivity (increasing the value of the millivolt scale) until pacing output occurs. Sensing thresholds should be greater than 6 mV and 1 mV for the ventricle and atrium, respectively. Sensitivity is maintained at 25% to 50% of the sensing threshold. AV intervals between 100 and 200 milliseconds are usually optimal during AV sequential pacing. Small changes in the AV interval can significantly influence hemodynamics in some patients.

After initiation of ventricular pacing, the position of the catheter should be confirmed by anteroposterior and lateral chest radiograph *and* electrocardiography. On the anteroposterior chest radiograph, a catheter tip in the right ventricular apex should cross to the left of the spine near the lateral cardiac border and point slightly inferiorly. On lateral projections, the catheter tip should be directed anteriorly only a few centimeters posterior to the sternum. Even with

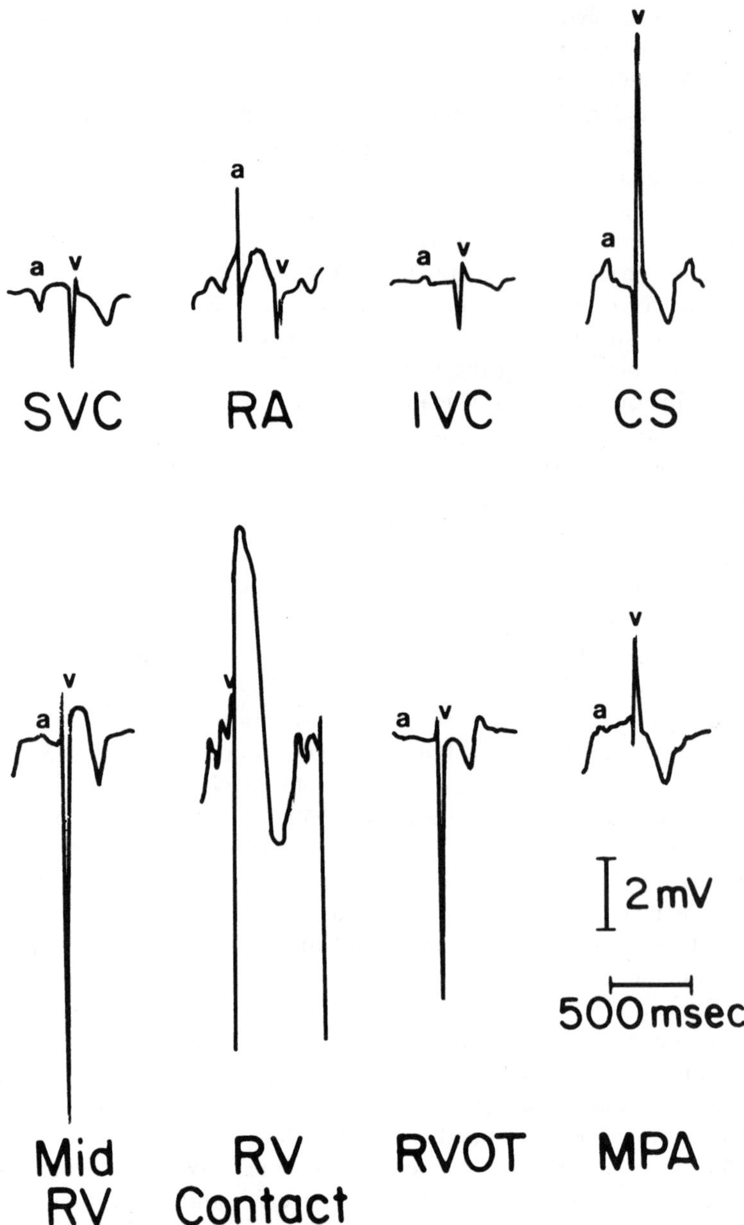

Figure 4.9. Unipolar electrograms obtained from the distal electrode of a temporary pacing catheter. Note the marked ST segment elevation with right ventricular endocardial contact and predominantly positive ventricular electrogram morphologies with the pulmonary artery and coronary sinus electrograms. a = atrial electrogram; v = ventricular electrogram; SVC = superior vena cava; RA = right atrium; IVC = inferior vena cava; CS = coronary sinus; Mid RV = mid-right ventricular cavity; RV Contact = contact with right ventricular endocardium; RVOT = right ventricular outflow tract; MPA = main pulmonary artery.

these findings, the chest x-ray cannot completely exclude malposition of the catheter into the coronary veins, left ventricle, or pericardial space.[28]

Electrocardiographically paced QRS complexes originating from the right ventricular apex should demonstrate left bundle branch block morphology with a superior axis. A right bundle branch block pattern during temporary ventricular pacing usually indicates coronary sinus pacing or lead perforation into the left ventricle or pericardial space. Rarely, apical pacing can produce a pattern of right bundle branch block due to preferential activation of the interventricular septum or delayed activation of the right ventricle.[29] In this situation, the QRS axis maintains a left superior orientation and the precordial transition occurs by lead V_3.[30] Various paced QRS morphologies may localize the catheter tip to other locations (Table 4.3).

Unipolar electrograms of intrinsic depolarizations recorded from the right ventricular apex (through lead V_1 of a standard ECG recorder) should demonstrate ST segment elevation acutely and a predominantly negative QRS morphology (see Fig. 4.9). The absence of acute ST elevation and the presence of a predominantly positive or biphasic electrogram morphology strongly suggests coronary sinus or extracardiac location of the electrode. Coronary sinus pacing is also suggested by high pacing thresholds, atrial or simultaneous atrial and ventricular pacing, absence of ventricular ectopy with catheter manipulation, posterior course of the catheter on a lateral chest radiograph, and recording both atrial and ventricular electrograms from the electrode. Although associated with unreliable ventricular capture, coronary sinus pacing may allow ventricular capture in the presence of impassible tricuspid valve anatomy (such as a mechanical tricuspid prosthesis).

Once it is in a satisfactory position, the lead is sutured securely to the skin, covered with a protective dressing, and examined daily for infection. The generator is affixed to the patient or bed with its controls shielded from inadvertent manipulation. Threshold testing and paced 12-lead ECGs should be performed daily.

For most emergency and prophylactic pacing situations, single-chamber ventricular pacing is preferred. Temporary atrial pacing is restricted to those patients with primarily sinus node dysfunction, absence of atrial dysrhythmias, and intact AV nodal function, as documented by 1:1 AV conduction at rates of

Table 4.3. Paced QRS Morphology from Various Electrode Positions

Lead Position	QRS Morphology	QRS Axis
Right ventricular apex	LBBB	Superior
Right ventricular inflow tract	LBBB	Normal
Right ventricular outflow tract	LBBB	Inferior or right
Mid or high left ventricle	RBBB	Inferior or right
Inferior left ventricle	RBBB	Superior
Coronary sinus	RBBB	Inferior

125 ppm. The instability of atrial leads and unpredictable effects of autonomic tone and ischemia on AV nodal conduction frequently preclude its use.

Although patients without underlying cardiac disease usually demonstrate similar hemodynamic responses to atrial and ventricular pacing, the maintenance of AV synchrony through atrial or dual-chamber pacing is beneficial in patients with left ventricular systolic and/or diastolic dysfunction.[31,32] In these patients, AV sequential pacing may augment cardiac output by 20% to 30% over ventricular pacing alone, while also maintaining higher systemic arterial pressures, lower mean left atrial pressures, lower pulmonary artery pressures, and enhanced ventricular end-diastolic filling. Patients with acute myocardial infarction (especially right ventricular infarction), hypertensive heart disease, hypertrophic or dilated cardiomyopathies, aortic stenosis, or recent cardiac surgery are known to benefit from AV sequential pacing.[33] AV sequential pacing should also be considered in any patient who has inadequate hemodynamic responses to ventricular pacing alone (for example, retrograde VA conduction producing pacemaker syndrome).

Initiating and sustaining myocardial capture depends on obtaining a stable catheter position, the viability of the paced myocardial tissue, and the electrical integrity of the pacing system. With fluoroscopy, a satisfactory catheter position should be obtainable in virtually all patients. The reported incidence of ventricular capture without fluoroscopy using flow-directed or semi-floating catheters ranges from 30% to 90%.[34,35] Capture is least likely during emergency situations, especially during asystole, without fluoroscopy.[34] Catheter coiling in the right atrium poses the most frequent obstacle to ventricular access and may be minimized by using the right internal jugular vein approach, using flow-directed catheters, or by advancing preformed J catheters from subclavian approaches.[36] These catheters have a tendency to prolapse into the ventricle when advanced beyond the typical atrial position.

Ventricular capture is adversely affected by hypoxia, myocardial ischemia, acidosis, alkalosis, marked hyperglycemia, and hypercapnia. In emergency situations, electrical capture is least likely in the setting of ventricular asystole, probably as a reflection of profound underlying myocardial dysfunction and/or severe metabolic derangement.[34] Electrode contact with previously infarcted or fibrotic myocardium may also prevent capture. Pharmacologic interventions such as administration of type Ia and Ic antiarrhythmics, hypertonic saline, glucose and insulin, and mineralocorticoids may also increase ventricular capture thresholds by up to 60%.[37] Conversely, thresholds may be decreased by epinephrine, ephedrine, glucocorticoids, and hyperkalemia.[37] Isoproterenol may initially decrease and subsequently increase the threshold by 20% to 80%.[37] Electrolyte effects tend to be transient. Digitalis, calcium gluconate, morphine sulfate, lidocaine, and atropine have minimal effects on ventricular thresholds. Ventricular thresholds may rise by 40% during sleep and, conversely, may decrease with activity.[38] Lead fractures, unstable electrical connections, generator failure, and battery depletion may also preclude myocardial capture.

After successful implementation, malfunction of the pacing system manifesting as inconsistent pacing or sensing may occur in 14% to 43% of

Table 4.4. Loss of Capture during Transvenous Cardiac Pacing

Cause	Evaluation	Solution
Catheter dislodgment/ perforation	Check position on chest radiograph, paced QRS morphology, or electrograms	Reposition catheter under fluoroscopy, increase output
Poor endocardial contact	Check position on chest radiograph, check electrograms	Reposition catheter, increase output
Local myocardial necrosis/ fibrosis	Check electrograms, evaluate for previous infarction	Reposition catheter, possibly increase output
Local myocardial inflammation/edema	Document adequate catheter position (chest radiograph and electrograms)	Increase output, possibly reposition
Hypoxia/acidosis/electro-lyte disturbance/drug effect (type Ia and Ic)	Check appropriate laboratory values/drug levels	Correct disturbance, reduce drug levels, increase output
Electrocautery/DC cardioversion damaging electrodes and/or tissue interface	Recent exposure to current source	Increase output, replace or reposition catheter, possibly replace generator
Lead fracture	Check unipolar pacing thresholds	Unipolarize functional electrode or replace catheter
Generator malfunction/ battery depletion	Document adequate catheter position, check battery reserve	Replace batteries and/ or generator
Unstable electrical connections	Document adequate catheter position, check connections	Secure connections

patients.[39–41] The possible etiologies are numerous; Tables 4.4 to 4.6 show the recommended solutions. By far the most common cause of loss of capture is catheter dislodgment or poor initial catheter position. Dislodgment is most common with brachial pacing sites and bears an inconsistent relationship to catheter size and stiffness.[39] Most failures occur within the first 48 hours of pacing and are usually corrected by adjusting generator output or sensitivity but up to 38% of malfunctions require catheter replacement or repositioning.[40] Stability is greatly enhanced by the use of temporary screw-in electrodes.[20,21] Lead fractures in bipolar catheters may be overcome by converting the functional electrode to a unipolar configuration or by replacing the lead. As mentioned, numerous physiologic variables and pharmacologic interventions can also affect pacing threshold.[37,38] Local inflammatory response at the electrode–tissue interface commonly elevates pacing thresholds within hours to days after lead insertion. Similarly, loss of sensing is most frequently related to catheter dislodgment or poor myocardial contact (see Table 4.5). Oversensing is a relatively uncommon problem with temporary pacing systems (see Table 4.6).

Table 4.5. Loss of Sensing during Transvenous Cardiac Pacing

Cause	Evaluation	Solution
Lead dislodgment or perforation	Check position on chest radiograph, check unipolar or bipolar electrograms	Reposition lead under fluoroscopy
Local tissue necrosis/fibrosis	Check unipolar or bipolar electrograms	Reposition lead, increase sensitivity
Electrodes perpendicular to depolarization wavefront, low amplitude electrograms, and/or low d*V*/d*t*	Check unipolar or bipolar electrograms	Unipolarize lead or reposition
Lead fracture	Check unipolar electrograms from each electrode	Unipolarize functional electrode or replace lead
Electrocautery/DC current damaging electrode or tissue interface	Exposure to current source, check electrograms	Replace or reposition lead, increase sensitivity
Spontaneous QRS during refractory period of generator	Analyze appropriate ECG tracings	No intervention, or replace with generator having shorter refractory period
Generator malfunction	Confirm adequate electrograms and generator sensitivity settings	Replace generator or reset sensitivity
Unstable electrical connections	Confirm adequate electrograms	Secure connections

Table 4.6. Oversensing during Transvenous Cardiac Pacing

Cause	Evaluation	Solution
P wave sensing	Catheter tip near tricuspid valve on chest radiograph, check electrograms	Reposition further into right ventricular apex, reduce sensitivity
T wave sensing	Check electrograms	Reduce generator sensitivity, possibly reposition catheter
Myopotential sensing	Check electrograms during precipitating maneuvers	If unipolar, replace with bipolar system or reduce sensitivity
Electromagnetic interference	Check proper electrical grounding and isolation of patient and pacer system, possibly check electrograms	Properly ground equipment, electrically isolate patient, turn off unnecessary equipment, reduce sensitivity
Intermittent electrical contacts, unstable connections, or lead fracture	Monitor sensing during manipulation connections/lead	Secure connections, replace lead

The complications of transvenous pacing are related to acquisition of venous access, intravascular catheter manipulation, and maintenance of an intravascular foreign body. In large series, the reported incidence of clinical complications ranges from virtually zero for prophylactic pacemaker insertion in the catheterization laboratory[42] to 20% of cases in coronary intensive care units.[40] Complications tend to be more common with brachial or femoral pacing sites. Arterial trauma, air embolism, or pneumothorax may complicate 1% to 2% of insertions.[43] Significant bleeding may be seen in 4% of patients.[40]

One of the most common complications of temporary pacing is the induction of ventricular tachycardia or fibrillation.[44] Non-sustained ventricular tachycardia is most common during catheter manipulation (3% to 10% incidence) and is usually terminated by withdrawal of the catheter.[45,46] Ventricular tachyarrhythmias are more common in the setting of myocardial ischemia, acute infarction, hypoxia, general anesthesia, vagal stimulation, drug toxicity, and catecholamine administration and during coronary artery catheterization.[47,48] Ventricular fibrillation may complicate up to 14% of acute myocardial infarctions requiring temporary pacemaker insertion.[48] Supraventricular tachycardias may result from catheter manipulation within the atrium.

Myocardial perforation may complicate temporary pacing in 2% to 20% of cases and is probably underdiagnosed clinically.[49,50] Perforation is more common with brachial or femoral catheters. Immobilization of the extremities is recommended to prevent excessive motion of the catheter. Diagnostic signs and symptoms of myocardial perforation are listed in Table 4.7. Loss of pacing or sensing, changes in paced QRS morphology, and diaphragmatic or skeletal muscle pacing are the most common manifestations; however, perforation to intracardiac and extracardiac locations can be clinically silent.[50] Penetration *into* the myocardium may occur in up to 30% of patients and is suggested by ventricular arrhythmias with the same morphology as paced complexes.[43] Perforation of the interventricular septum is usually hemodynamically inconsequential; however, extracardiac migration of the catheter can produce pericardial tamponade in approximately 1% of perforations.[43] Pericarditis may be seen in 5% of patients with perforated temporary pacing catheters.[43]

In the absence of hemodynamically significant pericardial effusion, myocardial perforation is managed by catheter withdrawal until effective capture is restored. Careful patient monitoring follows. Unipolar electrograms recorded from the catheter tip will demonstrate a pathognomonic transition from R wave to S wave morphology with ST elevation upon withdrawal from extracardiac to intracardiac locations (Fig. 4.10), thereby confirming the diagnosis.[51]

Thromboembolic events from temporary pacing appear to be more frequent than are clinically recognized. Venograms or ultrasound in patients with femoral pacing catheters reveal evidence of femoral venous thrombosis in up to 39% of the patients despite their receiving subcutaneous or systemic heparin.[52,53] Of the patients with thrombosis, 60% may have evidence of pulmonary emboli on ventilation perfusion scans.[52] Thrombosis is rarely suspected clinically. The incidence of thrombosis with other pacing sites has not been systematically

Table 4.7. Diagnostic Features of Myocardial Perforation by Temporary Pacing Catheter

Symptom	Pericardial chest pain, dyspnea (if pericardial tamponade present), skeletal muscle pacing, shoulder pain
Signs	Pericardial rub, intercostal muscle or diaphragmatic pacing, presystolic pacemaker "click" with bipolar systems, failure to pace and/or sense, pericardial tamponade
Chest radiograph	Change in lead position, extracardiac location of tip,* "fat-pad" sign,† new pericardial effusion
Surface ECG	Change in paced QRS morphology and/or axis, pericarditis pattern
Echocardiography	Extracardiac position of catheter tip,* pericardial effusion, loss of paradoxical anterior septal motion or rapid initial left posterior septal motion characteristic of right ventricular apical stimulation
Intracardiac electrogram	Change in morphology of unipolar electrograms; biphasic or predominantly positive (R wave) unipolar QRS morphology recorded from tip; change in QRS morphology from biphasic, R, or Rs morphology to rS or S configuration with ST elevation and T wave inversion during catheter withdrawal*

* Pathognomonic of perforation.
† Catheter tip < 3 mm from apical fat pad on lateral chest radiograph.

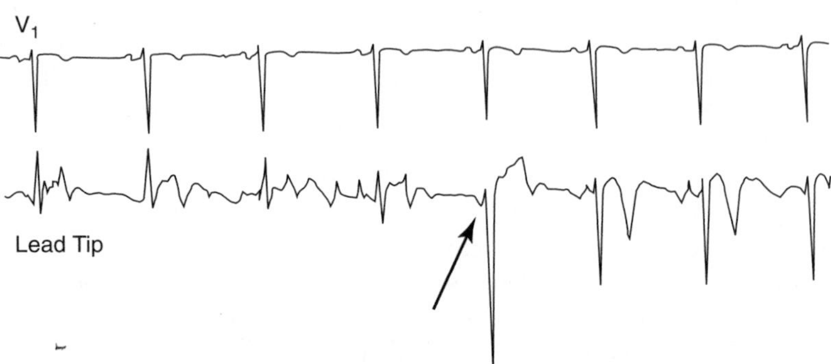

Figure 4.10. Continuous unipolar recording from the distal electrode of a perforated ventricular pacing catheter in an elderly women. Surface ECG lead V_1 is also shown. Perforation into the pericardial space was suspected clinically 24 hours after catheter placement. The first three complexes show a predominantly positive morphology to the unipolar electrogram recorded from the distal electrode. As the catheter is withdrawn the fourth unipolar electrogram becomes biphasic and afterward is negative (*arrow*) as the distal electrode moves from an epicardial to endocardial position. This finding confirms the diagnosis of myocardial perforation.

studied. Systemic anticoagulation with femoral pacing may reduce but does not eliminate venous thrombosis.[53]

Clinical infection or phlebitis complicates temporary pacing in 3% to 5% of patients and is most common with femoral sites.[40] Bacteremia has been demonstrated in 50% of patients by the third day of temporary pacing.[43] Sepsis is much less frequent, however. In general, pacing sites should be changed every 72 hours.

Other complications include knotting of catheters, induction of right bundle branch block (1%), and phrenic nerve or diaphragmatic pacing in the absence of myocardial perforation (10%).[43]

EPICARDIAL PACING

Transthoracic pacing is possible using temporary pacing wires passively fixed to the atrial and ventricular epicardium at the time of cardiac surgery or thoracotomy. The wires, usually paired to each chamber with or without a third subcutaneous lead for unipolar pacing. They are exposed through the skin in the subxiphoid region. Bipolar leads are also available. The wires should be appropriately marked as atrial or ventricular leads. If uncertain, the origin of the lead may be confirmed by pacing, timing unipolar electrograms from the lead with surface ECG signals, or chest radiograph examination. These leads are used in a similar fashion to transvenous leads; however, pacing and sensing thresholds tend to deteriorate progressively within days of implantation. Pacing thresholds in both chambers are elevated by the fourth postoperative day and sensing thresholds are lower on the second postoperative day (Fig. 4.11).[54] The use of bipolar electrodes may minimize sensing and pacing failures, especially for atrial pacing.[55] Reversal of bipolar lead polarity or unipolarization of the leads may circumvent high thresholds. Temporary biventricular pacing may improve hemodynamics in some patients following cardiac surgery.[56]

TRANSESOPHAGEAL PACING

The anatomic proximity of the esophagus to the posterior left atrium makes transesophageal *atrial* pacing possible in nearly all patients. The technique is relatively noninvasive and virtually free of serious complications. Furthermore, the technique requires minimal training to perform successfully. However, *ventricular* capture is inconsistent or often intolerably painful, which seriously limits the therapeutic and emergency applications of the technique. Transesophageal pacing is now used primarily to terminate supraventricular arrhythmias in patients under general anesthesia or pediatric patients. It has also been used as a substitute for pharmacologic provocation in stress testing.[57–61]

Transesophageal pacing uses an intraesophageal electrode positioned in proximity to the heart to deliver stimulating electrical current to the myocardial tissue. The necessary equipment includes a specialized bipolar electrode and a transesophageal pulse generator with unique output characteristics (Fig. 4.12). Dedicated transesophageal pacing catheters are 5 to 10F flexible designs for oral or nasal introduction (Fig. 4.13). Theoretically, the optimal interelectrode spacing

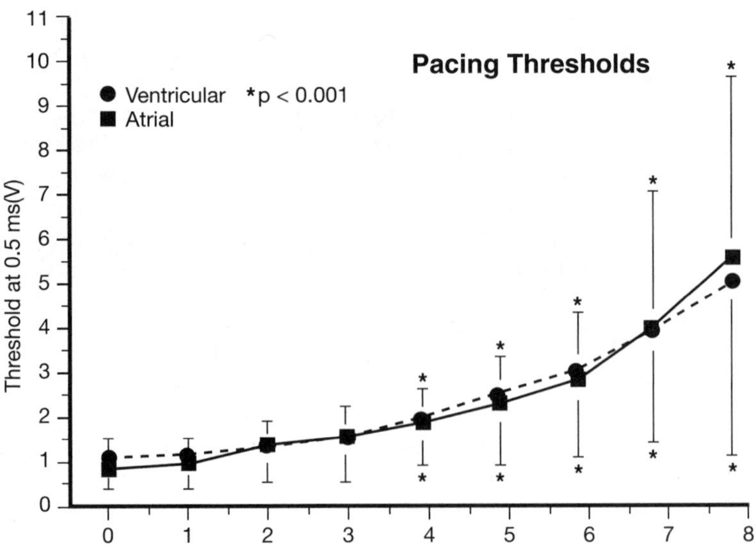

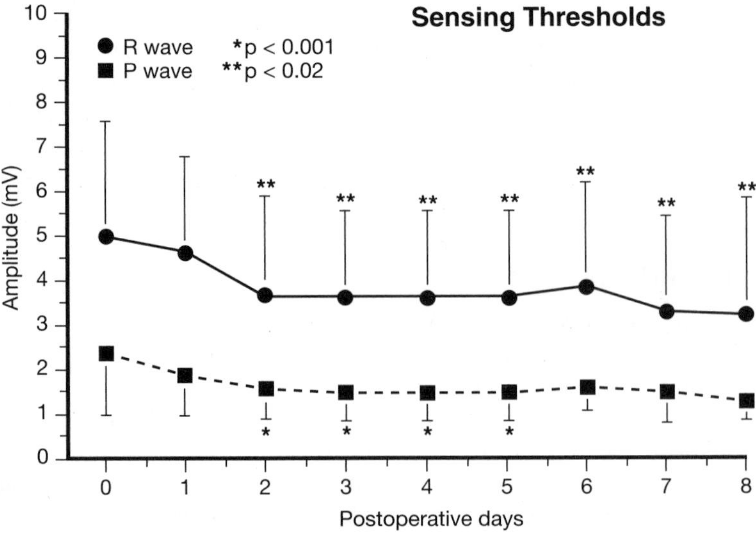

Figure 4.11. Pacing and sensing thresholds from paired unipolar temporary epicardial pacing wires placed in 60 patients at the time of cardiac surgery. Pacing and sensing thresholds are significantly worse compared to implant values by the 4th and 2nd postoperative days, respectively. *$P < .05$ compared to implant. (Reproduced by permission from Elmi F, et al. Natural history and predictors of temporary epicardial pacemaker wire function in patients after open heart surgery. Cardiology 2002;98:175–180.)

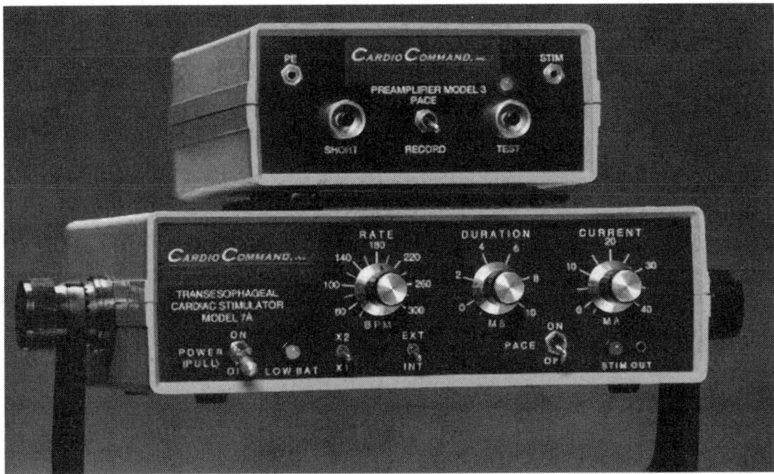

Figure 4.12. Specialized esophageal pacing generator and preamplifier for recording electrograms from the esophageal electrodes. (Courtesy of Cardiocommand, Inc.)

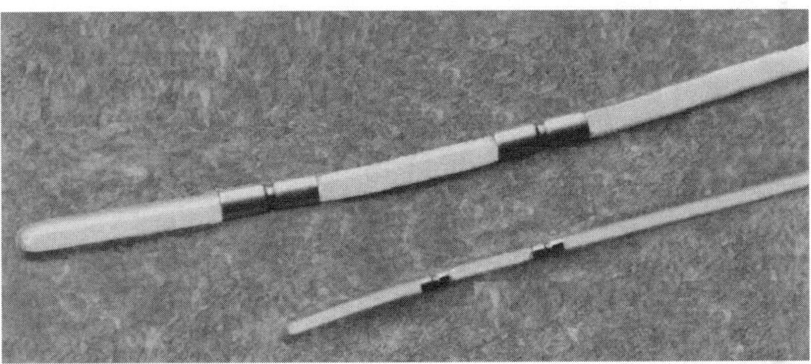

Figure 4.13. Specialized flexible 10-F **(top)** and 5-F **(bottom)** transesophageal pacing catheters. (Courtesy of Cardiocommand, Inc.)

for bipolar transesophageal pacing is directly proportional to 1.4 times the distance separating the excitable tissue from the midpoint between the pacing electrodes.[62] Fluoroscopic and anatomic studies reveal that the minimum distance from the esophagus to the left atrium in humans is 0.5 to 1.5 cm, regardless of left atrial size.[63] Clinically, spacings of 1.0 to 3.0 cm yield comparable atrial pacing thresholds.[64–66]

Transesophageal pacing generators must provide up to 25 to 30 mA of current output into high transesophageal impedances of 700 to 2600 ohms.[64] High-voltage outputs of 40 to 75 V are thereby mandatory for these devices. Stimulation pulse width should be up to 10 to 20 milliseconds to minimize pacing thresholds.[62,67] The short pulse width (1 to 2 milliseconds) and low voltages (12 to 15 V) provided by temporary transvenous pacing generators are not adequate for transesophageal pacing.

To initiate transesophageal pacing, the electrode is introduced orally or nasally, then advanced distally through the esophagus into proximity with the left atrium. Aspiration precautions should be observed during esophageal intubation, and other esophageal catheters should be removed if possible. Topical anesthesia to the nares and pharynx is recommended. The optimal esophageal site for atrial pacing is then identified by the esophageal electrode position recording the largest peak-to-peak atrial electrogram (Fig. 4.14).[67] Unipolar or bipolar electrograms may be used by connecting an electrode pole to lead V_1 (unipolar) or to each arm lead (bipolar) of a standard ECG recorder. After introduction to 30 to 40 cm from the teeth or nares, the lead is moved proximally and distally until the largest atrial electrogram is recorded.[68] This site averages 35 to 40 cm from the teeth or nares in most adult studies.[66,67] The most favorable electrode position for transesophageal ventricular pacing is less well defined but appears to lie 2 to 4 cm distal to the best site for atrial pacing.[69] A ventricular electrogram should be recorded from sites of attempted ventricular pacing; otherwise, the ventricular electrogram amplitude is not helpful.

Once positioned, the electrodes are connected to the transesophageal pacing generator. Capture thresholds are reduced by cathodal (negative) stimulation through the proximal electrode in bipolar systems.[66] Ventricular capture must be excluded before attempting rapid atrial pacing. Virtually all patients experience at least a mild thoracic burning sensation with effective current outputs. Once capture is achieved, the lead is taped securely to the patient's nose or chin.

In most large series, the incidence of atrial capture with transesophageal pacing equals or approaches 100% with mean current thresholds of 8 to 14 mA.[62,64,70] Atrial capture thresholds are not influenced by age, height, weight, body surface area, left atrial size, previous coronary bypass surgery, presence of structural heart disease, or size of recorded atrial electrograms in most studies.[71,72] Thresholds greater than 15 mA are frequently associated with increased patient discomfort.

Ventricular capture using transesophageal pacing is unreliable. Using conventional transesophageal electrodes and pacing generators, ventricular capture is successful only in 3% to 60% of patients.[70–73] Because the stimulating current density declines exponentially with distance from the bipolar current source, the ventricle, typically approximately 3 cm from the esophagus, receives only 20% of the current density achieved at the left atrium during transesophageal pacing.[62,71]

Serious complications of transesophageal pacing are limited to induction of ventricular tachyarrhythmias during rapid atrial pacing in three patients.[71,74] No long-term pacing complications have been reported. Virtually all patients experience mild chest or back pain, or a sensation of burning or indigestion during pacing at outputs less than 15 mA. Endoscopy following transesophageal pacing may reveal focal pressure necrosis typical of any indwelling esophageal

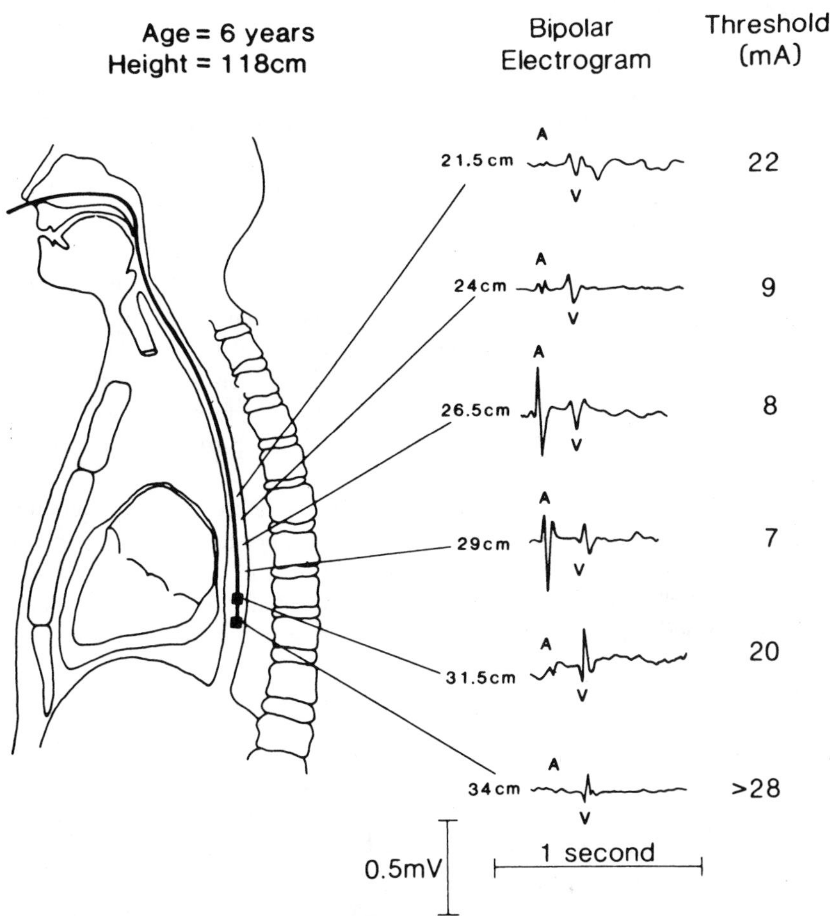

Figure 4.14. Illustration depicting transesophageal cardiac electrograms obtained from various catheter insertion depths in a 6-year-old child. A = atrial electrogram; V = ventricular electrogram. Minimal transesophageal atrial pacing thresholds correspond to electrode positions recording the atrial electrograms of largest amplitude. (Reproduced by permission from the American Heart Association from Benson DW. Transesophageal electrocardiography and cardiac pacing: state of the art. Circulation 1987;75 (suppl 3):86–90.)

catheter in up to 11% of patients.[71] No significant esophageal trauma had been reported in humans despite pacing up to 60 hours.[75] Aspiration is a potential complication of any esophageal intubation procedure. Diaphragmatic or phrenic nerve pacing may occur in 1% to 8% of patients, especially with distal esophageal catheter positions.[70,76] Coughing may be induced with proximal catheter positions due to tracheal stimulation, and brachial plexus stimulation has been reported in infants.[77]

MECHANICAL CARDIAC PACING

Mechanical cardiac pacing techniques stimulate myocardial tissue by direct or transmitted physical forces. Clinically, these techniques include percussion pacing (chest thumps) administered by a medical attendant and cough-induced cardiac resuscitation performed by patients themselves. Although they are lacking in technical sophistication, these techniques persist as useful clinical maneuvers by virtue of their sheer simplicity and immediacy of application.

Percussion pacing for bradyarrhythmias is performed by delivering sharp blows to the middle to lower two-thirds of the patient's sternum with the ulnar aspect of the fist.[78] The blows may be repeated serially at a rate of approximately 60 to 90 per minute, depending on the duration of bradycardia and the cardiac response (Fig. 4.15). True ventricular depolarization and mechanical response must be documented by palpitation of a pulse because percussion artifacts may convincingly simulate QRS complexes.[79] A true cardiac pulse must be differentiated from the transmitted percussion wave.

The myocardial response to external mechanical pacing depends on the duration of bradyasystolic arrest and the metabolic state of the myocardium. Percussion pacing is most successful very early in the course of witnessed arrests; in this setting it usually elicits a single myocardial depolarization for each blow delivered. As myocardial hypoxia and ischemia intervene, the evoked QRS

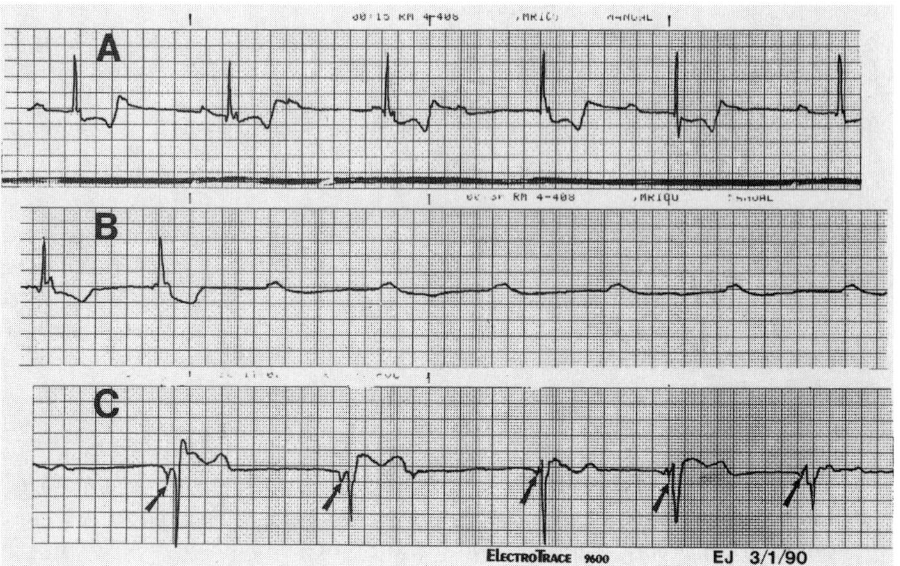

Figure 4.15. Percussion pacing during asystolic cardiac arrest. **A:** High-degree atrioventricular block with slow ventricular escape rhythm. **B:** Onset of ventricular asystole with continued atrial activity. **C:** Percussion pacing artifacts (*arrows*) each followed by ventricular depolarization.

complexes widen and occur in salvos or extended runs. Further metabolic compromise is associated with loss of QRS voltage, appearance of injury patterns, induction of ventricular fibrillation, and, eventually, failure of response.[80] If percussion pacing initially fails, repeated attempts after the administration of chest compressions and inotropic agents may be successful.[81]

Percussion pacing has sustained patients for up to 60 minutes as the sole mechanism of cardiac stimulation.[80] Single and serial chest blows have also been used to terminate ventricular tachycardia in humans.[82]

Cough-induced cardiac resuscitation is another mechanical means of generating cardiac output.[83,84] A forceful cough can generate up to 25 J of kinetic energy within the chest cavity.[84] It is unclear whether this energy induces myocardial contraction or whether cardiac output is produced by compression of intrathoracic structures with up to 250 to 450 mm Hg of pressure generated by the cough.[84]

To perform this maneuver, the conscious patient is instructed to cough *forcefully* every 1 to 3 seconds until an effective native rhythm returns or definitive treatment is administered. Paroxysms of coughing are ineffective. Clinically, cough-induced resuscitation has maintained aortic systolic blood pressures above 130 mm Hg during ventricular fibrillation as opposed to only 60 mm Hg during external chest compressions in the same patients.[83] Patients performing cough-induced resuscitation during ventricular fibrillation have remained conscious for up to 92 seconds.[83] The technique has the disadvantage of requiring a conscious patient who is able to immediately generate effective coughs within seconds of the onset of bradycardia.

SELECTION OF THE OPTIMAL TEMPORARY PACING TECHNIQUE

The urgency to initiate temporary cardiac pacing is the foremost consideration in selecting among the available techniques. For prophylactic and nonemergency applications, the duration of pacing, comfort of the patient, and desire to avoid specific complications also become significant. In emergency situations of bradyasystolic arrest, delayed recovery of an effective cardiac rhythm beyond 5 minutes virtually precludes successful resuscitation. In these situations, *rapid* initiation of *ventricular* pacing is paramount to other considerations. Although transvenous pacing has traditionally served as the mainstay of emergency temporary pacing, the significant time and operator skill needed to implement the technique are less than ideal. Transcutaneous pacing has provided an extremely rapid, simple, and noninvasive alternative to emergency transvenous pacing. The incidence of ventricular capture during arrest is quite variable for both techniques.

Given the narrow therapeutic time constraints in bradyasystolic arrest, one should proceed with the mode of pacing that will effect ventricular pacing *most rapidly*. Attempts at transcutaneous pacing neither interrupt nor impede performance of cardiopulmonary resuscitation (CPR), and it is usually feasible to attempt transcutaneous pacing while preparations are made for more invasive techniques.

Table 4.8. Comparison of Temporary Pacing Techniques

	Transvenous	Transcutaneous	Transesophageal	Epicardial	Percussion	Cough CPR
Time to initiate	3–10 min	<1 min	minutes	<1 min	immediate	immediate
Training	extensive	minimal	moderate	minimal	minimal	minimal
Chambers paced	atrium and/or ventricle	ventricle	atrium, possibly ventricle	atrium and/or ventricle	ventricle	none
Emergency use	+	+	–	+ if wires in	+	+
Prophylactic use	+	+	–	+	–	–
Prolonged use	+	–	–	+	–	–
Vascular injury	+	–	–	–	–	–
Arrhythmias	+	–	–	–	+	–
Infection	+	–	–	–	–	–
Discomfort	–	+	+	–	+	–
Comments	most versatile and reliable	fast, safe, easy	primarily atrial pacing	postoperative use only	witnessed brady-cardic arrest	cooperative patient, supports ventricular fibrillation

For prophylactic use, transcutaneous pacing is the method of choice, given its high efficacy combined with virtual absence of complications. Patient discomfort during pacing represents the only disadvantage. Temporary transvenous pacing, although invasive, provides well-tolerated and generally reliable atrial and/or ventricular pacing for extended periods of time. Transesophageal pacing is suitable for elective *atrial* pacing applications. Patient discomfort is sometimes a problem, but complications are exceptionally rare. Ventricular capture requires painfully high current outputs, but intraoperative use appears feasible.

Mechanical and cough-induced resuscitation techniques are limited to very brief applications. Nevertheless, cough-induced resuscitation is an effective and standard maneuver during asystole induced by coronary angiography. A comparison of the available temporary pacing techniques is shown in Table 4.8.

REFERENCES

1. Falk RH, Ngai STA. External cardiac pacing: influence of electrode placement on pacing threshold. Crit Care Med 1986;14:931–932.
2. Sado DM, Deakin CD, Petley GW, Clewlow F. Comparison of the effects for removal of chest hair with doing nothing before external defibrillation on transthoracic impedance. Am J Cardiol 2004;93:98–100.
3. Madsen JK, Pedersen F, Grande P, Meiborn J. Normal myocardial enzymes and normal echocardiographic findings during noninvasive transcutaneous pacing. Pacing Clin Electrophysiol 1988;11:1188–1193.
4. Klein LS, Miles WM, Heger JJ, Zipes DP. Transcutaneous pacing: patient tolerance, strength–interval relations and feasibility for programmed electrical stimulation. Am J Cardiol 1988;62:1126–1129.
5. Zoll PM, Zoll RH, Falk RH, et al. External noninvasive temporary cardiac pacing: clinical trials. Circulation 1985;71:937–944.
6. Falk RH, Ngai STA, Kumanki DJ, Rubinstein JA. Cardiac activation during external cardiac pacing. Pacing Clin Electrophysiol 1987;10:503–506.
7. Kelly JS, Royster RL, Angert KC, Case LD. Efficacy of noninvasive transcutaneous cardiac pacing in patients undergoing cardiac surgery. Anesth Analg 1989;70: 747–751.
8. Luck JC, Grubb BP, Artman SE, et al. Termination of sustained ventricular tachycardia by external noninvasive pacing. Am J Cardiol 1988;61:574–577.
9. Hedges JR, Syverud SA, Dalsey WC, et al. Threshold, enzymatic, and pathologic changes associated with prolonged transcutaneous pacing in a chronic heart block model. J Emerg Med 1989;7:1–4.
10. Feldman MD, Zoll PM, Aroesty JM, et al. Hemodynamic responses to noninvasive external cardiac pacing. Am J Med 1988;84:395–400.
11. Trigano JA, Remond JM, Mourot F, et al. Left ventricular pressure measurement during noninvasive transcutaneous cardiac pacing. Pacing Clin Electrophysiol 1989;12:1717–1719.
12. Murdock DK, Moran JF, Speranza D, et al. Augmentation of cardiac output by external cardiac pacing: pacemaker-induced CPR. Pacing Clin Electrophysiol 1986;9: 127–129.
13. Falk RH, Zoll PM, Zoll RH. Safety and efficacy of noninvasive cardiac pacing: a preliminary report. N Engl J Med 1983;309:1166–1168.

14. Altamura G, Bianconi L, Boccadamo R, Pistalese M. Treatment of ventricular and supraventricular tachyarrhythmias by transcutaneous cardiac pacing. Pacing Clin Electrophysiol 1989;12:331–338.
15. Zoll PM. Resuscitation of the heart in ventricular standstill by external electrical stimulation. N Engl J Med 1952;247:768–771.
16. Estes M, Deering TF, Manolis AS, et al. External cardiac programmed stimulation for noninvasive termination of sustained supraventricular and ventricular tachycardia. Am J Cardiol 1989;63:177–183.
17. Beland MJ, Hesslein PS, Rowe RD. Ventricular tachycardia related to transcutaneous pacing. Ann Emerg Med 1988;17:279–281.
18. Voorhees WD III, Foster KS, Geddes LA, Babbs CF. Safety factor for precordial pacing: minimum current thresholds for pacing and for ventricular fibrillation by vulnerable-period stimulation. Pacing Clin Electrophysiol 1984;7:356–360.
19. Francis GS, Williams SV, Achord JL, et al. Clinical competence in insertion of a temporary transvenous ventricular pacemaker. J Am Coll Cardiol 1994;23:1254–1257.
20. de Cock CC, Van Campen LC, Visser CA. Usefulness of a new active-fixation lead in transvenous temporary pacing from the femoral approach. PACE 2003;26: 849–852.
21. de Cock CC, Van Campen LC, In't Veld JA, Visser CA. Utility and safety of prolonged temporary transvenous pacing using and active-fixation lead: Comparison with a conventional lead. PACE 2003;26:1245–1248.
22. Simpson C, Yee R, Lee J, et al. Clinical evaluation of a new active fixation temporary cardiac pacing lead. Circulation 1998;98:I-427.
23. Syverud SA, Dalsey WC, Hedges JR, Hanseits ML. Radiologic assessment of transvenous pacemaker placement during CPR. Ann Emerg Med 1986;15:131–137.
24. Goldberger J, Kruse J, Ehlert FA, Kadish A. Temporary transvenous pacemaker placement: what criteria constitute an adequate pacing site? Am Heart J 1993;126: 488–493.
25. Kaemmerer H, Kochs M, Hombach V. Ultrasound-guided positioning of temporary pacing catheters and pulmonary artery catheters after echogenic marking. Clin Intensive Care 1993;4:4–7.
26. Lang R, David D, Klein HO, et al. The use of the balloon-tipped floating catheter in temporary transvenous cardiac pacing. Pacing Clin Electrophysiol 1981;4: 491–496.
27. Furman S, Hurzeler P, Mehra R. Cardiac pacing and pacemakers. IV. Threshold of cardiac stimulation. Am Heart J 1977;94:115–124.
28. Gulotta SJ. Transvenous cardiac pacing: techniques for optimal electrode positioning and prevention of coronary sinus placement. Circulation 1970;42:701–718.
29. Castellanos A, Maytin O, Lemberg L, Castillo C. Unusual QRS complexes produced by pacemaker stimuli with special reference to myocardial tunneling and coronary sinus stimulation. Am Heart J 1969;77:732–742.
30. Coman JA, Trohman RG. Incidence and electrocardiographic localization of safe right bundle branch block configuration during permanent ventricular pacing. Am J Cardiol 1995;76:781–784.
31. Befeler B, Hildner FJ, Javier RP, et al. Cardiovascular dynamics during coronary sinus, right atrial, and right ventricular pacing. Am Heart J 1971;81:372–380.
32. Benchimol A, Ellis JG, Dimond EG. Hemodynamic consequences of atrial and ventricular pacing in patients with normal and abnormal hearts. Am J Med 1965;39:911–922.

33. Hartzler GO, Maloney JD, Curtis JJ, Barnhorst DA. Hemodynamic benefits of atrioventricular sequential pacing after cardiac surgery. Am J Cardiol 1977;40:232–236.
34. Hazard PB, Benton C, Milnor JP. Transvenous cardiac pacing in cardiopulmonary resuscitation. Crit Care Med 1981;9:666–668.
35. Phillips SJ, Butner AN. Percutaneous transvenous cardiac pacing initiated at bedside: results in 40 cases. J Thorac Cardiovasc Surg 1970;59:855–858.
36. Davis MJE. Emergency ventricular pacing using a J-electrode without fluoroscopy. Med J Aust 1990;152:194.
37. Preston TA, Fletcher RD, Luccesi BR, Judge RD. Changes in myocardial threshold. Physiologic and pharmacologic factors in patients with implanted pacemakers. Am Heart J 1967;74:235–242.
38. Sowton E, Barr I. Physiologic changes in threshold. Ann NY Acad Sci 1969;167: 678–685.
39. Krueger SK, Rakes S, Wilkerson J, et al. Temporary pacemaking by general internists. Arch Intern Med 1983;143:1531–1533.
40. Austin JL, Preis LK, Crampton RS, et al. Analysis of pacemaker malfunction and complications of temporary pacing in the coronary care unit. Am J Cardiol 1982;49:301–306.
41. Lumia FJ, Rios JC. Temporary transvenous pacemaker therapy an analysis of complications. Chest 1973;64:604–608.
42. Harvey JR, Wyman RM, McKay RG, Baim DS. Use of balloon flotation pacing catheters for prophylactic temporary pacing during diagnostic and therapeutic catheterization procedures. Am J Cardiol 1988;62:941–944.
43. Silver MD, Goldschlager N. Temporary transvenous cardiac pacing in the critical care setting. Chest 1988;93:607–613.
44. Paulk EA, Hurst JW. Complete heart block in acute myocardial infarction. Am J Cardiol 1966;17:695–706.
45. Hynes JK, Holmes DR Jr, Harrison CE. Five-year experience with temporary pacemaker therapy in the coronary care unit. Mayo Clin Proc 1983;58:122–126.
46. Jowett NI, Thompson DR, Pohl JEF. Temporary transvenous cardiac pacing: a year's experience in one coronary care unit. Postgrad Med J 1989;65:211–215.
47. Lehmann MH, Cameron A, Kemp HG Jr. Increased risk of ventricular fibrillation associated with temporary pacemaker use during coronary arteriography. Pacing Clin Electrophysiol 1983;6:923–928.
48. Mooss AN, Ross WB, Esterbrooks DJ, et al. Ventricular fibrillation complicating pacemaker insertion in acute myocardial infarction. Cath Cardiovasc Diag 1982;8: 253–259.
49. Weinstein J, Gnoj J, Mazzara JT, et al. Temporary transvenous pacing via the percutaneous femoral vein approach. Am Heart J 1973;85:695–705.
50. Nathan DA, Center S, Pina RE, et al. Perforation during indwelling catheter pacing. Circulation 1966;33:128–130.
51. Van Durme JP, Heyndrickx G, Snoeck J, et al. Diagnosis of myocardial perforation by intracardiac electrograms recorded from the indwelling catheter. J Electrocard 1973;6:97–102.
52. Nolewajka AJ, Goddard MD, Broun TC. Temporary transvenous pacing and femoral vein thrombosis. Circulation 1980;62:646–650.
53. Sanders P, Farouque O, Ashby DT, Mahar LJ, Young GD. Effects of anticoagulation on the occurrence of deep venous thrombosis associated with temporary transvenous femoral pacemakers. Am J Cardiol 2001;88:798–801.

54. Elmi F, Tullo N, Khalighi K. Natural history and predictors of temporary epicardial pacemaker wire function in patients after open heart surgery. Cardiology 2002;98: 175–180.
67. Cohen SI, Smith KL. Transfemoral cardiac pacing and phlebitis. Circulation 1974;49:1018–1019.
68. Roe BB, Katz HJ. Complete heart block with intractable asystole and recurrent ventricular fibrillation with survival. Am J Cardiol 1965;15:401–403.
55. Scherhag A, Gulbins H, Lange R, Saggaw W. Improved reliability of postoperative cardiac pacing by use of bipolar temporary pacing leads. Eur JCPE 1995;5:101–108.
56. Janousek J, Hucin B, Tlaskai T, et al. Resynchronization pacing is a useful adjunct to the management of acute heart failure after surgery for congenital heart defects. Am J Cardiol 2001;88:145–152.
57. Anselmi M, Golia G, Rossi A, et al. Feasibility and safety of transesophageal atrial pacing stress echocardiography in patients with known or suspected coronary artery disease. Am J Cardiol 2003;92:1384–1388.
58. Hessling G, Brockmeier K, Ulmer HE. Transesophageal electrocardiography and atrial pacing in children. J Electrocardiol 2003;35(suppl):143–149.
59. Romano R, Ciccaglioni A, Rocco A, et al. Transesophageal atrial pacing in the management of re-entry supraventricular tachyarrhythmias occurring during general anesthesia. Minerva Anesthesiol 2003;68:825–829.
60. Atar S, Nagai T, Cecek B, et al. Pacing stress echocardiography: an alternative to pharmacologic stress testing. J Am Coll Cardiol 200;36:1935–1941.
61. Atar S, Nagai T, Cecek B, et al. Transthoracic stress echocardiography with transesophageal atrial pacing for bedside evaluation of inducible myocardial ischemia in patients with new-onset chest pain. Am J Cardiol 2000;86:12–16.
62. Arzbacher R, Jenkins JM. A review of the theoretical and experimantal bases of transesophageal atrial pacing. J Electrocardiol 2002;35(suppl):137–141.
63. Binkley PF, Bush CA, Kolibash AJ, et al. The anatomic relationship of the esophageal lead to the left atrium. Pacing Clin Electrophysiol 1982;5:853–859.
64. Kerr CR, Chung DC, Wickham G, et al. Impedance to transesophageal atrial pacing: significance regarding power sources. Pacing Clin Electrophysiol 1989;12:930–935.
65. Benson DW. Transesophageal electrocardiography and cardiac pacing: state of the art. Circulation 1987;75(suppl 3):86–92.
66. Nishimura M, Katoh T, Hanai S, Watanabe Y. Optimal mode of transesophageal atrial pacing. Am J Cardiol 1986;57:791–796.
67. Benson DW, Sanford M, Dunnigan A, Benditt DG. Transesophageal atrial pacing threshold: role of interelectrode spacing, pulse width, and catheter insertion depth. Am J Cardiol 1984;53:63–67.
68. Hammill SC, Pritchett ELC. Simplified esophageal electrocardiography using bipolar recording leads. Ann Intern Med 1981;95:14–18.
69. Andersen HR, Pless P. Transesophageal pacing. Pacing Clin Electrophysiol 1983;6: 674–679.
70. Gallagher JJ, Smith WM, Kerr CR, et al. Esophageal pacing: a diagnostic and therapeutic tool. Circulation 1982;65:336–341.
71. Dick M, Campbell RM, Jenkins JM. Thresholds for transesophageal atrial pacing. Cath Cardiovasc Diag 1984;10:507–513.
72. Buchanan D, Clements F, Reves JG, et al. Atrial esophageal pacing in patients undergoing coronary artery bypass grafting: effect of previous cardiac operations and body surface area. Anesth Analg 1988;69:595–598.

73. Lubell DL. Cardiac pacing from the esophagus. Am J Cardiol 1971;27:641–644.
74. Favale S, Di Biase M, Rizzo U, et al. Ventricular fibrillation induced by transesophageal atrial pacing in hypertrophic cardiomyopathy. Eur Heart J 1987;8: 912–916.
75. Burack B, Furman S. Transesophageal cardiac pacing. Am J Cardiol 1969;23:469–472.
76. Backofen JE, Schauble JF, Rogers MC. Transesophageal pacing for bradycardia. Anesth Analg 1984;61:777–779.
77. Benson DW, Dunnigan A, Benditt DG, Schneider SP. Transesophageal cardiac pacing: history, application, technique. Clin Prog Pacing Electrophysiol 1984;2:360–372.
78. Chester WL. Spinal anesthesia, complete heart block and the precordial thump: an unusual complication and a unique resuscitation. Anesth Analg 1988;69:600–602.
79. Skaaland K. Effect of chest pounding: electrocardiographic pattern. Lancet 1972;1: 1121–1122.
80. Scherf D, Bornemann C. Thumping of the precordium in ventricular standstill. Am J Cardiol 1960;5:30–40.
81. Iseri LT, Allen BJ, Baron K, Brodsky MA. Fist pacing, a forgotten procedure in bradysystolic cardiac arrest. Am Heart J 1987;113:1545–1550.
82. Margera T, Baldi N, Chersevani D, et al. Chest thump and ventricular tachycardia. Pacing Clin Electrophysiol 1979;2:69–75.
83. Criley JM, Blaufuss AH, Kissel GL. Cough-induced cardiac compression: self-administered form of cardiopulmonary resuscitation. JAMA 1976;236:1246–1250.
84. Wei JY, Greene HL, Weisfeldt ML. Cough-facilitated conversion of ventricular tachycardia. Am J Cardiol 1980;45:174–176.

Techniques of Pacemaker Implantation and Removal

Jeffrey Brinker and Mark G. Midei

5

A permanent pacing system consists of the pacemaker generator and the one or more leads that connect it to the endocardial or epicardial surface of the heart. Because of the initial mandate for epicardial lead placement, pacemaker implantation has traditionally been the task of the surgeon. Considerable evolution in technique and hardware has occurred over the past three decades, which has greatly simplified the implantation procedure. The introduction of relatively simple and safe methods of central venous access has facilitated the almost universal adoption of transvenous leads, which have proven to be the most reliable means of pacing the heart. Associated with this has been a miniaturization of the power source and circuitry of the generator such that its subcutaneous placement has become less demanding even in the very young or elderly.

Compared to the need to formulate optimal programming prescriptions and interpret complex electrocardiography (ECG)–pacer–patient interactions, the implantation of a modern sophisticated microprocessor based pacemaker may now be the least arduous aspect of pacing. Reflecting these changes has been the increasingly predominant role of the cardiologist, the electrophysiologist particularly, in the implantation process. It would be inappropriate however to give one the impression that all pacemaker implantation is easy, as any implanter faced with the challenges of biventricular pacemaking can attest to. This form of therapy, discussed in the chapter on cardiac resynchronization therapy, is designed to improve hemodynamics in certain patients with dilated cardiomyopathy. It requires left ventricular pacing, which is achieved by insertion of a lead into the coronary venous system. Establishing a stable lead position with good pacing characteristics in an appropriate coronary vein can be difficult requiring prolonged procedure times and considerable X-ray exposure. The learning curve, albeit truncated by the relatively rapid evolution of better leads and delivery systems, is remarkably similar to that of the early days of ventricular endocardial pacing.

In this chapter, transvenous pacemaker implantation for the typical indications (i.e., bradycardia) is examined from a broad perspective that emphasizes the practical considerations influencing the safety and efficacy of this procedure. In addition, because the physician must assume some long-term responsibility for the hardware he or she implants, the indications for and methodology of removing implanted pacing devices are reviewed.

PHYSICIAN QUALIFICATIONS

Although the practice of pacing overlaps a spectrum of the specialties of medicine and surgery, there has been a dramatic shift to non-surgeons with the evolution of technology. In general formal training in the implantation of arrhythmia control devices is confined to electrophysiology fellowship programs. There remains, however, a large number of non-electrophysiologists who implant devices either alone or as part of a team; for example, a surgeon obtains vascular access and makes a pocket while a physician places the lead, tests electrical parameters, and provides the follow-up evaluations. Although some nonsurgeons are becoming more aggressive in learning to perform certain procedural variations such as inframammary or subpectoral dissections, some still depend on their surgical colleagues for assistance in these more complicated situations.

Procedural success and safety is determined by the skill and experience of the operator. Although the degree of "surgery" required for a routine transvenous implantation is modest, good surgical technique is essential. Experience is also necessary to ensure proper positioning of leads so that optimal stability and performance are obtained. A physician wishing to implant pacing systems independently should perform a sufficient number of procedures under the supervision of an accomplished operator to gain the skill and confidence necessary for independent work. The minimal number of cases to credential a physician depends on the physician's prior familiarity with intravascular catheterization, surgical technique, and knowledge of the principles of pacing. This experience should include single-chamber and dual-chamber systems and use of both the subclavian and cephalic approaches for venous access. In addition to this initial exposure, there should be the expectation that a reasonable number of implantations will be performed over time to maintain a level of proficiency. Optimally, this number should be 30 procedures per year; a minimal number might be 10 to 15.[1] Guidelines for training in pacemaking have been published that, although directed at the fellowship experience, may serve as a more general model.[2] The guidelines acknowledge the special training necessary for those seeking credentials in biventricular pacing, defibrillator implantation, and lead extraction. Because fluoroscopic imaging is a necessary component of the implantation process, knowledge of the basics of radiation physics and safety is required to minimize risk to the patient and operator.

If a team approach to implantation is taken, the role of each member must be clearly delineated. Although this may be obvious during the procedure, the responsibility for performance of peri-procedural tasks such as writing orders, checking laboratory tests, adjusting the pacemaker, and arranging follow-up evaluations may be less clear.

Specialty assistance may be anticipated before a procedure in some cases, and appropriate consultation should be obtained. This might include enlisting the aid of a plastic surgeon for a procedure in a young woman or a pediatrician to help with a child. Implantation procedures are generally performed under conscious sedation, but on occasion there may be a need for support by anesthesiology. Operating physicians should be familiar with the principles of conscious sedation and the particular institutional guidelines under which they are employed, including the acceptable drugs (dosages, reversibility) and the necessary support personnel, monitoring equipment, and recovery procedures.

Quality assurance has become a necessary part of every hospital's activities; procedures and the physicians who perform them are most thoroughly scrutinized. It is the responsibility of all physicians to be conscious of the quality of their work; those in administrative positions must ensure that proper databases are maintained and performance evaluations are carried out. The objective of these practices is improved quality of care, which may be accomplished at many levels.[3]

LOGISTICAL REQUIREMENTS

The logistical requirements for pacemaker implantation are relatively modest. The procedure may be carried out in an operating room, a catheterization laboratory, or a special procedure room with no compromise of success rate or difference in complications.[4] Implantation by non-surgeons in the cardiac catheterization laboratory has been shown to result in a significant reduction in the cost and pre-implant hospital stay compared to implants in the operating room by surgeons.[5] This is likely due to the increased flexibility in scheduling in the catheterization laboratory as well as the use of conscious sedation administered by catheterization laboratory personnel instead of anesthesia staff. The procedure room should be adequate in size and well lighted, and it should comply with all the electrical safety requirements for intravascular catheterization. The radiographic equipment should function within accepted guidelines, and appropriate shielding must be available and used.

In addition to the operator, the staff should include qualified individuals to monitor the ECG and help with the imaging equipment. A nurse (who may perform one of the aforementioned tasks) is required to prepare and administer medications. Often a representative of a pacemaker company is present to provide technical assistance, such as operating the pacing system analyzer or device programming. These individuals may be a valuable source of information but should not be considered a substitute for a nurse or laboratory technologist during the implant procedure.

An adequate imaging system is an important requirement of the pacemaker laboratory. The image intensifier may be portable or fixed but must be capable of rotation so that oblique and lateral views of the areas of interest (which may extend from the neck to the groin) can be obtained. A mechanism for magnification is helpful for situations such as confirmation of extension of the helix of active-fixation leads, lead removal procedures, and the identification of problems such as fractures of a conductor or "J" retention wire. Digital acquisition and storage capabilities have proven to be advantageous. Such technology can be used to road-map or superimpose real-time fluoroscopy on a stored image. Thus, we can bring up a stored image of the subclavian venogram (obtained by injecting contrast into an ipsilateral upper extremity vein) to document the vein patency and to serve as a target for an exploring needle being advanced under fluoroscopic monitoring (Fig. 5.1). The use of pulsed digital fluoroscopy can reduce radiation exposure to patient and operator. Newer imaging systems may also increase patient safety by providing on-line measurements that more accurately reflect radiation exposure than does the traditional total fluoroscopy time.

The patient table should be flat, radiolucent, and configured in such a way that the operator may work on either side (and perhaps at either end). Movement of the imaging system about the support should be unhindered. A

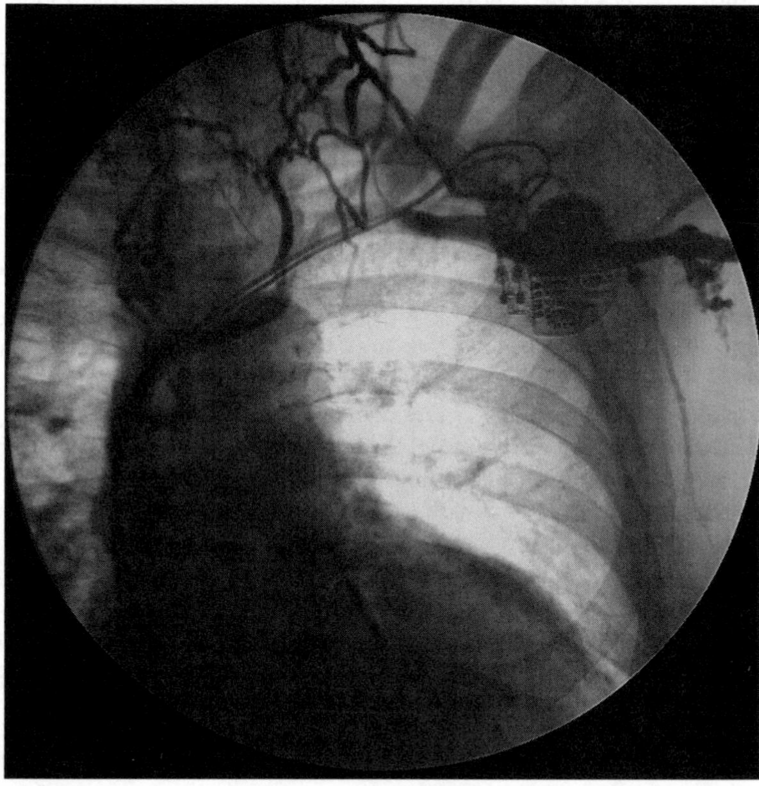

Figure 5.1. Venography may be helpful in documenting the patency of venous structures. This study shows complete occlusion of the subclavian vein with extensive collateral vein formation. This information would clearly be important when planning for procedures requiring new venous access.

mechanism to assume Trendelenburg and reverse Trendelenburg positions is advantageous, although in an emergency this can be quickly accomplished with the use of foam wedges.

It is essential that the ECG be continuously monitored; a simultaneous multi-lead display that is easily visualized is preferable. There should be an ability to obtain a hard copy of the monitored rhythm strip as well as a complete 12-lead tracing if necessary. Leads placed on the chest or back should consist of radiolucent electrodes and wires. Special electrodes having the capability of monitoring the ECG, delivering a direct current defibrillatory shock, or transcutaneously pacing the patient may be used. These should be connected to an appropriate device capable of performing these tasks so that the electrical therapies can be achieved expeditiously if necessary. A mechanism for monitoring blood pressure throughout the procedure is necessary; this may be achieved by using an automated noninvasive device. Pulse oximetry is now also considered essential in providing information about the respiratory status of a heavily sedated patient or one in whom a complication (e.g., air embolism or pneumothorax) may occur. A portable ultrasound device is helpful in identifying vascular structures and provide guidance for venous access.

The surgical instruments required for the procedure depend on the demands of the particular procedure and operator. A pacemaker tray may be derived from the hospital's surgical cutdown set and supplemented in accordance to the specifics of the case. Add-ons include tear-away vascular introducer sets, appropriate cables to connect to a pacing system analyzer (PSA), suction, and electrocautery. The operator should be familiar with the guidelines for electrocautery use to ensure safety, particularly when oxygen is being administered.

An adequate supply and variety of pacing hardware should be available, including not only pacemakers and leads but also sheaths, stylets, lead adapters, sterile lubricant, adhesive, and the like. It is good practice to have at least two of every item on hand in case of accidental damage or loss of sterility.

The PSA (Fig. 5.2) provides a mechanism to measure a variety of pacing parameters (capture and sensing threshold, lead impedance, electrograms, slew rate) that are essential in determining the adequacy of lead position and integrity. A direct digital readout and the capability to print a hard copy are desirable. Some manufacturers have consolidated products by configuring their programmers to act as PSAs when necessary. Equipment necessary for emergency pericardiocentesis and temporary endocardial pacing must be at hand, and it is advantageous to have prompt access to a two-dimensional echocardiography machine. A crash cart containing resuscitative supplies (including those necessary to establish endotracheal intubation), an adequate supply of all appropriate drugs, and experienced staff must be immediately available should complications occur.

ASSESSMENT OF THE PATIENT

The implantation process begins with a thorough evaluation of the patient. This should include reviewing medical records, obtaining a pertinent history (includ-

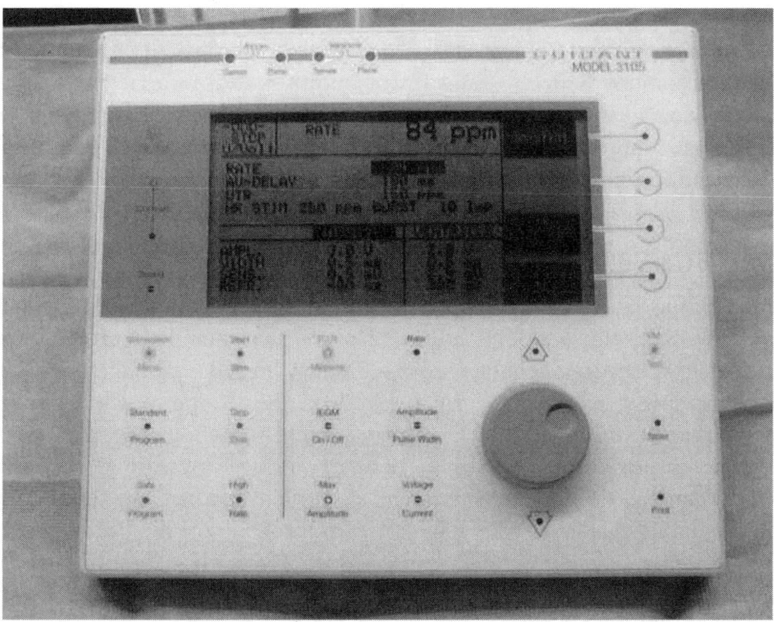

Figure 5.2. Guidant Pacing System Analyzer (PSA). This device can measure capture and sensing thresholds and display intracardiac electrograms. (Courtesy of Guidant.)

ing current medications, especially warfarin (Coumadin), and previous reactions to drugs and contrast material), performing a physical examination, and acquiring the basic laboratory tests.

The indication for pacing should be clear and characterized in accordance with the American College of Cardiology/American Heart Association guidelines.[6] In some situations, it may be reasonable to offer pacemaker therapy for conditions in which the indication for such therapy is controversial and evolving. Examples include, neurally mediated cardioinhibitory syncope, and atrial fibrillation prevention.[7] Documentation of the indication for a pacemaker implantation should be made in the patient's chart and supported by a relevant ECG tracing.

Consideration of the type of pacing system to be used should be part of the initial assessment so that a truly *informed* consent can be obtained. The decision on mode of pacing (e.g., atrial; ventricular; dual-chamber, single- or double-lead; rate-adaptive, biventricular) is made on the basis of the underlying conduction disturbance, the presumed immediate and future need for pacing, and the hemodynamic status of the patient. Other factors that might influence the method of implantation, the operative site, or the type of hardware needed should be delineated before the procedure. Examples include: the need for an unusual approach (e.g., iliac vein), a transatrial procedure, or an epicardial lead system in a patient with a previously documented venous anomaly; employment of an active-fixation ventricular lead in a patient with severe tricuspid regurgitation or corrected transposition of the great vessels; and the use of a steroid lead in a patient with a pacing history complicated by exit block. These factors comprise an extensive series of decisions that must be carefully made well before the patient enters the procedure room (Fig. 5.3). Thorough preparation is critical to minimizing problems at implant.

COST-EFFECTIVENESS

Great emphasis is currently being placed on the cost-effectiveness of medical care, especially those aspects of care that are procedurally centered. Ideally, attention to cost-effectiveness is accompanied by increased quality of care. Hospital administrators have increasingly focused on the throughput of patients, the cost of specific devices, and the level of patient satisfaction. Mechanisms of clinical practice improvement that may reduce cost yet increase the quality of care have been used.[8] Practice guidelines, critical paths, and other methods of standardizing care will likely become more widespread. Physicians must continue to play a leading role in cost constraint without compromising optimal patient care.

INFORMED CONSENT

It is the implanting physician's responsibility to obtain informed consent from the patient (or the patient's family) before the procedure. An honest appraisal of the anticipated risks and benefits, acute and long-term, must be given along with an explanation of alternatives. This should be relevant to the particular individual rather than the average patient. There should be a discussion not only of why pacing is being offered but also of why a particular mode of pacing is being considered. If the indication for pacing is controversial or investigational, more extensive counseling of the patient and documentation of such is necessary. Furthermore, the patients should be advised when there is reason to think that a third-party insurer may not cover the specific indications. The need for lifelong follow-up evaluations should be emphasized, and mention should be made of the eventuality of generator (and possibly lead) replacement. Finally, any physical or occupational restrictions imposed by the presence of a pacemaker should be thoroughly discussed with the patient.

It is good practice for the physician to establish a rapport with the patient and the patient's family. All their questions must be answered and their fears concerning the procedure should be allayed, although it is important that no guarantees regarding outcome be given. The participation of other physicians at the time of implantation or during the follow-up assessments should be described. The various members of the team should be in agreement about all aspects of the procedure so that the presentation to the patient is not confused.

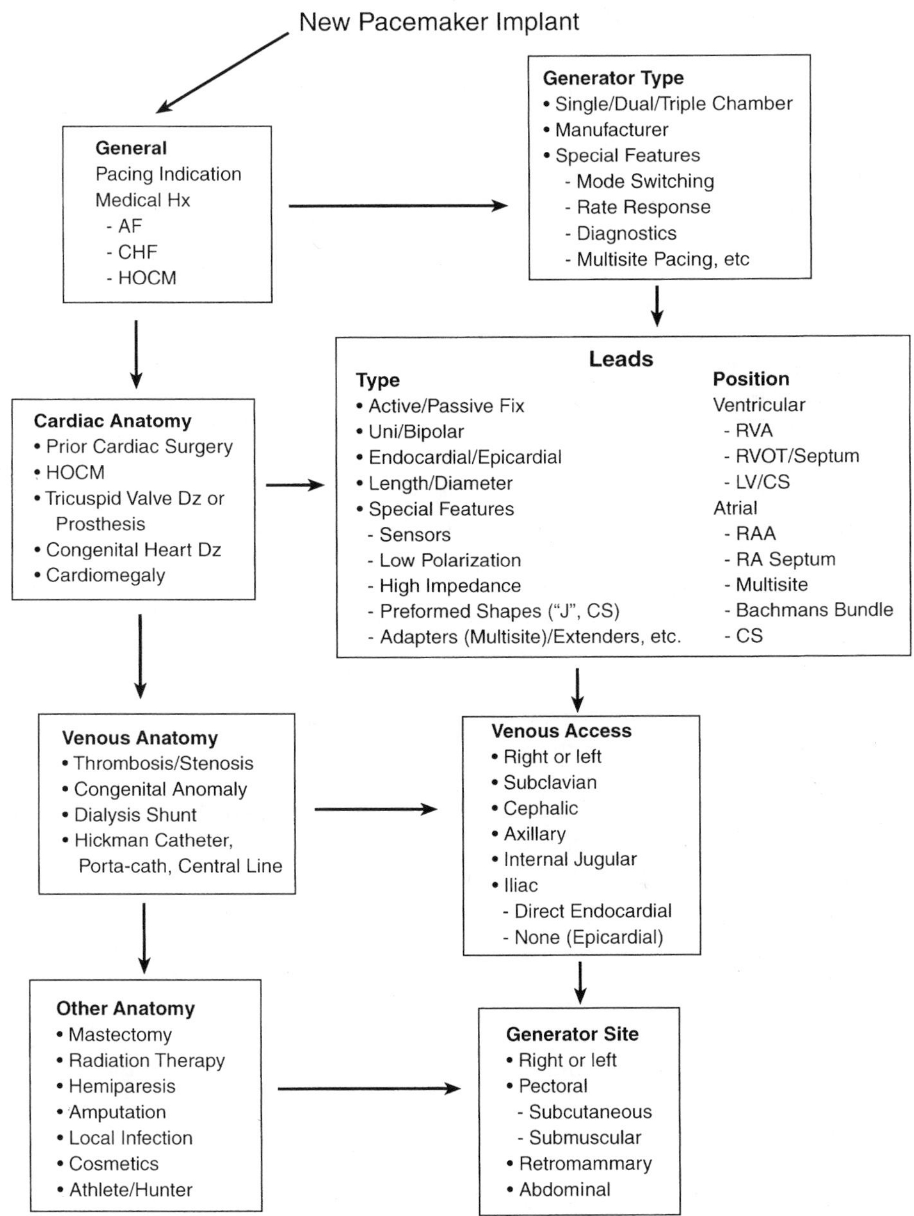

Figure 5.3. Flow chart for decision process surrounding a new pacemaker implant. All decisions should be thoroughly considered before the patient enters the operating room. AF = atrial fibrillation; CHF = congestive heart failure; CS = coronary sinus; Dz = disease; HOCM = hypertrophic obstructive cardiomyopathy; Hx = history; LV = left ventricle; RAA = right atrial appendage; RVA = right ventricular apex; RVOT = right ventricular outflow tract.

PREIMPLANTATION ORDERS

Although outpatient pacemaker implantation can be performed, the usual practice is to admit the patient to the hospital. This may be done on the day of the procedure if the patient's medical condition does not in itself mandate prior hospitalization. Routine pre-implant laboratory tests include a 12-lead ECG, a complete blood cell count (including platelet count), and measures of the prothrombin and activated partial thromboplastin times (aPTT), serum electrolytes, blood urea nitrogen (BUN), and creatinine. It may be valuable to have a recent posteroanterior and lateral chest radiograph to compare to the post-procedure radiographs.

Food is withheld for 6 to 8 hours before the procedure. Hydration is maintained by the establishment of an intravenous line, preferably with a large-bore cannula in a vein of the upper extremity *ipsilateral* to the intended implant site. This will facilitate the injection of contrast should difficulty be encountered in achieving venous access. In general, the patient is allowed to continue whatever medication he or she has been taking, with the obvious exception of anticoagulants, which are stopped prior to the procedure (see subsequent section). The dosage of insulin or oral hypoglycemic drugs may require temporary alteration.

As many as 45% of patients requiring a pacemaker implant may be on oral anticoagulation.[9] Their peri-implant management is often complicated and related to their indication for anticoagulation. There are three general options. The traditional approach has been to convert the patient on oral anticoagulation to intravenous unfractionated heparin. The latter can be stopped 4 to 6 hours before implant if there is concern about the duration of time during which the patient is not effectively anticoagulated (as for example, the presence of a mechanical mitral valve). Implantation is usually performed when the International Normalized Ratio (INR) is 1.2 or less. If necessary, heparin may be restarted 8 to 12 hours after the procedure and warfarin may be reinitiated the day of the procedure or even the night before. It should be understood that intravenous heparin administered within 24 hours after pacer or defibrillator implantation presents a significant risk (up to 20%) of pocket hematoma formation; this risk is five times that encountered in an unanticoagulated patient.[10] Resumption of intravenous anticoagulation should thus be deferred for as long as possible after implant and then only with careful attention to the PTT. Many operators now have abandoned intravenous heparin in favor of transitioning patients on oral anticoagulation to subcutaneously administered low-molecular-weight heparin (LMWH), which may be given up to 12 to 18 hours before planned implantation. This obviates pre-procedural hospitalization and is generally well tolerated. Resumption of warfarin at its maintenance dose post procedure with simultaneous LMWH for 3 to 5 days allows for the outpatient transition back to oral anticoagulation. The risk of post-procedure bleeding with LMWH is thought to be similar to that experienced with unfractionated heparin. There are, however, no randomized controlled trials demonstrating the safety and efficacy of LMWH compared to standard unfractionated heparin for this indication. The third option for managing the patient on warfarin is to perform the procedure without reversal of the anticoagulant. Recently Giudici and colleagues reported excellent results with this strategy in a series of 470 patients having a mean INR of 2.6.[9] The authors used meticulous implantation technique and suggest that the risk of pocket bleeding is not prohibitive because hemostasis in these procedures is primarily a function of capillary vasoconstriction and platelet activity. It should be emphasized, however, that this approach is associated with potential risk and is not, at this time, standard practice.

Antibiotic prophylaxis is controversial, but there has been a suggestion that its use, either systemic or local, decreases the incidence of infection.[11] A meta-analysis of randomized trials that used a systemic antibiotic supports the use of prophylactic antibiotic to prevent infection associated with permanent pacemaker implantation.[12] In an accompanying report, the same investigators suggested that contamination by local flora cultured at the site of implant can result in pacemaker-related infections presenting months later.[13] We routinely give a drug active against *Staphylococcus* (nafcillin, cephalosporin, vancomycin, etc.) before the procedure and for 24 hours after the procedure. Procedures that are prolonged, complicated by potential breaches in sterility, or are "redo" in nature are empirically given slightly longer courses of therapy (3 to 5 days).

The implant site (typically the area from above the nipple line to the angle of the jaw bilaterally) should be cleaned just before the patient's arrival in the pacemaker laboratory. Although shaving the surgical site is controversial, I continue to have this done. A reliable intravenous line is established in the prep area and intravenous fluids administered for hydration. Mild pre-procedural sedation (e.g., 5–10 mg of diazepam [Valium] and 25–50 mg of diphenhydramine [Benadryl], orally) is given in the prep area. This will be augmented by intravenous sedatives/analgesics during the procedure (e.g., 0.5–1 mg of midazolam, 25–50 μg fentanyl) as needed.

Care should be taken not to oversedate patients, especially the elderly. Drugs to reverse sedation should be readily available: intravenous flumazenil in 0.2-mg increments reverses midazolam; intravenous naloxone in 0.2-mg increments reverses fentanyl. On rare occasions for particular patients (such as children or emotionally disturbed patients), light general anesthesia may be needed. If such a situation is anticipated, appropriate arrangements with an anesthesiologist should be made in advance.

PATIENT PREPARATION

On entering the procedure room, the patient is placed on the support in such a way as to facilitate access to the specific operative site. Physiologic monitoring (ECG, automated blood pressure, and pulse oximetry) should be quickly established so that rhythm disturbances may be detected and treated. The operative site is prepared with an antiseptic solution, wiped dry, and a plastic adhesive sterile field is applied. Disposable towels and drapes are liberally applied to provide a large sterile workplace and to minimize the risk of accidental contamination. A separate adhesive plastic pocket is affixed to the lateral aspect of the procedure site to collect draining fluid and sponges. A sterile plastic cover is placed over the image intensifier and the leaded glass shield (if used) to avoid inadvertent contamination of the sterile field during the procedure.

IMPLANT PROCEDURE

Site

Access to the right heart for permanent pacing has been achieved by introducing leads into any of a number of veins, including the subclavian, cephalic, internal or external jugular, and iliofemoral.[14] Typically, the choice of venous entry site determines where the generator will be housed, although lead extenders can be used when necessary to allow a more remote positioning of the device. In most cases a cephalic, axillary, or subclavian vein is used, and the pacemaker is placed subcutaneously in the adjacent infraclavicular region. On occasion, however, the generator may be implanted under the pectoral muscle or in an abdominal position. For women in whom there is a concern about cosmetic appearance, an inframammary incision may be performed and the pacemaker placed under the breast.[15] In such circumstances, it may be wise to enlist the assistance of a plastic surgeon.

The site of implant is influenced by the factors listed in Figure 5.3. Most often the left side is chosen because most patients are right handed and there is a less acute angle between the left subclavian and the innominate vein than exists on the right side. A disadvantage of using the left side is the small (0.3% to 0.5%) incidence of persistent left superior vena cava with drainage into the coronary sinus, which complicates lead positioning. Suspicion of this anomaly may be raised by finding greater distension and a double A wave in the left jugular vein compared with that of the right vein, a left paramediastinal venous crescent on the chest radiograph, and an enlarged coronary sinus on echocardiography.[16] Contrast echocardiography or venography will confirm the diagnosis. Although both single-chamber ventricular and dual-chamber systems[17] have been placed through a persistent left superior vena cava via the coronary sinus, it is preferable to approach implantation from the right side when this anomaly exists (Fig. 5.4). Rarely, there is a coexistent absence of the right superior vena cava with all brachycephalic flow entering into the coronary sinus. Such a condition should be excluded before implantation is attempted from the right side in patients with a persistent left superior vena cava. The increasing experience with pacing from the coronary venous system coupled with the relative ease of entering these vessels in the case of persistent left superior vena cava suggests that this is a reasonable alternative in the latter patients. Other options for patients with anomalous venous drainage include an ilio-femoral approach or a traditional epicardial implantation, which now may be performed through a subxyphoid or thorascopic approach.

Venous Access

Figure 5.5 illustrates the two major easily identifiable landmarks (clavicle and deltopectoral groove) for implantation in a left infraclavicular site. Venous access

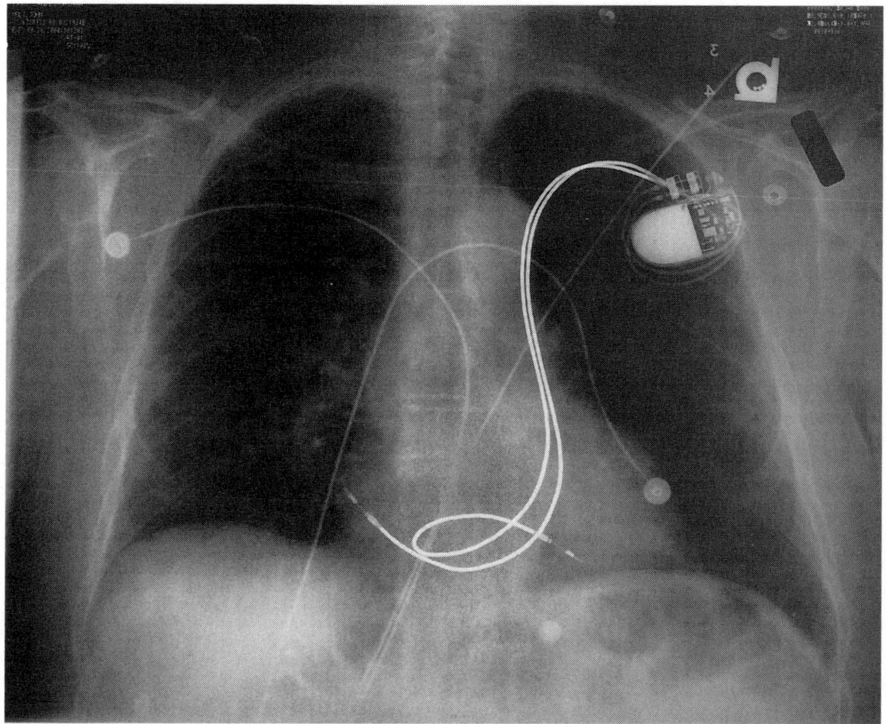

Figure 5.4. Anteroposterior chest radiograph of a patient with a dual-chamber pacemaker placed through a congenital persistent left superior vena cava. Given the circuitous course of the ventricular lead, long lead lengths are sometimes needed to reach the right ventricle.

into either the subclavian or cephalic vein is usually achieved through an incision that will also serve as the portal for subcutaneous generator placement. Local anesthetic is injected through a small-gauge needle along a line 4 to 6 cm long and two fingerbreadths below and parallel to the clavicle. If the cephalic vein is used, the incision begins about 0.5 cm lateral to the deltopectoral groove and is extended medially; otherwise, the incision may be placed just medial to the groove. This method provides adequate exposure for access to either the subclavian or cephalic vein.

Some operators begin with a smaller incision specifically located to achieve venous access, after which the incision is extended or a new one is made for the pocket. This is obviously necessary when a supraclavicular approach to the subclavian vein or a jugular venous access is contemplated. In the latter situations, the leads are tunneled over the clavicle to the generator, which is placed in the usual ipsilateral infraclavicular position.

Pacing leads may be introduced through a venotomy in an exposed vein (cephalic, jugular, iliofemoral), or venous access may be achieved using the Seldinger technique. The latter approach provides easy access to a relatively large

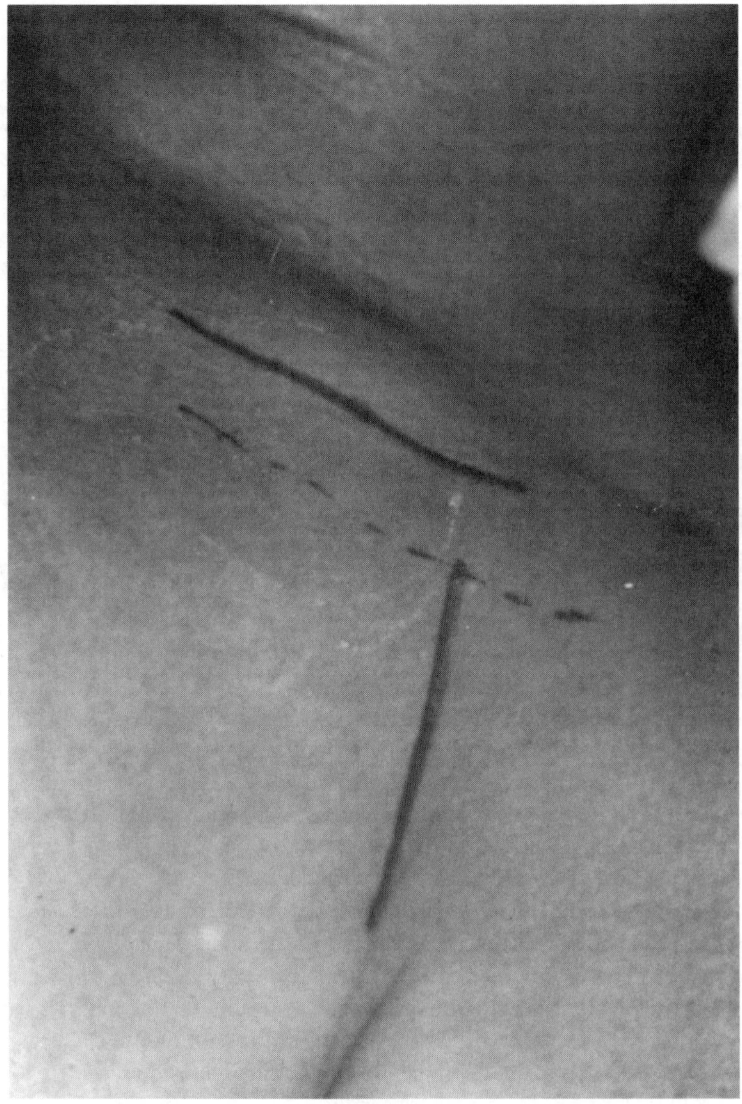

Figure 5.5. Surface landmarks in a patient about to undergo pacemaker implantation. The top solid line indicates the inferior margin of the left clavicle. The dashed line 2.0 cm beneath indicates the site of incision, from which access to the subclavian, axillary, and cephalic veins is possible. The more vertical solid line indicates the deltopectoral groove in which the cephalic veins are found. Incision at this site allows access to the cephalic, axillary, and subclavian veins.

central vein, obviating the need for surgical dissection. In addition, the use of the dilator-sheath technique facilitates the introduction of multiple large leads and provides a means (via a retained guidewire) to reenter the venous system should that be necessary (e.g., if change from a passive to an active-fixation lead is needed because a stable position is not found with the former). Nevertheless, the blind subclavian stick poses the risk of injury to nearby structures, including the artery, lung, thoracic duct, and nerves, and it is the most hazardous part of the implantation procedure.[1]

The Subclavian Method

The Seldinger approach to the subclavian vein has long been a popular method of gaining rapid access to the central venous circulation. The introduction of the tear-away sheath provided an effective means for the insertion of permanent pacemaker leads, and this method is now the most frequently used. The efficacy and safety of subclavian entry are increased by taking measures to distend the vein (proper hydration, leg elevation) and place it in the proper position (by placing a wedge under the patient's shoulders and by adduction of the ipsilateral upper extremity).

The traditional approach to the subclavian "stick" uses an 18-gauge exploring needle. My current practice is to use a smaller gauge micropuncture system for all percutaneous vascular access. I think that this is a bit safer and perhaps less painful. The needle, attached to a 10-mL syringe containing a few milliliters of local anesthetic, is introduced through an incision that has been bluntly dissected to the underlying prepectoral fascia. The tip of the needle is advanced, bevel down, along this tissue plane at the level of the junction of the medial and middle thirds of the clavicle and directed toward a point just above the sternal notch. Small amounts of anesthetic may be injected along this course. On reaching the clavicle, the needle's angle of entry with respect to the thorax is increased until the tip slips under the bone. Negative pressure is exerted on the syringe as the needle is advanced so that blood is aspirated on entrance into the vein.

Once under the clavicle, the needle should not be redirected; doing so may lacerate underlying structures. If venous entry is not obtained, the needle should be withdrawn, cleared of any obstructing tissue, and reinserted in a slightly different direction. Inadvertent arterial entry is apparent with the appearance of pulsatile bright red blood. Prompt withdrawal of the needle and compression at its entry site under the clavicle is usually all that is necessary to close the entry point. Repeated unsuccessful attempts to enter the vein suggest a deviation in anatomy or occlusion of the vessel. In either situation, the risk of complication is increased with additional blind needle insertions; no more than three such attempts should be made, at which point one should consider a contrast injection to determine vessel patency and to provide a road map to its site.

Adequate opacification of the subclavian vein is achieved by the injection of a bolus of 20 to 40 mL of iodinated contrast through a large-bore cannula in an ipsilateral arm vein. This should be followed immediately by injection of a saline "chaser" to hasten the transit of the contrast solution. The amount of fluid and rate of injection is gauged by fluoroscopic observation of the course of dye into the central veins. It is important that enough contrast be used and that adequate time be given for the contrast to fill the subclavian vein or collateral vessels. If the vessel is patent, there is often enough lingering contrast to allow an exploring needle to be directed at it.

It is helpful to record the injection on videotape or digitally so that the procedure may be reviewed. Some digital systems allow superimposition of real-time fluoroscopy on a stored contrast-filled image, which greatly facilitates the procedure. This technique may be especially useful in device upgrade procedures as a way to avoid needle damage to a preexisting lead. On occasion, a formal venogram may be obtained to document the status of the venous system before or after implantation (see Fig. 5.1).

On successful entry of the needle into a vessel, the character of the aspirated blood is examined. Dark nonpulsatile flow suggests a venous location; however, nonpulsatile flow does not exclude arterial entry, and pulsatile flow is sometimes noted from a vein (e.g., tricuspid regurgitation, right heart failure, cannon waves). Once vascular access is achieved, the syringe is detached (taking care to prevent air from entering the venous system) and a J-tipped guidewire is inserted through the needle (or small introducer sheath in the case of micropuncture access) and advanced under fluoroscopy to the inferior vena cava (IVC). If this is accomplished, inadvertent aortic entry is precluded; merely observing the guidewire coursing to the right of the sternum or even into a ventricular chamber does not exclude its presence in a tortuous ascending aorta or its passing retrograde into the left ventricle.

If resistance to advancement of the guidewire is encountered, the guidewire should be withdrawn through the needle with great care to prevent shearing off the distal wire by the needle tip. If any difficulty is encountered with withdrawal, either the wire and the needle should be withdrawn together or, if enough wire has been passed into the vein, the needle may be withdrawn and a small lumen plastic catheter advanced over the wire and into the vein. In the latter situation, contrast may then be injected through the catheter to identify the problem and a more torqueable wire capable of being directed appropriately can be introduced.

Once the guidewire is positioned in the IVC, a commercially available peel-away sheath-dilator combination (7 to 12F depending on lead(s) size) may be advanced over the wire into the superior vena cava, which will provide access for the introduction of pacing leads. The relatively stiff, straight dilator may be molded into a gentle curve by the operator before insertion. Advancement of the device under the clavicle may be facilitated by torquing it as if it were being screwed into place. Considerable resistance may be encountered if the subclavian vein has been entered medially through a fibrous or calcified ligament. The use of a stiffer guidewire may be advantageous in such a situation, as might the passage of initially small, then progressively larger dilators. Entrance into such a location may be a marker for future lead entrapment, thus one may consider seeking a more lateral entry site (see subsequent discussion). Excessive force should not be necessary once the sheath has entered the vein. Fluoroscopic confirmation of proper alignment of dilator and wire is necessary if resistance is encountered. On occasion, countertraction on the wire while advancing the dilator is helpful. The sheath should not be allowed to slide over the tapered tip of the dilator, nor should the dilator be unprotected by a guidewire at any time during advancement.

Once it is properly positioned in the superior vena cava, the dilator is removed while the guidewire is retained within the sheath to allow for the introduction of a second sheath if necessary. A clamp should be applied to the end of the guidewire to prevent its accidental migration into the vein. Care should be taken to limit the possibility of the aspiration of air through the large-bore open sheath by pinching its orifice until the lead is inserted. The patient should not be heavily sedated and should be instructed to avoid deep inspiration during this process. The use of tear-away sheaths with hemostatic valves are now often used and are helpful in limiting bleeding and preventing air embolism. The pacing lead is introduced alongside the guidewire and advanced into the right atrium or IVC, at which time the sheath is withdrawn and peeled apart proximal to the venous entry site to prevent injury to the vessel. If a dual-chamber device is to be employed, the retained wire is used to introduce a second sheath. If only one lead is to be used, it is still wise to retain the guidewire so that venous reentry is facilitated should the lead prove inadequate. It has been suggested that the use of a larger single sheath may be beneficial by allowing the two leads to be introduced simultaneously, but the risk of air embolism would seem greater in this situation. An alternative technique has been described in which two guidewires are inserted through a single introducer and then each used separately to insert an introducer sheath. Some implanters prefer to use two separate subclavian punctures when placing a dual chamber pacing system to limit lead interaction at the access site. This potential benefit does not, in my opinion, justify the risk of a second needle access.

The Axillary Vein Approach

There is evidence that the traditional percutaneous subclavian approach results in access to the medial aspect of the vein, which may result in entrapment of the lead between the subclavius muscle and the costoclavicular ligament.[18,19] Forces exerted on leads in this position may predispose them to insulation failure. This may be most problematic for some polyurethane leads (especially those made with Pellethane 80A) which appear to be particularly susceptible to failure when placed via the subclavian route.[20] These observation have led to the development of techniques to access the axillary vein by direct needle stick, which have yet to be widely adopted. The cephalic venotomy (see subsequent discussion) avoids the effects of the medial subclavicular musculotendinous complex. Our group has derived a technique of lateral access using a micro-puncture system and contrast venography (Fig. 5.6).[21] This method appears to be safe and effective; in the hands of non-surgeons, it is more likely to be successful than cephalic vein cutdown.[22]

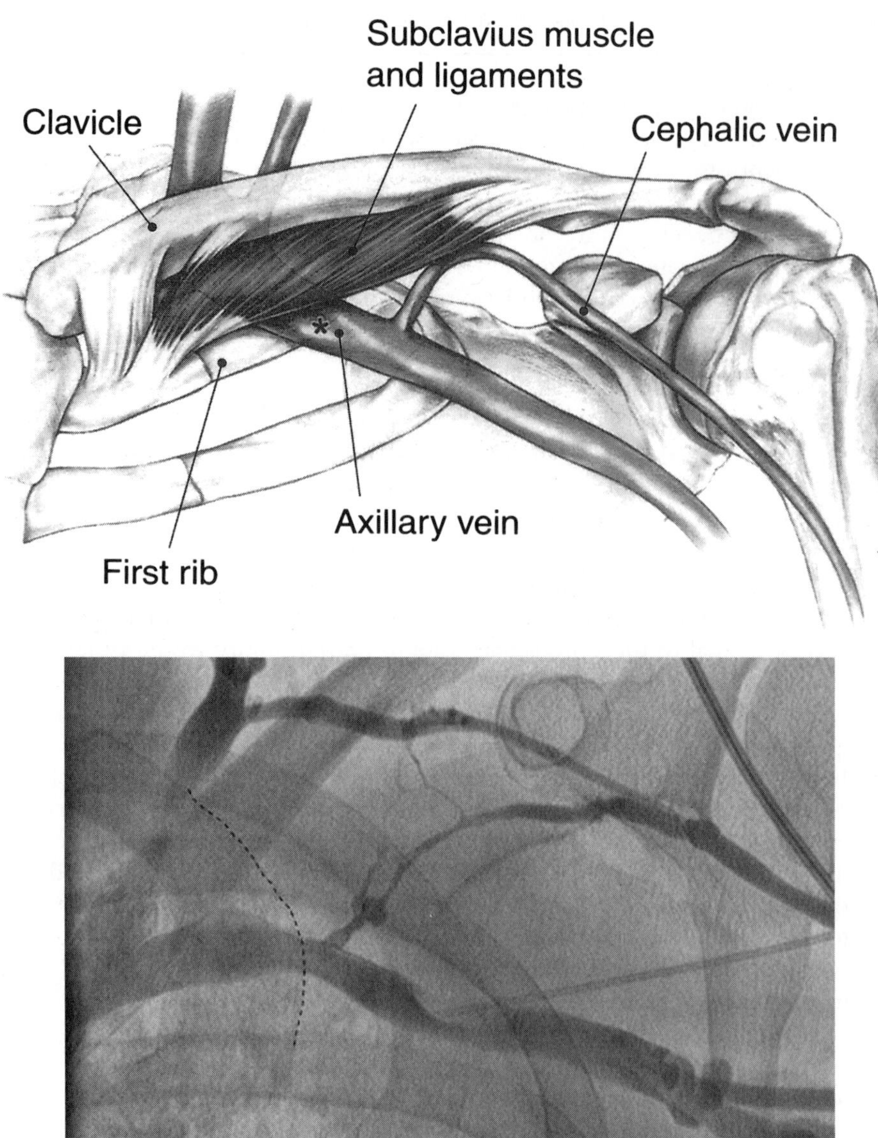

Figure 5.6. Anatomy of the subclavian venous system. **A:** Anatomy of the subclavian venous system and skeletal landmarks relevant to percutaneous access. The subclavius muscle and costoclavicular ligament complex are shown between the clavicle and first rib. Accessing the subclavian vein medially requires the lead to pass through these structures. This may be associated with a higher risk of lead fracture due to compressive forces on the lead. By accessing the cephalic vein or axillary vein (*asterisk*) extrathoracically it eliminates the problems of lead entrapment. **B:** Fluoroscopic guidance of introducer needle into the axillary vein. The peripheral venogram delineates the axillary vein as it crosses the first rib (*dotted line*) in anteroposterior projection. The introducer needle is seen indenting the axilllary vein just before puncture at a site that is far outside the thoracic cage.

Briefly, the axillary vein can be accessed by "blind" venipuncture without venography by entering the pectoral muscle with the access needle just medial to the acromion process on anteroposterior fluoroscopy. The needle is then directed under fluoroscopy to the point at which the lateral border of the first rib appears to cross the inferior margin of the clavicle (Fig. 5.6). The needle approach is angulated to a degree that the first rib is struck with the needle if the vein is not entered. By walking the needle up and down the first rib on repeated passes, the axillary vein is eventually entered. Alternatively, venography readily delineates the course of the vein and may allow for access of the vein far lateral to the first rib (see Fig. 5.6). The most common problem is too shallow an approach to the vein so that the needle passes anteriorly to the vein without entering it. The routine use of venography is valuable when learning this technique.

The Cephalic Vein Approach

The cephalic vein resides in the sulcus between the deltoid and pectoral muscles. This area is readily identified by palpation and is occupied by loose connective tissue and fat, which is easily separated to reveal the underlying vein that sometimes lies fairly deep in this groove. The consistent course of this vessel, its reasonable size, and the direct path it takes to the central venous system recommend it for lead placement. On occasion, however, this vessel is small, consists of a plexus of tiny veins rather than a larger single channel, or takes a circuitous route to the subclavian vein. These conditions may make lead insertion difficult or impossible. In addition, the occasional difficulty in inserting two leads into the cephalic vein may limit the opportunity of using this approach for dual-lead systems in some patients. The vein is isolated along a 1 to 2 cm length within the groove and ligated distally (Fig. 5.7). A ligature is placed around the proximal aspect of the vein for hemostasis. The vein can be entered by venotomy or with a 16- or 18-gauge peripheral IV catheter (Jelco). It is recommended that a guidewire then be passed into the vein to secure access and allow for lead introduction by peel away sheaths. A dilator-introducer sheath combination may then be used as described previously for the retained wire method in the subclavian approach.

The greatest benefit of the cephalic approach is its margin of safety compared with that of the subclavian stick—there is almost no risk of pneumothorax or hemothorax. Although the cephalic vein itself may be sacrificed by this hybrid procedure, it often dilates to accommodate the leads and remains intact. In either case, the guidewire provides virtually unlimited access to the central venous system. Tearing of the vein may result in significant bleeding from tributaries into the pocket, which may be controlled with a purse string suture around the venous access site.

Rarely, the cephalic vein takes an aberrant course or a pectoral vein is inadvertently accessed. In such cases the guidewire may easily enter the subclavian vein; however, it may not be possible to manipulate a sheath over the wire successfully, which necessitates abandoning the technique. In other cases the vein may spasm or be invaginated by passage of the sheath essentially grasping it

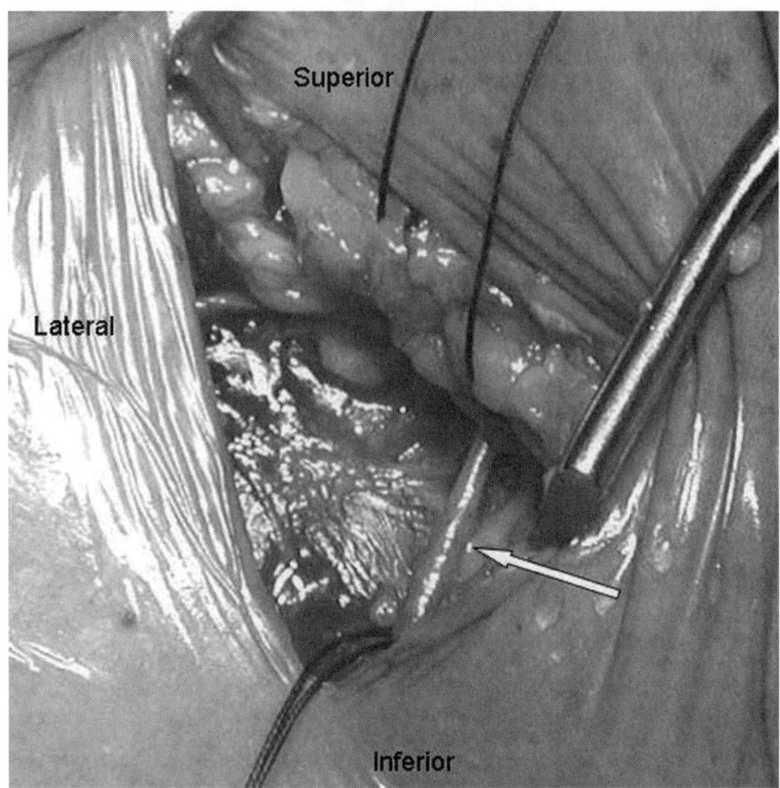

Figure 5.7. Surgical access to the right cephalic vein at pacemaker implant. The orientation of the patient in the figure is given. The moderately large cephalic vein (*arrow*) lies in the dissected deltopectoral groove and has ligatures placed proximally and distally. This vein can be accessed directly with venotomy or with a peripheral IV catheter to introduce a guidewire and peel away sheath.

and preventing its advancement or removal. Application of a vasodilator (e.g., nitroglycerine) or actually cutting the constricting vein, exposed by pulling back on the dilator, may be necessary to fully insert the sheath. Despite these potential limitations of the cephalic technique, an experienced operator can successfully implant leads by this approach in most cases when it is attempted. Occasionally, a floppy or hydrophobically coated wire is necessary to negotiate the cephalic-axillary vein junction. Pulling the arm caudally will flatten the shoulder and facilitate passage through the acute angle formed by this juncture.

THE PACEMAKER POCKET

The pacemaker is usually placed in a subcutaneous position near the site of venous entry. Generators have continued to decrease in size and can be placed quite easily in most patients, including those having a paucity of subcutaneous tissue. Most often, the device is placed in the infraclavicular area through the incision used to obtain venous access. Local anesthesia is applied to the subcutaneous tissue, which is then dissected down to the prepectoral fascia. Placing the pocket too superficially in a subcuticular pocket may lead to a pain syndrome requiring re-operation.[23] A pocket directed inferomedially over the pectoral fascia and large enough to accommodate both the generator and redundant lead is made in this tissue plane by blunt dissection using the fingers. Too small a pocket may result in tension exerted on the overlying tissue by the implanted hardware; too large a pocket invites future migration or "flipping over" of the generator. Augmentation of anesthesia with a rapidly acting parenteral agent is recommended during the brief time it takes for pocket creation because this may be the most uncomfortable part of the procedure. Attention to hemostasis is necessary, but significant bleeding rarely accompanies blunt dissection and Bovie cautery in the proper tissue plane. Stripping away the pectoral fascia during the dissection often leads to excessive bleeding from the denuded muscle. On completion of its formation, the pocket may be copiously flushed with antibacterial solution and temporarily packed with radiopaque sponges. Care should be taken to account for all sponges used in this fashion. Even a radiopaque sponge may be missed by fluoroscopy if it is under the generator and only casual observation is made.

In some circumstances (e.g., sparse subcutaneous tissue, large generator/defibrillator, impending erosion from a previous device, concerns about cosmetic appearance) the generator may be placed subpectorally or under the breast. These procedures should be well planned ahead of time and, when necessary, arrangements made with appropriate specialists (such as a plastic surgeon). The subpectoral site is best accessed by dissecting the natural plane between the pectoralis major and minor muscles. This plane is identified by blunt dissection in the deltopectoral groove and carried inferiorly and medially. Alternatively, a muscle-splitting incision can be made in the body of the pectoralis major itself. Care should be taken to note when a subpectoral position has been chosen so that operators will be aware of such should future generator exchange be necessary. An "intra-pectoral" pocket has been recently described by Kistler and colleagues[24] that appears easy to access and safe to create.

Pockets located at a distance from the site of lead insertion require that the leads (with or without extenders) be tunneled through subcutaneous tissue to its location. A simple method for tunneling leads from the infraclavicular site to a submammary pacemaker pocket by the use of a long needle, guidewire, and dilator–introducer set has been described by Roelke and colleagues.[25]

LEAD IMPLANTATION

A variety of leads are available for endocardial placement. They differ in composition, shape, electrode configuration, and method of fixation. Special leads that contain steroid-eluting collars or biosensors have been developed. Passive fixation leads have tines or fins that anchor them in the trabeculated right ven-

Box 5.1. Lead Characteristics

1. Active fixation lead
   - Easy passage
   - Low acute dislodgment rate
   - Unrestricted positioning
   - Easier removal of chronic implant
   - Higher capture thresholds
2. Passive fixation lead
   - Greater electrode variety
   - Lower thresholds
   - More difficult passage
   - More difficult chronic removal
   - Higher early dislodgment rate

tricle or atrial appendage; active-fixation leads employ a helix that provides a mechanism for actually fixing the lead to the endocardium. The helix may be extrudable and retractable, or may be fixed at the tip. In the latter situation, the helix is covered with an absorbable agent to facilitate passage of the lead to its site of implantation, by which time absorption of the material exposes the helix and allows it to be fixed to the heart. I prefer the extrudable devices, which are easier to remove if necessary. Both active and passive types of leads have advantages and disadvantages (Box 5.1) and may be used for either atrial or ventricular placement. Steroid-eluting active-fixation leads may offer some benefit in terms of lowered subacute and possibly chronic thresholds. Despite the progress in lead design and their overall excellent performance, the failure over time of several models of these devices remains a cause for concern.[26]

Before introduction, leads should be inspected for imperfections and, if they are to be inserted through a sheath, to confirm that this can be done easily in the presence of a retained guidewire. Active-fixation leads should be tested to ensure that the helix extrudes and retracts appropriately. Care should be taken to ensure that the screw does not pick up debris during this process. It is important to confirm that the connector pin of the lead is appropriate for the generator that has been selected. The suture sleeve should be positioned at the proximal portion of the lead and prevented from migrating distally during lead placement.

Stylets are used to supply a degree of stiffness and shapeability to the lead. The stylets may vary in stiffness and length and in some cases are specially configured to engage an active-fixation mechanism. They must be matched for a specific purpose to the lead. Stylets should be kept clean and dry to facilitate insertion and withdrawal from the lead. Torque applied to a shaped stylet may help rotate the lead. Special stylets are now available that allow for in situ alteration of the degree of curve they provide to the lead tip, which may facilitate atrial placement. Although not required to retract the lead, the stylet provides "body" to the lead and may be needed to advance it to an optimal position.

Leads may be inserted directly into a venotomy or through a peel-away sheath. The central venous system is usually traversed easily and the lead advanced and "parked" in the low right atrium or inferior vena cava, pending introduction of a second lead or removal of the sheath. On occasion there may be difficulty in advancing the lead through the sheath. This is more common when there is a sharp angle to be negotiated and the sheath kinks. The temptation to force the lead through the sheath should be resisted to avoid damage to the lead. Withdrawing the sheath slightly, advancing the retained guidewire along with the lead, and sometimes withdrawing the stylet to soften the lead tip may prove helpful.

Although the retained-guidewire approach facilitates the insertion of the two leads required for dual-chamber pacing, manipulation of one lead may affect the position of the other. There is also a potential for a lead or guidewire to be withdrawn accidentally if they are not attended to closely. Some implanters feel that two independent sheaths be used and not withdrawn until both leads have been positioned, or that separate venous sites (e.g., cephalic and subclavian or two separate subclavian entry sites) be accessed for each lead. If a modicum of care is taken, however, two leads may be inserted and positioned by using the retained-guidewire technique, which is quicker and probably safer than the alternative approaches.

Good fluoroscopic imaging is a key to successful lead implantation, however in unusual situations, such as with a pregnant patient, echocardiography has been used to help position leads to limit radiation exposure.[27]

Ventricular Lead Positioning

In dual-chamber systems, the right ventricular lead is usually positioned first because it may supply back-up pacing, its position is usually a bit less tenuous than that of the atrial lead, and it is usually considered the most important of the leads. Left ventricular lead placement is described in the chapter on cardiac resynchronization therapy. On occasion the lead may seem to enter the right ventricle with little assistance from the operator, but more often some manipulation is necessary. Withdrawing the straight stylet a few inches allows one to catch the lead tip in the right atrium; further advancement of the lead will cause its distal portion to form a J shape, which may then be rotated toward the tricuspid valve. Slight retraction results in prolapse into the right ventricle, at which time the lead can be either advanced into the pulmonary artery or directed down toward the apex by advancing the stylet while the lead is slowly pulled back. Prolapsing the lead ino the ventricle ensures that the lead is not in the coronary sinus and is not passing through the tricuspid valve apparatus. Entrance into the pulmonary artery confirms that the lead has traversed the right ventricle and is neither in the atrium nor in the coronary sinus. The lead may then be pulled back as the stylet is advanced (as described previously).

Once the lead tip falls toward the apex, the patient is asked to inspire deeply and the lead is advanced into place. This procedure is often accompanied by ventricular ectopy, the absence of which suggests that the lead is not in the ventricle. An alternative method of gaining entry to the ventricle is to form the stylet into a dogleg or a J shape and use it to direct the lead across the tricuspid valve.

Once it is in the right ventricle, the shaped stylet may be replaced with a straight one to facilitate positioning at the apex. The proper fluoroscopic appearance of the right ventricular apical lead is one in which the lead's tip is well to the left of the spine and is pointing anteriorly and slightly caudal (Fig. 5.8).

In the anteroposterior projection it may not be possible to distinguish whether a lead is in a posterior coronary vein, the left ventricle, or the right ventricular apex. Oblique views and the electrocardiographic pattern of ventricular activation during pacing may be helpful (Fig. 5.9). In patients with left ventricular prominence and/or counterclockwise rotation of the heart, the lead tip may not appear to extend far enough to the left border of the cardiac silhouette. Imaging in the right anterior oblique position may be helpful in such circumstances; observing the position of the lead with respect to the tricuspid valve allows an estimation of how far the lead is in the ventricle. Pacing at 10 V output is performed to exclude diaphragmatic stimulation by the lead.

Once in place, the tip should maintain a relatively stable position and not appear to be bouncing with cardiac contraction. A slight loop of lead is left in the atrium to avoid tension at the tip during deep inspiration. Too large a loop may result in ectopy, lead displacement, and possible chronic perforation at the tip. Lead position should be checked with the stylet withdrawn.

Although an apical position is preferred for reasons of stability, there are occasions when another location in the right ventricle is required (e.g., a retained ventricular lead, which might result in electrical potentials being generated between it and the new lead). Efforts to obtain a more physiologic activation sequence and, presumably, contraction from ventricular stimulation have led some to advocate positioning the lead in the right ventricular outflow tract[28] or at the ventricular septum (Fig. 5.8). In these circumstances, the use of an active-fixation lead is required. The hemodynamic benefits of routinely seeking such a position compared with the stability of the traditional apical location are unproven but this position eliminates the risk of extracardiac perforation and diaphragmatic stimulation.

When a reasonable position is obtained, preliminary measurements of the electrical parameters are made. This is usually accomplished with the stylet withdrawn about halfway so as not to interfere with the position of the lead tip and to facilitate movement of the lead body should that be necessary. When active-fixation leads are used, such measurements may be taken before extensions of the helix, as a screen of the implant site prior to fixing the leads. If the parameters are not good an alternative position may be tried. Once a reasonable site is established the helix is extruded and the parameters re-measured. Failure to record a large current of injury after fixing active-fixation leads suggests an unstable lead position. Active-fixation leads vary in the ways they interface with the heart; the helix may be electrically active, the distal electrode may be active, or both the helix and a distal electrode may be active. Adequate pacing characteristics may not be found immediately after extension of the helix: the screw may not have entered the myocardium, the site may be inadequate, or local tissue injury may have occurred consequent to entry of the helix. To place

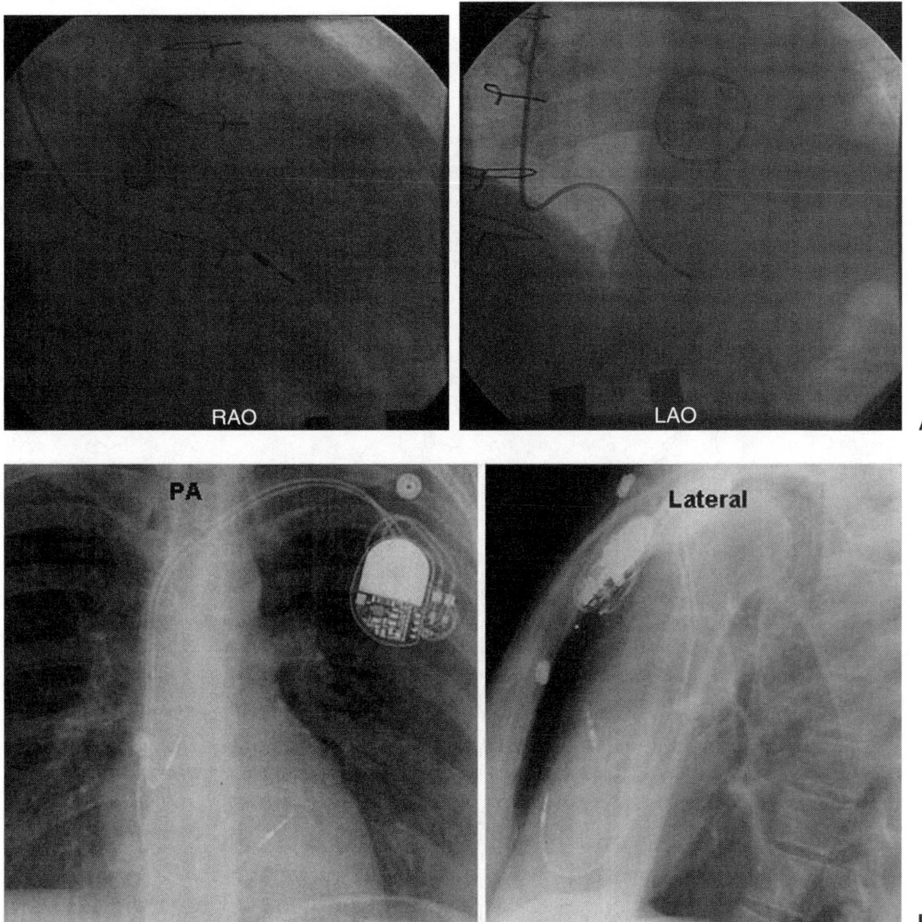

Figure 5.8. **A:** RAO and LAO views of right ventricular apical lead position at the time of implant. The patient has a prosthetic mitral valve in place. The ventricular lead is positioned with the tip at the right ventricular apex, well beyond the spine shadow, as shown here. The slight downward position of the tip is desirable. Some indentation of the ventricular lead at the level of the tricuspid valve is common. In LAO the lead lies against the ventricular septum. **B:** PA and lateral views of dual chamber system after implant. The right ventricular lead is positioned in the midright ventricular septum. Note the anterior direction of this lead in the lateral projection. The atrial lead is positioned in the right atrial appendage and is also oriented anteriorly.

a lead in the outflow tract or septum, the lead is prolapsed into the pulmonary artery as described. By withdrawing the lead with a curved stylet and torque to drive the tip into the septum, the septum can be mapped and the lead fixed. All lead positions should be confirmed by both left anterior oblique and right anterior oblique views in the laboratory. It is common for capture thresholds to decrease significantly 15 to 30 minutes after active fixation.[29] If parameters are

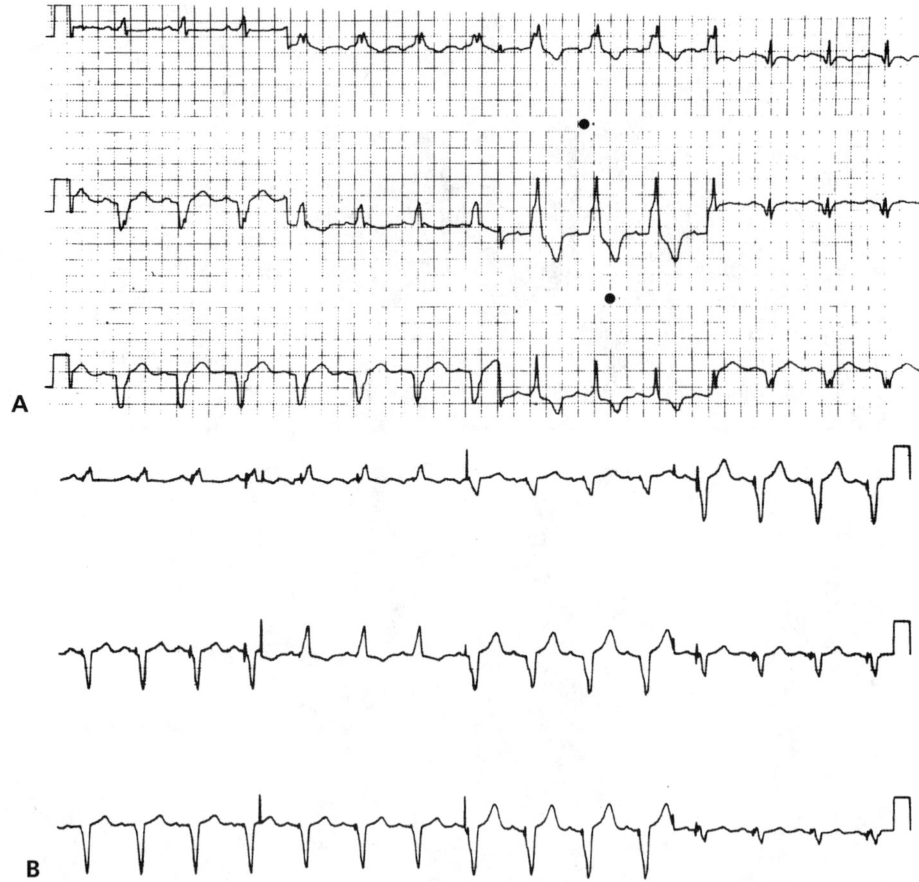

Figure 5.9. **A:** ECG demonstrated pacing with right bundle branch block morphology. The anteroposterior chest radiograph was consistent with right ventricular apical position; however, the lateral radiograph demonstrated the lead in the left ventricle (see Fig. 5.13). **B:** Left bundle branch block pattern with paced events was seen following repositioning of the lead into the right ventricle.

unacceptable, the helix may be retracted and a new site tested. It has been suggested that serial measurements of lead impedance be used to confirm fixation of helical screw electrodes, because with fixation the impedance may increase approximately 200 ohms in the ventricle and 50 ohms in the atrium.[30] At times one may be unable to retract the screw either because the mechanism has been damaged or because tissue has become impacted in the helix. It might still be possible to reposition the lead and fix it to the myocardium by rotating the entire lead (indeed, some active-fixation leads have nonretractable screws); however, replacement of the lead with a new one is probably a better option.

Threshold parameters tested with a PSA define the electrical adequacy of lead position. This is accomplished using a set of connector cables, which can be configured for unipolar or bipolar leads. When testing unipolar leads, the anode is connected to tissue in the pacemaker pocket using a disk electrode or a clamp. Electrograms may be obtainable from the PSA or may be recorded directly from the lead using the chest (V) lead of a standard ECG machine. If satisfactory parameters (Table 5.1) are not obtained, alternative lead positions should be sought. It is important to confirm that diaphragmatic pacing does not occur by temporarily testing the lead at high output energy (10 V).

Capture threshold may be influenced by a number of factors.[31] On occasion (such as with diseased myocardium or certain medications) optimal parameters may not be achieved, and acceptance of a position most closely approximating ideal is necessary. However, because the short- and long-term success of the pacing system is related to the initial lead position, effort should be expended to obtain the best possible initial location in terms of both stability and electrical performance. Rarely, a cardiac vein may prove the only site from which one may pace the ventricle reliably despite elevated thresholds.[32]

Atrial Lead Implantation

The right atrial appendage has become the preferred implant site for atrial leads because of its trabeculated nature. Studies have shown that reasonably good pacing parameters may be obtained and maintained from this location.[33] There has long been a perception, especially among physicians in the United States, that the atrium is a less reliable site for endocardial pacing. A number of studies have suggested that dislodgment is not more common with atrial leads, but reliance on an atrial appendage location may mandate the acceptance of less than ideal pacing characteristics that become unacceptable over time.[34] Active fixation leads (especially those with steroid-eluting capabilities) appear to be beneficial in this regard by allowing further exploration of the right atrium in the search for an optimal position. There is no evidence that the atrial stimulation site influences hemodynamics per se although atrial septal pacing near Bachman's bundle may be of some importance when atrial tachycardia algorithms are applied (Fig. 5.10).

A variety of leads (active, passive, J-shaped, straight) may be used for atrial pacing. A stylet can be used to impart a "J" configure to a routine ventricular

Table 5.1. Acceptable Electrical Parameters for New Lead Placement

Parameter	Atrium	Ventricle
Capture threshold*	<1.5 V	<1.0 V
Sensed P/R wave	>1.5 mV	>4.0 mV
Slew rate	>0.2 V/sec	>0.5 V/sec
Impedance	400–1000 ohms†	400–1000 ohms†

* At 0.5-msec pulse duration.

† High-impedance leads typically exceed these values; check with manufacturer for acceptable values.

lead, which facilitates its entry into the appendage. When using active-fixation leads, there are advantages and disadvantages to preformed devices. The non-J lead may be easier to place in areas other than the appendage; however, dislodgment may result in the lead's falling into the right ventricle and causing competitive pacing or ectopy (Fig. 5.11). The J-shaped active-fixation lead may also be positioned almost anywhere in the atrium, but in some sites (e.g., low

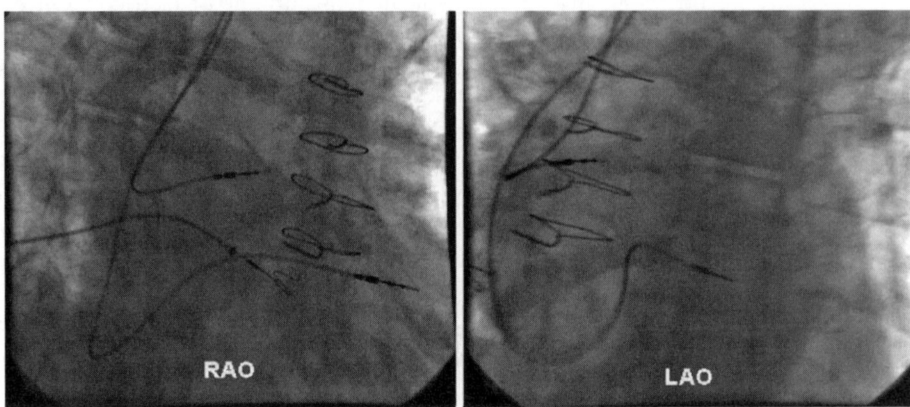

Figure 5.10. RAO and LAO views of atrial lead in the high right atrial septum (Bachman's bundle) at the time of implant. Note that in the LAO view the lead tip is directed posteriorly as opposed to anteriorly for right atrial appendage positions (compare with Fig. 5.8B). The unique position of the lead is difficult to appreciate in the RAO view. The ventricular lead is fixed to right ventricular septum.

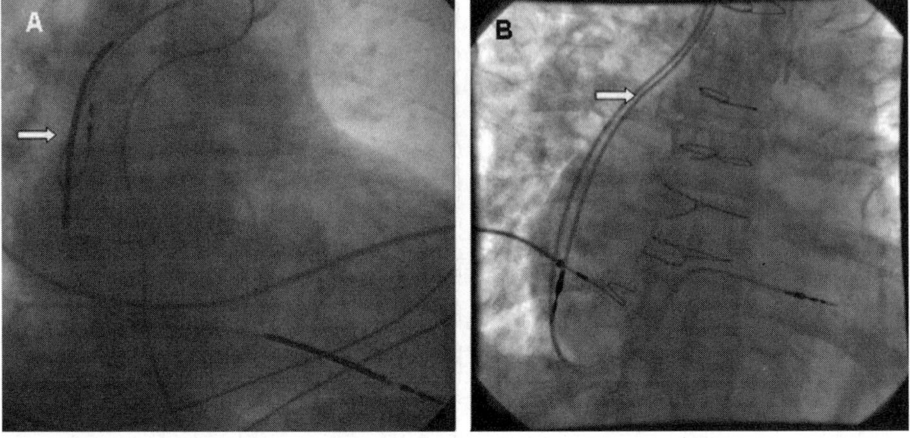

Figure 5.11. AP views of atrial lead dislodgments in two patients. The arrows represent the approximate location of the vena cava-atrial junctions. **A:** This preformed atrial "J" lead dislodged within 24 hours of implant and retracted into the superior vena cava producing phrenic nerve stimulation. **B:** This straight active fixation lead dislodged during implant to fall into the low lateral right atrium.

atrium) its shape may cause undue tension at the site of attachment to the endocardium increasing the risk of dislodgment (see Fig. 5.11).

The atrial lead is inserted into the venous system with a straight stylet to facilitate negotiation of the central veins. Positioning in the atrial appendage is attempted first. The lead is directed toward the high anterior atrium and allowed to take its J shape either by withdrawing the straight stylet (in preformed leads) or by inserting a J stylet (see Fig. 5.8B). Slow retraction of the "J" shaped lead results in the tip's entering the appendage, where it will appear to catch and take on a characteristic to-and-fro motion with atrial activity. When it is well positioned, slight rotation of the lead should not dislodge the tip, and deep inspiration opens the curve to an L configuration but no further. In some patients the atrial appendage may be quite large and trabeculae may be attenuated; in others, who have received cardiopulmonary bypass, the appendage may be oversewn. In either circumstance, placement of a preformed J lead may be difficult. Although some implanters feel that amputation of the right atrial appendage at the time of previous cardiac surgery is a mandate for an active-fixation atrial lead, others find passive fixation devices to be acceptable.[35] We are most comfortable recommending the routine use of active-fixation, steroid-eluting leads with normal or high impedance for patients with prior cardiac surgery. To place a lead on the atrial septum, allow the curve of the active fixation lead to form free in the body of the atrium and directed anteriorly. Rotate the lead to the septum in LAO view and pull the lead up until the roof of the atrium is encountered (see Fig. 5.10). Opening the stylet to a curve less than 180 degrees facilitates reaching the septum.

Acceptable electrical parameters for atrial pacing are listed in Table 5.1. As seen when positive fixation leads are used in the ventricle, there may be a significant improvement of the parameters during the first half hour; if borderline values are obtained initially, it may be worthwhile to remeasure them after a short wait. If poor values are obtained initially, however, it is best to search for a new position. The better the electrical characteristics, the more probable that long-term pacing will be successful. As with the ventricular lead, it is important to test for diaphragmatic pacing by temporarily stimulating the atrium at high output (10 V).

Epicardial and Transmyocardial Lead Placement

Permanent epicardial leads can be placed on the atrium and ventricles at thoracotomy. Newer steroids eluting active fixation and atraumatic suture-on electrodes provide the best long-term thresholds. Chronic epicardial atrial lead performance remains problematic, however. These leads must be passed between or beneath the ribs and then tunneled subcutaneously to the pocket.

When no venous access is available and the superior performance of endocardial lead placement is desired, transmyocardial placement may be indicated (Fig. 5.12). By thoracotomy, one or two leads can be passed through the right atrial wall and positioned in the atrium and ventricle with use of fluoroscopy. Purse string sutures around the atriotomies prevent bleeding. The leads are then tunneled to the pocket.

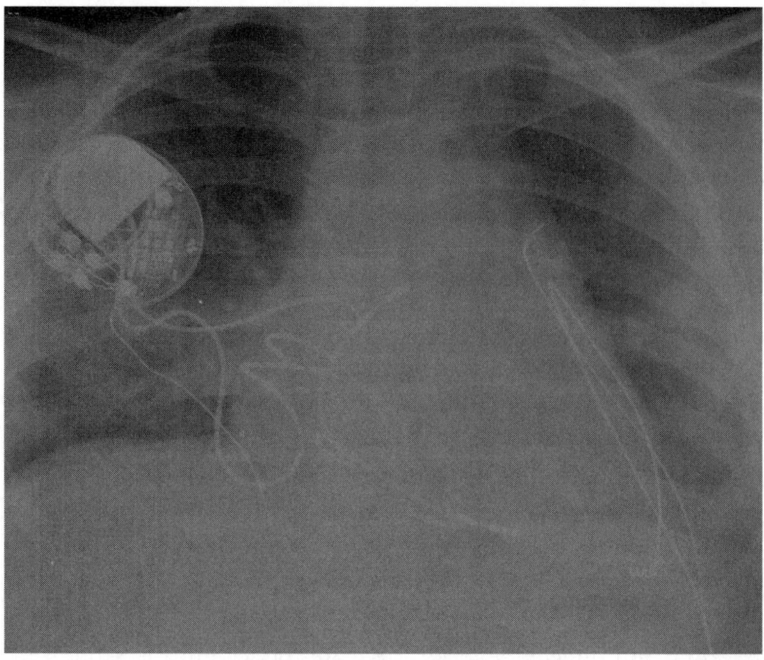

Figure 5.12. Transvenous active fixation leads placed in the right atrium and right ventricle through a left atriotomy in a 10-year-old boy. The patient had symptomatic heart block and had fractured multiple leads placed transvenously. These leads were extracted. The unipolar epicardial leads had exit block.

SINGLE-LEAD VDD PACING

The general principles of lead insertion are similar for the dual-chamber VDD systems that use specially arrayed proximal atrial sensing electrodes as well as a tip electrode to sense and pace the ventricle on a single lead. These devices have some attraction as a means of pacing patients with A-V block who have a normal sinus mechanism because they obviate the need for a separate atrial lead. Many implanters, myself among them, feel uncomfortable however with the limited functionality of these devices. When used it is important to have the atrial electrodes at an optimal position in the right atrium; one may have to choose among leads with varying distances between the tip and atrial electrodes. Care is necessary to ensure that there is a chronotropically intact sinus mechanism before implantation and that atrial activity is consistently sensed by the lead at implantation. Testing for atrial sensing during extremes of respiration and during cough is necessary. Although it may be necessary to accept low-amplitude P waves and program the device to be very sensitive, reasonable results are reported over a moderately long follow-up period.[36]

Inappropriate atrial sensing still may be a problem for a significant portion of patients implanted with single-lead VDD systems. Because atrial capture is rarely possible with VDD leads, the device provides only single-chamber VVI(R) function if the atrial rhythm slows below the lower rate limit. Of course the system is at a disadvantage if there is chronotropic incompetence, unless one is willing to sacrifice atrial synchronization and revert to VVIR. Some attention has to be directed toward the development of a single-lead DDD device.[37]

GENERATOR INSERTION

After the lead(s) have been placed in an acceptable electrical position, stability is confirmed with fluoroscopic observation during deep inspiration and cough. There should be just enough intravascular lead to prevent undue tension at the tip with inspiration. The suture sleeve is carefully advanced distally, with care not to pull on the lead. Frequent fluoroscopic checks are important during this process. The lead is tied down to the underlying muscle with two or three sutures of nonreabsorbable 2-0 or 3-0 material. Sutures should never be tied around the unprotected lead; and even with the suture sleeve, too tight a suture may compromise lead integrity. The sutures should be tight enough, however, to avoid lead migration. Electrical parameters and fluoroscopic position should be rechecked after suturing; if they are not optimal, the sutures may be removed and the lead repositioned.

Once the leads have been secured, the sponges that had been placed in the subcutaneous pocket are removed and the area is irrigated and checked for hemostasis and foreign matter. Fluoroscopy of the pocket area will reveal any radiopaque foreign body (such as sponges or needles) that was not removed before the generator insertion. The pacemaker should be preprogrammed to the desired initial settings while still in its sterile package, after which it is given to the operator for implantation. For dual-chamber devices it is important that the atrial and ventricular leads be identified easily and connected properly to the generator. Bifurcated leads are marked to ensure that the distal electrode is inserted into the cathodal portion of the connector block.

The proximal connector pin of the lead should be seen to pass the set screw(s) of the generator and remain there after tightening. Care should be taken that the screws are not overtorqued when tightened. A slight tug on the lead will confirm a tight connection. For in-line bipolar leads, both screws (when present) must be set correctly. Some pacemakers (i.e., unipolar, minute-ventilation) may not function as programmed until placed within the pocket.

The generator is carefully placed in the pocket. Redundant leads may be looped along the sides of the device or underneath it to avoid acute angulations. Once in place, the pacemaker should function as programmed. Fluoroscopic examination of the entire system may be done before pocket closure.

The pocket is closed in layers using 2-0 to 4-0 resorbable suture, subcutaneously. Care must be taken to avoid piercing a lead with the suture needle. The skin edges may be approximated with skin sutures, resorbable subcuticular sutures or staples. An antibiotic ointment and dressing are then applied.

Before leaving the pacemaker laboratory, a final fluoroscopic check of the generator pocket and the course of the leads is made. The system is noninvasively interrogated to confirm adequacy of function and is programmed so that it temporarily overdrives the intrinsic heart rate. A 12-lead electrocardiogram is obtained (to demonstrate the configuration of the a paced rhythm), and an over-penetrated anteroposterior and lateral (shot through the ipsilateral upper extremity) chest radiographs are performed to document the lead position and the absence of a pneumothorax. A sling may help discourage excessive movement of the ipsilateral upper extremity during the first 12 to 24 hours. A thorough operative report should be generated immediately to include the manufacturer, model, and serial numbers of all devices implanted, abandoned, or explanted as well as any difficulties encountered during the case.

Revision of the Implanted Pacemaker System and Pulse Generator Change

Revision of an implanted pacing system may involve replacement of the pulse generator, the pacing leads, or both (Fig. 5.13). The uncomplicated generator change is usually a simple procedure; however, the preparation is in many ways

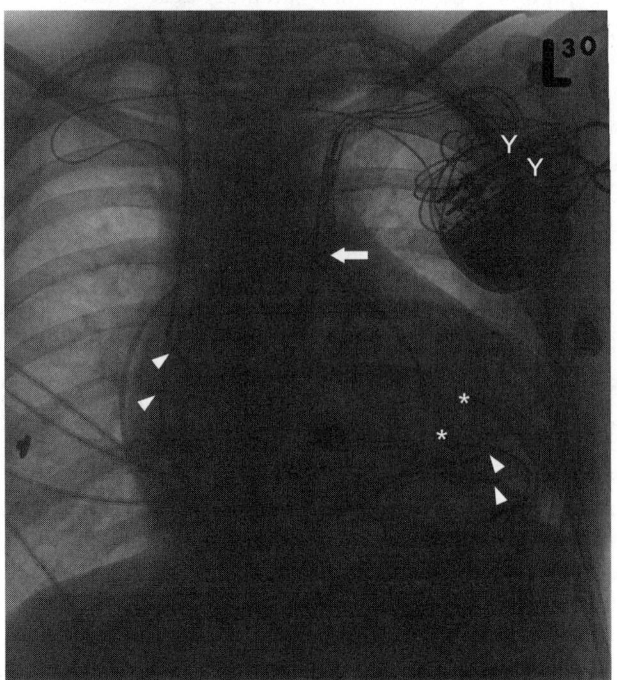

Figure 5.13. PA chest radiograph of woman with congenital heart disease referred for biventricular pacing system upgrade. She has a dual chamber pacing system comprising two separate sets of unipolar transvenous leads (*arrowheads*) to both the atrium and ventricle. These leads pass through a persistent left superior vena cava and the superior vena cava. The leads are adapted to the pacemaker header with "Y" adapters (Y). A separate ICD system is implanted in the abdomen using two screws in epicardial leads (*), an epicardial apical ventricular patch electrode, and a coil electrode in the left superior vena cava. The logistical aspects of any revision to these systems are enormous.

more involved than a new implant (Fig. 5.14). First, the indication for generator change should be confirmed and the system evaluated as thoroughly as possible noninvasively to identify any problems with the leads. For lead failure, the procedure itself is often more complex than a new implant (usually due to issues of venous access) and again requires extensive preoperative investigation into the cause of the lead failure to prevent its recurrence. If a lead replacement is anticipated, the patency of the ipsilateral venous system must be confirmed by venography. The decision to extract malfunctioning leads should be made beforehand so that appropriate preparations can be made (see subsequent discussion). Even if the leads are known to function preoperatively, they may be damaged or found to be compromised on surgical exposure and must be dealt with.

One of the most critical aspects to preparing for a lead or generator change is ensuring the mechanical and electrical compatibility between the new and retained components (Fig. 5.14). Over the years pacemaker systems have been manufactured with a variety of lead connector pins and generator header ports that may not be interchangeable. Currently, all new pacing systems conform to standard designs for these components. Older systems may have pacemaker lead designs that are incompatible with new generators or have a serviceable generator that is not compatible with new leads. For the lead to fit into the generator, the lead diameter, pin length, and presence or absence of sealing rings must be accommodated by the pulse generator (Table 5.2). In addition, at least one manufacturer (Guidant, Inc.) has introduced a proprietary LV-1 pin configuration for coronary sinus leads. Certain leads can be made compatible with new generators by the use of adapters. Most manufacturers continue to provide generator models to fit some of the discontinued lead styles. In addition, some pacemakers require unique leads to perform specialized functions or special tools to free the leads from the device. The importance of identifying the lead and pacemaker connector configuration *before* surgery cannot be overstated. This is especially true for implantable defibrillator revisions because even greater variability exists in the lead and header configurations of these devices. Manufacturers can provide the needed information about compatibility between components.

During the operative procedure, electrosurgical cautery can cause failure of output in generators near their end-of-life. For this reason and because leads can be damaged during generator removal, temporary pacing should be established in pacemaker-dependent patients. Meticulous attention to surgical technique is mandatory to prevent damage to implanted hardware and to reduce the risk of infection. If lead replacement is required but the ipsilateral venous access is occluded, abandoning the entire system for another site or recanalization of the vein by lead extraction (see subsequent discussion) will be necessary. Occasionally, isolated outer insulation defects in silicone leads can be repaired, but the integrity of the conductors is usually left in question. If leads are capped and abandoned in the pocket it is advisable to suture the lead to the floor of the pocket to prevent migration of the free end, causing erosion.

Finally, replacement of a lead or generator provides the opportunity to also revise the pocket, reimplant the generator submuscularly, or revise the surgical

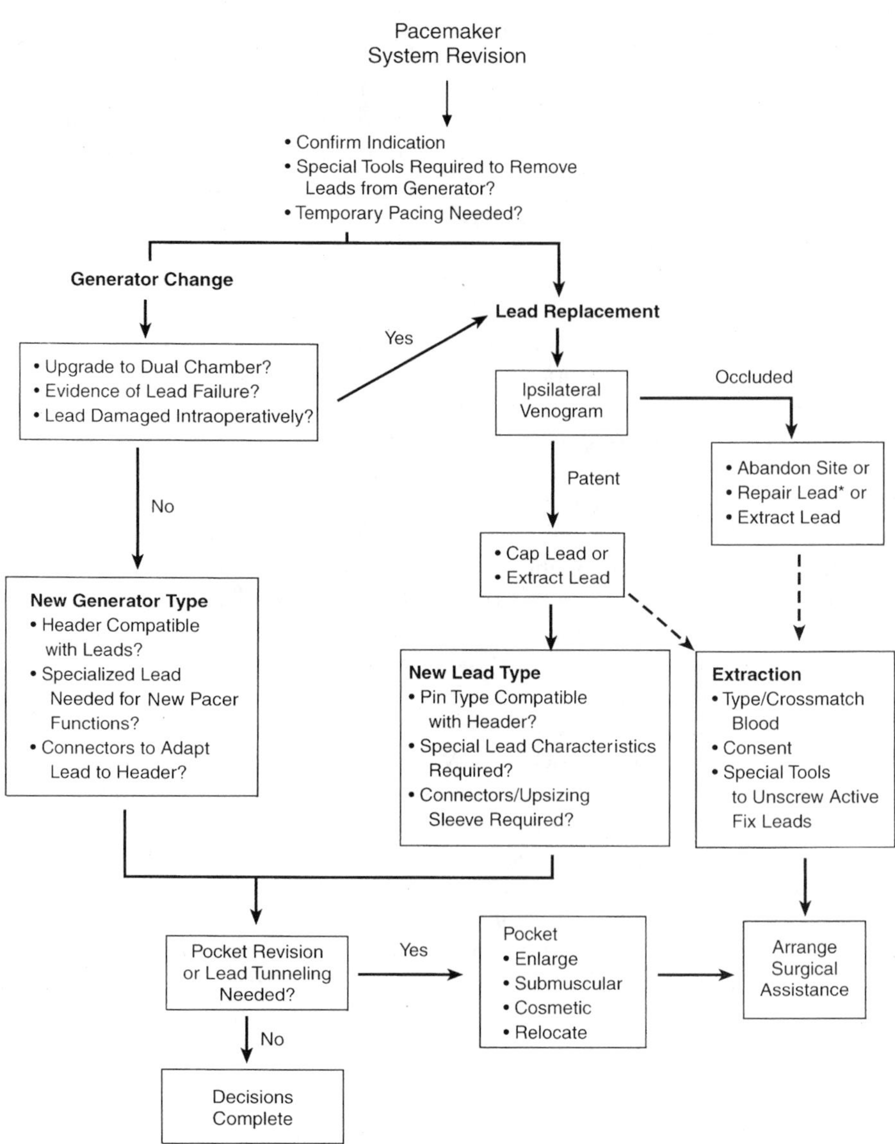

Figure 5.14. Flow chart for decisions surrounding revision of a previously implanted pacemaker system. All decisions should be thoroughly considered and the necessary equipment secured before the patient enters the operating room. (*Repair of isolated outer insulation defect can be performed on an exposed section of some silicone insulation leads using a repair kit. The integrity of the lead conductors is not assured, however.)

Table 5.2. Lead and Header Compatibility for Pacemakers

Lead Type	Header							
	IS-1 (short pin)	**VS-1 (short pin)**	**VS-1A (LP)**	**VS-1B★ (LP)**	**3.2-mm Lp★**	**3.2-mm LP Cordis**	**6-mm Unipolar**	**LV-1**
IS-1 (short pin)★ Unipolar or Bipolar	Yes	Yes	Yes	No[‡]	No[c]	Yes	Yes[†]	No
IS-1 (short pin)★ Unipolar or Bipolar	Yes	Yes	Yes	No[‡]	No[c]	Yes	Yes[†]	No
VS-1 (short pin)★ Unipolar or Bipolar	Yes	Yes	Yes	No[‡]	No[‡]	Yes	Yes[†]	No
3.2-mm LP Unipolar or Bipolar	No	No	No	Yes	Yes	No	Yes[†]	No
3.2-mm Cordis★ Unipolar or Bipolar	No	No	No	No[‡]	No	Yes	Yes[†]	No
6-mm Inline Bipolar	No[§]	No[§]	No[§]	No[§]	No[§]	No[§]	Yes (to Unipolar)	No
6-mm Unipolar	No[§]	No[§]	No[§]	No[§]	No[§]	No[§]	Yes	No
5-mm Bifurcated Bipolar	No[§]	No[§]	No[§]	No[§]	No[§]	No[§]	Yes[||] (to Unipolar)	No
5-mm Unipolar★	No[§]	No[§]	No[§]	No[§]	No[§]	No[§]	Yes[||]	No
LV-1 Unipolar	No	No	No	No	No	No	No	Yes

★ Has sealing rings.

† Compatible with use of nonconducting upsizing sleeve but availability must be verified with manufacturer.

‡ Both lead and header have sealing rings, but there may be compatibility depending on header tolerances; check with manufacturer.

§ Not compatible without electrically conductive downsizing adapter; check manufacturer for availability.

|| May require nonconducting upsizing sleeve.

LP = long pin.

scar as indicated. All of these factors should be evaluated and plans made for any contingency before the surgical procedure begins.

POST-PROCEDURE MANAGEMENT

Elective generator replacement is most often accomplished on an outpatient basis. While there has been some enthusiasm for performing same-day pacemaker implantation, most procedures involving lead placement continue to involve hospitalization for at least one night. For such new implants telemetry of the electrocardiogram is usually obtained for 12 to 24 hours. Longer hospitalization may be required because of ancillary medical problems or as a result of complication. Analgesia may be necessary but it is rarely needed after the first few days. The patient is advised to limit motion of the ipsilateral upper extremity for a time—specifically, to avoid raising it above the shoulder level or subjecting it to marked abduction for approximately 2 weeks. Patients should not, however, completely immobilize the arm as this may delay ultimate rehabilitation. The incision should be kept completely dry for 5 to 7 days.

Before the patient's discharge, the device is programmed in accordance with the patient's specific needs and a complete noninvasive assessment of the pacing system is performed. Programming of the pacemaker is guided by two principles: 1) optimization of the patient's hemodynamic state, and 2) maximal conservation of battery-energy expenditure. When these two factors are in opposition, the first should rule; however, opportunities to achieve the second should not be overlooked. This might include programming a longer AV interval to avoid fusion beats, a low resting minimal heart rate, and lower stimulation outputs (within an acceptable safety margin). Rate-adaptive parameters may be set before the patient is discharged or during a follow-up visit. This is commonly done empirically and is tested by having the patient perform walking exercises.[38] The adequacy of pacing response may be judged by real-time telemetry or by using rate histograms stored in the pacer. Follow-up evaluation and possibly adjustment of programmed parameters, including rate adaptation, will be necessary. An increase in capture threshold over the first 2 to 6 weeks after implantation is to be expected with non–steroid-eluting leads, but even if steroid-eluting devices are used, an adequate safety margin should be programmed into the generator to ensure successful pacing during this time. This is usually achieved with a voltage output of three to five times threshold at implant. Some of the newer devices have a mechanism for automatic capture threshold detection. These devices may allow for the programming of a lower pacing output with the recognition that the unit will increase pacing output if it detects a rise in threshold. Care should be taken to ensure that these devices have acceptable evoked response amplitudes acutely and at follow-up assessments. Older patients, interestingly, seem to have less of a rise in threshold over time presumably because they exhibit less of a reaction to the leads. A copy of the programmed parameters should be given to the patient to keep, in addition to the device registry card. Importantly, the implant site should be kept completely dry for 5 to 7 days to reduce the risk of infection.

It is important that the physician register the generator and leads appropriately so that the patient may be tracked should recall of a device occur. Arrangements for follow-up care must be made by the implanting physician, and the patient should be counseled as to the importance of having the system checked at regular intervals. There is some controversy as to the need for endocarditis prophylaxis in patients with endocardial leads. Although there is a potential for infective endocarditis to occur, this has been reported infrequently and rarely is the offending organism oral flora. Most implanters do not routinely recommend antibiotic prophylaxis although results of pending studies may change practice in the future.

COMPLICATIONS OF IMPLANTATION

Inherent with pacemaker therapy is the potential for the occurrence of an untoward event. Skill, experience, and technique are all mitigating factors, but every operator should anticipate that eventually he or she will have to deal with a complication. Thus, the implanting physician must be concerned not only with measures to avoid complications but also with their recognition and treatment. Such untoward events associated with the introduction and physical presence of the generator and lead may be classified according to their etiology (Boxes 5.2 and 5.3).

In the Pacemaker Selection in the Elderly (PASE) study, 6.1% of the 407 patients receiving dual chamber pacing systems had a complication of implantation.[39] There were nine lead dislodgments, eight instances of pneumothorax, and four cardiac perforations. A repeat surgical procedure of some sort was required in 18 (4.4%) of the patients. In a single center study of over 1300 permanent pacemaker implants reported by Tobin and colleagues,[40] complications were noted in 4.2% of patients. Lead displacement occurred in 2.4%, significant pneumothorax in 1.5%, pericardial tamponade in 0.2%, and hemothorax leading to death in one patient (0.08%). The economic consequences of a complication were substantial with the average incremental cost of $14,547 for a lead dislodgment; $10,052 for a pneumothorax; and $32,472 for a tamponade. There was an inverse relationship between the incidence of acute complication and operator case volume and experience. While the acute implant complications associated with DDD pacing is not different than that with single chamber pacing, the total complication rate associated with dual-chamber pacing over time is higher than that with VVI or single lead VDD due to the presence of the additional lead.[41]

Box 5.2. Acute Complications of Pacemaker Implantation

1. Venous access
   - Secondary to Seldinger technique
     Pneumothorax
     Hemothorax
     Other (e.g., injury to thoracic duct, nerves, etc.)
   - Secondary to sheath insertion
     Air or foreign body embolism
     Perforation of the heart or central vein
     Inadvertent entry into artery
2. Lead placement
   - Brady-tachyarrhythmia
   - Perforation of heart or vein
   - Damage to heart valve
   - Damage to lead
3. Generator
   - Improper or inadequate connection of lead
   - Pocket hematoma

Box 5.3. Delayed Complications of Pacemaker Therapy

1. Lead-related
   - Intravascular thrombosis (embolization)
   - Intravascular constriction (i.e., SVC obstruction)
   - Macro- or micro-lead dislodgment
   - Fibrosis at electrode-myocardial interface
   - Infection—endocarditis
   - Lead failure
     Insulation failure (inner/outer)
     Conductor fracture
   - Retention wire fracture
   - Chronic perforation
   - Pericarditis
2. Generator-related
   - Pain
   - Erosion
   - Infection-pocket
   - Migration
   - Premature failure
   - Damage from extrinsic energy (e.g., radiation, electrical shock, etc.)
3. Patient-related
   - Twiddler syndrome

Although neither elective generator replacement nor upgrading of a VVI system to a dual-chamber device is usually considered to be a risky procedure, both are associated with the potential of complication. Harcombe and co-workers found that the rate of late complications (those occurring later than 6 weeks after the procedure) was higher for elective replacement (6.5%) than for initial system implantation (1.4%).[42] These were primarily erosion and infection related to the pacemaker pocket. As might be expected, complications were more common with inexperienced operators who were relegated to the elective replacements suggesting that technique as well as physiologic substrate play important etiologic roles. Upgrade of a VVI device to a dual chamber or biventricular system carries the potential for all the complications associated with venous access and lead placement (which may be confounded by the preexisting lead), as well as a slight increase in risk of late pocket infection and skin erosion. Upgrade procedures are often longer in duration than a de novo dual-chamber implantation.[43] This may be related to difficulty isolating the generator and lead in the pocket due to adhesion formation, difficulty with venous access, interference with the existing lead, or a combination of these factors.

Venous Access

By its very nature, the blind subclavian venous puncture has a potential for complication, the risk of which depends on both operator skill and the patient's anatomy. Inadvertent damage by the exploring needle to structures that lie in proximity to the vein (e.g., lung, subclavian artery, thoracic duct, and nerves) is the most frequent cause of significant complications encountered during the implantation process. Such complications may be evident immediately, or they may be recognized only after the procedure has been completed. It has been suggested that knowledge of subclavian venous anatomy by digital cinefluoroscopic venography might be helpful in accessing the vessel and avoiding complication.[44]

Pneumothorax is often asymptomatic and discovered on the routine post-procedure chest radiograph. Rarely, it may be the cause of severe respiratory distress intraprocedurally. Pleuritic pain, cough (especially if productive of blood-tinged sputum), and difficulty in breathing suggest the diagnosis. The aspiration of air into the syringe during attempted venous puncture may also raise concern about this possibility, but it has been neither a sensitive nor specific sign. The presence of apical cystic lung disease, variations in the relationship between the clavicle and subclavian vein, and an uncooperative (poorly sedated) patient may increase the risk for this complication—and repeated unsuccessful attempts at venous puncture certainly do. Respiratory symptoms arising during the procedure should prompt assessment of pulse, blood pressure, oximetry, and perhaps blood gas analysis. Fluoroscopic examination of both lung fields should also be performed.

Treatment of pneumothorax depends on its severity and associated symptoms. Respiratory distress during the procedure may necessitate the urgent/emergency insertion of a chest tube. The completion of the implantation will depend on the patient's status and the progress already made. Although there may be some controversy as to the need for evacuation of an asymptomatic pneumothorax seen on chest radiograph, if its extent is greater than 10%, a chest tube should be considered. If a small pneumothorax does not resolve or enlarges on serial radiographs, evacuation is indicated. Inspiration of 100% oxygen by face-mask may help shrink a small pneumothorax.

Hemothorax, a less common complication of the subclavian approach, results from injury to the subclavian artery, vein, or other intrathoracic vessel. Penetration of the subclavian artery by the exploring needle is usually not productive of sequelae if the needle is withdrawn and slight pressure is applied at the site of entry under the clavicle. Significant complication may occur, however, if the artery is lacerated by the cutting edge of the needle or if a large-bore dilator or sheath is inadvertently introduced. If a large sheath is mistakenly inserted into the artery, it should probably be left in place, pending a prompt definitive management decision since removal may result in significant bleeding. Options include surgical repair; endovascular treatment using a prolonged balloon inflation[45] or a stentgraft[46]; or an attempt at sheath withdrawal with external compression. Opinions from an interventional radiologist and a vascular surgeon should be obtained if possible. A quick angiogram may determine whether an important branch vessel (e.g., internal mammary graft or vertebral artery) is involved or might be excluded by a covered stent. Because of the risk of thrombus formation around the sheath, it should be withdrawn to the subclavian artery itself to prevent embolization of clot to the cerebrovascular system. The likelihood of a bleeding complication is increased if the coagulation system is impaired either intrinsically by co-existing disease or by pharmacologic therapy. Angiographic evaluation and possible repair should be considered for severe or persistent bleeding from an uncertain source. A symptomatic hemothorax should be drained.

Air embolism can occur when a central vein is accessed by a sheath, regardless of the technique used to introduce it. This complication may be signaled by a hiss as air is sucked into the sheath by negative intrathoracic pressure and may occur suddenly when a heavily sedated, snoring patient deeply inspires at a time when control over the sheath's orifice is not adequate. Air may be fluoroscopically tracked into the right ventricle and pulmonary outflow tract.[47] In most instances, the amount of air introduced is small and well tolerated, but respiratory distress, chest pain, hypotension, and arterial oxygen desaturation may occur if there is significant blockage of pulmonary flow. Treatment of symptomatic air embolism includes supplemental oxygen, attempted catheter aspiration, and inotropic cardiac support if necessary. These supportive measures will usually suffice until the air embolism breaks up and absorption occurs. Postural changes to prevent migration of air trapped in the right atrium or ventricle from reaching the pulmonary arteries may be considered, although usually the latter occurs too rapidly for these maneuvers to be of much success. Preventive measures are listed in Box 5.4.

Infrequent complications of venous access include laceration of the thoracic duct leading to chylothorax, and damage to the internal mammary artery which may cause acute ischemia when this conduit has been used as a graft. Percutaneous repair has been reported in a case of acute occlusion of the origin of a left internal mammary graft caused by compression resulting from pacemaker lead implantation.[48]

Lead Placement

Arrhythmia: The introduction, manipulation, and positioning of the pacemaker leads in the heart may give rise to a number of complications. Arrhythmia may be a manifestation of the patient's underlying disease, or it may be procedurally

Box 5.4. Avoidance of Air Embolism

1. Increase central venous pressure.
   - Hydrate well.
   - Elevate legs (Trendelenburg position).
   - Have patient perform Valsalva maneuver when sheath is open.
2. Awaken patient and caution against deep inspiration.
3. Use smallest sheath compatible with task.
4. Pinch or occlude neck of sheath when appropriate.
5. Consider the use of sheaths with hemostatic valves.

Box 5.5. Causes of Arrhythmia during Pacer Implantation

1. Bradyarrhythmia
   - Patient's underlying electrophysiologic disorder
   - Vagal reaction
   - Lead trauma to the conduction system
   - Inadvertent disruption of a pacing system
   - Suppression of escape rhythm by anesthetic
2. Tachyarrhythmia
   - Atrial/ventricle
     Underlying electrophysiology
     Irritation by lead/wire
     Ischemia, anesthesia, hypoxia

related (Box 5.5). In a pacemaker-dependent patient, accidental interference with a preexisting pacing system—whether temporary or permanent—may cause asystole or symptomatic bradycardia. Other causes of a bradyarrhythmia include a vagal reaction, excessive local anesthesia, and injury to the conduction system during lead manipulation (e.g., trauma to the right bundle branch in a patient with left bundle branch block). The use of transcutaneous pacing and or the administration of atropine or isoproterenol may be helpful in these situations until a means of effective pacing can be established.

Tachyarrhythmia may also occur during implantation; it is usually the result of stimulation of myocardium by a lead or guidewire. Supraventricular arrhythmias are most likely to occur in patients with atrial enlargement, heart failure, pulmonary disease, or other predisposing conditions such as sick sinus syndrome; they are usually transient. Atrial fibrillation occurring before or during atrial lead placement may be problematic in that atrial parameters cannot be tested unless the rhythm terminates either spontaneously or by cardioversion. It has been suggested that an atrial lead may be placed in the presence of atrial fibrillation occurring at the time of implantation using the criteria of an intracardiac fibrillatory amplitude of 1.0 mV or greater. This reduces implantation time compared to the option of intraprocedural cardioversion.[49] Ventricular dysrhythmia is common as the lead is manipulated in this chamber; but it is rarely sustained. Predisposing factors to more malignant arrhythmia include hypoxia, ischemia, pharmacologic therapy (e.g., sympathomimetics), and asynchronous pacing. Removal of the lead from an irritating position almost always terminates the ectopy. On occasion a retained guidewire or a temporary ventricular pacing lead is displaced and serves as an occult source of ventricular irritation that is not resolved by retraction of the permanent pacing lead.

Because the attention of the implanter may be focused on the fluoroscopic image during lead placement, another individual should be assigned to monitor the ECG during this time. Rarely, a permanent ventricular (or prolapsing atrial) pacing lead will be the cause of recurrent ventricular tachycardia post implantation.

Perforation: The heart may be perforated internally (into another cardiac chamber) or externally (into the pericardial space) by the pacing lead. Right ventricular perforations are probably more common than reported because clinical sequelae may not occur. Poor sensing or capture thresholds may prompt withdrawal of the lead back into the ventricle with "self-sealing" of the perforation. On occasion, however, life-threatening tamponade may occur, and progressive hypotension during or after lead placement should be considered tamponade until proven otherwise by echocardiography. Old age, female gender, steroid therapy, recent right ventricular infarction, and the use of stiff leads (or stylets) may be considered risk factors for perforation. Pericarditis, tamponade, and even pneumothorax have been reported as complications caused by active fixation atrial lead placement due to the helix protruding through the atrial myocardium.[50,51]

Interference with normal coagulation predisposes the patient to tamponade. Anticoagulants should be withheld for at least 8 to 12 hours if there is no suspicion of perforation, and reinstituted with extreme caution if there is any cause for concern. Thrombolytics should be considered contraindicated in the immediate postimplant period. If symptoms suggestive of tamponade occurs, echocardiographic confirmation should be obtained unless the condition dictates emergency pericardiocentesis prior to the availability of the ultrasound equipment. Every effort should be made to obtain an echocardiogram in the latter situation as soon as possible. Pericardiocentesis with catheter drainage will rapidly reverse the pathophysiology of tamponade and may be the only therapy necessary since the perforation frequently is self-sealing. In some cases tamponade may occur with the acute accumulation of only a small amount of pericardial fluid. In such cases it may be difficult to access the pericardial space with a needle, necessitating emergency surgical consultation. Less frequently, a more slowly accumulating effusion may develop over several days as reaction to a relatively small amount of bleeding into the pericardial space. This may follow signs and/or symptoms of pericarditis or present as de novo tamponade. Drainage may be necessary if hemodynamics are threatened; otherwise, nonsteroidal anti-inflammatory agents may be used and the patient observed over time.

Suspicion of perforation without tamponade may be aroused by an extreme distal location of the lead tip at the cardiac apex (especially if it seems to curve around the apex, tenting up the cardiac silhouette), or by the presence of a pericardial friction rub, chest pain, an ECG-pacing pattern of right bundle branch block, or an upright unipolar electrogram recorded from the lead tip.[52] Poor pacing and sensing thresholds may be seen. In such situations, two-dimensional echocardiography may be helpful in localizing the lead tip. If perforation is confirmed, the lead should be withdrawn under hemodynamic monitoring at a time and facility capable of emergent surgical drainage if necessary.

A transvenous pacing lead may enter the left heart through a communication between the atria, through the membranous septum separating the right atrium from the left ventricle, or through the muscular intraventricular septum. The permanent pacing lead may also be inadvertently introduced into an artery and passed retrograde across the aortic valve into the left ventricle. The anteroposterior radiographic image of a lead positioned in the left ventricle may not be distinguishable from an image of one placed in the right ventricular apical position. Oblique or lateral views, however, will demonstrate the posterior location of a left ventricular lead (Fig. 5.15). In addition, pacing from the left ventricle will result in a right bundle branch block pattern (see Fig. 5.9). Two-dimensional echocardiography can be used to trace the course of a lead.

Early recognition of a lead in a systemic chamber should prompt its immediate repositioning because of the danger of thrombus formation and systemic embolization.[53] A review of the literature found that 10 of 27 patients had thromboembolic complications, including three patients on antiplatelet drugs.[54] Options for management of patients with chronically implanted left heart endocardial leads include long-term anticoagulation, lead removal at thoracotomy, or percutaneous lead removal. The latter has been thought to be associated with excessive risk of systemic embolization but a number of successful procedures have been reported usually in patients thought to be at increased risk for surgery.[55]

Other Lead Complications: Ordinarily, the presence of a pacing lead across the tricuspid orifice results in little or no valvular dysfunction. On occasion, however, this structure may be interfered with or damaged. During insertion, the tines of a passive fixation lead may become entangled with the chordae tendineae, and rupture of the latter may result if vigorous lead withdrawal is attempted. Occasionally, extrication of the lead from the tricuspid apparatus may require use of a locking stylet (with or without extraction sheath) to transmit

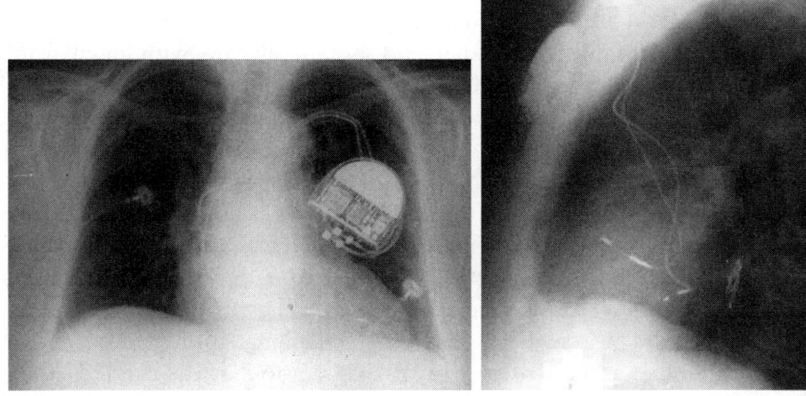

Figure 5.15. **A:** Anteroposterior chest radiograph of a patient after implantation of a dual-chamber pacemaker. Right bundle branch pattern was noted on ECG (see Fig. 5.9). The ventricular lead appears to be positioned near the right ventricular apex and the atrial lead appear to be in a suitable position in this view. **B:** Lateral chest radiograph shows a posterior diversion of the ventricular lead at the atrial level. Echocardiography studies showed evidence of the lead within the left ventricle; and passage of the lead across a patent foramen ovale, across the mitral valve, and into the left ventricular apex was confirmed.

the force of traction to the lead tip rather than merely stretching the lead. The valve may be chronically injured by the lead's lying across it; clot and adhesions may form between the two and serve as a nidus for infection. Recurrent endocarditis on a right ventricular lead has been associated with the development of tricuspid stenosis.[56]

The pacing lead itself may be damaged by the physical forces exerted upon it during the process of implantation, by entrapment by the muscular-skeletal system, by retention ligatures, and by the stresses placed on it by the beating heart. Loss of integrity of the insulation (either inner or outer) is manifested by a low lead impedance that causes a high current drain; conductor fracture is associated with a high impedance. Lead fracture may be recognized radiographically. A defect in the insulation between the conductor wires of a bipolar lead may produce potentials resulting in transient inhibition of the pacemaker. Detection of such intermittent dysfunction may require the performance of provocative maneuvers such as raising, abducting, or adducting the ipsilateral upper extremity. Prolonged contact between the conductors can result in a short circuit, preventing current from reaching the electrodes and depleting the power supply. Both lead fracture and loss of insulation integrity can lead to clinical symptoms including death in pacemaker-dependent patients.

The most common complication of lead placement is its subsequent displacement. This may be obvious on fluoroscopy or radiography (macro-) or accompanied by no obvious change in position (micro-) and usually occurs early, before clot and fibrosis act to further anchor the device. Dislodgment rates are inversely related to the experience of the implanter, which suggests that inadequate initial positioning is a major risk factor. A unique cause of lead dislodgment is known as *Twiddler's syndrome*.[57] In these cases, the (usually elderly) patient unwittingly "plays" with the pacemaker in the pocket, turning it in such a way that the lead(s) are wound around it and, potentially, are withdrawn from the heart (Fig. 5.16). Two other situations in which traction on a lead may result in dislodgment relate to the generator. If not sutured to underlying structures, a generator lying in the subcutaneous tissue may gradually descend through this space and pull on the lead. Similarly a "sagging heart syndrome" (postural descent of heart resulting in tension on the lead and displacement) has accompanied marked weight loss in morbidly obese patients.[58]

The incidence of lead dislodgment has been reduced with refinement of both active and passive fixation devices; it is now less than 2% or 3%. The risk of this complication is lessened by ensuring a stable position at implant, leaving a proper amount of intravascular lead so that tension is not exerted at the tip by respiration or arm motion, adequately anchoring the suture sleeve to underlying tissue, and by limiting abduction and elevation of the ipsilateral upper extremity for a time after implantation.

Early recognition of lead dislodgment (often by deterioration in pacing parameters or the occurrence of ectopy) should result in attempts at repositioning. This is usually accomplished with minimal effort because the lead has not fibrosed to endocardium or venous endothelium. Deterioration of the

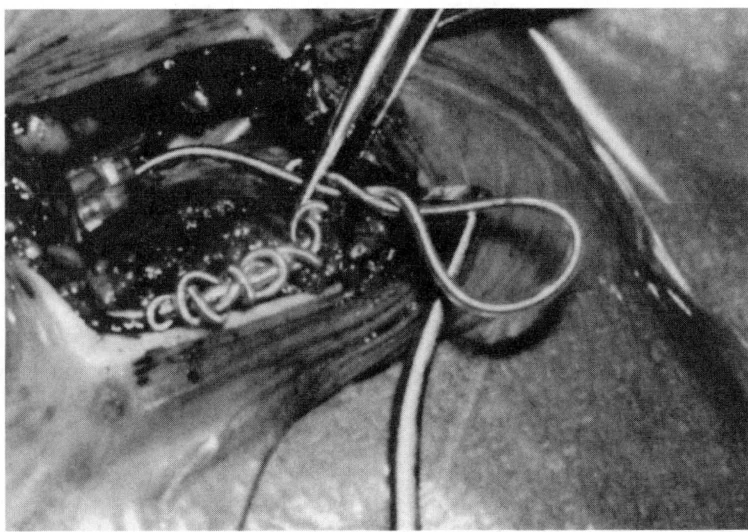

Figure 5.16. Photograph obtained at the time of operative intervention to reposition a lead dislodged due to Twiddler's syndrome. The lead can be seen to be tightly twisted upon itself. Although this tangle can be straightened, the stresses imparted to both the conductor and the insulation make it unsafe to reuse this lead. A new lead should be inserted. (Courtesy of Dr. Paul Levine.)

performance of one or more chronic leads may present a more difficult problem and it is often necessary to use a new lead. If exit block is a problem, a short course of steroid therapy may be tried, but more often than not a repositioning or insertion of a new lead is necessary. Steroid-eluting leads (including those configured with an active-fixation mechanism) are beneficial in this regard.

Venous Thrombosis: It should not be surprising that the presence of one or more intravascular leads may incite thrombosis of the subclavian vein. While asymptomatic thrombus appears to be quite common (see subsequent discussion), its relationship with the number and type of leads remains controversial. Clinically significant pulmonary embolization is surprisingly rare but may occur. Symptomatic thrombosis of the brachiocephalic veins occurs on occasion and presents as a swollen, painful upper extremity, usually within a few weeks of implant. Extension of the clot to involve the innominate vein, superior vena cava, contralateral structures or the cerebral venous sinus may occur. Venography will reveal the extent of thrombus and the state of development of collateral pathways.

Symptomatic thrombosis that is limited to the subclavian or axillary veins may be treated conservatively, with heparin acutely and then warfarin for 3 to 6 months, or more aggressively with thrombolytic drugs (Fig. 5.17). Thrombolytic therapy may be given in a large dose for a short time (e.g., 1 million units streptokinase during 1 hour) or during 12 to 24 hours (e.g., 200 to

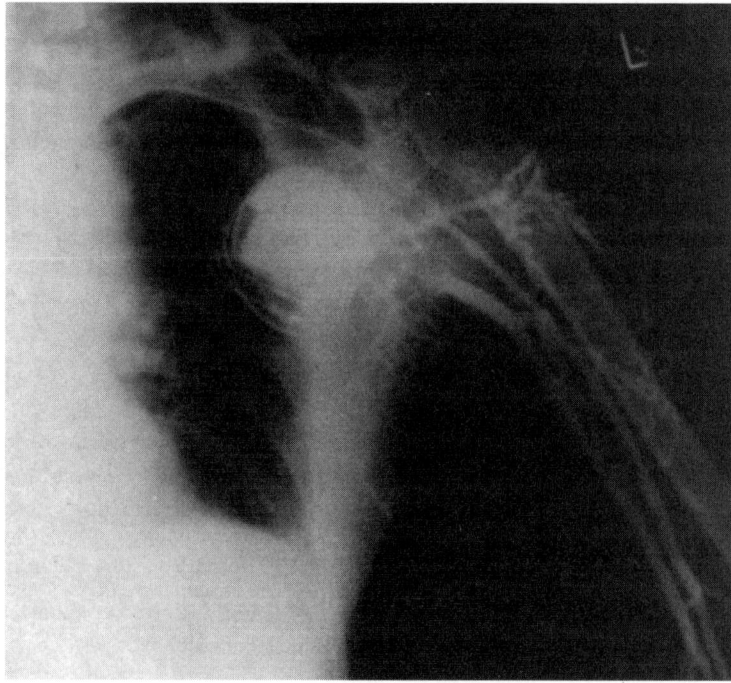

Figure 5.17. Venogram 1 week after dual-chamber pacemaker implantation. The patient presented with swelling and pain in the left arm. Left axillary vein thrombosis is noted. The patient was treated with streptokinase, and a repeat venogram showed restoration of venous patency and disappearance of collateral vessels. (Reproduced by permission from Platia EV, ed. Management of Cardiac Arrhythmias. Philadelphia: JB Lippincott, 1987.)

500,000 units urokinase during 1 hour followed by 100,000 units per hour) with or without concomitant heparin. The newer thrombolytic agents such as tissue plasminogen activator and Retavase may also be used. Thrombolytics need not be delivered directly into an ipsilateral arm vein.

In our experience, thrombolytic therapy has been associated with rapid symptomatic and angiographic improvement. Prolonged therapy with either aspirin or oral anticoagulants may then be considered. We have not observed a bleeding complication or clinical recurrence in patients treated in either fashion. Conservative therapy with heat and upper extremity elevation may also be satisfactory. This may allow for the development of adequate collateralization.

Silent venous thrombosis is not uncommon; routine venography at the time of elective generator replacement revealed stenosis in 11% and total occlusion in 12% in 100 asymptomatic patients.[59] Duplex sonography showed either pathologic changes in the vessel wall (46%) or occlusion (11%) in 56 patients 41 months after implant.[60] No significant risk factors for thrombosis have been identified, although more recently it has been suggested that in patients presenting for lead extraction, those with systemic infection are more likely to have occlusion of the access vein.[61] Further evidence supporting the concept that venous occlusion may be related to the patient substrate is supplied by Oginosawa and colleages.[62] They performed digital subtraction venography before device implantation in 131 patients without symptoms of central venous disease. They found venous obstruction in 14%, half of which had totally occluded veins. Obstruction was more common on the left compared to the right side, 12% vs 1.5%. The most common site of obstruction was in the left innominate vessel. Repeat venography was performed a mean of 44 months after pacer implant, at which time 33% of the patients had obstructions, 38% of which were total occlusions. There were no specific identifiable risk factors either before or after pacemaker insertion. In most patients, asymptomatic thrombosis becomes a problem only when attempts are made to reenter the vessel (e.g., for upgrade to a dual-chamber unit). It is not necessary to treat asymptomatic occlusions. Pacemaker leads inserted via the transfemoral route may be associated with femoroiliac thrombosis and significant pulmonary embolization, necessitating lead extraction and possibly insertion of an IVC filter.

Complete or partial occlusion of the superior vena cava has been reported as a complication of pacemakers.[63] This has been attributed to both thrombosis and fibrosis and may be treated with balloon dilatation or surgical reconstruction if it becomes symptomatic. Acute or subacute occlusion may be treated with anticoagulants and thrombolytic agents. Chronic occlusion is more problematic and is, in general, resistant to pharmacotherapy. In some situations of total occlusion of the superior vena cava, endovascular reconstruction may be complicated by an inability to pass a guidewire through the obstruction. In such cases it may be possible to remove the existing leads and use the extraction sheath as a means of gaining entrance through the occluded venous system. Dilatation and stenting may then be considered; stenting should not be performed over indwelling pacemaker leads. In cases in which endovascular repair is not possible, a surgical approach that enlarges the venous channel with a patch grafting has been used with some success.

The incidence of lead associated thrombus is uncertain since TEE is usually performed only if there is a clinical indication. Such thrombus in the presence of infection would be termed a "vegetation." In general the chance finding of a clot on a lead does not, in itself mandate therapy; however, if it was very large, consideration would probably be given to anticoagulation. Obviously such therapy would be indicated if there is evidence of thromboembolism. A pedunculated clot on a pacing wire may occlude the tricuspid orifice and cause profound symptoms. Treatment of lead-associated atrial thrombus with thrombolytic therapy has been reported.[64, 65]

Generator: The function of a pacing system depends on a proper connection between the leads and the generator. The terminal lead pin(s) are inserted into the connector block of the generator and are fixed into position by some mechanism, most commonly set screws. If this is not done properly, the pin may either

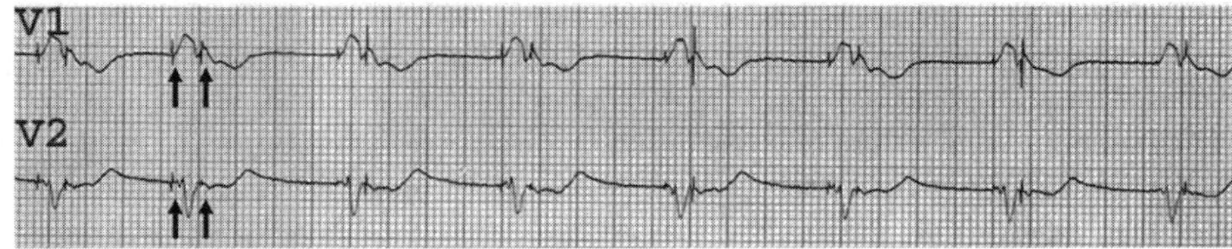

Figure 5.18. Continuous rhythm strip of a patient with a dual-chamber pacemaker in whom the leads were inadvertently reversed at the generator. There is AV sequential output from the generator (*arrows*) with the first stimulus capturing the ventricle and the second stimulus to the atrium occurring late in the QRS complex.

lose contact altogether (i.e., have no electrical continuity, an "open circuit") or intermittently contact the pacemaker terminal and produce spurious potentials that may be sensed by the pacemaker as intrinsic electrical activity, which will cause inhibition of pacer output. When dual-chamber systems are used, it is essential that the atrial and ventricular leads be connected correctly to their corresponding terminals (Fig. 5.18).

Care should be exercised when using electrocautery; its application in the vicinity of the generator may lead to inhibition of pacing or to abnormal tracking—reprogramming of the device to a reversion mode or the induction of a runaway pacemaker may also result. Exposure to other sources of energy—such as direct-current defibrillation, magnetic resonance imaging, security systems, high-dose radiation therapy, and cellular telephones—may also affect pacemaker function. In some cases, pacemaker function can be restored by use of a special engineering programmer; in other situations, the device may be permanently damaged and require removal.

The generator is usually well tolerated in its subcutaneous pocket, but on occasion its presence may be associated with pain. Most often this occurs because the pocket is small and tension is exerted on the overlying tissue. A low-grade infection not productive of significant effusion may also be a source of pain. Pain attributed to neuralgia has been treated successfully with steroid injections, and more recently with lipoinjection.[66] Movement of the pacemaker may occur if the pocket is large, the surrounding tissue lax, and the device not secured. Swelling of pocket may be caused by infection, seroma, or hematoma. Aspiration of the effusion should be discouraged because of the possibility of introducing infection, however, the strong suspicion of infection should prompt exploration.

Migration of the pacemaker under the breast or into the axilla may place tension on the leads or result in the assumption of a position (e.g., in the axilla) that is uncomfortable or is predisposed to erosion. Internal erosion evidenced by the migration of a generator into the urinary bladder from an implantation site in the posterior rectus muscle has also been reported.[67]

Erosion of pacing hardware is caused by pressure necrosis of overlying tissue or infection. This is usually signaled by a preceding period of "pre-erosion,"

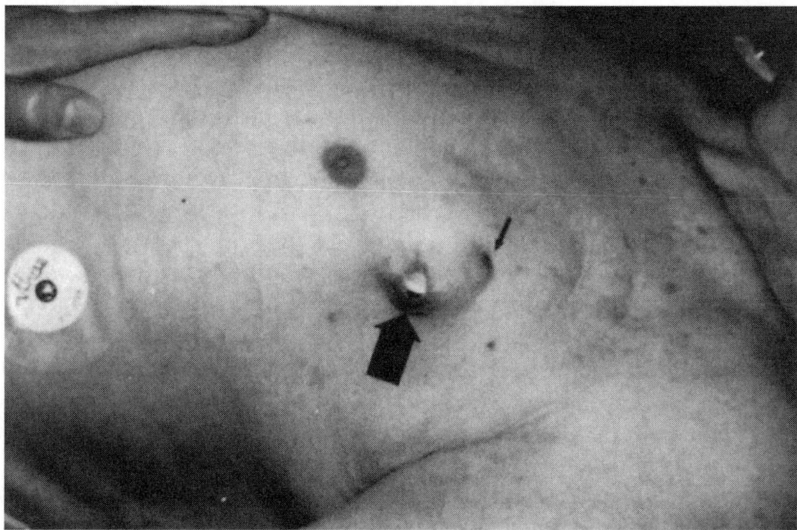

Figure 5.19. Patient with a permanent pacemaker in whom areas of pre-erosion (*small arrow*) and erosion (*large arrow*) are present.

during which there is discomfort and discoloration of thinning tissue tensely stretched over a protrusion of the pacing apparatus (Fig. 5.19). The risk factors for erosion include a paucity of subcutaneous tissue, the mass and configuration of the pacemaker, need for extra hardware (e.g., lead adapter) in the pocket, the pocket's construction, and irritation caused by the patient or by articles of clothing. Identification of pre-erosion allows the salvage of the pacing system, as the hardware can be repositioned under the pectoralis muscle or in an abdominal location.

If erosion occurs, the system is considered contaminated and current opinion favors removal of the generator and leads. There has been the suggestion that extensive débridement of the pocket and prolonged irrigation and antibiotic therapy may provide an alternate option to removal in cases of both erosion and frank infection, but this approach is not generally accepted. For localized erosions, some have suggested removing the generator, débriding the site, and cutting the leads but leaving them in situ. However, now that percutaneous lead removal has advanced to a relatively high degree, it would appear appropriate to try to remove leads rather than to leave them if there is any question concerning sterility.

Bleeding into the pocket may occur when hemostasis is inadequate, when there is a coexistent coagulopathy, or when anticoagulant or thrombolytic therapy is begun prematurely. On occasion this may compromise the pocket's integrity and may be a risk factor for infection. Hematoma progression, excessive pain, and stress on the suture line may require hematoma evacuation and search for a bleeding site.

While not a complication of implantation per se, a generator may prematurely and without warning fail or may revert to an unsafe pacing mode. The former may relate to a defect in the power supply and the latter a function of unrecognized problems with circuit design. Pacemakers are also subject to electromagnetic interference if the field is strong enough. There is a potential risk of exposing pacemaker patients to magnetic resonance imaging equipment.

Infection

A non-eroded pacemaker implantation site may become infected. Diabetes mellitus and postoperative hematoma appear to be predisposing factors.[68] Acute infections (usually with *Staphylococcus aureus*) become manifest within the first few weeks of implantation and are often associated with the accumulation of pus. A more indolent infection caused by a less virulent agent such as *S. epidermidis* may present months or years after implantation. A fungal infection may also occur in the pocket and present as an indolent process with relatively scant growth of the organism. Infections with less virulent organisms can present as a small area of erythema, a pimple-like lesion, or a draining sinus. In some cases they appear as cellulitis or pre-erosions. One-third to one-half of infections complicate new implants; the rest are associated with reoperation for generator replacement or lead repositioning.[69] Pocket infections are generally considered to result from organisms introduced from the skin's surface. Superficial infections of the suture line that do not extend to the pocket itself may be treated conservatively.

Staphylococci and presumably other pathogens, adhere to the plastic insulation of pacing hardware and form colonies that become covered with a secreted substance protecting the organism from host defense and antimicrobial drugs. Antibiotic therapy alone is rarely sufficient to cure these infections, and removal of the pacing system is usually indicated. In patients with erosions or localized pocket infections who have been on antimicrobial therapy and have negative blood cultures, it may be possible to place a new pacing system at a different site at the time of removal of the suspect hardware. Most of the time however it would seem prudent to take a two-step approach with temporary pacing (if pacer dependent) used to bridge the time between explantation and new device implant a few days later. After device removal the infected pocket may be partially closed and a drain inserted or packed with wet-to-dry dressings and left open to heal by secondary intention.

Less frequently, a pacemaker patient may develop sepsis without localizing signs, in which case endocarditis associated with a pacing lead should be excluded. Lead endocarditis generally occurs later than pocket infection. It may be related to an organism introduced at implantation but is more often thought to be secondary to a transient bacteremia often from an undefined source. The diagnosis of lead endocarditis is made when a vegetation is detected by ultrasound. In the absence of a positive transthoracic echocardiogram a transesophageal is necessary to rule the diagnosis in or out. A recent report suggests pacemaker associated endocarditis constitutes 4.6% of the entire population with infective endocarditis and occurs with an incidence of about 0.6% in pacer recipients. Staphylococci species predominate with about two-thirds being coagulase negative.[70]

The presence of a vegetation should mandate the removal of all pacing hardware after antibiotics have been started. In these situations, time between explant and implantation of a new permanent system is necessary for antibiotic therapy to sterilize the blood. Generally this interval is related to the duration of previous antibiotic treatment and the confirmation of negative blood cultures, usually 3 to 10 days. Patients are usually capable of being discharged thereafter on continued antibiotics. The antibiotic therapy is selected on the basis of the organism cultured from the blood or hardware, and treatment duration should be similar to that of non–pacemaker associated infective endocarditis with the same organism.

In the absences of a positive echocardiogram, a first episode of sepsis without an identifying cause should be treated with antibiotics and the pacing system retained. A recurrence of sepsis after a course of antibiotic therapy in a patient without a demonstrable etiology should prompt consideration of removal of the entire pacing system even if there is no clinical evidence that the leads or generator are infected.

Complications of Biventricular Pacing

Implantation of a coronary venous lead is the major procedural difference between biventricular and simple dual-chamber pacemaking. It is subject to all the complications associated with dual-chamber systems plus those unique to left ventricular pacing.[71] The left ventricular lead must be placed in a lateral wall vein that has been a challenge especially in the early experience with this modality. Inability to achieve a left ventricular lead placement by a transvenous approach has been reported to be as high as 9%. Unique complications include extensive coronary sinus dissection (4% to 7%) and coronary venous perforation (2%). The latter may lead to tamponade requiring urgent drainage. With better tools and more experience lead placement has been facilitated and the long procedure times as well as the significant complication rate reduced. Extracardiac stimulation from the left ventricular lead (diaphragm and phrenic nerve) may also be problematic and should be tested for at the time of implant. Its occurrence should prompt search for another lead implant site. Appropriate programming of these devices is a concern since the patient population is hemodynamically fragile and sensitive to changes in the A-V interval.

Lead Extraction

General Principles: On occasion, consideration is given to the removal of implanted endocardial leads (Box 5.6). The ease of accomplishing this task and the risk associated with lead removal is related to the time the lead has been implanted. Thus, a lead that has been in place for 3 months or less should be easily removed whereas one in place for longer than a year may well present difficulties due to fibrosis, which may occur at any of a number of sites in the

Box 5.6. Indications for Lead Extraction

Class I

Sepsis (including endocarditis) involving the pacing system

Life-threatening arrhythmias due to retained lead fragment

Retained lead or fragment that poses imminent physical threat to patient

Clinically significant thromboembolic event caused by a lead or lead fragment

Occlusion of all useable veins with need to implant a new pacer system

Lead that interferes with the operation of another device

Class II

Localized pocket infection or erosion that does not involve transvenous portion of leads when lead can be separated from infected area

Occult infection with no clear source but pacer system suspected

Chronic pain at pocket or lead insertion sites unresponsive to other management

Lead failure or design flaw that may pose a future risk to the patient

Lead that interferes with treatment of a malignancy

Leads preventing vascular access for new implantable device

Nonfunctional lead in a young patient

Class III

Risk of lead removal significantly higher than benefit

Single nonfunctional lead in older patient

Normally functioning lead that may be reused at the time of generator replacement

heart and central veins, which the lead had contact with. Non-isodiametric leads and those with anchoring appendages (tines or fins) present additional problems. When we speak of lead extraction we are generally concerned with the special challenges presented by a chronically implanted lead, i.e., one with an implant duration greater than 1 year. This definition may also be used in situations in which specialized tools (e.g., sheaths, locking stylets, snares, etc.) are needed and/or when the lead is removed from a site other than that of original venous access. The term "lead explant" is used for the removal of leads having an implant duration of less than 1 year with only the tools used in a typical implantation and manual traction. These definitions have some importance in terms of the requisite qualifications of physicians performing the respective procedures (see subsequent discussion).[72] While most of this discussion is directed at lead "extraction," it is relevant to physicians performing lead "explantation" as well.

There are two general approaches for the removal of pacing leads: percutaneous or transthoracic. Most pacing physicians think that if extraction is to be performed it should be done percutaneously; others however may still argue the benefits of surgery as a primary approach. Certainly simple traction on the lead is easy, straightforward, and logistically undemanding. If all leads would yield to this treatment there would be little debate as to the threshold for lead extraction and even less support for the more invasive surgical option. Unfortunately, chronic leads are not so readily removed and, even with the variety of tools available to assist us in the percutaneous technique, the procedures may be long, difficult, and associated with a finite mortality and a significant morbidity.

The risks of lead removal correctly influence the aggressiveness with which one should pursue this approach. Postmortem pathologic studies of the hearts of patients with permanent pacemakers have revealed intense fibrosis and encapsulation, especially involving the ventricular portion of the lead. This includes the tricuspid valve and its supporting apparatus. Attempts to remove these leads ex vivo are associated with myocardial avulsion, valve damage, and disruption of the lead.[73] Implants of longer duration tend to have more extensive fibrosis, but we have observed significant encapsulation of an atrial lead at post mortem examination 6 weeks after implantation.

Contemporary leads used in the United States are of low profile and primarily coaxial bipolar in configuration; they do not, in general, tolerate the physical forces that may be necessary to extract them by simple traction in the presence of significant fibrosis. Thus, a great variety of tools have been developed to facilitate the extraction of these devices via the process of countertraction. These include a stylet that "locks" in the distal lead, and sheaths that are passed over the lead body, stripping it of fibrous attachments.

The specific events that might complicate lead extraction pertain to the physical forces used to strip away fibrous adhesions to the lead body, and those used to extricate the tip of the lead from the heart. Catastrophic events, when they occur, usually result from either a laceration of a central vein by an extraction tool or perforation of the heart at the site of tip fixation. Embolization of a large vegetation to the pulmonary artery may also cause death. Damage to the tricuspid valve, or embolization of lead fragment or clot to the lung or, through a patent foramen ovale to the systemic circulation, may also occur. While most complications become evident during or shortly after the extraction procedure, some such as a retroperitoneal bleed, pulmonary embolism, or pericardial tamponade may be delayed in presentation. Because of the risks involved it is essential that an adequate informed consent be obtained from the patient and that the reasons for performing lead extraction, the potential risks and benefits, and alternatives are thoroughly discussed with the patient and family by the operator.

Indications

Lead extraction has inherent risks, thus the decision to undertake the procedure must be weighed against the risk of not extracting the lead. Indications for lead removal based on the latter have been classified in the ACC/AHA guideline format as: class I, general agreement for removal; class II, situations in which leads are often removed but with some divergence of opinion; class III, general agreement that removal is unnecessary.[72] This classification primarily addresses the nature of the risk to the patient of *not removing* a lead, but it does not approach the risk *of extracting* a chronically implanted lead in a specific patient. Thus, an infected lead is often surprisingly easy to remove, whereas elective removal of a nonfunctioning passive-fixation lead in place for a number of years may be extremely difficult and result in complications. A number of modifying factors based on clinical parameters thought to influence the risk of lead extraction have been included in the indication guidelines for the extracting physician to consider. These parameters relate to the patient (age, gender, overall health); anatomy (presence of calcification and vegetations associated with the lead); lead (number of leads, their construction and condition); operator (physician training, experience, and case volume); and the wishes of the patient. These factors are not absolutes but rather supply a context in which to assess the risks for each specific situation and weigh these against the perceived benefit of extraction. Their consideration may be especially important for class II indications for which the clinical necessity of removal may be debated.

An infected lead heads all hierarchical classifications of indications for lead removal, whereas retained nonfunctioning hardware is the least aggressively pursued. The latter poses little risk to the patient[74] but may complicate the placement of additional pacing leads either by adding to the venous obstruction (and the risk of thrombosis/embolization) or by generation of spurious electrical potentials between leads. Rarely a functionless retained lead may, if not properly sutured down in the pacer pocket, retract into the venous system and migrate into the heart, pulmonary artery, or even into the left heart via a patent foramen ovale. The likelihood of any of the latter is small and the routine removal of superfluous noninfected leads probably forms the dividing line between the aggressive lead extractor and those who are more conservative.

Lead failure is almost always defined in terms of electrical performance (e.g., ability to pace and or sense appropriately; or impedance changes suggesting insulation or conductor failure). The danger to the patient is not due to the physical presence of the lead but to the potential inability of the device to do its job. In these cases, removal of the problem lead is of much less concern than the insertion of a new device with normal electrical function. There are leads, however, which may exhibit normal electrical function but offer a physical risk to the patient. The Accufix J lead presents a unique risk to the patient in that a small metal wire placed within the lead only to maintain a J shape is subject to fracture under the stress and strain of clinical use. The fractured ends may wear through the insulation and potentially perforate the heart causing cardiac tamponade or mediastinal hemorrhage. In this situation of "lead failure," electrical function is normal but the physical presence of the lead places the patient at risk. Alleviation of this risk at the time of recognition of the problem would have required lead extraction in the some 45,000 patients in whom the device was implanted. A critical concern for those suggesting guidelines for patient management is whether the risk of lead extraction is less than the mortality and morbidity from the Accufix J lead itself. Indeed a registry established to study this issue concluded that the risk of death from elective lead extraction of non-fractured leads is higher than the risk of injury from the lead.[75] This information has resulted in a recommendation of conservative management of these patients with periodic cinefluoroscopy to screen for retention wire fracture. If fracture occurs options include removal of the lead itself or snaring of the protruding wire fragment using a percutaneous catheter technique.

Risks

Lead extraction using modern tools was associated with a 0.6% risk of death and a 2.5% risk of potentially life-threatening complications in the multicenter Cook Extraction Registry.[76] The same group subsequently found a lower risk of death and major complication (0.04% and 1.4%, respectively), attributed to increasing experience, with no deaths reported by high volume operators.[77] Risk of a major complication was associated with the female gender and number of leads in place while risk of any complication was related to less experienced operators (<50 procedures). The risk of death may have been understated by this registry since the Accufix J lead registry[75] (which was contemporaneous with the former) revealed a 0.4% risk of death. The availability of new extraction tools, such as the laser sheath, has facilitated the extraction procedure and the overall success rate, but has not reduced complications. A recent multicenter report of the use of the laser sheath in the removal of over 2500 leads revealed an in-hospital death rate of 0.8%.[78] Extraction of any chronically implanted lead should be undertaken only after careful consideration of the risk-benefit ratio including patient age, overall health, presence of calcification or vegetations involving the leads, duration of implant, and patient preference to assume additional risk.

TECHNIQUE

Extraction of chronically implanted endocardial leads should only be undertaken by experienced physicians and surgeons skilled in the required techniques. Unfortunately this procedure is not frequently performed and there are few opportunities even in fellowship programs to receive adequate formal training. Acknowledging the well documented association with complications and inexperienced operators, guidelines for the qualification of physicians have been proposed.[2,72] The performance of a minimum of 20 procedures under the supervision of an experienced (more than 100 procedures) operator is recommended before independent practice of these techniques.

The extraction process begins with the gathering and collating of knowledge about the patient and implanted system (Box 5.7) from the patient's history and medical records. This may be augmented from information from the manufacturers of the implanted devices. A chest radiograph is recommended before the procedure to exclude the presence of undocumented hardware. Recent laboratory data, such as complete blood cell count, platelet count, INR and aPTT, electrolytes, BUN, creatinine, and basic chemistries, should be confirmed acceptable. Blood should be typed and cross-matched. It is necessary to know if

Box 5.7. Pre-explant Information

Device:
1. Site(s) of venous access
2. Number and types of leads
3. Method used for retention of leads (e.g., sleeve, number of sutures)
4. Difficulties encountered in prior procedures
5. All information on previously abandoned leads

Patient:
1. Degree of pacemaker dependency
2. Risk for sedation/anesthesia
3. Co-morbidities/medications
4. Special considerations (e.g., vascular anomaly or occlusion; IVC filter)

Laboratory:
1. Complete blood cell count, INR, aPTT, platelet count, sample to blood bank
2. Blood chemistries
3. ECG
4. Chest radiograph (PA and LAT) and/or lead fluoroscopy

complete removal of all devices is essential and whether a new device will be implanted as part of the same procedure. Based on the aggregate of these data, a plan of action is devised. The availability of all the tools and equipment that may be needed must be confirmed before the patient is taken to the procedure room.

Most operators perform the procedure in the pacemaker laboratory at a time when cardiovascular surgical support is available if it is needed. Some surgeons prefer to do the procedure in an operating room so that they can immediately address a complication should it occur or revert to a thoracotomy if attempts to remove the lead percutaneously are unsuccessful. In either case adequate fluoroscopy must be available. The patient is prepared as for an implantation, although some surgeons scrub the chest as in preparation for a thoracotomy. We routinely prep both groin areas and place a venous line (6F sheath) in the right femoral vein and a small arterial line in the left femoral artery. Sterile drapes are liberally placed so that a sterile field is maintained from the neck to the toes. If the patient is pacemaker-dependent, a temporary pacing wire is inserted through either a femoral or an internal jugular vein. If such a patient is not to receive a new implant as part of the same procedure I have been using an active fixation permanent lead as the temporary device for added security against lead dislodgment before a new system can be placed. A commercially available lead-extraction kit (Cook Vascular, Leechburg, PA) supplemented by a variety of other tools (such as snares, wires, locking stylets, biopsy forceps, guidewires, and laser extraction sheaths) must be available. The operator should have on hand all of the tools that he or she may feel qualified to use in a complex case, whether their use is anticipated or not—nothing is as frustrating as to be lacking the tool that might turn a failed procedure into a successful one. A pericardiocentesis tray should be readily available and an echocardiography machine should be accessible. The operator must have a step-by-step approach to the specific problems offered by the case in mind, and always be prepared to meet exigencies as they might arise.

The pocket is usually entered through the previous incision line although this may be altered to include a site of erosion. With a combination of sharp and blunt dissection, the generator and lead(s) are freed. Electrocautery is extremely helpful in freeing leads that are often extensively fibrosed to themselves and subcutaneous tissue. The lead is traced to the venous entry point, the suture sleeve is identified, and all retention sutures are cut. The lead is disconnected from the generator and its internal integrity is accessed by passing a routine stylet to the tip. In all cases an initial attempt at gentle traction is probably worthwhile, but care must be taken not to damage the lead during this process.

Passive leads are usually more difficult to extract than active leads presumably because the appendages incorporated on the former devices provide a greater surface area for fibrous adhesion. It is necessary to attempt to unscrew an active fixation lead before removal. If the retraction mechanism is not effective (or if this is a non-retractable helix) an attempt should be made to rotate the entire lead counterclockwise to unscrew the tip from the heart. This may be impossible in situations where the body of the lead is extensively fibrosed to the heart and veins. In this case stripping the lead with telescoping extraction sheaths prior to rotation of the lead may be of help. Pulling out such a lead without retracting the helix, especially when in an atrial position may result in the removal of a full thickness plug of myocardium and a pericardial bleed.

TOOLS FOR EXTRACTION

The Superior Approach

If a lead is not easily removable by gentle traction, the stylet should be withdrawn and the lead cut close to the terminal pin with lead cutter. Care must be taken not to damage the distal lead, which may be held by a specially designed soft clamp. The central lumen of the lead is identified and carefully dilated with a coil-expander tool. The diameter of the lumen is then determined by the insertion of a series of gauge pins. A locking stylet (Fig. 5.20) of a size corresponding to the largest gauge pin accepted by the lead is then advanced through the lumen to the lead tip. This device is essential to focus the force of traction as close to the lead tip as possible. There are now a number of types of locking stylets available, which vary in the way they grip the inner core of the lead. Because current generations of these devices have a greater flexibility in adapting to a range of inner-core diameters, fewer different types and sizes need to be stocked. The operator however needs to be familiar with the specific directions for each of the locking stylets he uses. It may be

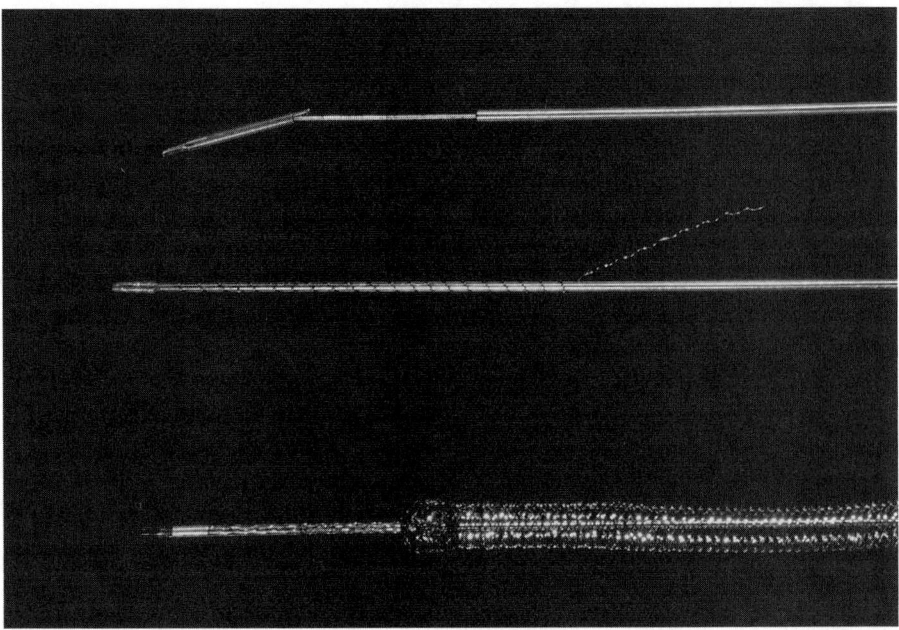

Figure 5.20. Locking stylets for lead extraction. Three types are shown. **Top:** The Wilkoff stylet (Cook Vascular, Leechburg, Penn.) has a sliding distal segment that retracts to form an angulated barb that binds to the lumen of the lead at its tip. **Middle:** The Cook stylet (Cook Vascular) has a small wire "whisker" wound at the tip that unravels and binds the lumen when the stylet is rotated counterclockwise in the lead. **Bottom:** The Spectranetics stylet (Spectranetics, Colorado Springs, CO) has an expandable mesh over the stylet body that when expanded binds the lumen of the lead along its length. Shown here the mesh is fully expanded. With the mesh retracted, the entire length of the stylet is isodiametric with the stylet tip for insertion.

difficult or impossible to reverse the locking mechanism and remove these devices once they are inserted into the lead. In patients with inner conductor failure, the inner lumen of the lead may be interrupted, making it impossible to pass a locking stylet. In this case the femoral approach may be required.

A variety of plastic and metal dilating sheaths (both "powered" by laser or cautery or unpowered) are available to advance over the lead body and free it from fibrous adhesions. These dilating devices have been used coaxially in a telescoping fashion to provide support and allow for a slightly larger device to be used when necessary. In many cases, applying considerable force and torque to the sheath is necessary to separate the lead from fibrous adhesions. To minimize the risk of perforation by the stiff sheaths, fluoroscopic monitoring must be used to ensure that the proper alignment of the dilator sheath and the lead is maintained. Traction upon the lead via the locking stylet facilitates the processes. Correct positioning of the sheath near the tip of the lead provides a mechanism for countertraction to be applied to the lead to facilitate extraction. By advancing the outer sheath to the lead tip at the endocardial surface, the sheath pins the myocardium in place and allows traction on the lead without invaginating or tearing the myocardium (Fig. 5.21).

If the lead(s) are removed successfully, a new pacing system may be implanted at the same site (if circumstances permit) by using a guidewire inserted through the extraction sheath to facilitate venous entry. This technique allows access through even chronically occluded veins.

The process of lead extraction with the use of early generation tools is labor intensive and time consuming: Complete removal of a lead was achieved 81% to 87% of the time and inability to remove the lead was encountered in 6% to 7% of cases.[76] The evolution of technology and introduction of the excimer laser sheath has greatly facilitated lead extraction by the superior approach (see Fig. 5.21). The latter device has optical fibers arrayed circumferentially in the lining of the sheath, which is attached to the Spectranetics excimer laser generator (Spectranetics Colorado Springs, CO). Laser energy ablates the fibrous adhesions as the sheath is advanced. Complete removal of leads using this approach may be anticipated 90% of patients and partial removal in another 3%.[78] An electrosurgical cutting sheath is also available for lead extraction. This device is less expensive but may not be as effective in the more difficult cases as is the laser although there are no adequate comparison trials. It should be re-emphasized that neither of these adjunct energy devices have increased the safety of lead extraction.

Femoral Approach

On occasion, a lead cannot be removed from its original venous access site using the techniques described above due to inadequate lead remnant in the pocket or inability to pass a locking stylet. In these cases the femoral venous approach is often successful. With this method, a large (16F) sheath with a hemostatic valve is used as a "workstation" through which any of a number of devices designed to grasp the lead body may be introduced. These devices may include smaller sheaths, a Dotter retrieval basket, a tip-deflecting guidewire, a "Needle's eye" device (all Cook Vascular, Leechburg, PA), or a variety of other catheters, snares, and bioptomes (see Fig. 5.21). With the femoral technique, one must grasp the lead body which can be done with a single device (the Needle's eye snare) or with two devices such as a tip deflecting wire and an Amplatz gooseneck snare. The Needle's eye device is contained in a 12F sheath. There are two independently moving mechanisms that can be advanced from the sheath: a hook shaped wire loop (needle's eye) and a more narrow "threader," which is designed to pass within the hook of the needle's eye. The goal is to place the device so that the lead body is trapped between the needle's eye and threader. This is usually accomplished by first placing the sheath in the low right atrium with the devices retained inside. The needle's eye is advanced out of the sheath and rotated so that it "hooks" around a lead body. The threader is then advanced so that it passes through the distal portion of the needle's eye such that the lead is between the devices (Fig. 5.22). The sheath is then advanced over the

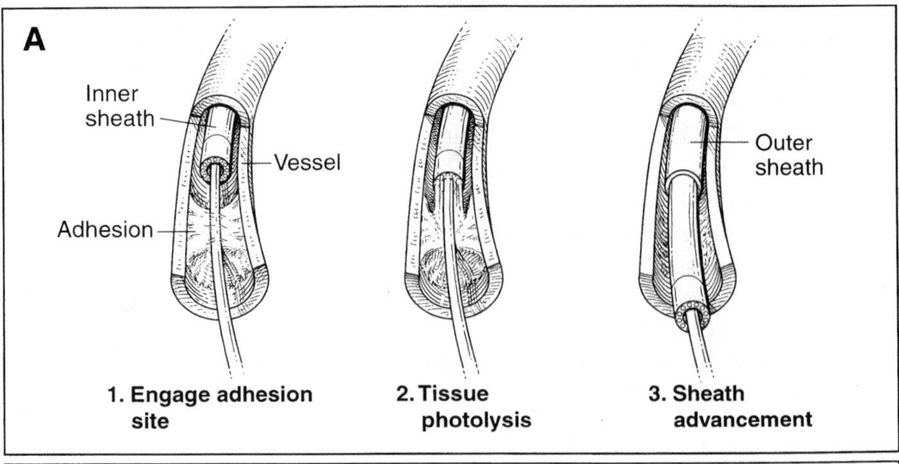
A
Inner sheath
Vessel
Adhesion
Outer sheath
1. Engage adhesion site
2. Tissue photolysis
3. Sheath advancement

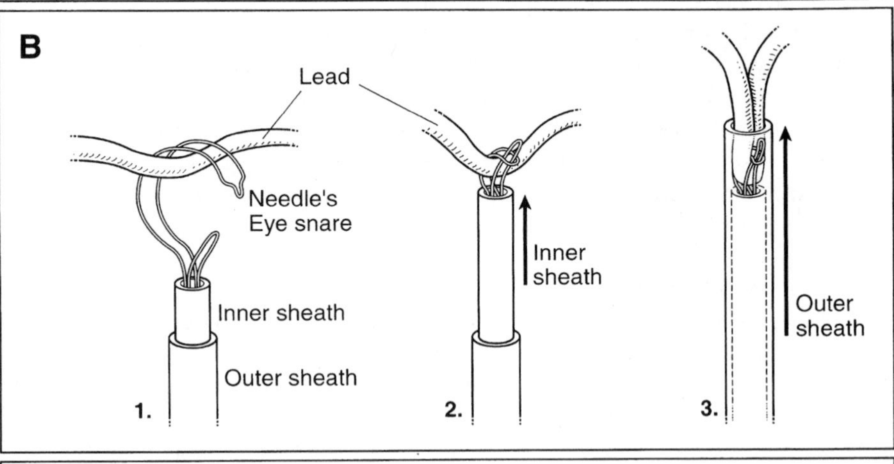
B
Lead
Needle's Eye snare
Inner sheath
Outer sheath
1.
Inner sheath
2.
Outer sheath
3.

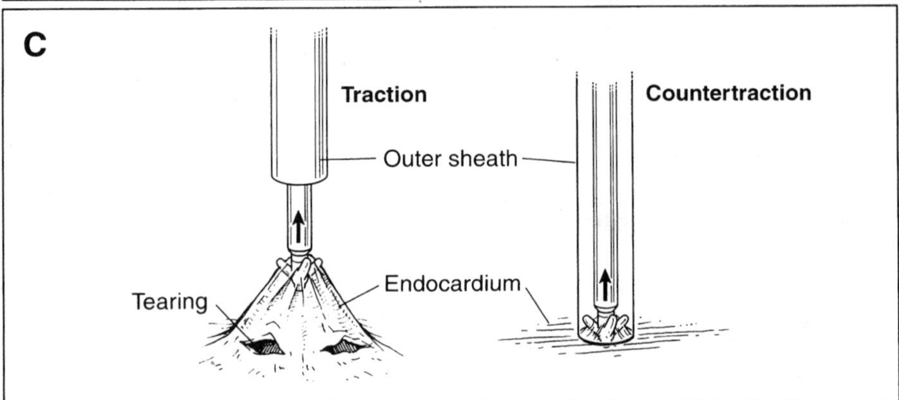
C
Traction
Outer sheath
Countertraction
Tearing
Endocardium

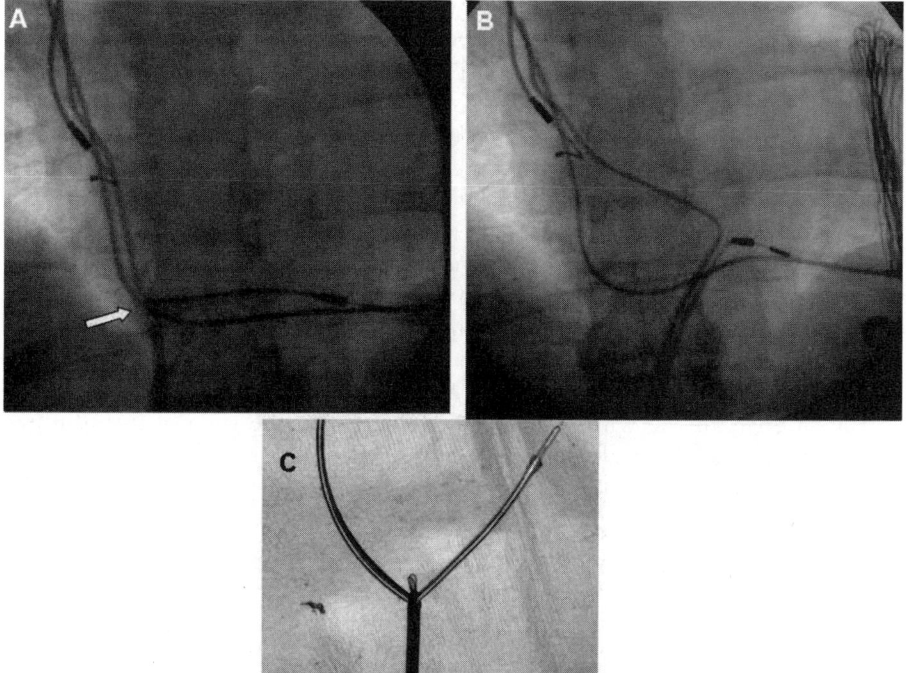

Figure 5.22. Fluoroscopic images of ventricular lead extraction by the femoral approach. **A:** The ventricular lead has been captured with the Needle's eye snare apparatus at the point of the arrow and the redundancy of the lead retracted into the low atrium. **B:** With traction the lead tip is dislodged from the ventricle and the folded lead body is withdrawn into the large outer sheath. **C:** The completely extracted lead.

Figure 5.21. Basic techniques of lead extraction. **A:** Lead extraction from the superior approach using the Spectranetics laser sheath apparatus. As the telescoping sheath apparatus encounters fibrous adhesions, the inner end-firing laser sheath is used to lyse the fibrosis. The larger outer sheath may then be advanced to apply countertraction at the lead tip. **B:** Lead extraction from the femoral approach using the Cook Intravascular Needle's Eye Snare apparatus. The snare is deployed from telescoping sheaths in the femoral vein. The lead is entrapped in the snare and then secured against the inner sheath. The larger outer sheath may then be advanced to apply countertraction at the lead tip. **C:** The concept of countertraction is illustrated. When unmodified traction is applied to the lead, the heart wall may invaginate and tear the myocardium around the lead tip. Using countertraction, the outer sheath holds the myocardium in place, thus minimizing deformity and tearing of the myocardium.

ensemble fixing the captured lead. Once this is accomplished the proximal lead is cut near its original insertion site and traction applied by the sheath pulling the proximal lead into the heart. The captured lead may be prolapsed into the workstation, which can be used as a countertraction device as it is advanced over the distal lead; this however may not be feasible with many larger leads. In the latter instance just withdrawing the proximal free end of the lead into the heart or IVC and then disengaging the Needle's eye, will allow it to be captured by a gooseneck snare and more easily removed through the workstation. The workstation may be advanced over the lead into the ventricle to supply countertraction if necessary. The Needle's eye technique has been found safe and effective with a complete extraction success rate of 87% in a population that included patients who had failed prior extraction from the cephalic approach.[79] A similar procedure may be performed with a deflecting wire and snare. In this situation both the wire and snare are situated in the right atrium through the workstation. A "J" curve is placed on the deflector wire, which is used to "catch" the lead body. The snare is then advanced to tightly grasp the tip of the deflecting wire. This effectively forms a loop around the lead body, which can act to retract the lead after the proximal portion is cut from the original access site. Once captured, the lead can be removed as described previously for the Needle's eye device.

While it is always best to withdraw the lead through the workstation, there are times when this cannot be done and the workstation has to be removed with the lead inside. This could be a problem if there is more than one lead to be removed. In such situations we sometimes leave a "buddy" wire in the femoral vein at the time of original access. This allows us to re-enter the same entry site with a second workstation if it has been necessary to remove the first. Once all of the leads are out it is safe to remove the workstation and apply manual pressure to the femoral access site for hemostasis.

The femoral workstation technique appears to be reasonably safe (perhaps safer than the superior approach outlined previously) and quite successful. It avoids having to free up adhesions in the central veins because the proximal lead is usually more easily pulled through fibrous sheath from below. On occasion however the proximal lead appears trapped within the subclavian vein and will not yield to femoral traction. In these cases the laser sheath can be very helpful in freeing up the proximal lead allowing it then to be extracted via the femoral workstation. The workstation has a large lumen and blood in it easily clots; if care is not taken a large thrombus may form and be pushed into the circulation during the manipulation of devices through the sheath. We routinely attach a pressurized continuous flush to the sidearm of the device to help prevent thrombus formation.

Variations on the femoral approach include a hybrid procedure in which the femoral workstation is used as described above to pull the proximal lead into the heart. At this point a snare introduced from the internal jugular vein is used to catch the free end of the lead and pull it out using countertraction from a long sheath placed in the internal jugular. The entire procedure might be performed using an internal jugular approach which has been favored by some since the direction of force exerted during countertraction is parallel to the course of the lead.

Accufix Wire Fragment Retrieval

As noted previously, fracture of the "J" retention wire in the Accufix family of atrial leads may produce protrusion of a wire fragment (Fig. 5.23), which has the potential to lacerate the heart and other mediastinal structures. It may be possible to selectively retrieve the protruding fragment if it is the distal portion of the proximal part of the wire. This is achieved using an Amplatz gooseneck snare passed through an 8F coronary guide catheter of a shape matching the specifics of the case. Since the proximal portion of the retention wire lies free under the outer insulation of the lead, traction on its protruding end results in the fragment's removal from the lead into the guide catheter without disrupting the lead itself. Detection of a protruding fragment (so-called class III fracture) by screening fluoroscopy should prompt consideration of this form of therapy as an option to lead extraction.[80]

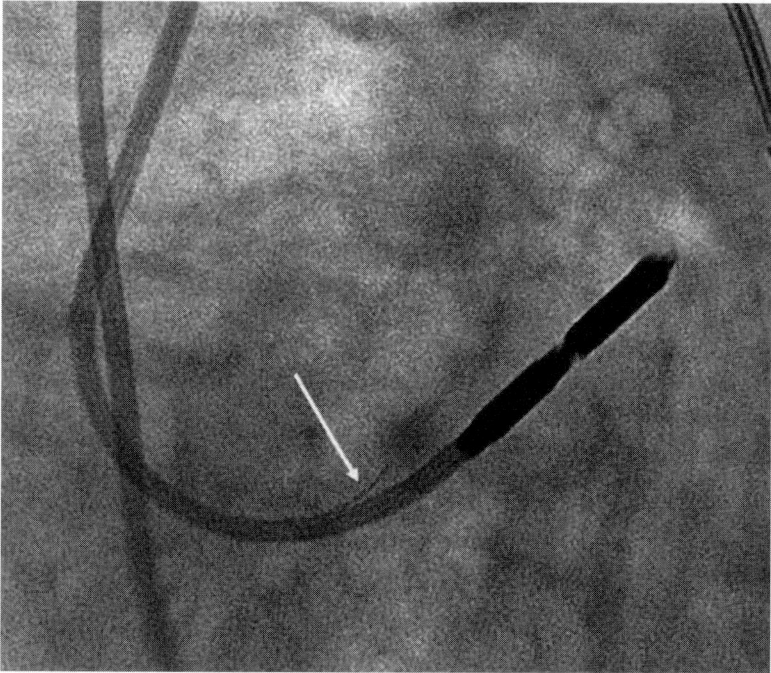

Figure 5.23. Cinefluoroscopy of the Telectronics Pacing Systems model 330–801 Accufix atrial J lead. This right anterior oblique projection shows the protruding segment of the retention wire fragment (*arrow*).

Extraction of Coronary Venous Leads

With the increased use of biventricular pacing, there has been some concern that removal of chronically implanted leads from the coronary venous system will be associated with high complication rates because of the risk of disruption of the thin-walled coronary veins. While there is limited experience thus far, removal of these devices has not been associated with complication. This however includes only a very small number of leads with long implant duration.[81]

Thoracotomy for Lead Extraction

There has been a natural reticence even among surgeons to remove leads at thoracotomy. While there is no randomized data comparing the two techniques, the Accufix experience suggests no clinically significant difference in the incidence of death or major complications. This is not surprising considering the advanced age and co-morbidity of many pacemaker patients. Surgery however may be the only alternative in situations in which percutaneous techniques have failed and there is an absolute indication for lead removal.

Lead Abandonment

The alternative to extraction is lead abandonment and (usually) insertion of a new lead. This is not an option in cases of infection where failure to remove all hardware results in an unacceptable risk of re-infection despite vigorous treatment with antibiotics. One may abandon the lead by detaching it from the generator and applying an insulating cap to the connector pin. The lead may then be placed under the generator or elsewhere in the pocket reserving an option for future use in some situations as well as lead extraction should that prove necessary (e.g., the occurrence of infection). Many operators now prefer to cut the lead and electrically isolate it by pulling the insulation over the exposed end and tying a ligature tightly around the insulation cuff. The lead is then sutured to the underlying tissue to prevent its retraction into the vascular space. Enough lead is left in the pocket to allow for future extraction if that proves necessary. Active fixation leads however should not be cut because this precludes retraction of the helix of the lead if extraction should ever be needed.

MEDICAL-LEGAL ASPECTS OF IMPLANTATION

As with many invasive procedures, the patient's expectations for pacemaker therapy may exceed the results obtained. As noted above, there is ample opportunity for even the most skilled and experienced operator to encounter a misadventure. The risk of litigation[82] is real and may be focused on any of several areas of physician responsibility (Box 5.8). Avoiding litigation requires not only that the highest of standards be maintained but also that a rapport be established with the patient and the patient's family.

The best defense against successful litigation is full documentation in the patient's medical record of every aspect of the implantation (or extraction)

Box 5.8. Responsibilities of an Implanting Physician

1. Establish and document accepted indications.
2. Obtain a fully informed consent.
3. Implant an indicated system.
4. Avoid undo delay.
5. Conform to accepted technique and standards.
6. Obtain expert consultation when appropriate.
7. Provide for follow-up care.

process. This should include the indication for the procedure, the informed consent, a complete procedure note to include the pacing parameters achieved and any difficulties encountered, evidence of postprocedure evaluation, and arrangements for follow-up care. The removal of preexisting hardware and its disposition (e.g., returned to manufacturer for evaluation) must also be documented.

Pacemaker implantation implies a great deal of physician responsibility. As with any implantable device, there is a continued risk to the patient as long as he or she has the device. Somewhat unique to implantable antiarrhythmic devices is the knowledge that the power source has limited life and will eventually need to be replaced. The recent extension of pacemaker therapy to patients without dysrhythmia (e.g., those with hypertrophic obstructive and dilated cardiomyopathies) further complicates the picture. The North American Society of Pacing and Electrophysiology (NASPE) as well as the American College of Cardiology and the American Heart Association have provided a service to physicians by creating guidelines to assist in patient treatment.

REFERENCES

1. Parsonnet V, Bernstein AD, Lindsay B. Pacemaker-implantation complication rates: an analysis of some contributing factors. J Am Coll Cardiol 1989;13:917–921.
2. Hayes DL, Naccarelli GV, Furman S, et al. NASPE training requirements for cardiac implantable electronic devices: selection, implantation, and follow-up. PACE 2003; 26:1556–1562.
3. Schoenfeld MH. Quality assurance in cardiac electrophysiology and pacing: a brief synopsis. Pacing Clin Electrophysiol 1994;17:267–269.
4. Garcia-Bolao I, Alegria E. Implantation of 500 consecutive cardiac pacemakers in the electrophysiology laboratory. Acta Cardiol 1999;54:339–343.
5. Yamamura KH, Kollsterman EM, Alba J, et al. Analysis of charges and complications of permanent pacemaker implantation in the cardiac catheterization laboratory versus the operating room. Pacing Clin Electrophysiol 1999;22:1820–1824.
6. Gregoratos G, Cheitlin MD, Conill A, et al. ACC/AHA guidelines for implantation of cardiac pacemakers and antiarrhythmia devices: executive summary—a report of the American College of Cardiology/American Heart Association Task Force on

Practice Guidelines (Committee on Pacemaker Implantation). Circulation 1998;97: 1325–1335.
7. Hayes DL. Evolving indications for permanent pacing. Am J Cardiol 1999; 83:161D–165D.
8. National Quality of Care Forum. Bridging the gap between theory and practice: exploring clinical practice guidelines. J Qual Improve 1993;19:384–400.
9. Giudici MC, Barold SS, Paul DL, Bontu P. Pacemaker and implantable cardioverter defibrillator implantation without reversal of warfarin therapy. PACE 2004;27: 358–360.
10. Michaud GF, Pelosi F Jr, Noble MD, et al. A randomized trial comparing heparin initiation 6h or 24h after pacemaker or defibrillator implantation. J Am Coll Cardiol 2000;35:1915–1918.
11. Mounsey JP, Griffith MJ, Tynan M, et al. Antibiotic prophylaxis in permanent pacemaker implantation: a prospective randomized trial. Br Heart J 1994;72:339–343.
12. DaCosta A, Kirkorian G, Cucherat M, et al. Antibiotic prophylaxis for permanent pacemaker implantation: a meta-analysis. Circulation 1998;97:1796–1801.
13. Da Costa A, Lelievre H, Kirkorian G, et al. Role of the preaxillary flora in pacemaker infections: a prospective study. Circulation 1998;97:1791–1795.
14. Mathur G, Stables RH, Heavens D, Ingram A, Sutton R. Permanent pacemaker implantation via the femoral vein: an alternative in cases with contraindications to the pectoral approach. Europace 2001 Jan;3(1):56–59.
15. Bellot PH, Bucko D. Inframammary pulse generator placement for maximizing cosmetic effect. Pacing Clin Electrophysiol 1983;6:1241–1244.
16. Spearman P, Leier DV. Persistent left superior vena cava: unusual wave contour of left jugular vein as a presenting feature. Am Heart J 1990;120:999–1022.
17. Zardo F, Nicolosi GL, Burelli C, Zanuttini D. Dual chamber transvenous pacemaker implantation via anomalous left superior vena cava. Am Heart J 1986;112:621–622.
18. Jacobs DM, Fink AS, Miller RP, et al. Anatomical and morphological evaluation of pacemaker lead compression. Pacing Clin Electrophysiol 1993;16:434–444.
19. Magney JE, Flynn DM, Parsons JA, et al. Anatomical mechanisms explaining damage to pacemaker leads, defibrillator leads, and failure of central venous catheters adjacent to the sternoclavicular joint. Pacing Clin Electrophysiol 1993;16:445.
20. Antonelli D, Rosenfeld T, Freedberg NA, et al. Insulation lead failure: is it a matter of insulation coating, venous approach, or both? Pacing Clin Electrophysiol 1998;21:418–421.
21. Ramza BM, Rosenthal L, Hui R, et al. Safety and effectiveness of placement of pacemaker and defibrillator leads in the axillary vein guided by contrast venography. Am J Cardiol 1997;80:892–896.
22. Calkins H, Ramza BM, Brinker J, et al. Prospective randomized comparison of the safety and effectiveness of placement of endocardial pacemaker and defibrillator leads using the extrathoracic subclavian vein guided by contrast venography versus the cephalic approach. PACE 2001;24:456–464.
23. Furman S, Curtis AB, Conti JB. Recognition and correction of subcuticular malposition of pacemaker pulse generators. PACE 2001;24:1224–1227.
24. Kistler PM, Eizenberg N, Fynn SP, Mond HG. The subpectoral pacemaker implant: it isn't what it seems! PACE 2004;27:361–364.
25. Roelke M, Jackson G, Harthorne JW. Submammary pacemaker implantation: a unique tunneling technique. Pacing Clin Electrophysiol 1994;17:1793–1796.

26. Brinker JA. Endocardial pacing leads: the good, the bad, and the ugly. Pacing Clin Electrophysiol 1995;18:953–954.
27. Jordaens LJ, Vandenbogaerde JF, VandeBruquene P, DeBuyzere M. Transesophageal echocardiography for insertion of a physiological pacemaker in early pregnancy. Pacing Clin Electrophysiol 1990;13:955–957.
28. Giudici MC, Thornburg GA, Buck DL, et al. Comparison of right ventricular outflow tract and apical lead permanent pacing on cardiac output. Am J Cardiol 1997;79:209–212.
29. deBuitleir M, Kou WH, Schmalz S, Morady F. Acute changes in pacing threshold and R- or P-wave amplitude during permanent pacemaker implantation. Am J Cardiol 1990;65:999–1003.
30. Roelke M, Bernstein AD, Parsonnet V. Serial lead impedance measurements confirm fixation of helical screw electrodes during pacemaker implantation. Pacing Clin Electrophysiol 2000;23:488–492.
31. Dohrmann ML, Goldschlager NF. Myocardial stimulation threshold in patients with cardiac pacemakers: effect of physiologic variables, pharmacologic agents, and lead electrodes. Cardiol Clin 1985;3:527–537.
32. Bai Y, Strathmore N, Mond H, et al. Permanent ventricular pacing via the great cardiac vein. Pacing Clin Electrophysiol 1994;17:678–683.
33. Timmis G, Westveer D, Gadowski G, et al. The effect of electrode position on atrial sensing for physiologically responsive cardiac pacemakers. Am Heart J 1984;108: 909–916.
34. Parsonnet V, Crawford CC, Bernstein AD. The 1981 United States survey of cardiac pacing practices. J Am Coll Cardiol 1984;3:1321–1332.
35. Connelly DT, Steinhaus DM, Handlin L, et al. Atrial pacing leads following open heart surgery: active or passive fixation? Pacing Clin Electrophysiol 1997;20:2429–2433.
36. Antonioli GE. Single lead atrial synchronous ventricular pacing: a dream come true. Pacing Clin Electrophysiol 1994;17:1531–1547.
37. Tse HF, Lau CP. The current status of single lead dual chamber sensing and pacing. J Interv Card Electrophysiol 1998;2:255–267.
38. Hayes DL, Von Feldt L, Higano ST. Standardized informal exercise testing for programming rate-adaptive pacemakers. Pacing Clin Electrophysiol 1991;14:1772–1776.
39. Link MS, Estes NA 3rd, Griffin JJ, et al. Complications of dual chamber pacemaker implantation in the elderly. Pacemaker Selection in the Elderly (PASE) Investigators. J Interv Card Electrophysiol 1998;2:175–179.
40. Tobin K, Stewart J, Westveer D, Frumin H. Acute complications of permanent pacemaker implantation: their financial implications and relation to volume and operator experience. Am J Cardiol 2000;85:774–777.
41. Weigand UKH, Bode F, Bonnemeier H, Eberhard F, Schlei M, Peters W. Long-term complication rates in ventricular, single lead VDD, and dual chanber pacing. PACE 2003;26:1961–1969.
42. Harcombe AA, Newell SA, Ludman PF, et al. Late complications following permanent pacemaker implantation or elective unit replacement. Heart 1998;80:240–244.
43. Hildick-Smith DJ, Lowe MD, Newell SA, et al. Ventricular pacemaker upgrade: experience, complications and recommendations. Heart 1998;79:383–387.
44. Smith DE, Doherty TM, Reynolds GT, et al. Subclavian vein anatomic subtypes defined by digital cinefluoroscopic venography prior to permanent pacemaker lead insertion. Cathet Cardiovasc Diagn 1996;37:252–257.

45. Oude Ophuis AJ, Van Doorn DJ, van Ommen VA, et al. Internal balloon compression: a method to achieve hemostasis when removing an inadvertently placed pacemaker lead from the subclavian artery. PACE 1998;21:2673–2676.
46. Hilfiker PR, Razavi MK, Kee ST, et al. Stent-graft therapy for subclavian artery aneurysms and fistulas: single-center mid-term results. J Vasc Interv Radiol 2000;11:578–584.
47. Rotem CE, Greig JH, Walters MB. Air embolism to the pulmonary artery during insertion of transvenous endocardial pacemaker. J Thorac Cardiovasc Surg 1967;53:562–565.
48. Chou TM, Chair KM, Jim MH, Boncutter A, Milechman G. Acute occlusion of left internal mammary artery graft during dual-chamber pacemaker implantation. Catheter Cardiovasc Interv 2000;51:65–68.
49. Wiegand UK, Bode F, Bonnemeier H, et al. Atrial lead placement during atrial fibrillation. Is restitution of sinus rhythm required for proper lead function? Feasibility and 12-month functional analysis. Pacing Clin Electrophysiol 2000;23: 1144–1149.
50. Glikson M, Von Feldt LK, Suman VJ, et al. Clinical surveillance of an active fixation, bipolar, polyurethane insulated pacing lead. Part I: The atrial lead. Pacing Clin Electrophysiol 1994;17:1399–1404.
51. Ho WJ, Kuo CT, Lin KH. Right pneumothorax resulting from an endocardial screw-in atrial lead. Chest 1999;116:1133–1134.
52. Barold SS, Center S. Electrocardiographic diagnosis of perforation of the heart by pacing catheter electrode. Am J Cardiol 1969;24:274–278.
53. Sharifi M, Sorkin R, Lakier JB. Left heart pacing and cardioembolic stroke. Pacing Clin Electrophysiol 1994;17:1691–1696.
54. Van Gelder BM, Bracke FA, Oto A, et al. Diagnosis and management of inadvertently placed pacing and ICD leads in the left ventricle: a multicenter experience and review of the literature. Pacing Clin Electrophysiol 2000;23:877–883.
55. de Cock CC, van Campen CMC, Kamp O, Visser CA. Successful percutaneous extraction of an inadvertently placed left ventricular pacing lead. Europace 2003;5:195–197.
56. Hagers Y, Koole M, Schoors D, Van Camp G. Tricuspid stenosis: a rare complication of pacemaker-related endocarditis. J Am Soc Echocardiogr 2000;13:66–68.
57. Bayliss CE, Beanlands DS, Bair RJ. The pacemaker-Twiddler's syndrome: a new complication of implantable transvenous pacemakers. Can Med Assoc J 1968;99: 371–373.
58. Iskos D, Lurie KG, Shultz JJ, et al. "Sagging heart syndrome": a cause of acute lead dislodgment in two patients. Pacing Clin Electrophysiol 1999;22:371–375.
59. Goto Y, Aabe T, Sekine S, Sakurada T. Long-term thrombosis after transvenous permanent pacemaker implantation. Pacing Clin Electrophysiol 1998;21:1192–1195.
60. Zuber M, Huber P, Fricker U, et al. Assessment of the subclavian vein in patients with transvenous pacemaker leads. Pacing Clin Electrophysiol 1998;21:2621–2630.
61. Bracke F, Meijer A, Van Gelder B. Venous occlusion of the access vein in patients referred for lead extraction: influence of patient and lead characteristics. PACE 2003;26:1649–1652.

62. Oginosawa Y, Abe H, Nakashima Y. The incidence and risk factors for venous obstruction after implantation of transvenous pacing leads. PACE 2002;25: 1605–1611.
63. Blair RP, Seibel J, Goodreau J, et al. Surgical relief of thrombotic superior vena cava obstruction caused by endocardial pacing catheter. Ann Thorac Surg 1982;33: 511–515.
64. Cooper CJ, Dweik R, Gabbay S. Treatment of pacemaker-associated right atrial thrombus with 2-hour rTPA infusion. Am Heart J 1993;126:228–229.
65. Lamas GA, Ellenbogen KA, Hennekens CH, Montanez A. Evidence base for pacemaker mode selection: from physiology to randomized trials. Circulation 2004;109: 443–451.
66. Gubner RE, Sands MP, Gross JR. Lipoinjection as a treatment on pacemaker pocket neuralgia. Pacing Clin Electrophysiol 1998;21:624–626.
67. Baumgartner G, Nesser HJ, Jurkovic K. Unusual cause of dyspnea: migration of a pacemaker generator into the urinary bladder. Pacing Clin Electrophysiol 1990;13: 703–704.
68. Kaul Y, Mohan JC, Gopinath N, Bhatia ML. Permanent pacemaker infections: their characterization and management—a 15-year experience. Indian Heart J 1983;35: 345–349.
69. Choo MH, Holmes DR, Gersh BJ, et al. Permanent pacemaker infections: characterization and management. Am J Cardiol 1981;48:559–564.
70. del Rio A, Anguera I, Miro JM, et al. Surgical treatment of pacemaker and defibrillator lead endocarditis: the impact of electrode lead extraction on outcome. Chest 2003;124:1451–1459.
71. Bhatta L, Luck JC, Wolbrette DL, Naccarelli GV. Complications of biventricular pacing. Curr Opin Cardiol 2003;19:31–35.
72. Love CJ, Wilkoff BL, Byrd CL, et al. Recommendations for extraction of chronically implanted transvenous pacing and defibrillator leads: indications, facilities, training. North American Society of Pacing and Electrophysiology Lead Extraction Conference Faculty. Pacing Clin Electrophysiol 2000;23:544–551.
73. Kozlowski D, Dubaniewicz A, Kozluk E, et al. The morphological conditions of the permanent pacemaker lead extraction. Folia Morphol 2000;59:25–29.
74. de Cock CC, Vinkers M, Van Campe LC, et al. Long-term outcome of patients with multiple (> or =3) noninfected transvenous leads: a clinical and echocardiographic study. Pacing Clin Electrophysiol 2000;23:423–426.
75. Kay GN, Brinker JA, Kawanishi DT, Love CJ, et al. Risks of spontaneous injury and extraction of an active fixation pacemaker lead: report of the Accufix multicenter clinical study and worldwide registry. Circulation 1999;100:2344–2352.
76. Smith HJ, Fearnot NE, Byrd CL, U.S. Lead Extraction Database Investigators. Five-year experience with intravascular lead extraction. Pacing Clin Electrophysiol 1994;17:2016–2020.
77. Byrd CL, Wilkoff BL, Love CJ, Sellers TD, et al. Intravascular extraction of problematic or infected permanent pacemaker leads: 1994–1996. Pacing Clin Electrophysiol 1999;22:1348–1357.
78. Byrd CL, Willkoff BL, Love CJ, Sellers TD, Reiser C. Clinical study of the laser sheath for lead extraction: the total experience in the United States. PACE 2002;25:804–808.

79. Klug D, Jarwe M, Messaoudene SA, et al. Pacemaker lead extraction with the needle's eye snare for countertraction via the femoral approach. PACE 2002;25:1023–1028.
80. Lloyd MA, Hayes DL, Stanson AW, Holmes DR. Snare removal of a Telectronics Accufix atrial J retention wire. Mayo Clin Proc 1995;70:376–379.
81. Tyers GF, Clark J, Yang Y, Mills P, Bashir J. Coronary sinus lead extraction. PACE 2003;26:524–526.
82. Dreifus LS, Cohen D. Implanted pacemakers: medicolegal implications. Am J Cardiol 1975;36:266–268.

Pacemaker Timing Cycles

David L. Hayes and Paul A. Levine

6

Understanding various pacing modes and paced electrocardiograms (ECGs) requires a thorough understanding of pacemaker timing cycles. Pacemaker timing cycles include all potential variations of a single complete pacing cycle—the time from paced ventricular beat to paced ventricular beat; the time from paced ventricular beat to an intrinsic ventricular beat, whether it is a conducted R wave or a premature ventricular contraction (PVC); the time from paced atrial beat to paced atrial beat; the time from intrinsic atrial beat to paced atrial beat; the time from intrinsic ventricular beat to paced ventricular beat; and so forth. These cycles include events sensed, events paced, and periods when the sensing circuit or circuits are refractory. Each portion of the pacemaker timing cycle should be considered in milliseconds and not in pulses per minute (ppm). Although thinking of the patient's pacing rate in paced beats per minute may be easier, portions of the timing cycle are too brief to consider in any unit but milliseconds.

Knowledge of the relation between elements of the paced ECG enhances understanding of pacemaker rhythms. Although multiple unknown factors may affect a native rhythm, each timing circuit of a pacemaker can function in only one of two states. A given timer can proceed until it completes its cycle; completion results in either the release of a pacing stimulus or the initiation of another timing cycle. Alternatively, a given timer can be reset, at which point it starts the timing period again.

To make this chapter more readable and to facilitate clarity, a series of abbreviations is used to designate native and paced events and portions of the timing cycle. These abbreviations are listed in Box 6.1. P indicates native atrial depolarization, A an atrial paced event, R native ventricular depolarization, and V a ventricular paced event. I represents an interval. From this, PR refers to a native complex that completely inhibits the pacemaker on both the atrial and the ventricular channels. AV refers to pacing sequentially in both the atrium and the ventricle. If an atrial paced complex is followed by native ventricular depolarization that inhibits the ventricular output of the pacemaker, the designation is AR. If a native atrial complex is followed by a paced ventricular depolariza-

Box 6.1. Abbreviations for Native and Paced Events and Portions of the Timing Cycle

P	Native atrial depolarization
A	Atrial paced event
R	Native ventricular depolarization
V	Ventricular paced event
I	Interval
AV	Sequential pacing in the atrium and ventricle
AVI	Programmed atrioventricular pacing interval
AR	Atrial paced event followed by intrinsic ventricular depolarization
ARP	Atrial refractory period
PV	Native atrial depolarization followed by a paced ventricular event, P-synchronous pacing
AEI	Interval from a ventricular sensed or paced event to an atrial paced event, the VA interval
LRL	Lower rate limit
URL	Upper rate limit
MTR	Maximum tracking rate
MSR	Maximum sensor rate
PVARP	Postventricular atrial refractory period
RRAVD	Rate-responsive atrioventricular delay
VA	Ventriculoatrial interval: interval from a sensed or paced ventricular event to an atrial paced event
VRP	Ventricular refractory period

tion, P-synchronous pacing, the designation is PV. Because the pacemaker timing cycle in dual-chamber pacing has more portions to consider than single-chamber pacing, more discussion is devoted to understanding dual-chamber timing cycles, specifically those of universal (DDD) pacing systems.

Multiple programmable features may affect device behavior (Box 6.2). These are discussed throughout the chapter.

PACING NOMENCLATURE

A three-letter code describing the basic function of the various pacing systems was first proposed in 1974 by a combined task force from the American Heart Association and the American College of Cardiology. Since then, the code has been updated periodically.[1] It is a generic code and, as such, does not describe specific or unique functional characteristics of each device. The code has five positions.

The first position reflects the chamber or chambers in which stimulation occurs. A refers to the atrium, V indicates the ventricle, and D means dual chamber, or both atrium and ventricle.

The second position refers to the chamber or chambers in which sensing occurs. The letter designators are the same as those for the first position. Man-

Box 6.2. Features That May Affect Device Behavior*

Intrinsic rate *slower* than programmed base rate
- Hysteresis
- Sleep or rest rate
- Special algorithms (+PVARP on PVC)

Base rate (AV, AR) *higher* than programmed base rate
- Sensor driven
- Rate smoothing
- Mode-switching response rate
- Special algorithms (+PVARP on PVC)

Intrinsic AV conduction interval (PR, AR) *longer* than programmed paced or sensed AVI
- AV or PV hysteresis
- Sinus rate with intact AV conduction exceeding MTR

Paced or sensed AVI *shorter* than programmed paced or sensed AVI
- Rate-responsive AV delay
- Negative AV or PV hysteresis
- Safety pacing
- NCAP (noncompetitive atrial pacing)
- Auto-threshold test

Loss of atrial tracking (DDD mode)
- Automatic mode switch
- MSR > MTR

* Not necessarily continuously; the effect can be on single cycles or during a brief period.

ufacturers also use S in both the first and the second positions to indicate that the device is capable of pacing only a single cardiac chamber. Once the device is implanted and connected to a lead in either the atrium or the ventricle, S should be changed to either A or V in the clinical record to reflect the chamber in which pacing and sensing are occurring.

The third position refers to the mode of sensing, or how the pacemaker responds to a sensed event. An I indicates that a sensed event inhibits the output pulse and causes the pacemaker to recycle for one or more timing cycles. T means that an output pulse is triggered in response to a sensed event. D, in a manner similar to that in the first two positions, means that there are dual modes of response. This designation is restricted to dual-chamber systems. An event sensed in the atrium inhibits atrial output but triggers ventricular output. Unlike the single-chamber triggered mode, in which an output pulse is triggered immediately on sensing, a delay occurs between the sensed atrial event and the triggered ventricular output to mimic the normal PR interval. If a native ventricular signal or R wave is sensed, it inhibits ventricular output and possibly even atrial output, depending on where sensing occurs.

The fourth position of the code reflects rate modulation. An R in the fourth position indicates that the pacemaker incorporates a sensor to control the rate independently of intrinsic electrical activity of the heart.

The fifth position indicates whether multisite pacing is not present (O) or present in the atrium (A), ventricle (V), or both (D). Multisite pacing is defined for this purpose as stimulation sites in both atria, both ventricles, more than one stimulation site in any single chamber, or any combination of these.

PACING MODES

Ventricular Asynchronous Pacing, Atrial Asynchronous Pacing, and AV Sequential Asynchronous Pacing

Ventricular asynchronous (VOO) pacing is the simplest of all pacing modes because there is neither sensing nor mode of response. The timing cycle is shown in Figure 6.1. Irrespective of any other events, the ventricular pacing artifacts occur at the programmed rate. The timing cycle cannot be reset by any intrinsic event. In the absence of sensing, there is no defined refractory period.

Atrial asynchronous (AOO) pacing behaves exactly like VOO, but the pacing artifacts occur in the atrial chamber.

Dual-chamber, or AV sequential asynchronous (DOO), pacing has an equally simple timing cycle. The interval from atrial artifact to ventricular artifact (atrioventricular interval, AVI) and the interval from the ventricular artifact to the subsequent atrial pacing artifact (ventriculoatrial interval, VAI, or atrial escape interval, AEI) are both fixed. The intervals never change, because the pacing mode is insensitive to any atrial or ventricular activity, and the timers are never reset (Fig. 6.2).

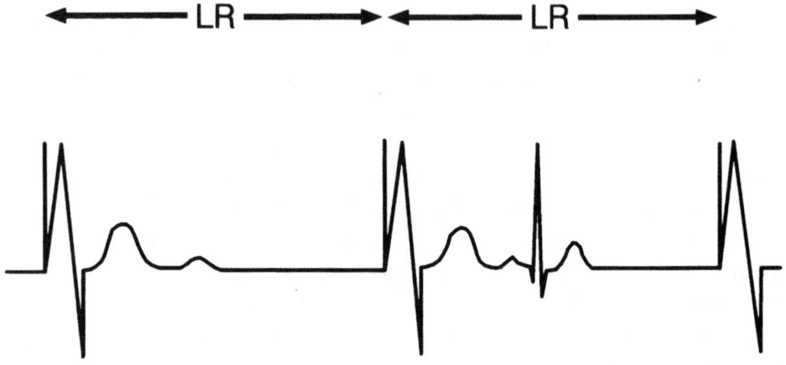

Figure 6.1. The VOO timing cycle consists of only a defined rate. The pacemaker delivers a ventricular pacing artifact at the defined rate regardless of intrinsic events. In this example, an intrinsic QRS complex occurs after the second paced complex, but because there is no sensing in the VOO mode, the interval between the second and the third paced complex remains stable.

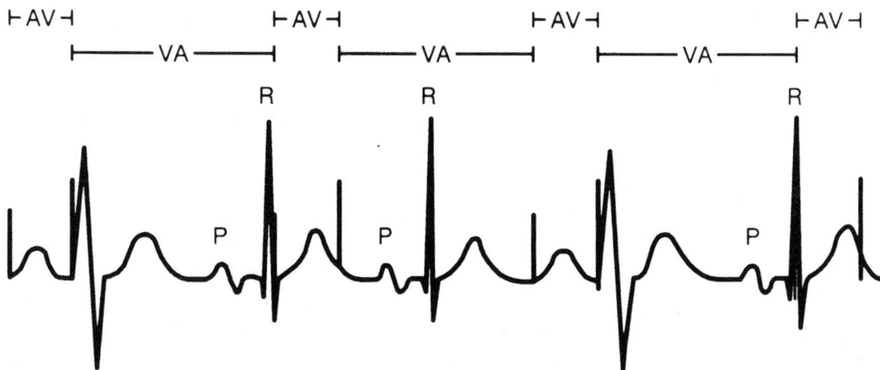

Figure 6.2. The DOO timing cycle consists of only defined AV and VV intervals. The VAI is a function of the AV and VV intervals. An atrial pacing artifact is delivered, and the ventricular artifact follows at the programmed AVI. The next atrial pacing artifact is delivered at the completion of the VAI. The intervals do not vary because no activity is sensed; that is, nothing interrupts or resets the programmed cycles.

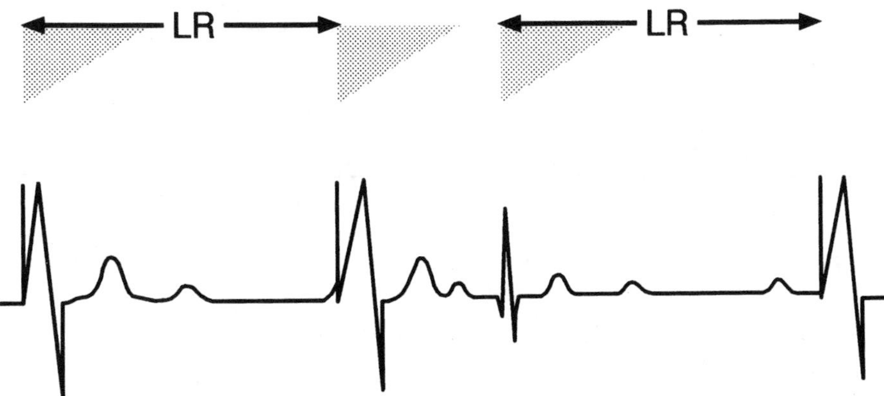

Figure 6.3. The VVI timing cycle consists of a defined LRL and a VRP *(shaded triangles)*. When the LRL timer is complete, a pacing artifact is delivered in the absence of a sensed intrinsic ventricular event. If an intrinsic QRS occurs, the LRL timer is started from that point. A VRP begins with any sensed or paced ventricular activity.

Ventricular Inhibited Pacing

By definition, ventricular demand inhibited (VVI) pacing incorporates sensing on the ventricular channel, and pacemaker output is inhibited by a sensed ventricular event (Fig. 6.3). VVI pacemakers are refractory after a paced or sensed ventricular event, a period known as the ventricular refractory period (VRP). Any ventricular event occurring within the VRP is not sensed and does not reset the ventricular timer (Fig. 6.4).

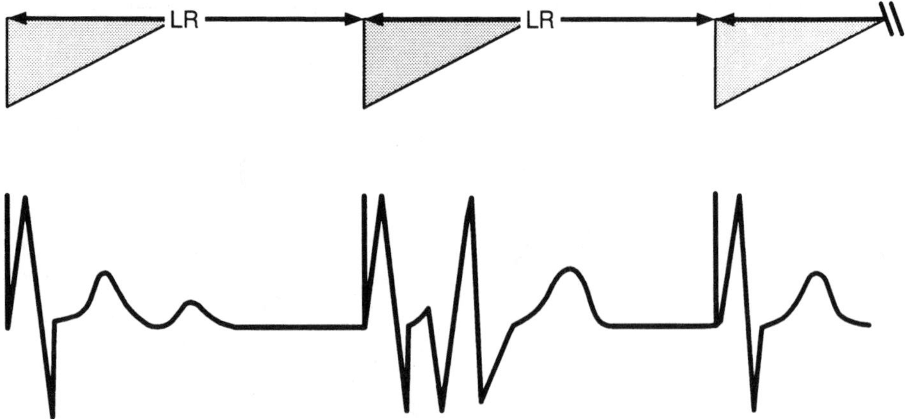

Figure 6.4. If, in the VVI mode, a ventricular event occurs during the VRP *(shaded triangles)*, it is not sensed and therefore does not reset the LRL timer.

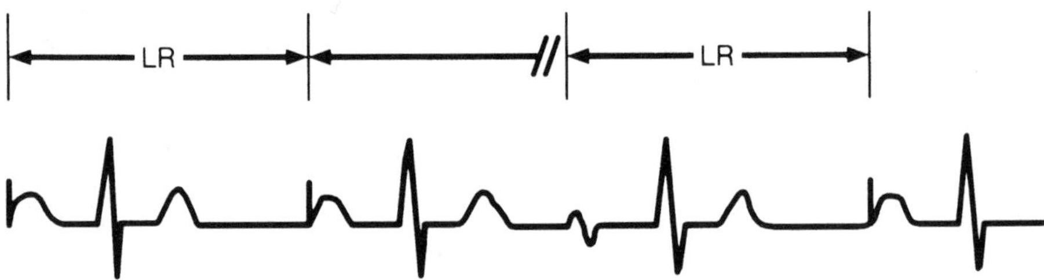

Figure 6.5. The AAI timing cycle consists of a defined LRL and an ARP. When the LRL timer is complete, a pacing artifact is delivered in the atrium in the absence of a sensed atrial event. If an intrinsic P wave occurs, the LRL timer is started from that point. An ARP begins with any sensed or paced atrial activity.

Atrial Inhibited Pacing

Atrial inhibited (AAI) pacing, the atrial counterpart of VVI pacing, incorporates the same timing cycles, with the obvious differences that pacing and sensing occur from the atrium and pacemaker output is inhibited by a sensed atrial event (Fig. 6.5). An atrial paced or sensed event initiates a refractory period during which the pacemaker senses nothing. Confusion can arise when multiple ventricular events occur during atrial pacing. For example, a premature ventricular beat following the intrinsic QRS that occurs in response to the paced atrial beat does not inhibit an atrial pacing artifact from being delivered (Fig. 6.6). When the AA timing cycle ends, the atrial pacing artifact is delivered regardless of ventricular events, because an AAI pacemaker should not sense anything in the ventricle. The single exception to this rule is far-field sensing; that is, the ventricular signal is large enough to be inappropriately sensed by the

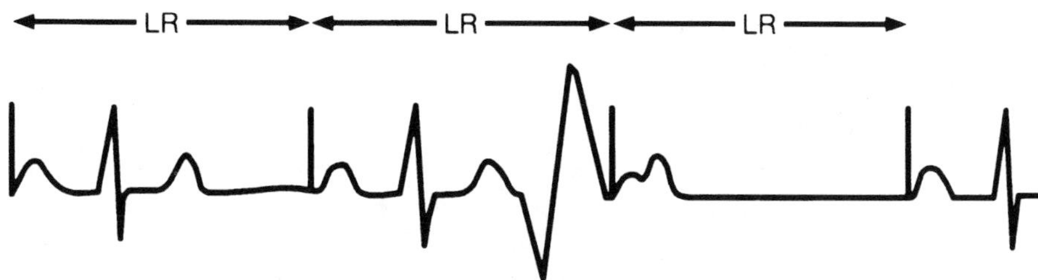

Figure 6.6. In the AAI mode, only atrial activity is sensed. In this example, it may appear unusual for paced atrial activity to occur so soon after intrinsic ventricular activity. Because sensing occurs only in the atrium, ventricular activity would not be expected to reset the pacemaker's timing cycle.

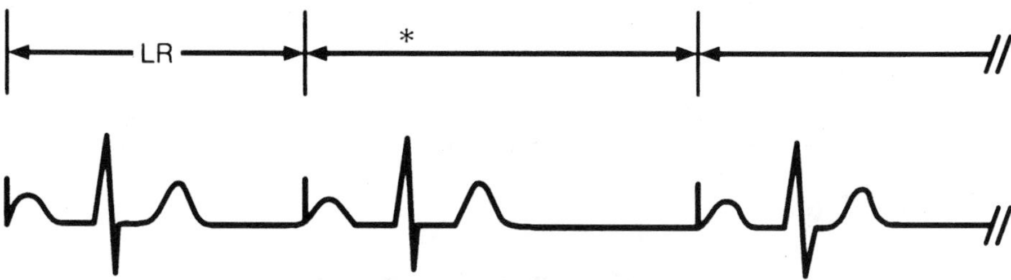

Figure 6.7. In this example of AAI pacing, the AA interval is 1000 milliseconds (60 ppm). The interval between the second and third paced atrial events is greater than 1000 milliseconds. The interval from the second QRS complex to the subsequent atrial pacing artifact is 1000 milliseconds. This occurs because the second QRS complex *(asterisk)* has been sensed on the atrial lead (far-field sensing) and has inappropriately reset the timing cycle. LR = lower rate.

atrial lead (Fig. 6.7). In this situation, the atrial timing cycle is reset. Sometimes this anomaly can be corrected either by making the atrial channel less sensitive or by lengthening the refractory period.

Single-Chamber Triggered-Mode Pacing

In single-chamber triggered-mode pacing, the pacemaker releases an output pulse every time a native event is sensed. This feature increases the current drain on the battery, accelerating its rate of depletion. This mode of pacing also deforms the native signal, compromising ECG interpretation. However, it can serve as an excellent marker for the site of sensing within a complex. It can also prevent inappropriate inhibition from oversensing when the patient does not have a stable native escape rhythm. In addition, it can be used for noninvasive electrophysiologic studies, with the already implanted pacemaker tracking chest wall stimuli created by a programmable stimulator. One special requirement to use the triggered mode for noninvasive electrophysiologic studies is shortening the refractory period intentionally, thereby allowing the implanted pacemaker to track external chest wall stimuli to rapid rates and close coupling intervals.

Rate-Modulated Pacing

The "sensor function of the pacemaker" refers to modulation of the paced rate in response to an input signal other than the presence or absence of native depolarization. The most widely used sensors include those that sense motion, either acceleration or vibration, impedance signals that measure minute ventilation and the measured interval from pacemaker stimulus to the T wave, i.e., a QT-interval sensor. Many other sensors have been used but not widely.

Single-Chamber Rate-Modulated Pacing: Single-chamber pacemakers capable of rate-modulated (SSIR) pacing can be implanted in the ventricle (VVIR) or atrium (AAIR). The timing cycles for SSIR pacemakers are not markedly different from those of their non–rate-modulated counterparts. The timing cycle includes the basic VV or AA interval and a refractory period from the paced or sensed event. The difference lies in the variability of the VV or AA interval (Fig. 6.8). Depending on the sensor incorporated and the patient's level of exertion,

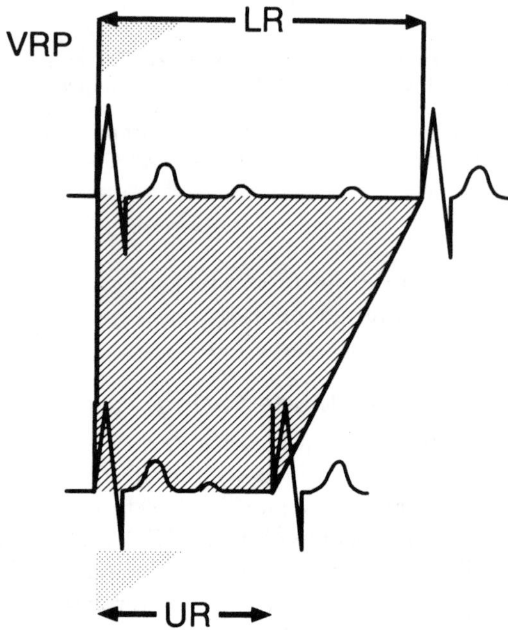

Figure 6.8. The VVIR timing cycle consists of an LRL, an upper rate limit (UR), and a VRP, represented by shaded triangles. As indicated by sensor activity, the VV cycle length shortens accordingly. (The *striped area* represents the range of sensor-driven VV cycle lengths.) In most VVIR pacemakers, the VRP remains fixed despite the changing VV cycle length. In selected VVIR pacemakers, the VRP shortens as the cycle length shortens.

the basic interval is shorter than the programmed lower rate limit (LRL). Shortening requires that an upper rate limit (URL) be programmed to define the absolute shortest cycle length allowable. Most approved SSIR pacemakers incorporate a fixed refractory period; that is, regardless of whether the pacemaker is operating at the LRL or URL, the refractory period remains the same. Thus, at the higher rates under sensor drive, the pacemaker may effectively become SOOR, because the alert period during which sensing can occur is so abbreviated. Native beats falling during the refractory period are not sensed. Hence, in SSIR pacing systems, if the refractory period is programmable, it should be programmed to a short interval to maximize the sensing period at both the low and the high sensor-controlled rates. In some pacemakers, when the cycle length shortens, the refractory period shortens correspondingly; this is referred to as the *rate-variable refractory* period. This event is analogous to the QT interval of the native ventricular depolarization.

Single-Chamber and Dual-Chamber Rate-Modulated Asynchronous Pacing: The asynchronous pacing modes (that is, AOO, VOO, and DOO, as explained previously) have fixed intervals that are insensitive to all intrinsic events and have timers that are never reset. If rate modulation is incorporated in an asynchronous pacing mode, the basic cycle length is altered by sensor activity. In the single-chamber rate-modulated asynchronous (AOOR and VOOR) pacing modes, any alteration in cycle length is attributable to sensor activity and not to the sensing of intrinsic cardiac depolarizations. In the dual-chamber rate-modulated asynchronous (DOOR) pacing mode, the pacing rate changes in response to the sensor input signal but not to the native P or R wave. In some pacemakers, the AVI may be programmed to shorten progressively as the rate increases, whereas in other units, it remains fixed at the initial programmed setting.

Atrioventricular Sequential, Ventricular Inhibited Pacing

AV sequential, ventricular inhibited (DVI) pacing is rarely used. However, this pacing mode is a programmable option in most available dual-chamber pacemakers. For this reason, it is important to understand the timing cycles for DVI pacing.[2,3]

By definition, DVI provides pacing in both the atrium and the ventricle (D) but sensing only in the ventricle (V). The pacemaker is inhibited and reset by sensed ventricular activity but ignores all intrinsic atrial complexes. The DVI units in the first generation were large and bulky and had two relatively large bipolar leads. The bipolar design produced small output pulses and generated a highly localized sensing field. In this setting, the ventricular sense amplifier remained alert when the atrial stimulus was released and throughout the AVI. Thus, a native R wave during the AVI was sensed so that ventricular output was inhibited and the AEI was reset (Fig. 6.9A). For both atrial and ventricular stimuli to be inhibited, the sensed R wave must occur during the AEI.

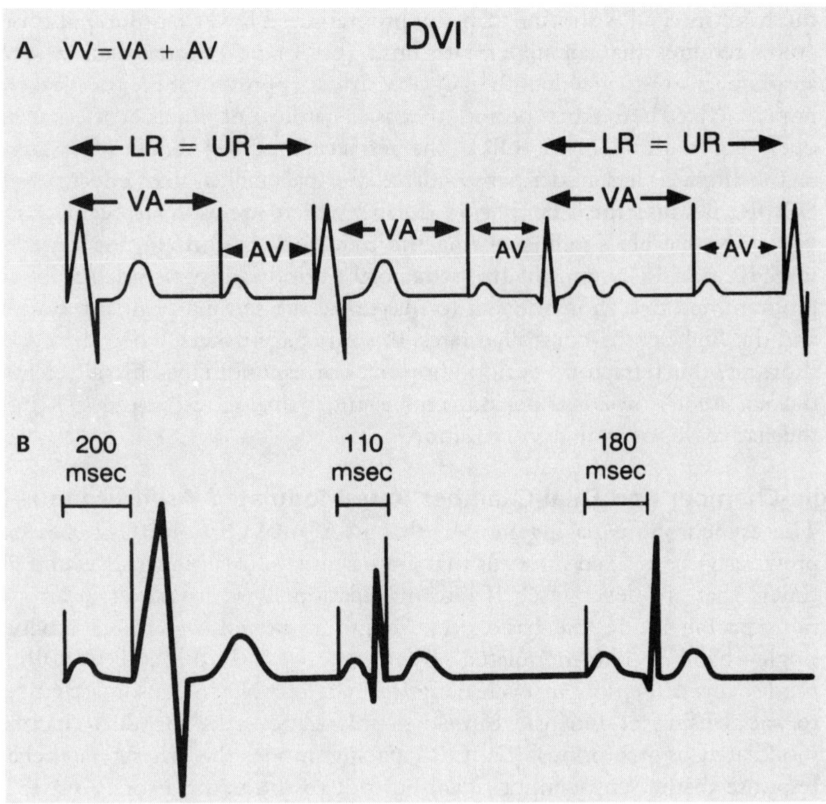

Figure 6.9. A: In the noncommitted version of DVI, the components of the timing cycle are the same as those for DVIC (see Fig. 6.10). However, if ventricular activity is sensed after the atrial pacing artifact, ventricular output is inhibited; that is, a ventricular pacing artifact is not committed to the previous atrial pacing artifact. **B:** In the modified or partially committed version of DVI, ventricular events sensed within the nonphysiologic AVI do not inhibit ventricular output, and a ventricular pacing stimulus occurs at the end of the interval. Ventricular events occurring within the physiologic AVI inhibit pacemaker function. In this example, the first paced atrial and ventricular events represent normal DVI pacing. The second paced atrial and intrinsic ventricular complex demonstrates a spontaneous ventricular event occurring within the nonphysiologic AVI and resulting in a ventricular pacing stimulus. In the third event shown, after an atrial paced event, a spontaneous ventricular event falls within the physiologic AVI, resulting in inhibition of ventricular pacing function.

Improvements in circuit design enabled the manufacturers to reduce the size of the pulse generator. They also made the next generation unipolar to facilitate venous access for the two leads. The large unipolar atrial stimulus could be sensed on the ventricular channel. It would be sensed by the pacemaker as a ventricular event and inhibit ventricular output. This occurrence is known as *crosstalk*, which is potentially catastrophic if concomitant AV block is present. To prevent crosstalk, the second generation of DVI pacemakers initiated the VRP on completion of the AEI timer. Thus, once an atrial output pulse occurred, the ventricular sense amplifier was refractory, and the pacemaker was obligated to release a ventricular output pulse, regardless of whether it was physiologically necessary. This event was termed *committed AV sequential pacing* (Fig. 6.10). It caused significant confusion because a normally functioning system might demonstrate functional undersensing and functional noncapture in both atrium and ventricle simultaneously.

The present generation of devices still requires a period of ventricular refractoriness, a "ventricular blanking period," to minimize the chance of crosstalk, but this interval is brief, lasting from 12 to 125 milliseconds. In many pacemakers the duration of this interval is programmable. If the atrial stimulus were to coincide with a native R wave, for example, a PVC, and the intrinsic deflection of the native complex fell outside the blanking period, the R wave would be sensed, and ventricular output would be inhibited. In this situation, the pacemaker would behave like the earlier noncommitted systems. If, however, the intrinsic deflection coincided with the blanking period, the R wave would not be seen, and the pacemaker would release a ventricular output pulse at the end of the AVI in a manner analogous to that of the committed systems. This operation has been termed *modified* or *partially committed* to reflect the fact that the devices may demonstrate both noncommitted and committed functions as part of their normal behavior[4] (Fig. 6.9B).

The timing cycle (VV) consists of the AVI and VAI. The basic cycle length (VV), or LRL, is programmable, as is the AVI. The difference, VV–AV, is the VAI,

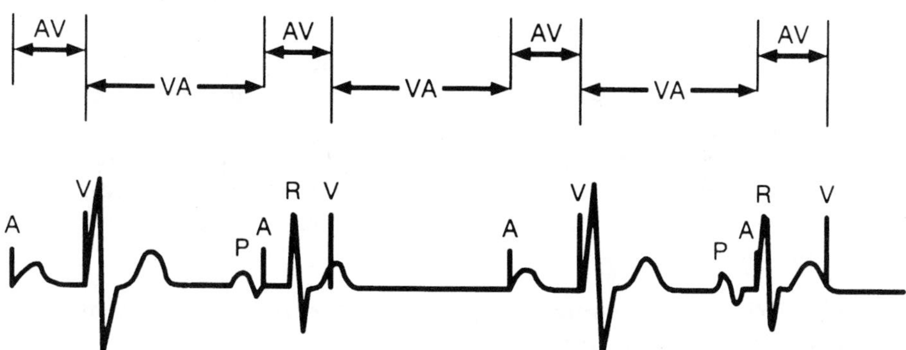

Figure 6.10. The timing cycle in committed DVI consists of an LRL, an AVI, and a VRP. The VRP is initiated with any sensed or paced ventricular activity. (By definition, there is no atrial sensing and, therefore, no defined ARP.) The VAI is equal to the VV or LRL interval minus the AVI. In a committed system, a ventricular pacing artifact follows an atrial pacing artifact at the AVI regardless of whether intrinsic ventricular activity has occurred. In this example, the LRL is 1000 milliseconds, or 60 ppm, and the AVI is 200 milliseconds. At the end of the VAI, 800 milliseconds after a ventricular event, if no ventricular activity has been sensed, the atrial pacing artifact is delivered. A ventricular pacing artifact occurs 200 milliseconds later, irrespective of any intrinsic events. This is functional undersensing, because the ventricular pacing artifact is delivered as a function of the DVI pacing mode.

or AEI. During the initial portion of the VAI, the sensing channel is refractory. (The refractory period is almost always a programmable interval.) After the refractory period, the ventricular sensing channel is again operational, or "alert." If ventricular activity is not sensed by the expiration of the VAI, atrial pacing occurs, followed by the AVI. If intrinsic ventricular activity occurs before the VAI is completed, the timing cycle is reset. (Additional discussion of crosstalk, the ventricular blanking period, and ventricular safety pacing can be found in the section that specifically discusses AVI.)

Atrioventricular Sequential, Non–P-Synchronous Pacing with Dual-Chamber Sensing: AV sequential pacing with dual-chamber sensing, non–P-synchronous (DDI) pacing can be thought of as either an upgrade of DVI noncommitted pacing or a downgrade of DDD pacing—that is, DDD pacing without atrial tracking.[5] The difference between DVI and DDI is that DDI incorporates atrial sensing as well as ventricular sensing. This prevents competitive atrial pacing that can occur with DVI pacing. The DDI mode of response is inhibition only; that is, no tracking of P waves can occur. Therefore, the paced ventricular rate cannot be greater than the programmed LRL. The timing cycle consists of the LRL, AVI, postventricular atrial refractory period (PVARP), and VRP. The PVARP is the period after a sensed or paced ventricular event during which the atrial sensing circuit is refractory. The atrial sensing circuit does not sense any atrial event occurring during the PVARP. If a P wave occurs after the PVARP and is sensed, no atrial pacing artifact is delivered at the end of the VAI. The subsequent ventricular pacing artifact cannot occur until the VV interval has been completed; that is, the LRL cannot be violated (Fig. 6.11).

It bears repeating that, because P-wave tracking does not occur with the DDI mode, the paced rate is never greater than the programmed LRL. A slight exception to this statement may occur when an intrinsic ventricular complex takes place after the paced atrial beat (AR) and inhibits paced ventricular output before completion of the programmed AVI; that is, AR is less than AV. In this situation, the cycle length from A to A is shorter than the programmed LRL by the difference between the AR and the AVI (Fig. 6.12).

Atrioventricular Sequential, Non–P-Synchronous, Rate-Modulated Pacing with Dual-Chamber Sensing

The timing cycles for non–P-synchronous, rate-modulated AV sequential (DDIR) pacing are the same as those described previously for DDI pacing except that paced rates can exceed the programmed LRL through sensor-driven activity. Depending on the sensor incorporated and the level of exertion of the patient, the basic cycle length shortens from the programmed LRL. This cycle length change requires that a URL be programmed to define the absolute shortest cycle length allowable.

Even though no P-wave tracking occurs in a DDIR system, an intrinsic P wave may inhibit the atrial pacing artifact and give the appearance of P-wave

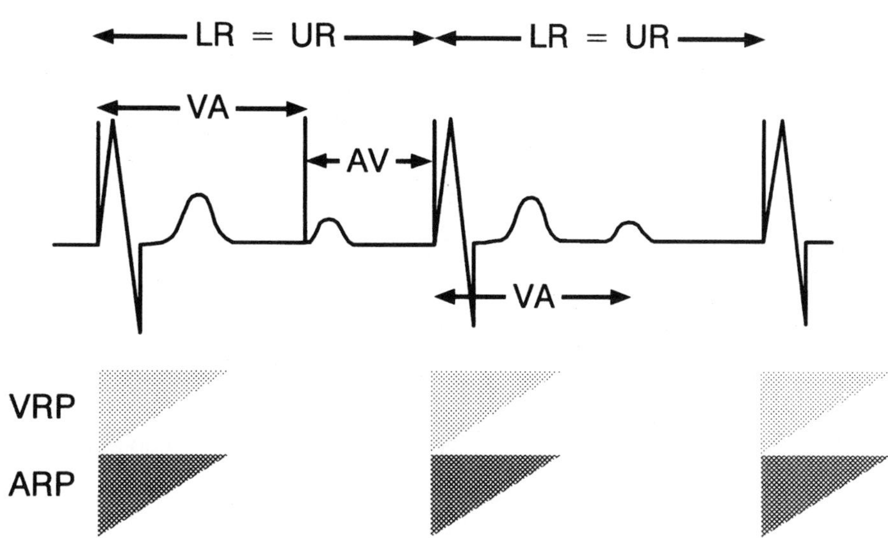

Figure 6.11. The timing cycle in DDI consists of an LRL, an AVI, a VRP, and an ARP. The VRP is initiated by any sensed or paced ventricular activity, and the ARP is initiated by any sensed or paced atrial activity. DDI can be thought of as DDD pacing without the capability of P-wave tracking or DVI without the potential for atrial competition by virtue of atrial sensing. The LRL cannot be violated even if the sinus rate is occurring at a faster rate. For example, the LRL is 1000 milliseconds, or 60 ppm, and the AVI is 200 milliseconds. If a P wave occurs 500 milliseconds after a paced ventricular complex, the AVI is initiated; but at the end of the AVI, 700 milliseconds from the previous paced ventricular activity, a ventricular pacing artifact cannot be delivered, because it would violate the LRL.

tracking if an appropriately timed intrinsic atrial depolarization falls within the atrial sensing window (ASW).[6] This phenomenon is coincidental.

In a DDDR pacing system in which the programmed maximum sensor rate (MSR) is greater than the maximum tracking rate (MTR), AV sequential pacing occurs when the sensor function drives the ventricular rate above the programmed maximum rate. The actual mode at this time is DDIR. If the intrinsic atrial rate also exceeds the MTR so that the native atrial signal is sensed, atrial output is inhibited. Meanwhile, the ventricular paced complex is controlled by the sensor. The appearance may be of PV pacing (atrial-sensed ventricular pacing), with the ventricular rate violating the MTR. In actuality, the ventricular paced complex is a result of sensor drive, and if the sensor input to the pacemaker would not allow a paced rate this rapid, the ventricular rate would be limited by the MTR limit.

Atrial Synchronous (P-Tracking) Pacing: Atrial synchronous (P-tracking) (VDD) pacemakers pace only in the ventricle (V), sense in both atrium and ventricle (D), and respond both by inhibition of ventricular output by intrinsic ventricular activity (I) and by ventricular tracking of P waves (T). This mode of pacing

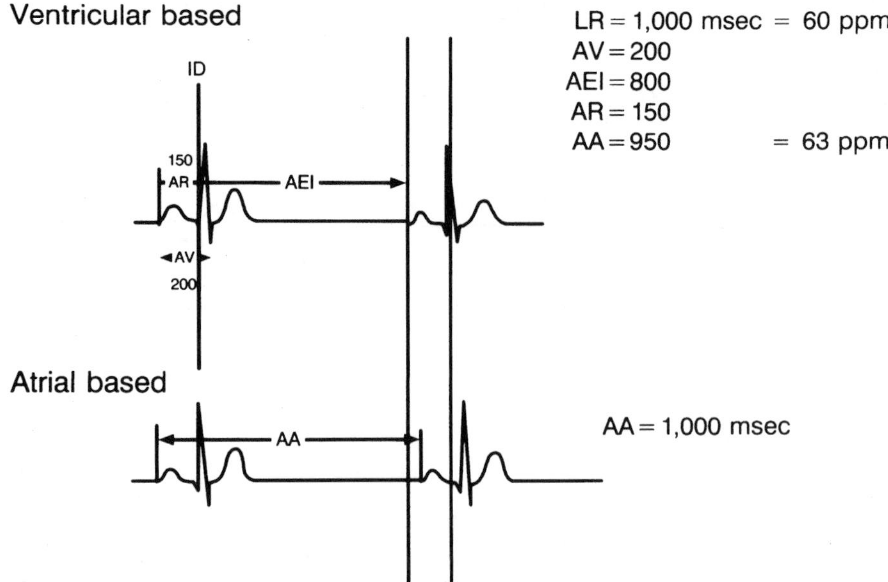

Figure 6.12. **Top:** With ventricular-based timing in patients with intact AV nodal conduction after AR pacing, the sensed R wave resets the AEI. The base pacing interval consists of the sum of the AR and the AEI; thus, it is shorter than the programmed minimum rate interval. **Bottom:** With atrial-based timing in patients with intact AV nodal conduction after AR pacing, the sensed R wave inhibits ventricular output but does not reset the basic timing of the pacemaker. There is atrial pacing at the programmed base rate. (From Levine PA, Hayes DL, Wilkoff BL, Ohman AE. Electrocardiography of rate-modulated pacemaker rhythms. Sylmar, CA: Siemens-Pacesetter, 1990. By permission of Siemens-Pacesetter.)

is a programmable option in many dual-chamber pacemakers.[7] The VDD mode is also available as a single-lead pacing system. In this system, a single lead is capable of pacing in the ventricle in response to sensing atrial activity by way of a remote electrode(s) situated on the intra-atrial portion of the ventricular pacing lead.

The timing cycle is composed of LRL, AVI, PVARP, VRP, and URL. A sensed atrial event initiates the AVI. If an intrinsic ventricular event occurs before termination of the AVI, ventricular output is inhibited, and the LRL timing cycle is reset. If a paced ventricular beat occurs at the end of the AVI, this beat resets the LRL. If no atrial event occurs, the pacemaker escapes with a paced ventricular event at the LRL; that is, the pacemaker displays VVI activity in the absence of a sensed atrial event (Fig. 6.13).

Dual-Chamber Pacing and Sensing with Inhibition and Tracking

Although the DDD timing cycle involves more intervals, standard dual-chamber pacing and sensing with inhibition and tracking (DDD) are reasonably easy to comprehend on the basis of the timing cycles already discussed.[7–12] The basic

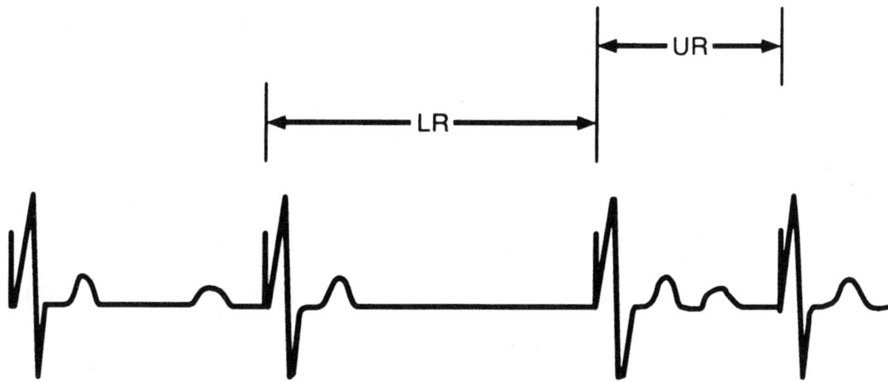

Figure 6.13. The timing cycle of VDD consists of an LRL, an AVI, a VRP, a PVARP, and a URL. A sensed P wave initiates the AVI (during the AVI, the atrial sensing channel is refractory). At the end of the AVI, a ventricular pacing artifact is delivered if no intrinsic ventricular activity has been sensed, that is, P-wave tracking. Ventricular activity, paced or sensed, initiates the PVARP and the VAI (the LRL interval minus the AVI). If no P-wave activity occurs, the pacemaker escapes with a ventricular pacing artifact at the LRL.

timing circuit associated with LRL pacing is divided into two sections. The first is the interval from a ventricular sensed or paced event to an atrial paced event and is known as the AEI, or VAI. The second interval begins with an atrial sensed or paced event and extends to a ventricular event. This interval may be defined by a paced AV, PR, AR, or PV interval. An atrial sensed event that occurs before completion of the AEI promptly terminates this interval and initiates an AVI, and the result is P-wave synchronous ventricular pacing.[8] If the intrinsic sinus rate is less than the programmed LRL, AV sequential pacing at the programmed rate or functional single-chamber atrial (AR) pacing occurs (Fig. 6.14A).

An option for "circadian response," or "sleep rate," in many contemporary pacemakers[1] allows a lower rate to be programmed for the approximate time during which the patient is sleeping. A separate, potentially faster LRL may then be programmed for waking hours. (For example, the LRL during waking hours may be programmed to 70 bpm, and the LRL during sleeping hours may be programmed to 50 bpm.) In some pacemakers, this feature is tied to a clock, and the usual waking and sleeping hours are programmed into the pacemaker. In other pacemakers, the sleep rate is also set on the basis of waking and sleeping hours, but verification by a sensor is required to allow rate changes to occur.

PORTIONS OF PACEMAKER TIMING CYCLES

Refractory Periods

Every pacemaker capable of sensing must include a refractory period in its basic timing cycle. Refractory periods prevent the sensing of known but clinically

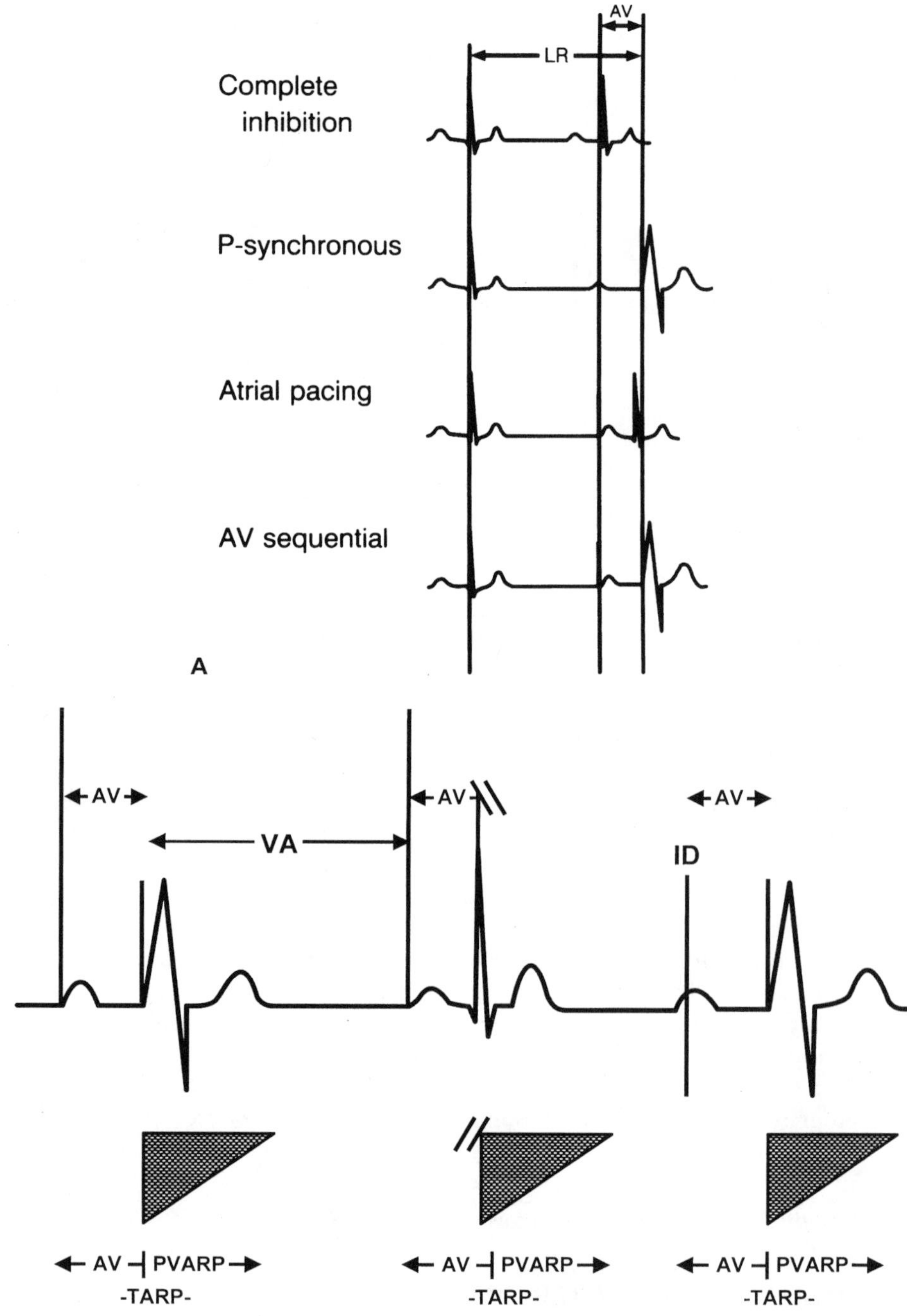
AV
LR
Complete inhibition
P-synchronous
Atrial pacing
AV sequential
A
AV
VA
AV
AV
ID
AV PVARP
-TARP-
AV PVARP
-TARP-
AV PVARP
-TARP-
B

inappropriate signals, such as the evoked potential and repolarization (T wave).

In a single-chamber system that is otherwise capable of sensing (either the inhibited or the triggered mode), each sensed or paced event is followed by a refractory period. Once this timing period ends, the sense amplifier becomes alert and is receptive to the detection of native signals. If an appropriate event, such as a PVC, coincides with the VRP, it is not detected, and competition between the pacemaker and the intrinsic activity may occur. The refractory period of a pacemaker is analogous to the refractory period of the heart (QT interval). During the cardiac refractory period, a stimulus delivered to the heart is ineffective because the myocardium is already depolarized and a subsequent depolarization cannot occur until the resting membrane potential is reestablished. Like the heart, the pacemaker has a refractory period consisting of two components. The first is the absolute refractory period, during which native activity cannot be detected. More recently, this has been called a *blanking period.* The terminal portion of the refractory period is relative when events can be detected, but they are not used to trigger or reset an output pulse. Rather, they are used to detect rapid signals. If these signals exceed 400 to 600 cycles per minute (which is above the physiologic range), they are labeled *electrical noise.* Rather than be inhibited by these inappropriate signals, the pacemaker is designed to adopt asynchronous behavior, which is termed *noise mode response.* In the recent generation of dual-chamber pacing systems, rapid events detected on the atrial channel, but not the ventricular channel, help the device detect pathologic atrial rates and initiate automatic mode switching (see "Mode Switching," below).

In a DDD system, a sensed or paced atrial event initiates an atrial refractory period (ARP) and also initiates the AVI (Fig. 6.14B). During this portion of the timing cycle, the atrial channel is refractory to another native atrial event; nor does atrial pacing occur during this period. Atrial pacing occurs only at the end of the AVI or later (see "Upper Rate Behavior," discussed subsequently). A

Figure 6.14. **A:** The timing cycle in DDD consists of an LRL, an AVI, a VRP, a PVARP, and a URL. There are four variations of the DDD timing cycle. If intrinsic atrial and ventricular activity occur before the LRL times out, both channels are inhibited and no pacing occurs **(first panel)**. If a P wave is sensed before the VAI is completed (the LRL minus the AVI), output from the atrial channel is inhibited. The AVI is initiated, and if no ventricular activity is sensed before the AVI terminates, a ventricular pacing artifact is delivered, that is, P-synchronous pacing **(second panel)**. If no atrial activity is sensed before the VAI is completed, an atrial pacing artifact is delivered, which initiates the AVI. If intrinsic ventricular activity occurs before the termination of the AVI, ventricular output from the pacemaker is inhibited, that is, atrial pacing **(third panel)**. If no intrinsic ventricular activity occurs before the termination of the AVI, a ventricular pacing artifact is delivered, that is, AV sequential pacing **(fourth panel)**. **B:** Potential pacing combinations that can occur in the DDD pacing mode. The intrinsic P wave is sensed during the early portion of the P wave. The AVI is initiated at the point of the intrinsic deflection (ID) of atrial activity, as seen on the atrial electrogram. (Modified from Medtronic, Minneapolis, MN.)

sensed or paced ventricular event initiates a VRP. (A VRP is always part of the timing cycle of any pacing system with ventricular pacing and sensing.) The VRP prevents sensing of the evoked potential and the resultant T wave on the ventricular channel of the pacemaker. A sensed or paced ventricular event also initiates a refractory period on the atrial channel (PVARP).[13,14] The PVARP may prevent atrial sensing of a retrograde P wave (see "Endless-Loop Tachycardia," below), but the PVARP alone may not prevent sensing of far-field ventricular events in devices with an automatic mode-switching algorithm. The combination of the PVARP and the AVI forms the total atrial refractory period (TARP). The TARP, in turn, is the limiting factor for the maximum sensed atrial rate that the pacemaker can sense and, hence, track. For example, if the AVI is 150 milliseconds and the PVARP is 250 milliseconds, the TARP is 400 milliseconds, or 150 ppm. In this case, a paced ventricular event initiates the 250-millisecond PVARP, and only after this interval has ended can an atrial event be sensed. If an atrial event is sensed immediately after the termination of the PVARP, the sensed atrial event initiates the AVI of 150 milliseconds. On termination of the AVI, in the absence of an intrinsic R wave, a paced ventricular event occurs, resulting in a VV cycle length of 400 milliseconds, or 150 ppm. Programming a long PVARP limits the upper rate by limiting the maximum sensed atrial rate (Fig. 6.15).[15,16] If the native atrial rate were 151 bpm, every other P wave would coincide with the PVARP, not be sensed, and hence not

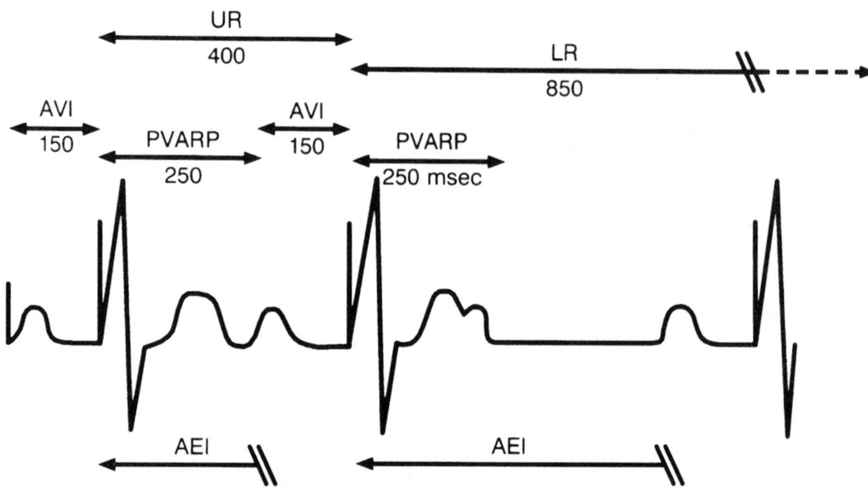

Figure 6.15. In the DDD pacing mode, the upper rate (UR) is limited by the AVI and the PVARP. In this example, the AVI is 150 milliseconds and the PVARP is 250 milliseconds, for a TARP of 400 milliseconds (this is equal to 150 ppm). As shown, after the first paced ventricular complex, a P wave occurs just after the completion of the PVARP. This P wave is sensed, initiates the AVI, and is followed by another paced ventricular complex. The subsequent P wave occurs within the PVARP and is therefore not sensed. The DDD response is to wait for the next intrinsic P wave to occur, as in this example, or for the AEI to be completed, whereupon AV sequential pacing occurs.

be tracked; so the effective paced rate would be approximately 75 ppm, or half the atrial rate.

In a pacemaker with a mode-switching algorithm "on," the pacemaker must be able to detect higher atrial rates, even if the native P waves coincide with the PVARP. Although these P waves may not be tracked, the pacemaker is capable of monitoring events that coincide with the refractory period to recognize rapid pathologic atrial rates. Thus, the system can switch from a tracking mode (DDD) to a nontracking mode (VVI or DDI), so that the first of the pathologic atrial events that occur during the atrial alert period is not tracked.

Atrioventricular Interval

The AVI, often poorly understood, should be considered a single interval with two subportions (Fig. 6.16A).[17] For most dual-chamber systems, the atrial

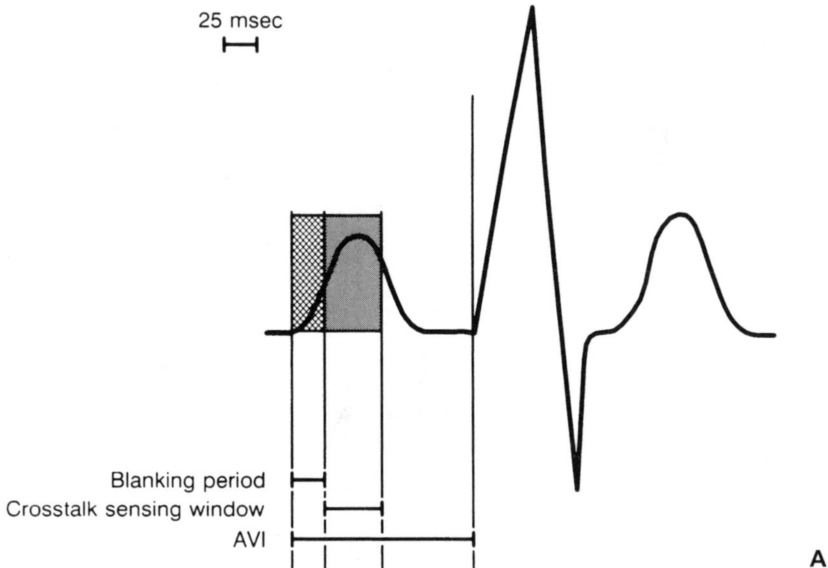

Figure 6.16. **A:** The AVI should be considered as a single interval with two subportions. The entire AVI corresponds to the programmed value, that is, the interval following a paced or sensed atrial beat allowed before a ventricular pacing artifact is delivered. The initial portion of the AVI is the blanking period. This interval is followed by the crosstalk sensing window. **B:** If the ventricular sensing circuit senses activity during the crosstalk sensing window, a ventricular pacing artifact is delivered early, usually at 100 to 110 milliseconds after the atrial event. This has been referred to as "ventricular safety pacing," "110-millisecond phenomenon," and "nonphysiologic AV delay." **C:** The initial portion of the AVI in most dual-chamber pacemakers is designated as the blanking period. During this portion of the AVI, sensing is suspended. The primary purpose of this interval is to prevent ventricular sensing of the leading edge of the atrial pacing artifact. Any event that occurs during the blanking period, even if it is an intrinsic ventricular event (as shown in this figure), is not sensed. In this example, the ventricular premature beat that is not sensed is followed by a ventricular pacing artifact delivered at the programmed AVI and occurring in the terminal portion of the T wave.

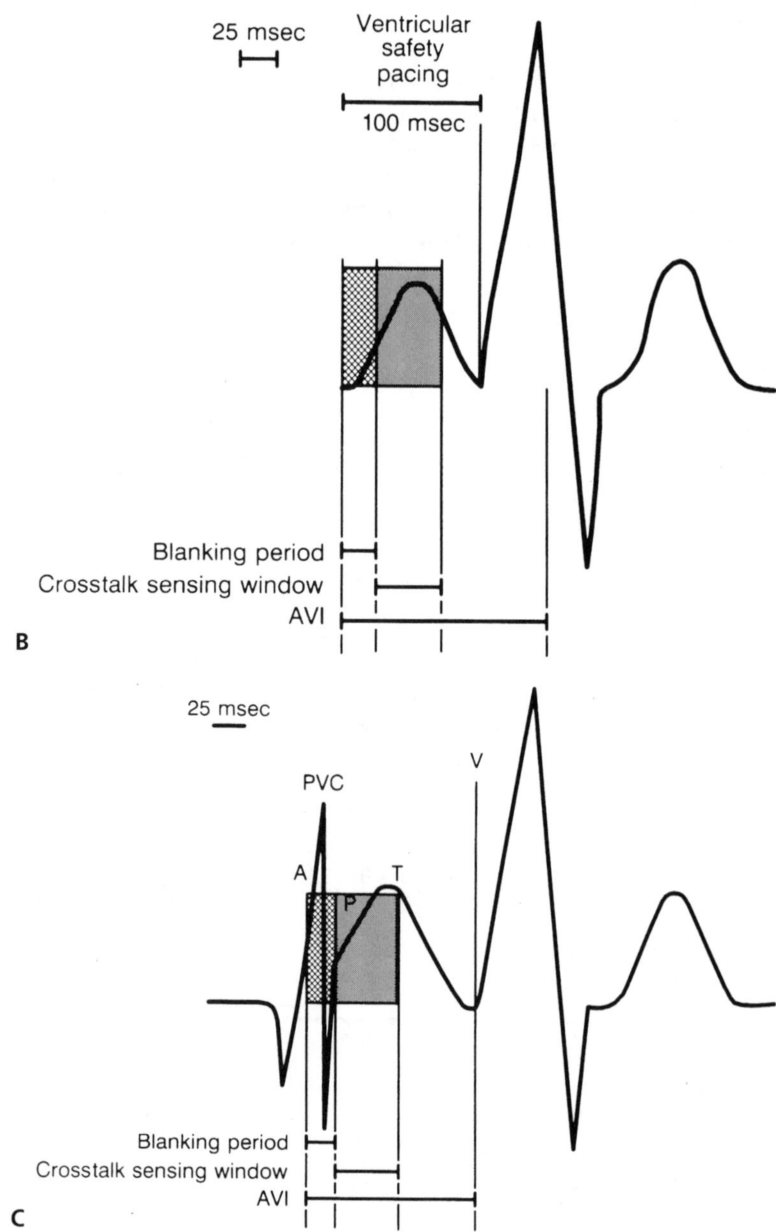

Figure 6.16. *Continued*

channel is totally refractory to the detection of other atrial signals that may occur during the AVI. In most devices, only the first portion of the AVI is absolutely refractory. The terminal portion is a relative refractory period, to assist in the detection of rapid pathologic atrial rhythms for purposes of mode switching (Fig. 6.17).

Atrial output also triggers a timing period on the ventricular channel, known as the *ventricular blanking period*. It coincides with the earliest portion of the AVI, and its purpose is to avoid sensing of an event or a stimulus of one channel in the opposite channel.[18–20]

If the atrial pacing artifact were sensed by the ventricular sensing circuit, ventricular output inhibition would result, i.e., crosstalk. To prevent crosstalk, the leading edge of the atrial pacing artifact is masked, or blanked, by rendering the ventricular sensing circuit absolutely refractory during the very early portion of the AVI (Fig. 6.16B). In DDD pacemakers, the blanking period may be programmable, ranging from 12 to 125 milliseconds. The blanking period is traditionally of short duration because it is important for the ventricular sensing circuit to be returned to the "alert" state relatively early during the AVI so that intrinsic ventricular activity can inhibit pacemaker output if it occurs before the AVI ends. The potential exists for signals other than those of intrinsic ventricular activity to be sensed and inhibit ventricular output. The greatest concern is crosstalk.[19,21] Even though the leading edge of the atrial pacing artifact is effectively ignored because of the blanking period, the trailing edge of the atrial pacing artifact occurring after the blanking period can occasionally be sensed on the ventricular channel. In a pacemaker-dependent patient, inhibition of ventricular output by crosstalk results in asystole. To prevent such an outcome, a safety mechanism is present.

If activity is sensed on the ventricular sensing circuit in a given portion of the AVI immediately after the blanking period (this second portion of the AVI

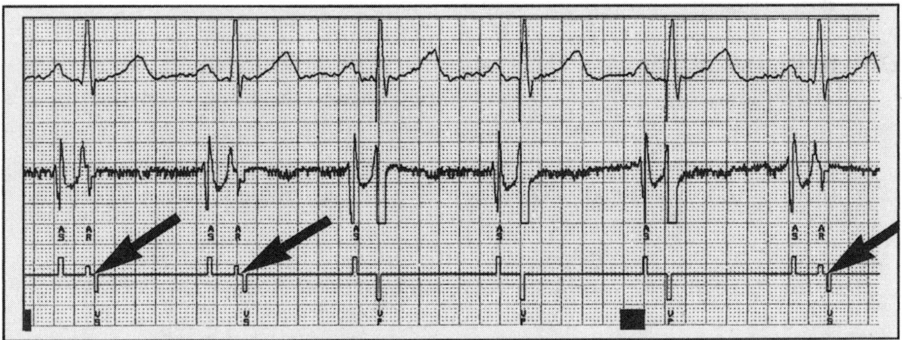

Figure 6.17. Surface ECG, atrial electrogram, and event markers *(arrows)* demonstrating occasional AR complexes, events that are occurring within the ARP. They coincide with the QRS complex but are detected on the atrial channel before being detected by the pacemaker on the ventricular channel.

has been called the "ventricular triggering period" or the "crosstalk sensing window"), it is assumed that crosstalk cannot be differentiated from intrinsic ventricular activity. To prevent catastrophic ventricular asystole, a ventricular pacing artifact is delivered early—at an AVI of 100 to 120 milliseconds, although in some pulse generators this interval is programmable for 50 to 150 milliseconds (Fig. 6.16C).[22] If the signal sensed is indeed crosstalk, a paced ventricular complex delivered at the abbreviated interval prevents ventricular asystole. In addition, AV pacing at a shorter-than-programmed AVI on the ECG indicates the occurrence of crosstalk and allows the pacemaker to be programmed to eliminate this behavior. Elimination of crosstalk may be accomplished by extending the ventricular blanking period, decreasing atrial output, or reducing the ventricular sensitivity. Or, if true intrinsic ventricular activity occurs during the early portion of the AVI, the safety mechanism results in delivery of a ventricular pacing artifact within or immediately after the intrinsic beat. This delivery is safe because the ventricle is refractory, no depolarization results from the pacing artifact, and the pacing artifact is delivered too early to coincide with ventricular repolarization or a vulnerable period. This event has been referred to as "ventricular safety pacing," "nonphysiologic AV delay," or the "110-millisecond phenomenon." Although the safety pacing phenomenon accompanying a late-cycle PVC has been interpreted as a sensing failure, it actually reflects normal sensing. Pacemaker behavior changes with respect to a ventricular event that is sensed during the "crosstalk sensing" window. The response is altered in comparison with an event sensed at any other time during the ventricular alert period. Sensing during this special brief timing period results in a triggered rather than an inhibited output. Unlike single-chamber function in which the triggered mode rapidly delivers an output pulse as soon as an event is detected, the R wave that occurs in the earliest portion of this special detection interval triggers an output at the end of the safety pacing interval.

After the blanking period and the crosstalk sensing window have timed out, the ventricular sensing circuit returns to the alert status, in which a detected event causes the output pulse to be reset.

Differential Atrioventricular Interval: If AVIs initiated by a sensed event and those initiated by a paced event show consistent differences, the most likely explanation is a differential AVI. As noted in the introduction to this section, a differential AVI is an attempt to provide an interatrial conduction time of equal duration whether atrial contraction is paced or sensed. The PV interval initiated with atrial sensing commences only when the atrial depolarization is detected by the pacemaker and commonly occurs 20 to 60 milliseconds after the onset of the P wave seen on a surface ECG. Conversely, the AVI initiated with atrial pacing commences immediately with the pacing artifact, not with atrial depolarization. The AVI that follows a sensed atrial event should therefore be shorter than one that follows a paced atrial event (Fig. 6.18) in an effort to achieve similar functional AVIs, whether the atrial event is paced or sensed. The AVI differential is programmable in some pacemakers and preset in others.

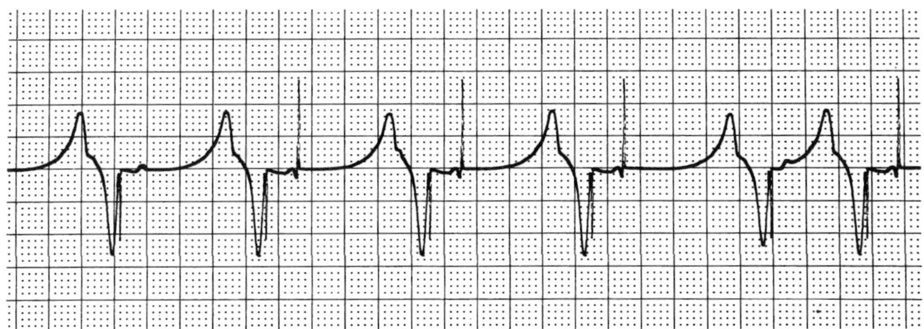

Figure 6.18. ECG tracing demonstrating differential AVI. The AVI is 50 milliseconds longer than the PV interval. (From Relay Models 293-03 and 294-03. Intermedics Cardiac Pulse Generator Physician's Manual. Angleton, Texas: Intermedics, 1992. By permission of Intermedics.)

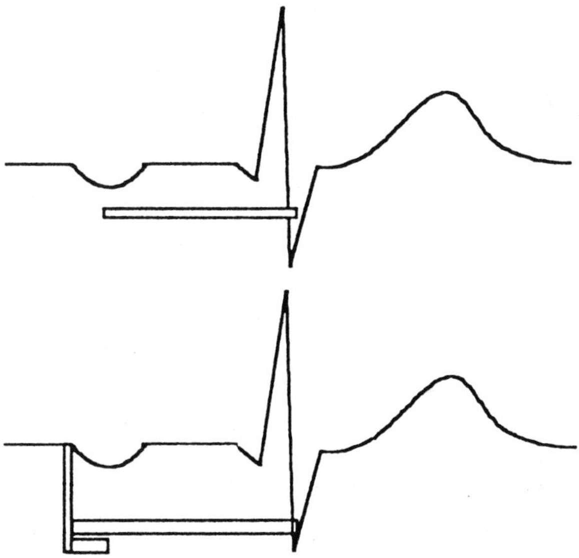

Figure 6.19. Schematic diagram of one manufacturer's differential AVI, designated "AV delay hysteresis." (Modified from Chorus II Model 6234, 6244 Dual Chamber Pulse Generator Physician's Manual. Minnetonka, Minnesota: ELA Medical, 1994.)

One DDD pacemaker automatically calculates the AVI differential between paced and sensed atrial events.[23] When an atrial paced event occurs, the AR interval is measured. When an atrial sensed event follows an atrial paced event, a new PR interval is measured. The AV delay hysteresis is set equal to the maximum value (AR or PR) minus the PR interval (Fig. 6.19).

Most dual-chamber pacemakers allow the paced and sensed AV delays to be programmed independently. Although the two may be nominally different, wider differences up to 100 milliseconds are programmable.

Rate-Variable or Rate-Adaptive Atrioventricular Interval: Most DDD and DDDR pacemakers can shorten the AVI as the atrial rate increases, either by an increase in sinus rate or by a sensor-driven increase in paced rate (Fig. 6.20). Rate-adaptive or rate-variable AVI is intended to optimize cardiac output by mimicking the normal physiologic decrease in the PR interval that occurs in the normal heart as the atrial rate increases.[24–26] The rate-related shortening of the AVI may also improve atrial sensing by shortening the TARP and thereby extending the time for the ASW.

Rate-adaptive AVI may be designed in several ways. The more common method is to allow linear shortening of the AVI from a programmed baseline AVI to a programmed minimum AVI. Another method allows a limited number of stepwise shortenings of the AVI. These steps may or may not be programmable.

Atrioventricular Interval Hysteresis: The term *AVI hysteresis* has been used variously but most commonly describes alterations in the paced AVI relative to the patient's intrinsic AV conduction. For example, a longer paced AVI is permitted, to allow maintenance of intrinsic AV conduction. However, once the intrinsic PR or AR interval triggers the programmed AVI hysteresis, consistent AV pacing at the programmed AVI occurs. Commonly, AVI hysteresis is programmed by selecting the desired AV delay during pacing with an additional programmable delta. If there is AV pacing, the system periodically extends the AV delay by the programmed delta. If a native R wave is detected within this extended interval, the longer interval remains in place and results in functional single-chamber atrial pacing. However, with the first cycle of AV pacing, which may occur with a transient increase in vagal tone or even intermittent pathologic AV block, the AV delay returns to the programmed value.

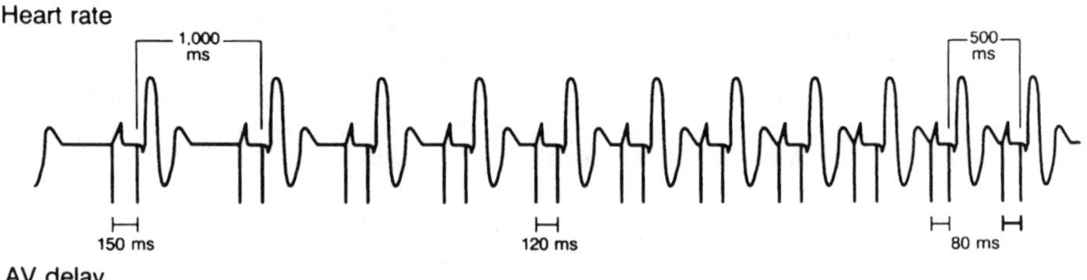

Figure 6.20. As heart rate increases, AV delay dynamically adapts to the change in cycle length. (From Hayes DL, Ketelson A, Levine PA, et al. Understanding timing systems of current DDDR pacemakers. Eur JCPE 1993;3:70–86. By permission of Mayo Foundation.)

This programming accomplishes two goals. In a patient with a normal ventricle, normal ventricular activation sequence (narrow QRS), and a normal PR interval, single-chamber atrial pacing provides hemodynamics superior to those of dual-chamber pacing. Ventricular stimulation causes a disordered ventricular activation sequence. However, an AV delay that is too long, as in first-degree AV block, may be hemodynamically deleterious. In this situation, hemodynamics may be superior with a shorter AV delay despite the disordered ventricular activation sequence. AVI hysteresis allows for both a longer AV delay when AV nodal conduction is intact and a shorter AVI when conduction is compromised.

Hysteresis Programming

Programming of hysteresis permits prolongation of the first pacemaker escape interval after a sensed event. A pacemaker programmed at a cycle length of 1000 milliseconds (60 bpm) and a hysteresis of 1200 milliseconds (50 bpm) allows 200 milliseconds more for another sensed QRS complex. If another QRS complex is not recognized, then the pacemaker continuously stimulates the heart at the programmed rate of 60 bpm, an escape interval of 1000 milliseconds (Fig. 6.21), until a sensed event restarts the cycle. The advantage of hysteresis in a single-chamber pacing mode is the ability to maintain spontaneous AV synchrony as long as possible.[2] This feature may prevent symptomatic retrograde VA conduction. In patients with VVI pacing and pacemaker syndrome, hysteresis provides reliable higher rate backup pacing while increasing the potential for maintaining the patient's intrinsic rhythm.

Several types of hysteresis may be programmable options in some dual-chamber pacemakers. In the first-generation algorithm, a native event had to be sensed to reestablish the hysteresis escape interval. The native complex had to occur at a rate faster than the basic pacing rate. If the basic pacing rate was relatively high, the system may have continued pacing long after the need for pacing had resolved. Therefore, *search hysteresis* was introduced. In search hysteresis, once a specific number of timing cycles at the more rapid rate (the number of cycles may be fixed or programmable) has occurred, the prolonged escape interval is permitted to allow manifestation of a slower intrinsic rate—that is, a rate higher than the programmed LRL. If intrinsic rhythm does not return at a rate exceeding the programmed lower rate, stimulation resumes at the more rapid rate for a given number of cycles (Fig. 6.22). This feature has been further modified in some systems to prevent an isolated PVC from resetting the basic dual-chamber pacing interval. Rather, resetting the hysteresis escape interval requires a sensed P wave to produce either a PR or a PV complex that inhibits the higher rate of pacing and reestablishes the hysteresis feature.

Another feature can be considered a refinement of search hysteresis.[3] A "sudden bradycardia response" or "rate drop response" (RDR) reacts to a defined drop in heart rate. When this occurs, the pacemaker feature intervenes by pacing at an elevated rate in both chambers for a specific, programmed duration (Fig. 6.23). At the conclusion of the programmed duration of more rapid

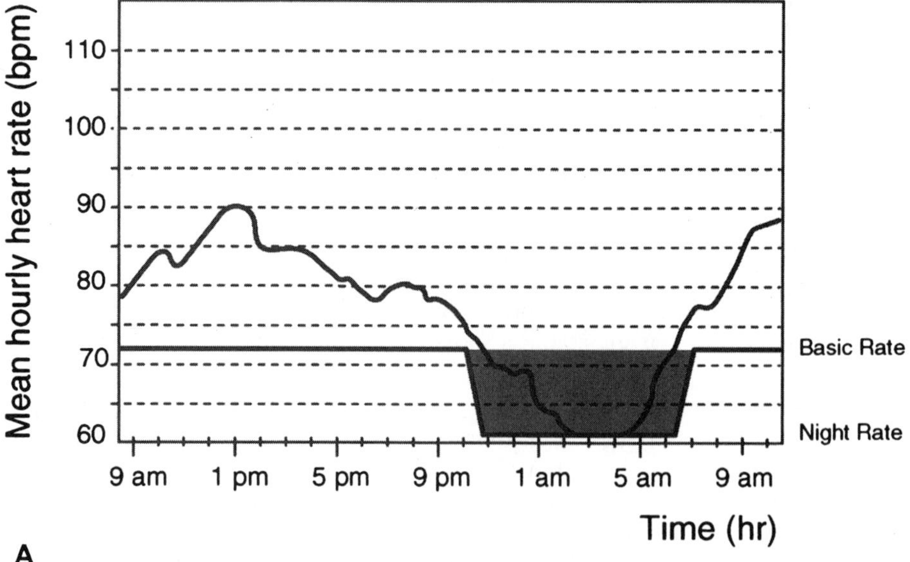

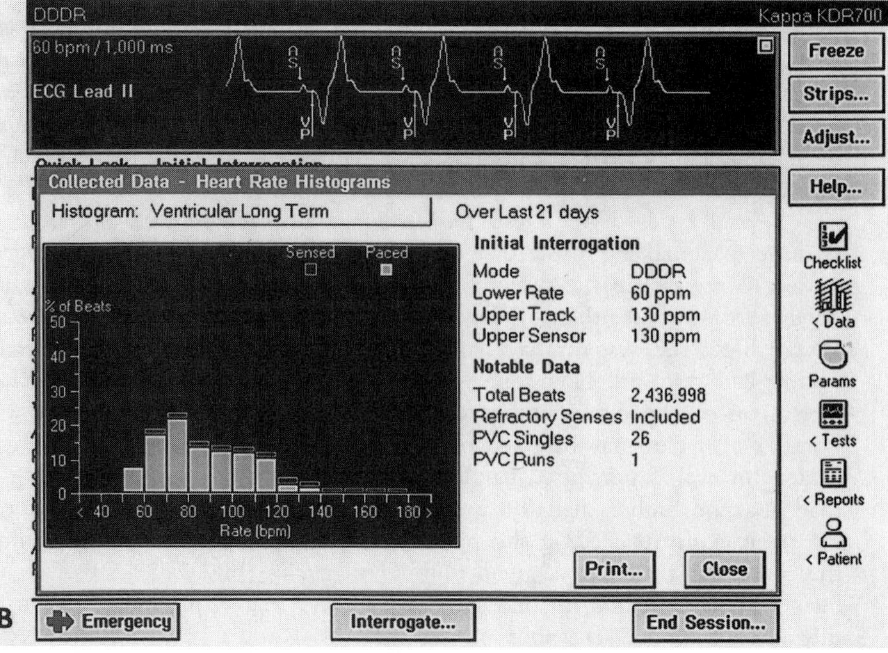

Figure 6.21. **A:** Printout of telemetric data of patient's mean hourly heart rate. The pacemaker is programmed to a lower, or basic, rate of 72 bpm and to a sleep rate, or night rate, of approximately 60 bpm. The graph demonstrates the slower rates allowed during night hours, in this example from 10 PM to 7 AM. **B:** Heart rate histogram from a patient with a DDDR pacemaker programmed to a lower rate of 60 bpm and an upper rate of 130 bpm. However, the histogram is compatible, with approximately 7% of the rates being less than 60 bpm. This can be explained by a sleep rate programmed to 50 bpm. (From Lloyd MA, Hayes DL, Friedman PA. Programming. In: Hayes DL, Lloyd MA, Friedman PA, eds. Cardiac Pacing and Defibrillation: A Clinical Approach. Armonk, NY: Futura, 2000:247–323. By permission of Mayo Foundation.)

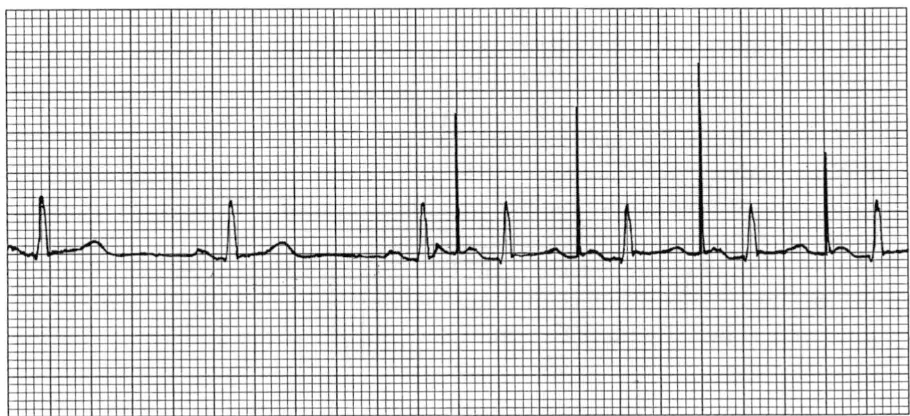

Figure 6.22. Onset of pacing in a DDDR pacemaker programmed to a lower rate of 100 bpm, hysteresis at 65 bpm, when the intrinsic rate has declined to 63 bpm. After 256 cycles of pacing at 100 bpm, pacing is suspended for the pacemaker to "search" for the intrinsic lower rate. If the lower rate is greater than the hysteresis rate, pacing is inhibited until the rate again falls below the hysteresis rate. (From Lloyd MA, Hayes DL, Friedman PA. Programming. In: Hayes DL, Lloyd MA, Friedman PA, eds. Cardiac Pacing and Defibrillation: A Clinical Approach. Armonk, NY: Futura, 2000:247–323. By permission of Mayo Foundation.)

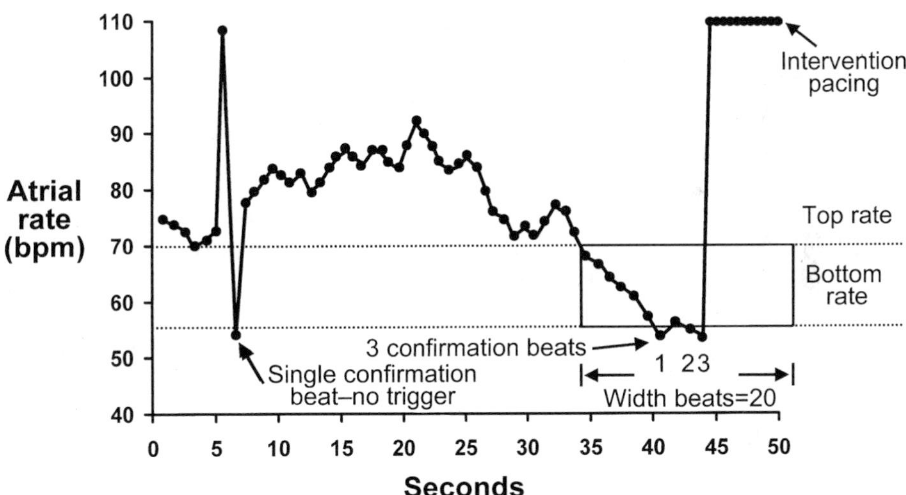

Figure 6.23. Diagrammatic representation of RDR. This algorithm requires that "top" and "bottom" rates be defined for rate drop detection, a specific number of beats, width over which the rate may drop, and the pacing rate that results if criteria are met, that is, the intervention rate. Three confirmation beats below the bottom rate must occur before therapy is triggered. In the early portion of this diagram, a single beat falls below the bottom rate but fails to trigger intervention because confirmation is not met. (From Lloyd MA, Hayes DL, Friedman PA. Programming. In: Hayes DL, Lloyd MA, Friedman PA, eds. Cardiac Pacing and Defibrillation: A Clinical Approach. Armonk, NY: Futura, 2000:247–323. By permission of Mayo Foundation.)

pacing, the pacing rate gradually returns to the programmed lower rate. Several programmable detection algorithms are available. The first algorithm available was "drop detect," in which the pacemaker monitors a drop in heart rate that must satisfy two programmable requirements to trigger an intervention, namely, the programmable "drop size," which is the number of beats the rate must fall, and the "detection window," which is the amount of time monitored for a rate drop (this is a programmable interval) (Fig. 6.24). The "nominal" values for RDR are not successful for everyone.

In the "low rate detect" algorithm, therapy is triggered when pacing occurs at the programmed lower rate for the programmable consecutive number of "detection beats." This detection method can be used as a backup to the "drop detect" method if the sudden drop in rate varies between slow and fast (Fig. 6.25).[4]

Dual-chamber rate hysteresis has multiple variations and different levels of complexity. Although the primary mode of therapy for vasovagal syncope is pharmacologic, it is not always 100% successful. Another treatment objective is dual-chamber pacing support at a relatively high rate during each spell, which may be effective in ameliorating if not totally eliminating the episodes. Because patients with neurocardiogenic syncope have a normal rhythm at other times, the hysteresis circuit allows for pacing at the higher rate only during the spell (when the native heart rate falls precipitously) and otherwise remains inhibited.[27,28]

BASE RATE BEHAVIOR

The way a pacemaker behaves in response to a sensed ventricular signal varies among manufacturers and even among devices from the same manufacturer. Dual-chamber pacemakers have historically been designed with a ventricular-based timing system, an atrial-based timing system, or a hybrid of these two systems.[3,29] Designation of a pacemaker's timing system as atrial-based or ventricular-based gained increased importance with the advent of rate-adaptive pacing. The difference between atrial-based and ventricular-based dual-chamber pacemakers was of little clinical importance in non–rate-adaptive pacemakers, although the difference created some minor confusion in interpretation of paced ECGs.

With the refinement of timing systems, use of a specific system has once again become less important. A description of pure atrial-based and ventricular-based timing systems appears below. However, few contemporary dual-chamber pacemakers are "pure" atrial-based or ventricular-based systems. The majority is in some way hybrid, designed specifically to avoid the potential rate variations or limitations that could occur with either pure timing system.

Ventricular-Based Timing

In a ventricular-based timing system, the AEI is "fixed." A ventricular sensed event occurring during the AEI resets this timer, causing it to start again (Fig.

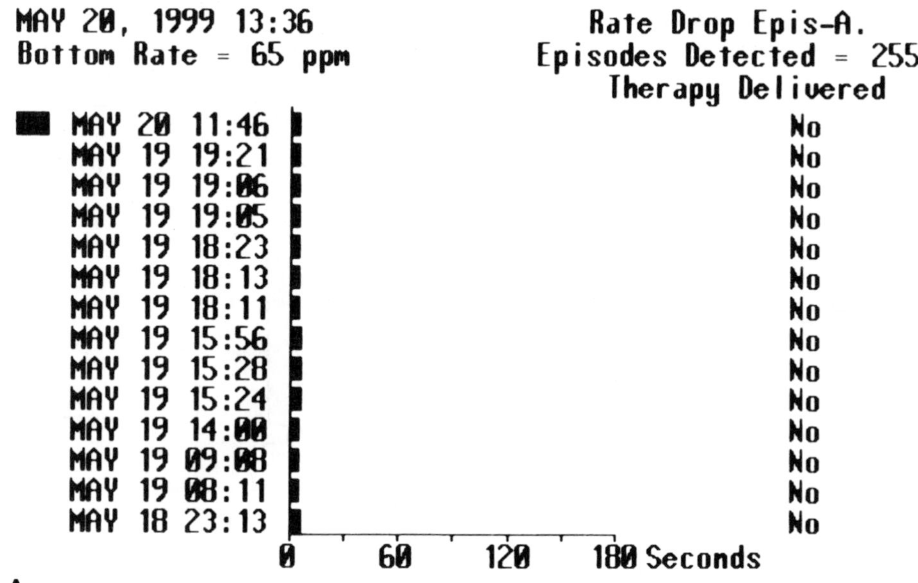

A

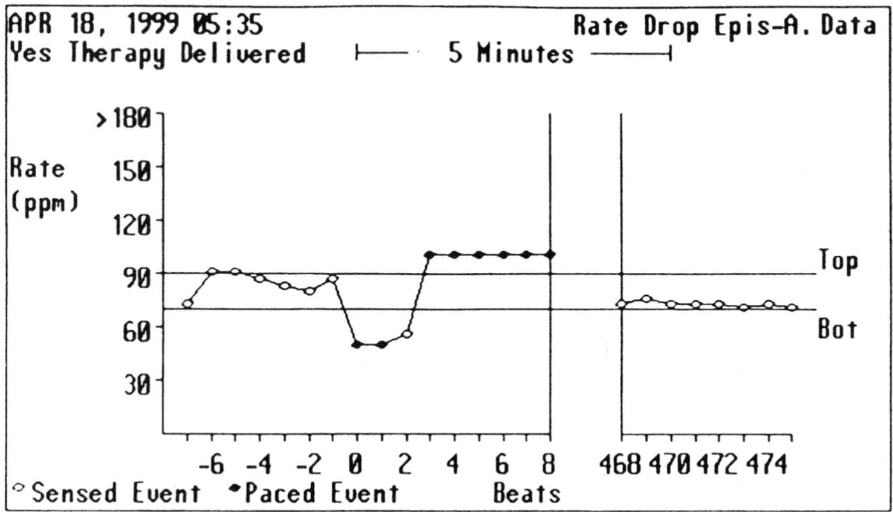

B

Figure 6.24. **A:** The RDR counters indicate that the pacemaker had documented multiple episodes of sudden rate drop. However, "therapy"—that is, a response to the sudden drop in rate with an increase in pacing rate for a programmed period—had not been initiated. **B:** With a pacemaker in place and RDR that had been programmed "on" but not initiated because of the programmed parameters, adjusting the RDR parameters would be reasonable. For this patient, the RDR criteria were programmed more sensitively. When the patient returned, the rate counter was again full, with 255 episodes detected and therapy delivered on two occasions. The second printout details the event on April 18 at 05:35 when therapy was delivered. The diagram documents a sudden decrease in rate; RDR was met and therapy delivered. (From Lloyd MA, Hayes DL, Friedman PA. Programming. In: Hayes DL, Lloyd MA, Friedman PA, eds. Cardiac Pacing and Defibrillation: A Clinical Approach. Armonk, NY: Futura, 2000:247–323. By permission of Mayo Foundation.)

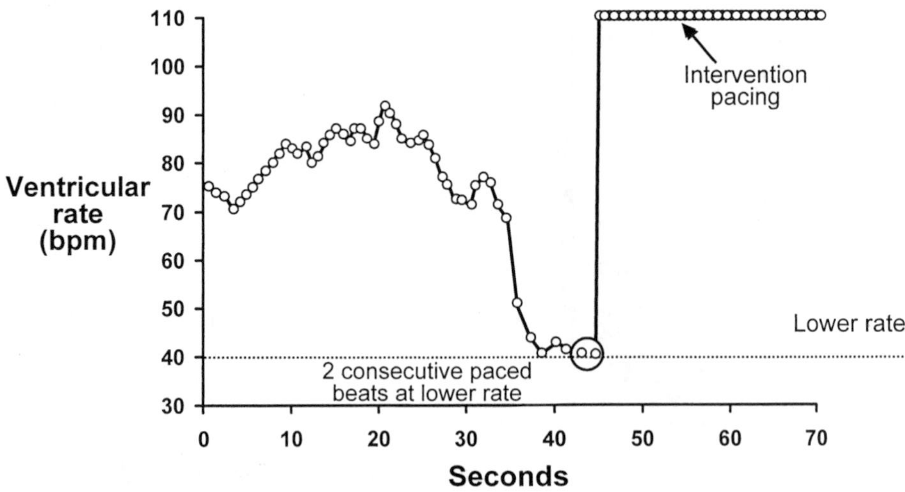

Figure 6.25. In the low rate detect algorithm (Medtronic, Inc.), when pacing occurs at the programmed lower rate for the programmable consecutive number of detection beats, therapy is triggered. Low rate detect may be used as a backup to the drop detect method if the sudden drop in rate varies between slow and fast. (From Lloyd MA, Hayes DL, Friedman PA. Programming. In: Hayes DL, Lloyd MA, Friedman PA, eds. Cardiac Pacing and Defibrillation: A Clinical Approach. Armonk, NY: Futura, 2000:247–323. By permission of Mayo Foundation.)

6.26, top). A ventricular sensed event occurring during the AVI both terminates the AVI and initiates an AEI (see Fig. 6.12, top). If there is intact conduction through the AV node after an atrial pacing stimulus such that the AR interval (atrial stimulus to sensed R wave) is shorter than the programmed AVI, the resulting paced rate accelerates by a small amount. This response is demonstrated in Figure 6.12 (top).

This phenomenon is best understood by example. In a pacemaker programmed to an LRL of 60 bpm (a pacing interval of 1000 milliseconds) that has a programmed AVI of 200 milliseconds, the AEI is 800 milliseconds (AEI = LRL − AVI). If AV nodal function permits conduction in 150 milliseconds (AR interval + 150 milliseconds), the conducted or sensed R wave inhibits ventricular output. This, in turn, resets the AEI, which remains stable at 800 milliseconds. The resulting interval between consecutive atrial pacing stimuli is 950 milliseconds (AEI + AR interval), which is equivalent to a rate of 63 bpm, a rate slightly faster than the programmed LRL. When a native R wave occurs—for example, a ventricular premature beat during the AEI—the AEI is also reset. The pacemaker then recycles, resulting in a rate defined by the sum of the AEI and AVI. This escape interval is therefore equal to the LRL (Fig. 6.26, top). In both cases, the sensed ventricular event, an R wave, regardless of where it occurs, resets the AEI.

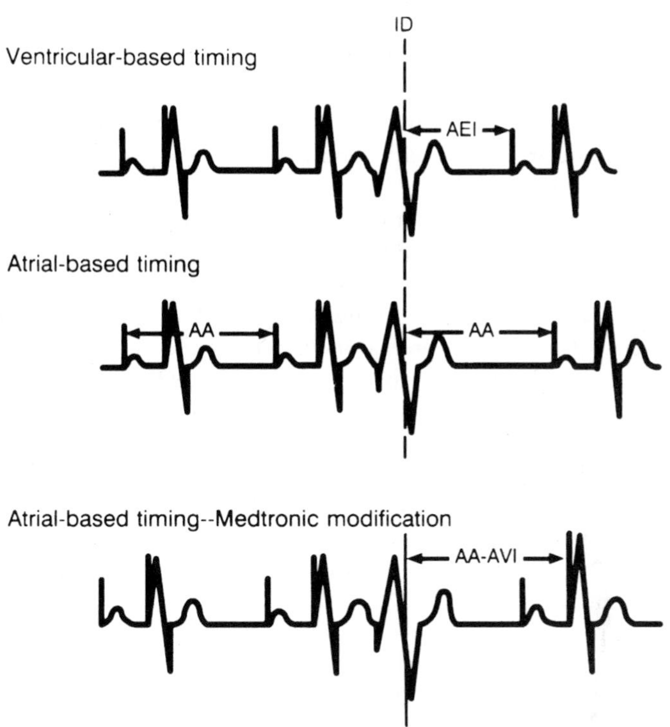

Figure 6.26. **Top:** Ventricular-based timing resets the AEI so that the recycled pacing interval is equal to the programmed base rate. **Middle:** Atrial-based timing resets the AA interval and then adds the AVI. Thus, the interval from the sensed R wave to the next paced ventricular beat exceeds the base rate interval, a form of obligatory hysteresis. **Bottom:** Medtronic modification of the AA timing subtracts the AVI from the AA interval. The resulting rhythm is identical to that seen with ventricular-based timing. (From Levine PA, Hayes DL, Wilkoff BL, Ohman AE. Electrocardiography of Rate-Modulated Pacemaker Rhythms. Sylmar, CA: Siemens-Pacesetter, 1990. By permission of Siemens-Pacesetter.)

Atrial-Based Timing

In an atrial-based timing system, the AA interval is fixed, whereas in a ventricular-based system, the AEI is fixed. As long as LRL pacing remains stable, there is no discernible difference between the two timing systems.

In a system with pure atrial-based timing, a sensed R wave occurring during the AVI inhibits ventricular output but does not alter the basic AA timing. Hence, the rate stays at the programmed LRL (see Fig. 6.12, bottom) during effective single-chamber atrial pacing. When a ventricular premature beat is sensed during the AEI, the timers are also reset, but the AA interval rather than the AEI is reset. The pacemaker counts out an AA interval and then adds the programmed AVI, in an attempt to mimic the compensatory pause commonly seen in normal sinus rhythm with ventricular ectopy—a form of obligatory hysteresis (Fig. 6.26, middle).

Other manufacturers have chosen to modify an atrial timing system. One DDDR pulse generator primarily uses modified atrial, or AA, timing, whereby an atrial sensed or paced event commonly resets the timing cycle of the device (much like the sinus node itself).[30] However, in certain situations (for example, after a PVC), an exception is made, and ventricular (VA) timing is used. Another manufacturer uses an atrial timing system that ignores the sensed R wave during stable AR pacing, which eliminates the rate acceleration that would be seen with ventricular-based timing designs.[31] This feature is modified when a native R wave or sensed premature ventricular event occurs after the VRP is completed. The AA interval is reset but only after the AVI is first subtracted (Fig. 6.27).

Comparison of Atrial-Based and Ventricular-Based Systems

When the heart rate is considered, usually the ventricular rate is paramount, because it, not the atrial rate, causes the effective (hemodynamic) pulse. During periods of 2:1 AV block at the lower rate, a ventricular-based timing system

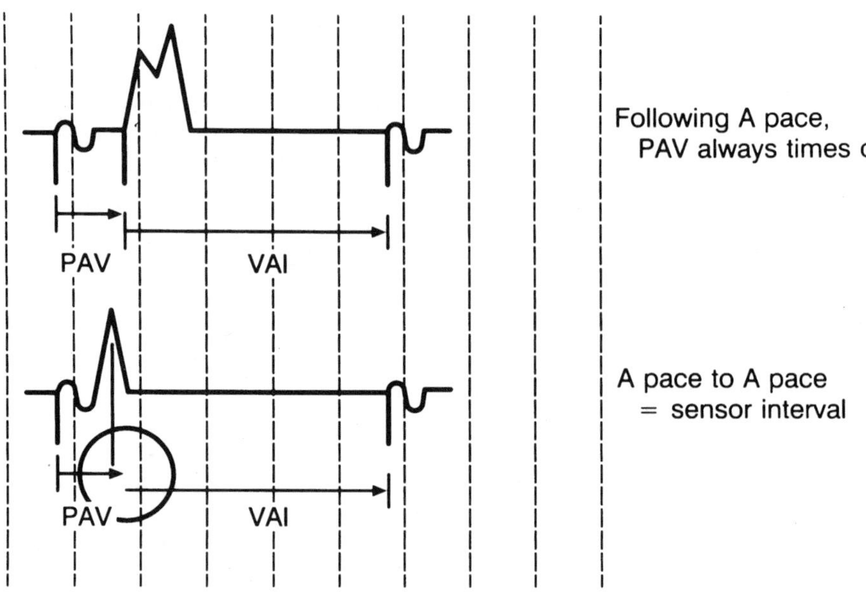

Figure 6.27. Ventricular-based versus atrial-based timing. The lower portion demonstrates atrial escape timing after an atrial (A) pace in atrial-based timing. With this timing, the AVI after atrial pacing (PAV) always times out, regardless of ventricular inhibition. The escape interval from one atrial pace to the next is equal to the sensor interval. VAI, interval from ventricular sensed or paced event to atrial paced event. (From Hayes DL, Ketelson A, Levine PA, et al. Understanding timing systems of current DDDR pacemakers. Eur JCPE 1993;3:70–86. By permission of Mayo Foundation.)

alternates between the programmed rate (AV pacing state) and a slightly faster rate (AR pacing state), as shown in Figure 6.28 (top).

In an atrial-based system, the alternation of the longer AVI with the shorter AR interval results in ventricular rates that are both faster and slower than the programmed base rate. This response is shown in Figure 6.28 (bottom).

Although ventricular-based timing may result in an increase in the paced rate during AR pacing (see "Effects of Ventricular- and Atrial-Based Timing Systems on DDDR Timing Cycles," below), the LRL is never violated. This is not the case with atrial-based timing. When an AV complex follows an AR complex, the effective paced ventricular rate for that cycle falls below the programmed LRL. A 2:1 AV block in an atrial-based timing system induces alternating cycles that are either faster or slower than, but never the same as, the programmed base rate (see Fig. 6.28, bottom).

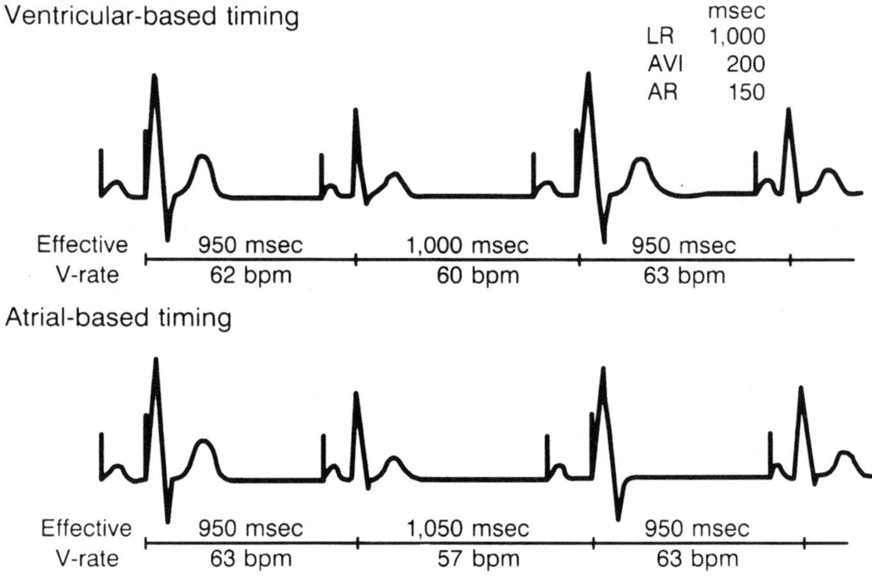

Figure 6.28. Diagrammatic representations of 2:1 AV block during base rate pacing. **Top:** With a ventricular-based timing system, the interval between consecutive AV and AR paced complexes is slightly shorter; hence, the rate is slightly faster than the programmed base rate. The interval between consecutive AR and AV paced complexes results in ventricular pacing at the base rate for that pacing cycle. **Bottom:** In an atrial-based timing system, the effective ventricular paced rate alternates between rates that are faster and slower than the programmed rate. The cycle between an AR and AV complex results in a ventricular rate that is slower than the programmed rate, a form of hysteresis. Meanwhile, the cycle between an AV and an AR complex causes the ventricular rate to be faster than the programmed rate. Atrial pacing is stable at the programmed rate, but it is the ventricular contraction that induces cardiac output. (From Levine PA, Hayes DL, Wilkoff BL, Ohman AE. Electrocardiography of Rate-Modulated Pacemaker Rhythms. Sylmar, CA: Siemens-Pacesetter, 1990. By permission of Siemens-Pacesetter.)

Interpretation of an ECG of a patient with a dual-chamber pacemaker is helped by knowing whether the pacemaker has atrial-based or ventricular-based timing. With a ventricular-based timing system, a pair of calipers set to the VAI can be used to measure backward from an atrial paced stimulus to the point of ventricular sensing, since a ventricular event, paced or sensed, always initiates the VAI.

A similar technique can be used in an atrial-based timing system, but only when a sensed ventricular complex occurs after the VRP ends. The calipers must be set to the AA interval before measuring backward from the atrial paced event that follows a ventricular sensed event. If one were to misidentify an atrial-based timing system as a ventricular-based system, an otherwise normal rhythm might be misinterpreted as T-wave oversensing or some other form of oversensing (see Fig. 6.26, middle).

Sensor Input to Base Rate Pacing

The sensor input to the pacing system temporarily adjusts the rate of the pacemaker. If the individual is active and rate modulation is enabled, the heart rate is determined by the faster of either the native rate or the sensor-determined rate. The sensor rate behaves in a manner identical to the programmed base rate. If the native rate is faster than the base rate, the pacemaker is either inhibited or tracks the atrial complexes. If the base rate is faster than the intrinsic rate, the heart rate is controlled by the pacemaker. Regardless of whether the programmed base rate or the sensor rate is in effect, pacing is always atrial in a dual-chamber pacing system. When the sensor input to the pacing system fluctuates, the rate changes.

Automatic Mode Switch Base Rate

On the basis of the older literature on lone atrial fibrillation,[32–35] higher heart rates are often needed to compensate for the loss of atrial transport. Thus, during paroxysmal atrial fibrillation in a patient with high-grade AV block and a pacemaker with mode-switching capability, the resting heart rate during the nontracking mode may be too low. This low intrinsic rate is of particular concern during protracted periods of pacing in the nontracking mode. For this reason, the ability to independently program a resting pacemaker rate in effect while the mode switch algorithm is engaged has been introduced to some devices. The programmed base rate might be 60 ppm during sinus rhythm and normal DDD function, whereas the base rate might be 80 to 90 bpm during atrial fibrillation with the system functioning in the DDI mode. If rate modulation were also activated, any increase in sensor-driven rates would start at the appropriate base for the functional pacing mode at the time.

Upper Rate Behavior

In the DDD mode of operation, acceleration of the sinus rate results in the sensed P wave terminating the AEI and initiating an AVI, an effect known as *P-wave synchronous ventricular pacing*. (If the PR interval is shorter than the PV interval—the time from an intrinsic P wave to a paced ventricular depolarization—the pacemaker is completely inhibited.) P-wave synchronous pacing occurs in a 1:1 relationship between the programmed LRL and the programmed URL. In other words, when the interval between consecutive native atrial events is longer than the TARP, each P wave occurs in the atrial alert period and is therefore sensed. Consequently, atrial output is inhibited while simultaneously triggering ventricular output after the AVI. However, when the interval between consecutive native atrial events is shorter than the TARP, some P waves are not sensed because, by definition, they fall into the TARP. The pacemaker goes into an abrupt fixed-block (2:1, 3:1, etc.) response, sensing only every other or every *n*th P wave, depending on the native atrial rate (Fig. 6.29). Programming a long PVARP results in the fixed-block response occurring at a relatively low tracking rate. The abrupt change in pacing rate when the fixed block occurs can result in serious symptoms, which frequently happened in early generation DDD pacemakers.

An additional timing circuit, known as the MTR interval,[9,15] better modulates the upper rate behavior. (The MTR interval has also been referred to as "upper rate limit" and "ventricular tracking limit.") This timing period defines the maximum paced ventricular rate or the shortest interval initiated by a sensed P wave at which a paced ventricular beat can follow a preceding paced or sensed ventricular event. The pacemaker has an upper rate behavior that mimics AV nodal Wenckebach behavior. The appearance is that of group beating, progressive lengthening of the PV interval, and intermittent pauses on the ECG when the native atrial rate exceeds the programmed MTR interval (Fig. 6.30). In these pacing systems, two timers must each complete their cycles for a ventricular stimulus to be released. These timing cycles are known as the AVI and the MTR interval. A sensed P wave initiates an AVI. If, on completion of the AVI, the

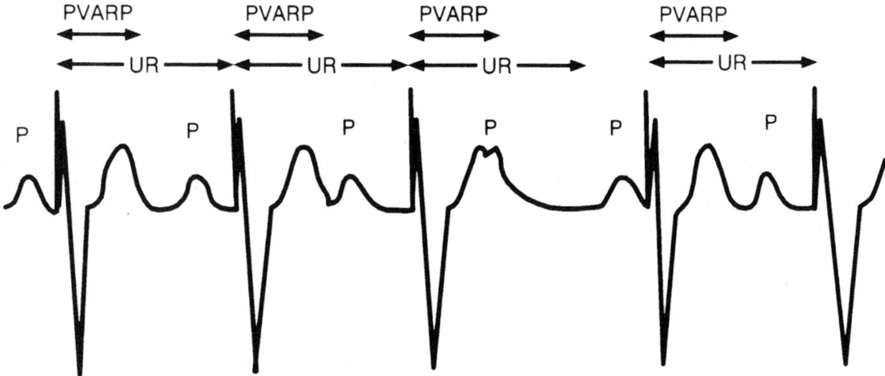

Figure 6.29. If the sinus rate becomes so rapid that every other P wave occurs within the PVARP, effective 2:1 AV block occurs; that is, every other P wave is followed by a ventricular pacing artifact.

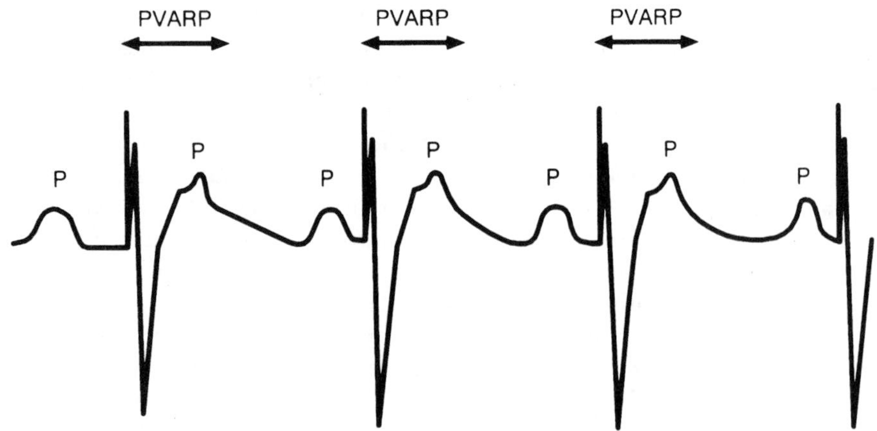

Figure 6.30. In the DDD pacing mode, the programmed upper rate limit (UR) cannot be violated regardless of the sinus rate. When a P wave is sensed after the PVARP, the AVI is initiated. If, however, delivering a ventricular pacing artifact at the end of the AVI would violate the UR, the ventricular pacing artifact cannot be delivered. The pacemaker would wait until completion of the UR and then deliver the ventricular pacing artifact. This action would result in a prolonged AVI.

MTR interval has been completed, a pacemaker stimulus is released at the programmed AVI. If the MTR interval has not yet been completed, the release of the ventricular output pulse is delayed until the MTR interval ends. This delay has the functional effect of lengthening the PV interval and places the ensuing ventricular paced beat closer to the next P wave. Both the PVARP and the MTR interval are initiated by a paced or sensed ventricular event. During Wenckebach upper rate behavior, a P wave eventually coincides with the PVARP, is not sensed, and is therefore ignored by the pacemaker, which results in a relative pause. The MTR interval is then able to complete its timing period, which depends on the atrial rate and programmed base rate, so that either the P wave that follows the unsensed P wave is tracked (restarting the cycle at the programmed AVI) or the pause is terminated by AV sequential pacing.

Thus, upper rate behavior can demonstrate Wenckebach-like behavior or go into abrupt fixed block (e.g., 2:1). It demonstrates 2:1 block behavior when the P wave falls into the TARP. If the MTR interval is longer than the TARP (TARP = AVI + PVARP), then Wenckebach-like behavior occurs. This can be summarized by the following equation: Wenckebach interval = MTR interval − TARP.

Therefore, if a positive number results, Wenckebach-like behavior occurs. In contrast, if a negative number results, fixed 2:1 AV block occurs. For example, if a patient's pacemaker is programmed to an AVI of 250 milliseconds, a PVARP of 225 milliseconds, and an MTR of 400 milliseconds, by the above equation the Wenckebach interval is 400 − (250 + 225), or a negative number. Therefore, when the atrial rate reaches 401 milliseconds, a 2:1 AV upper rate response is seen. If this patient's AVI is reprogrammed to 125 milliseconds, by the equation the Wenckebach interval is 400 − (125 − 225), or a positive number (+50 milliseconds). In the latter instance, when the atrial rate is 351 milliseconds, Wenckebach-like conduction is seen for a 50-millisecond interval. As the atrial rate increases further to 401 milliseconds, 2:1 AV block is noted.

Rate smoothing, a variation of upper rate behavior, was introduced by Cardiac Pacemakers, Inc. (Guidant, St. Paul, Minnesota) as a method of preventing marked changes in cycle length not only occurring at the URL of a DDD pacemaker but also any time the sinus rate is accelerating or decelerating.[36] (With rate smoothing, the pacemaker is programmed to a percentage change that is allowed between VV cycles, that is, 3%, 6%, 9%, or 12%. For example, if the VV cycle length is stable at 900 milliseconds during P-synchronous pacing, rate smoothing is "on" at 6%, and the sinus rate suddenly accelerates, the subsequent VV cycle cannot accelerate by more than 54 milliseconds, which is 6% of 900 milliseconds.) The ventricular rate is therefore relatively smooth, but sometimes at the expense of uncoupling AV synchrony (Fig. 6.31).

Because Wenckebach upper rate behavior results in the loss of a stable AV relationship and some patients may be symptomatic with both this and the resul-

Without rate smoothing

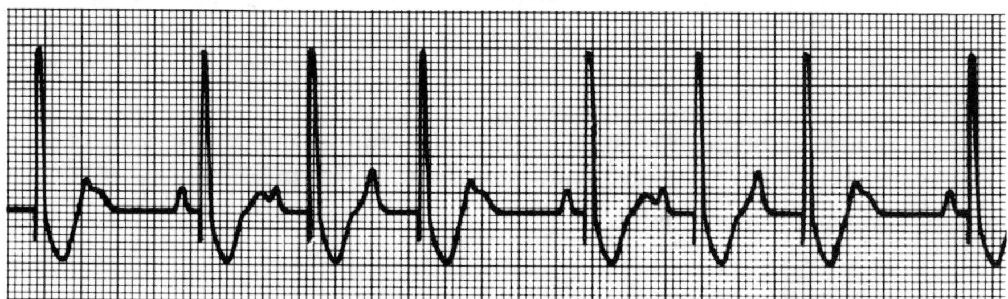

With rate smoothing (6%)

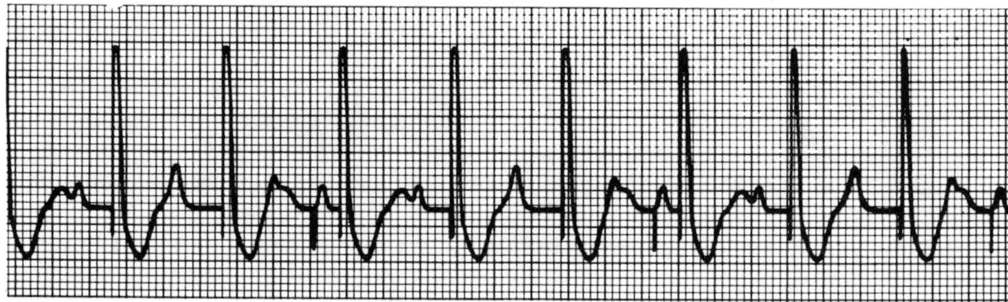

Figure 6.31. ECG demonstrating DDD pacing with true rate smoothing capabilities (6% of the preceding RR interval). With true rate smoothing, the Wenckebach interval is allowed to lengthen only 36 milliseconds over the preceding RR interval, at an MTR of 100 ppm. (Reprinted with permission from Cardiac Pacemakers, Inc., St. Paul, MN.)

tant pauses that occur when a P wave coincides with the PVARP and is not tracked, another upper rate behavior, fallback, is available in some devices. When the atrial rate exceeds the programmed MTR, the pacemaker continues to sense atrial activity but uncouples the native atrial rhythm from the ventricular paced complexes. The ventricular paced rate then slowly and progressively decreases to either an intermediate rate or the programmed base rate. This arrangement avoids the abrupt pauses that occur with both the Wenckebach and the fixed-block behaviors. When the atrial rate slows below either the MTR or the fall-back rate, depending on the design of the system, the desired AV relationship is restored.

Mode Switching

Mode switching refers to the ability of the pacemaker to automatically change from one mode to another in response to an inappropriately rapid atrial rhythm.[37] With mode switching, when the pacemaker is functioning in the DDDR mode, the algorithm automatically reprograms the pacemaker to the VVIR mode if specific criteria for a pathologic atrial rhythm are met. Mode switching is particularly useful for patients with paroxysmal supraventricular rhythm disturbances. In the DDD or DDDR pacing mode, if a supraventricular rhythm disturbance occurs and the pathologic atrial rhythm is sensed by the pacemaker, rapid ventricular pacing may occur (Fig. 6.32). Any pacing mode that eliminates tracking of the pathologic rhythm, for example, DDI, DDIR, DVI, or DVIR, also eliminates the ability to track normal sinus rhythm, which is usually the predominant rhythm. Mode switching avoids this limitation (Fig. 6.33).

Refinement of mode-switching algorithms has made this a successful feature (Fig. 6.34).[38] Mode switching functions by measuring intervals between

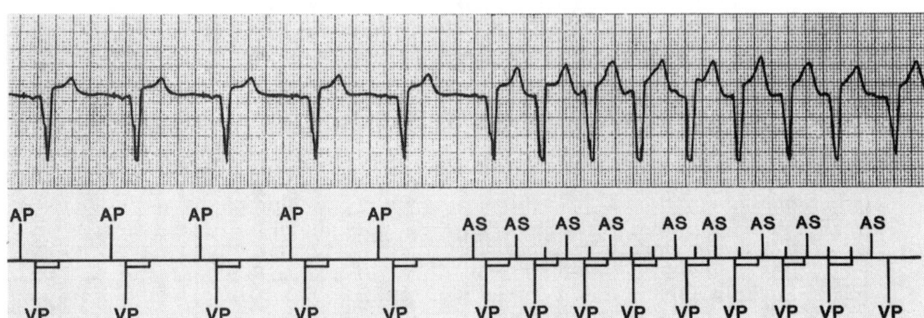

Figure 6.32. Resting ECG tracing demonstrating AV sequential pacing at lower rate (55 ppm) followed by paroxysmal atrial flutter with ventricular tracking at MTR (110 ppm). Diagram shows atrial paced events (AP), atrial sensed events (AS), and ventricular paced events (VP), with the PVARP noted by the rectangle. Short, unlabeled ticks represent atrial activity that occurs in the PVARP and is not sensed. (Diagram is based on Marker Channel, Medtronic, Inc., Minneapolis, MN.) (From Levine PA, Hayes DL, Wilkoff BL, Ohman AE. Electrocardiography of rate-modulated pacemaker rhythms. Sylmar, CA: Siemens-Pacesetter, 1990. By permission of Siemens-Pacesetter.)

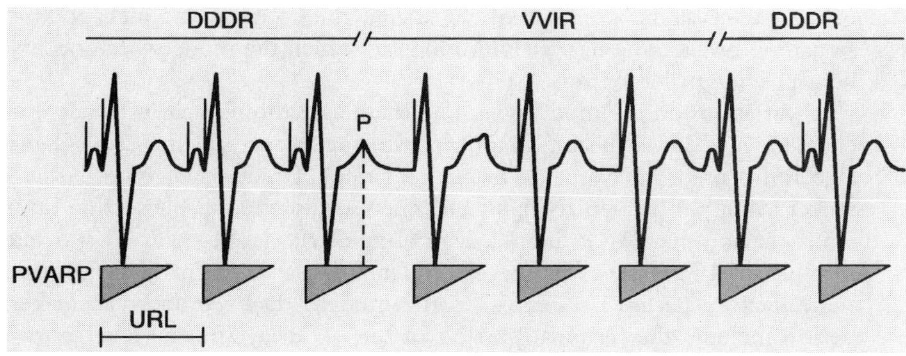

Figure 6.33. ECG appearance of mode switching. The first three cardiac cycles are due to sensor-driven AV sequential pacing, that is, DDDR pacing. After the third paced ventricular complex, a P wave occurs during the PVARP (*shaded triangles*) and initiates mode switching to the VVIR mode because the atrial rate has exceeded the URL. The pacing mode reverts to DDDR when the atrial rate falls below the programmed URL; that is, P waves fall outside the PVARP. (From Hayes DL. Timing cycles of permanent pacemakers. Cardiol Clin 1992;10:593–608. By permission of WB Saunders Company.)

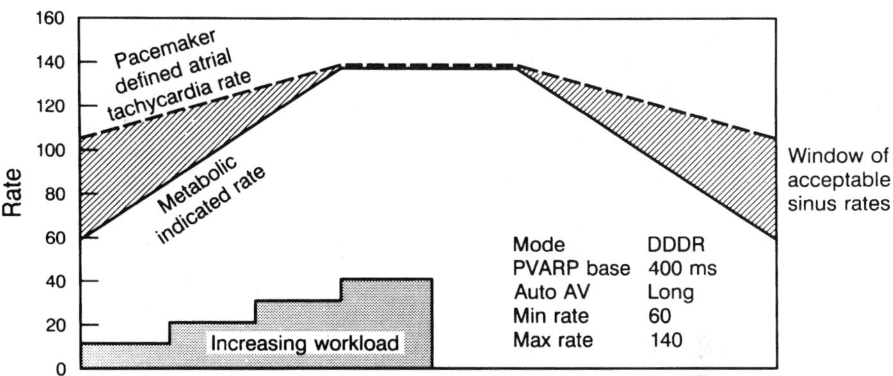

Figure 6.34. Diagram of the method by which a pacemaker monitors the atrial rate to determine whether it is physiologic or nonphysiologic. The shaded area identifies tracked sinus rates. Sinus rates below the metabolic indicated rate (*solid line*) elicit atrial pacing, sinus rates within the shaded area elicit atrial tracking, and sinus rates above the atrial tachycardia rate (*dashed line*) result in automatic switching of the mode to VVIR. Auto AV, automatic alteration of the AVI. (From Hayes DL, Ketelson A, Levine PA, et al. Understanding timing systems of current DDDR pacemakers. Eur JCPE 1993;3:70–86. By permission of Mayo Foundation.)

atrial events.[39] In most pacemakers, the rate at which mode switching occurs is a programmable feature. The pacemaker uses a counter that considers a short interval to be one that is shorter than the programmed mode-switching rate and a long interval to be one that is longer than the programmed rate. When the counter accrues a specified number of short intervals, the pacemaker reprograms to a nontracking mode and remains in this mode until a specified number of long intervals have occurred and altered the counter, at which point mode switching reverts. The nontracking mode to which the mode switch occurs may be a programmable option.

Variations on the mode-switching theme are too numerous to detail in this chapter. One should become familiar with the nuances of the mode-switching algorithms used.[40] Key to the implementation of mode switching is the pacemaker's ability to recognize high atrial rates. As discussed in the section on upper rate behavior, the TARP limits the atrial rate that can be detected and tracked. If rapid atrial rates are to be detected, identifying atrial events that occur during the refractory period is essential. In the modern dual-chamber pacemaker, this period includes the terminal portion of the AV delay and the latter portion of the PVARP. As noted for single-chamber refractory periods, the PVARP has absolute and relative portions. The absolute portion is the first part of the PVARP, and it is termed the *postventricular atrial blanking* (PVAB) period. The purpose of this timing period is to prevent sensing of the far-field R wave. The ventricular depolarization is a relatively large signal. To ensure sensing of pathologic atrial tachyarrhythmias whose signal amplitudes may fluctuate and may be very small, the atrial channel is usually programmed to a sensitive value. This combination predisposes to detection of ventricular signals on the atrial channel. The pacemaker may label these "P" waves and thus respond as if the atrial rate were high when the rhythm is actually normal sinus rhythm.[41–43] The result is a form of double counting, resulting in "false" mode switching. To prevent far-field R-wave sensing, a period of absolute refractoriness corresponding to the expected timing of this event forms the first portion of the PVARP. In devices with first-generation mode-switching algorithms, PVAB was not even mentioned because it was not programmable. In dual-chamber devices from virtually all manufacturers as of 2000, PVAB is programmable from 50 to 250 milliseconds. There is an inverse relationship between the duration of the PVAB and the detection of atrial arrhythmia, with the shorter PVABs allowing detection of higher atrial rates (increased sensitivity to atrial tachyarrhythmias). However, increasing the PVAB increases the specificity of rhythm detection and minimizes inappropriate mode switching.

Because a far-field R wave may be detected before the depolarization is sensed by the ventricular channel of the pacemaker (Fig. 6.35), another timing circuit, *preventricular atrial blanking* (pre-VAB), may be helpful. Although the site of native ventricular depolarization cannot be predicted, the algorithm sets up a monitoring interval following the detected atrial event. This programmable period varies from 0 to 60 milliseconds. If an R wave is detected during the pre-VAB interval, the atrial event is labeled a far-field R wave and is not used in the calculation of high atrial rates.

Atrial Flutter Response

An algorithm to specifically respond to atrial flutter is available in some pacemakers. Such an algorithm is designed to prevent pacing into the atrial vulner-

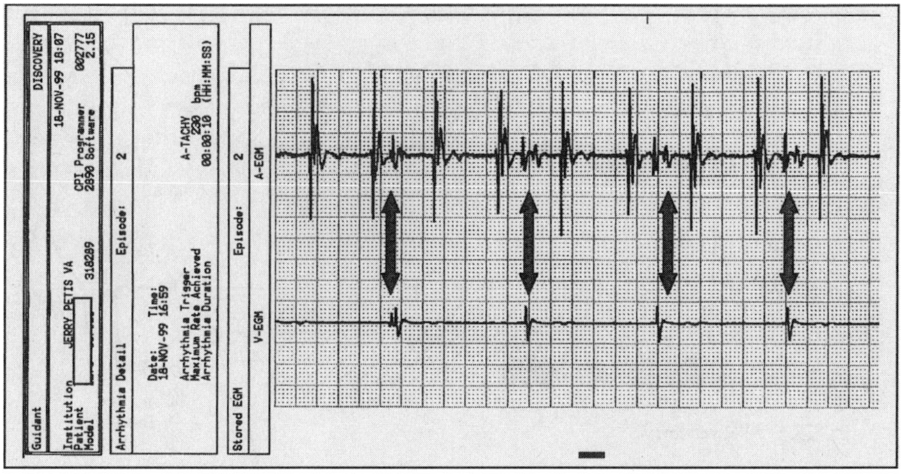

Figure 6.35. Stored electrogram from a pacemaker demonstrates mode-switching behavior (AV dissociation) during normal sinus rhythm with the pacemaker detecting an atrial rate higher than 200 bpm. The far-field R wave is identified by double arrows.

able period and to provide immediate fallback for atrial rates higher than the atrial flutter response (AFR) programmable rate. The fallback rate would be continued as long as atrial events continue to exceed the AFR programmable rate.[44,45]

For example, if the AFR were programmed to 250 bpm, an atrial event detected inside the PVARP or a previously triggered AFR interval would start an AFR timing window of 240 milliseconds (250 bpm). Atrial detection inside the AFR would be noted as "sensed" events within the refractory period and would not be tracked. The sensing window would begin only after both the AFR and the PVARP expire. If a paced atrial event is scheduled inside an AFR window, it is delayed until the AFR window expires (Fig. 6.36).

Sinus Preference

Another algorithm that may affect the timing cycle attempts to maintain sinus rhythm, i.e., sinus preference. The algorithm is programmed to search for the sinus rate, allowing a programmable number of beats per minute that the rate can be reduced as the search occurs. If sinus rhythm is detected within that programmable rate, the sinus rhythm is then allowed to predominate.[46]

Atrial Fibrillation Prevention Algorithms

Numerous atrial fibrillation prevention algorithms are available, and each of these may alter the pacemaker timing cycle. A complete discussion of these algorithms is beyond the scope of this chapter. Potential effects would include a shorter atrial pacing cycle after a premature atrial contraction to prevent the

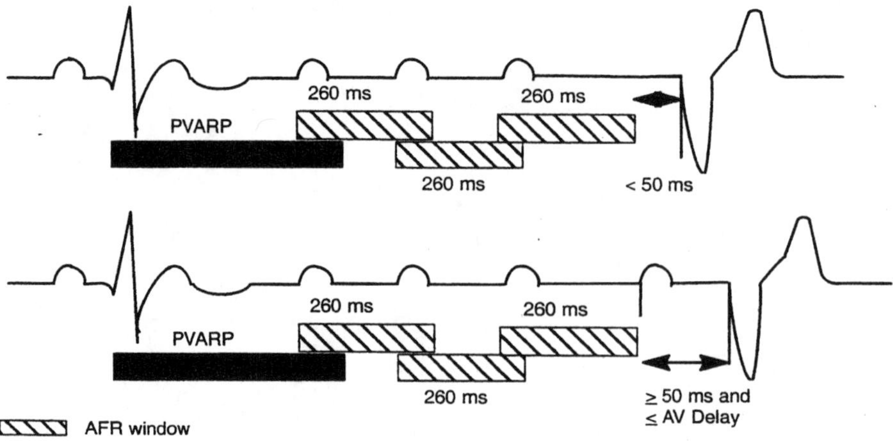

Figure 6.36. Artial Flutter Response. Atrial detection inside PVARP starts a 260-ms interval which will restart if another atrial event is detected. A ventricular pace will take place on the scheduled interval. An atrial pace will not occur unless there is at least 50 ms before the scheduled V pace. This prevents competitive pacing. (Courtesy of Guidant Corporation.)

"short-long" cycle that typically occurs, incremental atrial pacing rate to overdrive sinus rhythm and/or atrial premature contractions, and faster pacing following a mode switch episode.

Rate Smoothing and Ventricular Rate Regularization

Two additional algorithms may have an effect on the pacing rate and alter the rate from either the programmed lower rate, sinus-driven or sensor-driven rates. Rate smoothing, available for many years, is intended to prevent sudden changes in ventricular cycle length. Traditionally, rate smoothing operates between the LRL and the MTR (maximum pacing rate if in a single-chamber inhibited mode or DDI mode) in non–rate-adaptive pacing modes. Rate smoothing is programmable as a percentage, i.e., 3% to 24% in 3% increments, and can be programmed independently for increments and decrements in the paced rate. The pacemaker stores the most recent RR interval, whether intrinsic or paced, and uses this interval to calculate an allowable change in cycle length based on the rate smoothing percentage programmed. Figure 6.31 demonstrates rate smoothing.

Ventricular rate regularization (VRR) is a variant of rate smoothing. In patients with atrial fibrillation, the marked variation in RR intervals may, in part, be responsible for patient symptoms. VRR is used to minimize the cycle length variation during atrial fibrillation. It is similar to rate smoothing, with the exception that it may calculate the appropriate cycle length on the basis of a weighted sum of the current ventricular cycle length, as opposed to using the most recent ventricular cycle length with classic rate smoothing.[47]

Effect of Dual-Chamber Rate-Modulated Pacemakers on Timing Cycles

Dual-chamber rate-modulated (DDDR) pacemakers are capable of all the variations described for DDD pacemakers (see Fig. 6.14). In addition to using P-synchronous pacing as a method for increasing the heart rate, the sensor incorporated in the pacemaker may increase the heart rate. The rhythm may therefore be sinus driven (alternatively called "atrial driven" or "P synchronous") or sensor driven (Fig. 6.37).

An important difference in the timing cycle between DDD and DDDR pacing is the ability to pace the atrium during the PVARP in the DDDR mode (Fig. 6.38). This feature does not occur in the DDD mode, because paced atrial activity does not occur until the LRL has been completed, which, by definition, must be at some point after the PVARP. In the DDDR mode, however, even though the atrial sensing channel is refractory during the PVARP, sensor-driven atrial output can still occur (Fig. 6.38).[48]

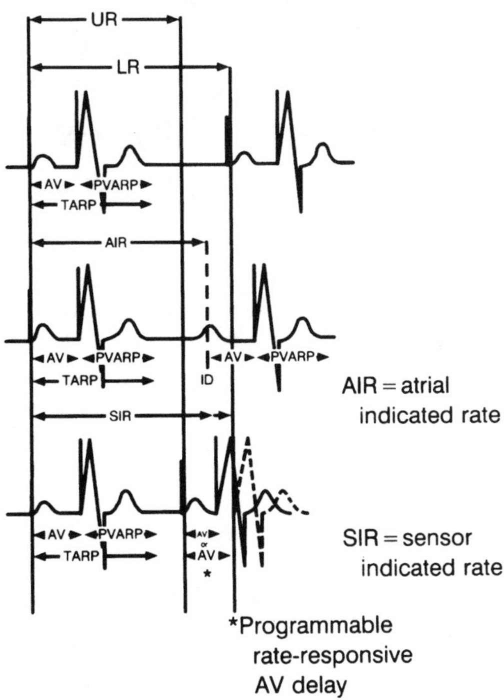

Figure 6.37. DDDR pacemakers are capable of all pacing variations previously described for DDD pacemakers (see also Fig. 6.14). When the device is functioning above the programmed LRL, it may increase the heart rate on the basis of the AIR or SIR. In most DDDR pacemakers, the PVARP remains fixed regardless of cycle length. Rate-adaptive or rate-variable AVI allows the length of the AVI to vary with the SIR; that is, as the SIR increases, the AVI shortens. Because an RRAVD is incorporated, the TARP may shorten by virtue of the changing AVI even though the PVARP does not change at faster rates.

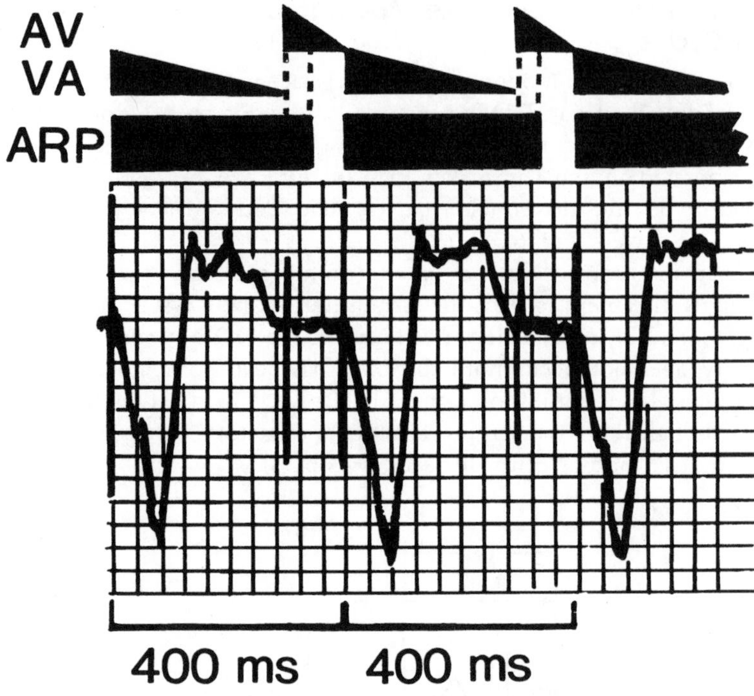

Figure 6.38. In this ECG example from a DDDR pacemaker, the MSR is 150 ppm (400 milliseconds), the ARP is 350 milliseconds, and the AVI is 100 milliseconds. As illustrated in the block diagrams above the ECG, the two sensor-driven atrial pacing artifacts both occur during the terminal portion of the PVARP. Even though no atrial sensing can occur during the PVARP, as can be seen in this example by the intrinsic P wave that occurs immediately after the first paced ventricular depolarization, a sensor-driven atrial pacing artifact is not prevented by the PVARP. Whether a sensor-driven atrial pacing artifact is delivered depends on the sensor-indicated rate at that time and not on the PVARP. (Reprinted by permission from Hayes DL, Higano ST. DDDR pacing: follow-up and complications. In: Barold SS, Mugica J, eds. New Perspectives in Cardiac Pacing, 2. Mount Kisco, NY: Futura, 1991:473–491.)

DDDR pacing systems further increase the complexity of the upper rate behavior. The pacemaker can be driven by intrinsic atrial activity to cause PV pacing or by a sensor with an input signal that is not identifiable on the ECG, or by both, to result in AV or AR pacing.[3,29] The eventual upper rate also depends on the type of sensor incorporated in the pacemaker and how the sensor is programmed.[49] Between the programmed LRL and the programmed URL, there may be stable P-wave synchronous pacing, P-wave synchronous pacing alternating with AV sequential pacing, or stable AV sequential pacing at rates exceeding the base rate (Fig. 6.39).[50] AV sequential pacing rates may increase as high as the programmed MSR.

Although the MSR and MTR are closely related, they are not identical. The tracking rate refers to the rate at which the pacemaker is sensing and track-

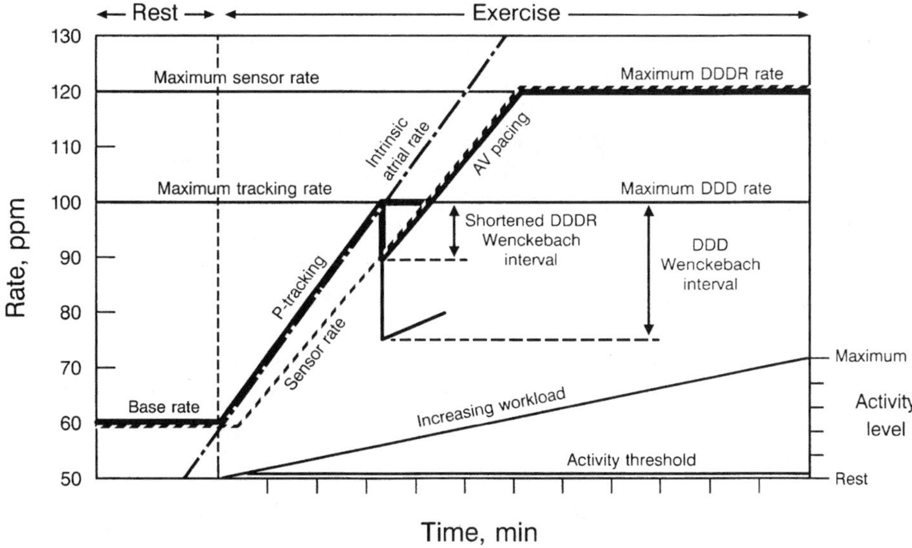

Figure 6.39. Diagram illustrating the rate response of the DDDR pacemaker and its behavior at both maximum tracking and the MSR. The *dashed-dotted line* represents the intrinsic atrial rate, and the *diagonal dashed line* represents the sensor rate during progressively increasing workloads. The *heavy black line* shows the ventricular paced rate, assuming complete heart block, as it progresses from the P-tracking mode to AV sequential pacing through a period of Wenckebach-type block. The DDD Wenckebach interval is shortened by sensor-driven pacing, that is, "sensor-driven rate smoothing." Maximum shortening of the Wenckebach period is accomplished by optimal programming of the sensor rate-response variables (threshold and slope programming for an activity-driven sensor). (From Higano ST, Hayes DL, Eisinger G. Sensor-driven rate smoothing in a DDDR pacemaker. Pacing Clin Electrophysiol 1989;12:922–929. By permission of Futura Publishing Company.)

ing intrinsic atrial activity. The MTR is the maximum ventricular paced rate that is allowed in response to sensed atrial rhythms. The MTR may result in fixed-block, Wenckebach, fallback, or rate-smoothing responses, depending on the design of the system. The sensor-controlled rate is the rate of the pacemaker that is determined by the sensor-input signal. The MSR is the maximum rate that the pacemaker is allowed to achieve under sensor control.

Whether at the MTR or during rate acceleration below the MTR, the rhythm that results may be in part sensor driven and in part sinus driven (P-wave tracking) and not purely one or the other (see Fig. 6.37). Which of these mechanisms predominates depends on the integrity of the sinus node and the sensor and how the pacemaker is programmed. DDDR pacing can result in a type of rate smoothing. If the sensor is optimally programmed, then as the atrial rate exceeds the MTR, the RR interval displays minimal variation between sinus-driven and sensor-driven pacing.[50] As shown in Figure 6.40, the variation in RR interval is markedly lessened with the sensor "on" (DDDR) rather than "passive" (DDD) mode. In the DDDR mode, the RR interval is allowed to lengthen only as much as the difference between the MTR and the activity sensor rate interval. For example, if a device is programmed to a P-wave tracking limit of 120 ppm and the patient's atrial rate exceeds this, then the pacemaker operates in a Wenckebach-type block. If the sensor-indicated rate at this time is 100 ppm, the paced rate decreases from 120 ppm (500 milliseconds) to an AV sequential paced rate of 100 ppm (600 milliseconds) for the Wenckebach cycle and then returns to P-wave tracking at a rate of 120 ppm. This situation usually shortens the DDD Wenckebach interval, but this interval depends on the atrial rate and the programmed values for the MTR and the TARP.

Maximal sensor-driven rate smoothing requires optimal programming of the sensor variable. If the rate-responsive circuitry is programmed to mimic the native atrial rate, the paced ventricular rate cannot demonstrate the 2:1 or Wenckebach-type behavior. Conversely, if the rate-responsive circuitry is programmed to low levels of sensor-driven pacing, little or no rate smoothing occurs (Figs. 6.39 and 6.41). Figure 6.40 shows the sensor "passive" (DDD)

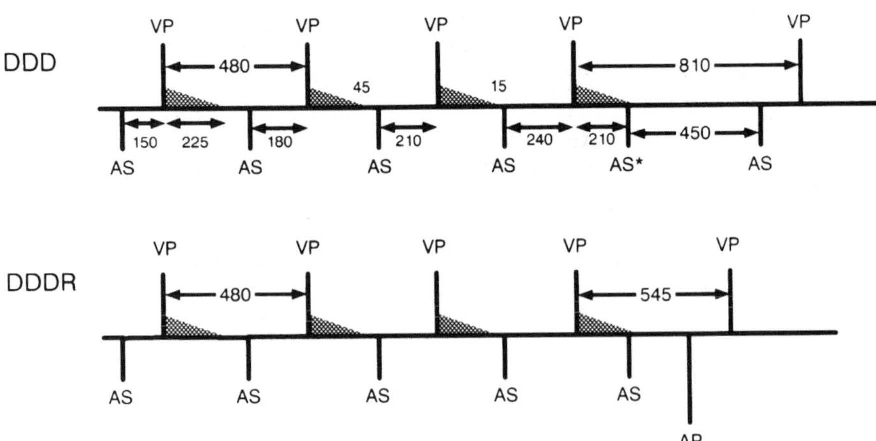

Figure 6.40. This diagram illustrates the difference in DDD and DDDR behavior when the intrinsic atrial rate increases. In the **upper panel,** DDD pacing is illustrated. The sensed atrial events (AS) occur increasingly closer to the PVARP, which is programmed to 225 milliseconds (shown by the shaded triangles) until the fifth AS event (*) occurs at 210 milliseconds after the preceding ventricular paced event (VP) and within the PVARP and is not sensed. This is followed by another AS and VP after the programmed AVI of 150 milliseconds. The resultant cycle length is 810 milliseconds, significantly longer than the preceding cycles of 480 milliseconds. In the **lower panel,** DDDR pacing is illustrated. The intervals are programmed to the same values as in the upper panel. When the fifth AS event occurs within the PVARP, it is, by definition, not sensed. However, the escape event is a sensor-driven atrial pacing artifact followed by a VP after the AVI. The sensor-indicated cycle length is 545 milliseconds. Therefore, only a 65-millisecond difference exists between the programmed URL and the sensor-indicated rate—a minor difference in cycle lengths. (Modified from Markowitz HT. Dual chamber rate responsive pacing [DDDR] provides physiologic upper rate behavior. PhysioPace 1990;4:1–4. By permission of Medtronic.)

response to exercise-induced increases in atrial rate, assuming complete heart block, an MTR of 100 ppm, and a Wenckebach-type response at the MTR. The ventricular and atrial rate responses to exercise are shown. As the MTR is exceeded, there is a transition from 1 : 1 P-synchronous function to Wenckebach upper rate behavior. Figure 6.39 shows the response that occurs with the sensor "on" (DDDR) and an MSR of 120 ppm. The ventricular rate response to exercise, along with the atrial and sensor rates, is shown. Below the maximum P-wave tracking rate, the ventricle is paced in a P-synchronous fashion, similar to sensor "passive" (DDD) function. However, with the sensor "on" (DDDR), there is a transition from P-synchronous to AV sequential pacing through a period of Wenckebach-type block as the atrial rate exceeds the MTR. The Wenckebach interval is shortened by sensor-driven pacing. The sensor rate response curve can be relocated almost anywhere on the graph by sensor parameter programming. Maximum sensor-driven rate smoothing requires optimal programming of these variables. Thus, sensor-modulated rate smoothing occurs only when the activity sensor is driving the pacemaker, when the intrinsic atrial rate exceeds the programmed MTR.

Another aspect of DDDR timing cycles is the ASW. The ASW is the portion of the RR cycle that is not part of the PVARP or the AVI. It is the

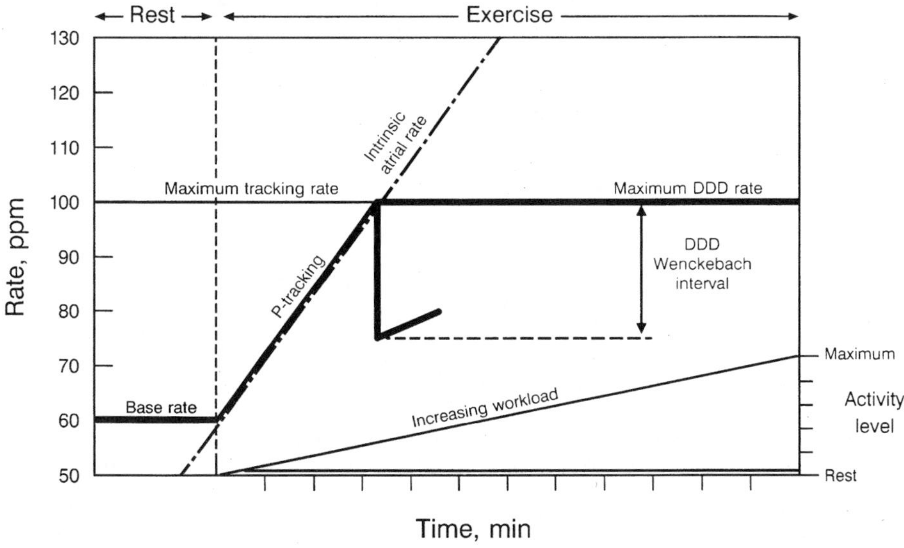

Figure 6.41. Diagram of the rate response of a DDD pacemaker with Wenckebach-type block at the URL (100 ppm). The *dashed-dotted line* represents the intrinsic atrial rate, and the *heavy black line* represents the ventricular paced rate, assuming complete heart block. The RR intervals during Wenckebach-type block vary as the atrial rate exceeds the MTR. (From Higano ST, Hayes DL, Eisinger G. Sensor-driven rate smoothing in a DDDR pacemaker. Pacing Clin Electrophysiol 1989;12:922–929. By permission of Futura Publishing Company.)

period during which the atrial sensing channel is alert. If the PVARP or AVI (or both) is extended, there may effectively be no ASW and even a DDD pacemaker functions as a DVI system. Conversely, if a DDDR pacemaker has exceeded the programmed MTR and is pacing at faster rates based on sensor activation, an appropriately timed intrinsic P wave can still inhibit the sensor-driven atrial pacing artifact and give the appearance of P-wave tracking at rates greater than the MTR (Fig. 6.42).[51] Although the MTR is programmed to a single value in DDDR pacing, it behaves as if it were variable and equal to the sensor-driven rate when the sensor-driven rate exceeds the programmed MTR

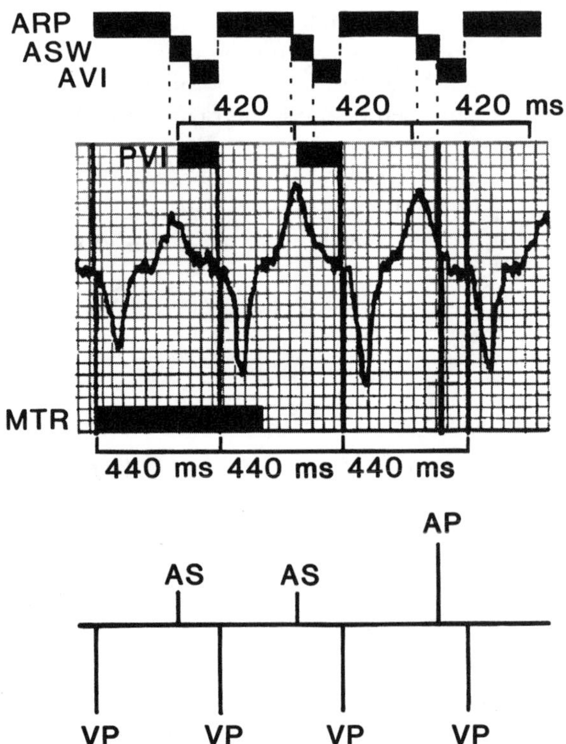

Figure 6.42. Diagram showing how an appropriately timed P wave can inhibit the sensor-driven A spike and result in apparent P-wave tracking above the MTR. In this example, the MTR is 100 ppm, or 600 milliseconds. The second and third complexes are preceded by intrinsic P waves that occurred during the ASW. This resulted in A-spike inhibition, or P-wave tracking above the MTR. The fourth complex was initiated by atrial pacing, because the preceding native P wave occurred outside the ASW in the ARP (ARP = 275 milliseconds). Note the short P-stimulus interval produced by the subsequent atrial spike. Also shown are the ASW (ASW = 65 milliseconds), AVI (AVI = 100 milliseconds), and variable PV interval (PVI). The intrinsic atrial rate is 143 bpm (420 milliseconds). The sensor rate is 136 ppm (440 milliseconds). A diagram in marker-channel fashion demonstrates the ECG findings. (From Higano ST, Hayes DL. P wave tracking above the maximum tracking rate in a DDDR pacemaker. Pacing Clin Electrophysiol 1989;12:1044–1048. By permission of Futura Publishing Company.)

if a P wave occurs during the ASW to inhibit output of an atrial pacing artifact.

Effects of Ventricular- and Atrial-Based Timing Systems on DDDR Timing Cycles

As noted previously, the "timing system" may affect the timing cycle. In a ventricular-based timing system, the effective atrial paced rate theoretically may be considerably higher than the programmed MSR if AR conduction were present (Fig. 6.43, top).[3] Assuming that the maximum sensor-controlled rate is 150 ppm (a cycle length of 400 milliseconds), the AEI with a programmed AVI of 200 milliseconds is also 200 milliseconds. If AV conduction were intact such that the AR interval was 150 milliseconds, the actual pacing interval would be ARI + AEI, or 150 + 200 milliseconds, or 350 milliseconds. A cycle length of 350 milliseconds equals 171 ppm, which is markedly higher than the programmed MSR of 150 ppm. Although this potentially achievable faster rate may not be a

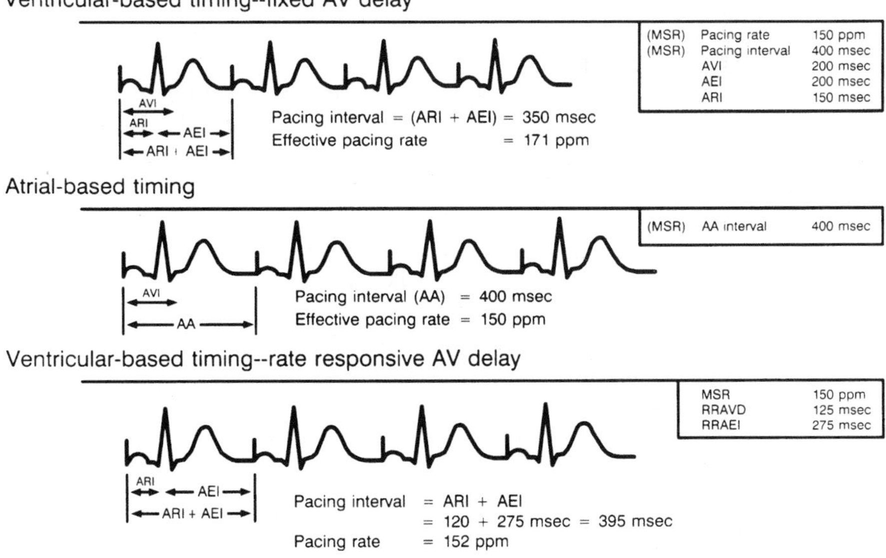

Figure 6.43. Effect of different timing systems on MSR with intact stable AV nodal conduction (AR pacing). **Top:** In a ventricular-based timing system, there is a considerable theoretical increase in the paced atrial rate exceeding that programmed by the physician. In the example shown, even though the MSR programmed is 150 ppm, or 400 milliseconds, the effective pacing rate achieved is 171 ppm, because the effective pacing rate is the sum of the ARI and the AEI; that is, 150 + 200 = 350 milliseconds (171 ppm). **Middle:** In an atrial-based system, the R wave sensed during the AVI alters the basic timing during stable AR pacing. This results in atrial pacing at the sensor-indicated rate. **Bottom:** The addition of an RRAVD to a ventricular-based timing system minimizes the increase in the paced atrial rate above the programmed sensor-indicated rate. (From Levine PA, Hayes DL, Wilkoff BL, Ohman AE. Electrocardiography of Rate-Modulated Pacemaker Rhythms. Sylmar, CA: Siemens-Pacesetter, 1990. By permission of Siemens-Pacesetter.)

problem or may even be advantageous for some patients, it could create problems for other patients (Fig. 6.43, middle).

Rate acceleration can also be minimized in a DDDR ventricular-based timing system by incorporating a rate-responsive AV delay (RRAVD).[29,52] As the sinus or sensor-driven rate progressively increases, RRAVD causes the PV and AVIs to progressively shorten (Fig. 6.43, bottom). Shortening the AVI with RRAVD results in a shorter TARP (shorter AVI + PVARP), which increases the intrinsic atrial rate that can be sensed and reduces the likelihood of both a fixed-block upper rate response and functional atrial undersensing. It also minimizes the chance of an inappropriately long PV interval at the higher rate, which may occur with a fixed AV delay when the fixed AV delay is programmed appropriately for lower rate behavior. In this case, the AV delay may be too long at higher rates. In a DDDR system, when the AVI shortens, the ventricular rate drive is held to that governed by the sensor so that the time subtracted from the AVI is added to the AEI. Thus, at a rate of 150 ppm and pacing interval of 400 milliseconds, if the RRAVD causes the AVI to shorten by 75 milliseconds from an initially programmed AVI of 200 milliseconds, then the AVI shortens to 125 milliseconds. Because the overall ventricular timing is held constant, the 75 milliseconds subtracted from the AVI is added to the AEI, increasing it to 275 milliseconds.

The RRAVD provides a more physiologic AVI at the faster rate and minimizes the degree of rate increase over the programmed MSR if AR conduction is intact. Assuming that the rate is 150 ppm and the initial AVI is 200 milliseconds, the RRAVD is 125 milliseconds, resulting in AV sequential pacing at the sensor programmed rate when the AR interval is 140 milliseconds. If intact AV conduction is present at 120 milliseconds, the overall shortening of the pacing interval is only 5 milliseconds more than that seen at 150 bpm, a rate of 152 bpm (Fig. 6.43, bottom).

Another option is extending the VAI as needed to control the AA pacing rate according to the programmed MSR (Fig. 6.44). This extension results in adaptive-rate pacing, regardless of AV conduction status, which is equal to, but does not exceed, the desired MSR.

ENDLESS-LOOP TACHYCARDIA

Endless-loop tachycardia (ELT) is not a portion of the timing cycle, but understanding the timing cycle of dual-chamber pacing is crucial to understanding ELT, and vice versa. ELT has also been referred to as "pacemaker-mediated tachycardia" (PMT), "pacemaker-mediated reentry tachycardia," and "pacemaker circus movement tachycardia."[9] ELT has been defined as a reentry arrhythmia in which the dual-chamber pacemaker acts as the anterograde limb of the tachycardia and the natural pathway acts as the retrograde limb.[53,54]

If AV synchrony is uncoupled—that is, if the P wave is displaced from its normal relation to the QRS complex—the subsequent ventricular event may result in retrograde atrial excitation if retrograde or VA conduction is intact.[53,54]

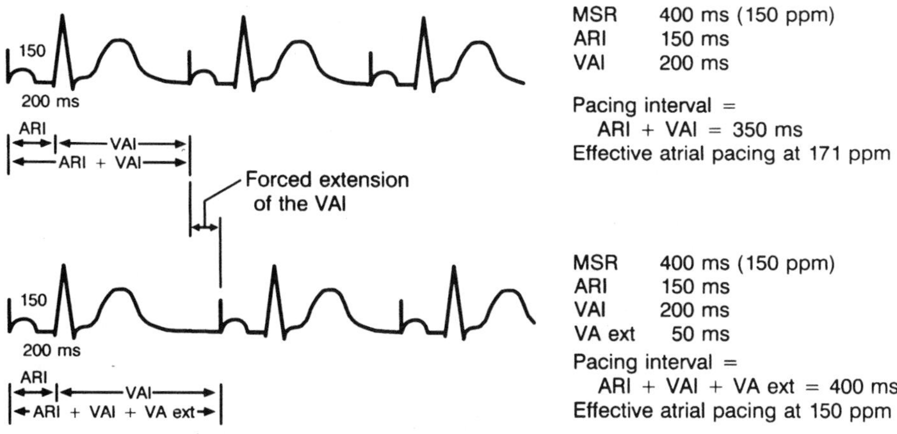

Figure 6.44. Pacing at MSR. Timing algorithm provides effective pacing at MSR with intrinsic conduction to the ventricle. ARI = interval from atrial stimulus to sensed R wave; VA = ventriculoatrial; VAI = ventriculoatrial interval. (From Hayes DL, Ketelson A, Levine PA, et al. Understanding timing systems of current DDDR pacemakers. Eur JCPE 1993;3:70–86. By permission of Mayo Foundation.)

If the retrograde P wave is sensed, the AVI of the pacemaker is initiated. On termination of the AVI and MTR interval, a ventricular pacing artifact is delivered, which could once again be conducted in a retrograde fashion. Once established, this reentrant mechanism continues until interrupted or until the retrograde limb of the circuit is exhausted. The paced VV interval cannot violate the programmed maximum or URL of the pacemaker, and the ELT often occurs at the URL. Many mechanisms have been adopted to prevent or minimize ELT.[55]

Among the early preventive algorithms was automatic PVARP extension following a PVC, because ventricular ectopic beats were the most common triggers for an ELT. ELT was not a major problem when the programmed base rate was low; however, if the base rate is intentionally programmed to a relatively high level or is functioning there due to sensor drive, PVARP extension blocks detection of either a retrograde or an anterograde P wave. Because of the high rate, however, the AEI may time out, resulting in delivery of an atrial output pulse when the atrial myocardium is still refractory from the native depolarization. In this circumstance, atrial output is ineffective. If the patient can sustain retrograde conduction, this sequence of events can result in a rhythm termed *repetitive nonreentrant ventriculoatrial synchrony*.

Algorithms for Termination of Pacemaker-Mediated Tachycardia

If ELT cannot be prevented, various recognition and termination algorithms are available. The simplest algorithm assumes that atrial-sensed ventricular pacing occurring at the MTR is a PMT and after a preset number of cycles either withholds ventricular output or extends the PVARP. If the rhythm is a true ELT, it is terminated by this mechanism. A further refinement to these algorithms allows the clinician to select an ELT rate that is below the MTR. This adjustment addresses the balanced ELTs in which the sum of the retrograde conduction (VA) interval plus the sensed AV delay is longer than the MTR interval, and, hence, the ELT rate is slower than the MTR. The limitation of both these algorithms is that they respond whether the rhythm is an ELT or an intrinsic atrial rhythm that is being appropriately tracked by the pacemaker. For a native atrial rhythm, repeated pauses are caused by the activation of the PMT termination algorithm.

Another approach is to monitor the retrograde conduction interval. If the VP interval is stable, the device labels the rhythm as a possible PMT and then varies the next PV interval. If the atrial rhythm is independent of the ventricular paced event, the VP interval on the next cycle is either lengthened or shortened by the same degree that the PV interval was changed. The rhythm is then labeled normal, and normal atrial synchronous ventricular pacing continues. If the VP interval is stable, the P wave was caused by retrograde conduction (related to the ventricular paced event), and the rhythm is probably a PMT. At that point, ventricular output is withheld following the detected P wave. An atrial alert period is initiated, and if another P wave is not detected, an atrial output pulse is delivered 330 milliseconds later. This interval was chosen as sufficient for recovery of the atrial myocardium. Successful atrial capture breaks the cycle and prevents retrograde conduction after the next ventricular paced complex. This algorithm also prevents some of the pauses occurring with an earlier generation of PMT algorithms (Fig. 6.45).

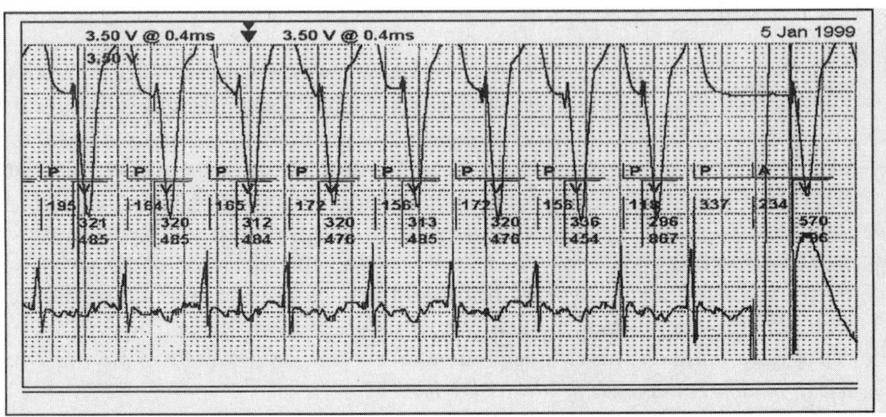

Figure 6.45. Endless-loop tachycardia was induced during an atrial capture threshold test (loss of atrial capture allowed for retrograde conduction). The PMT algorithm was enabled. The PV interval was shortened; the subsequent VP interval was stable, resulting in withholding of ventricular output and delivery of atrial output 330 milliseconds later.

Noncompetitive Atrial Pacing

Noncompetitive atrial pacing (NCAP) is used to minimize competition between the sensor (atrial pacing) and sinus rhythm. Implementation of this capability has been facilitated by microprocessors and the ability of pacemakers to detect events coinciding with the refractory period. If atrial depolarization is sensed within the alert period, it inhibits atrial output and triggers ventricular output. However, if the native atrial event coincides with the PVARP, it may be detected but does not otherwise alter the basic timing period of the pacemaker. With NCAP enabled, if atrial output is scheduled to be delivered within a given interval after the detected P wave, atrial output is delayed until a preset interval has timed out. A Medtronic device, for example, uses a fixed interval of 300 milliseconds (this may not always be sufficient, in our experience). Atrial output is delivered at that time. To maintain a stable ventricular rate, the paced AVI may be foreshortened for this one cycle (Fig. 6.46).

SUMMARY

A clear understanding of the components of pacemaker timing cycles is crucial to understanding and interpreting paced ECGs. The information in this chapter provides basic rules for timing cycles for pacing modes currently in use (VVI, AAI, VVIR, AAIR, DDI, DDD, DDDR, DDIR) and for pacing modes less fre-

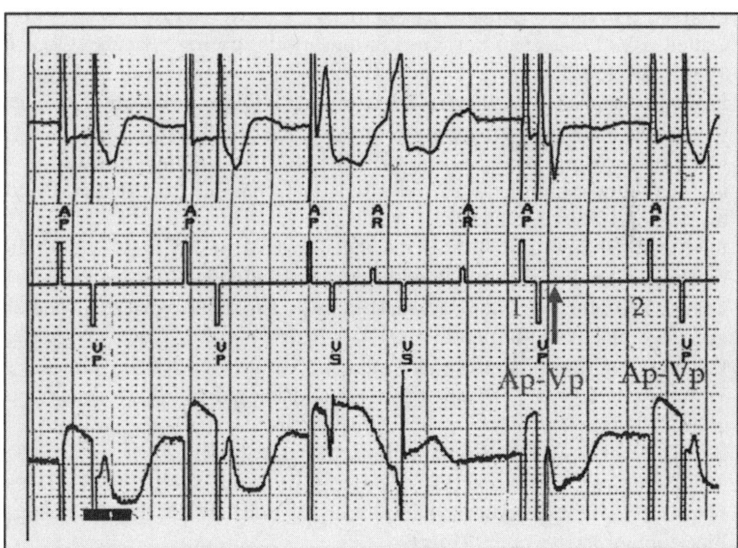

Figure 6.46. Premature ventricular contraction associated with a retrograde P wave. This P wave coincides with the PVARP and is not tracked. But it is sensed and labeled "AR." The scheduled atrial output is delayed 300 milliseconds. This results in a foreshortening of the AV delay. AP = atrial paced event; AS = atrial sensed event; VP = ventricular paced event; VS = ventricular sensed event. (Courtesy of S. Serge Barold, M.D.)

quently used or of historical interest but still important to understand how timing cycles have developed (VOO, AOO, DOO, DVIC, DVI, VDD).

Each pacemaker manufacturer may take license and alter or add some nuance to the timing cycle of a particular pacemaker. Although understanding basic timing cycles allows interpretation of most paced ECGs, manufacturers' alterations require familiarity with the design of each pacemaker to be interpreted. When unexpected behavior of the pacemaker occurs in a patient whose condition is clinically stable, the presumption should be that this reflects a unique behavioral eccentricity of the pacemaker. All manufacturers maintain a group of technical service engineers who are available 24 hours a day, 7 days a week. They should be contacted before any intervention, such as replacing the pulse generator, is attempted, for in all probability the device is behaving normally.

REFERENCES

1. Bernstein AD, Daubert J-C, Fletcher RD, et al. The revised NASPE/BPEG generic code for antibradycardia, adaptive-rate and multisite pacing. Pacing Clin Electrophysiol 2002;25:260–264.
2. Barold SS, Falkoff MD, Ong LS, Heinle RA. Interpretation of electrocardiograms produced by a new unipolar multiprogrammable "committed" AV sequential demand (DVI) pulse generator. Pacing Clin Electrophysiol 1981;4:692–708.
3. Levine PA, Sholder JA. Interpretation of Rate-Modulated, Dual-Chamber Rhythms: The Effect of Ventricular Based and Atrial Based Timing Systems on DDD and DDDR Rhythms. Sylmar, CA: Siemens-Pacesetter, 1990:1–20.
4. Calfee RV. Dual-chamber committed mode pacing. Pacing Clin Electrophysiol 1983;6:387–391.
5. Floro J, Castellanet M, Florio J, Messenger J. DDI: a new mode for cardiac pacing. Clin Prog Pacing Electrophysiol 1984;2:255–260.
6. Hanich RF, Midei MG, McElroy BP, Brinker JA. Circumvention of maximum tracking limitations with a rate modulated dual chamber pacemaker. Pacing Clin Electrophysiol 1989;12:392–397.
7. Levine PA, Lindenberg BS, Mace RC. Analysis of AV universal (DDD) pacemaker rhythms. Clin Prog Pacing Electrophysiol 1984;2:54–70.
8. Levine PA. Normal and abnormal rhythms associated with dual-chamber pacemakers. Cardiol Clin 1985;3:595–616.
9. Furman S. Comprehension of pacemaker timing cycles. In: Furman S, Hayes DL, Holmes DR Jr, eds. A Practice of Cardiac Pacing. 2nd ed. Mount Kisco, NY: Futura, 1989:115–166.
10. Furman S, Hayes DL. Implantation of atrioventricular synchronous and atrioventricular universal pacemakers. J Thorac Cardiovasc Surg 1983;85:839–850.
11. Hauser RG. The electrocardiography of AV universal DDD pacemakers. Pacing Clin Electrophysiol 1983;6:399–409.
12. Barold SS, Falkoff MD, Ong LS, Heinle RA. Timing cycles of DDD pacemakers. In: Barold SS, Mugica J, eds. New Perspectives in Cardiac Pacing. Mount Kisco, NY: Futura, 1988:69–119.
13. Levine PA. Postventricular atrial refractory periods and pacemaker mediated tachycardias. Clin Prog Pacing Electrophysiol 1983;1:394–401.

14. Barold SS. Management of patients with dual chamber pulse generators: central role of the pacemaker atrial refractory period. Learning Center Highlights 1990;5:8–16.
15. Furman S. Dual chamber pacemakers: upper rate behavior. Pacing Clin Electrophysiol 1985;8:197–214.
16. Barold SS, Falkoff MD, Ong LS, Heinle RA. Upper rate response of DDD pacemakers. In: Barold SS, Mugica J, eds. New Perspectives in Cardiac Pacing. Mount Kisco, NY: Futura, 1988:121–172.
17. Hayes DL, Osborn MJ. Pacing A. Antibradycardia devices. In: Giuliani ER, Fuster V, Gersh BJ, et al., eds. Cardiology: Fundamentals and Practice (Vol 1, 2nd ed.). St. Louis: Mosby-Year Book, 1991:1014–1079.
18. Hayes DL. Programmability. In: Furman S, Hayes DL, Holmes DR Jr, eds. A Practice of Cardiac Pacing. 2nd ed. Mount Kisco, NY: Futura, 1989:563–596.
19. Batey RL, Calabria DA, Shewmaker S, Sweesy M. Crosstalk and blanking periods in a dual chamber (DDD) pacemaker: a case report. Clin Prog Electrophysiol Pacing 1985;3:314–318.
20. Barold SS, Ong LS, Falkoff MD, Heinle RA. Crosstalk of self-inhibition in dual-chambered pacemakers. In: Barold SS, ed. Modern Cardiac Pacing. Mount Kisco, NY: Futura, 1985:615–623.
21. Brandt J, Fahraeus T, Schuller H. Far-field QRS complex sensing via the atrial pacemaker lead. II. Prevalence, clinical significance and possibility of intraoperative prediction in DDD pacing. Pacing Clin Electrophysiol 1988;11:1540–1544.
22. Barold SS, Belott PH. Behavior of the ventricular triggering period of DDD pacemakers. Pacing Clin Electrophysiol 1987;10:1237–1252.
23. Chorus II Model 6234, 6244 Dual Chamber Pulse Generator Physician's Manual. Minnetonka, MN: ELA Medical, 1994.
24. Daubert C, Ritter P, Mabo P, et al. Rate modulation of the AV delay in DDD pacing. In: Santini M, Pistolese M, Alliegro A, eds. Progress in Clinical Pacing 1990. New York: Elsevier, 1990:415–430.
25. Janosik DL, Pearson AC, Buckingham TA, Labovitz AJ, Redd RM. The hemodynamic benefit of differential atrioventricular delay intervals for sensed and paced atrial events during physiologic pacing. J Am Coll Cardiol 1989;14:499–507.
26. Mehta D, Gilmour S, Ward DE, Camm AJ. Optimal atrioventricular delay at rest and during exercise in patients with dual chamber pacemakers: a non-invasive assessment by continuous wave Doppler. Br Heart J 1989;61:161–166.
27. Sutton R, Brignole M, Menozzi C, et al, for the Vasovagal Syncope International Study (VASIS) Investigators. Dual-chamber pacing in the treatment of neurally mediated tilt-positive cardioinhibitory syncope: Pacemaker versus no therapy: a multicenter randomized study. Circulation 2000;102:294–299.
28. Connolly SJ, Sheldon R, Roberts RS, Gent M. The North American Vasovagal Pacemaker Study (VPS). A randomized trial of permanent cardiac pacing for the prevention of vasovagal syncope. J Am Coll Cardiol 1999;33:16–20.
29. Levine PA, Hayes DL, Wilkoff BL, Ohman AE. Electrocardiography of Rate-Modulated Pacemaker Rhythms. Sylmar, CA: Siemens-Pacesetter, 1990.
30. Relay Models 293-03 and 294-03. Intermedics Cardiac Pulse Generator Physician's Manual. Angleton, TX: Intermedics, 1992.
31. The Elite Activity Responsive Dual Chamber Pacemaker With Telemetry (Including DDDR, DDD, DDIR, DDI, DVIR, and VVIR). Models 7074, 7075, 7076, and 7077 Technical Manual. Minneapolis: Medtronic, 1991.

32. Brunner-La Rocca HP, Rickli H, Weilenmann D, Duru F, Candinas R. Importance of ventricular rate after mode switching during low intensity exercise as assessed by clinical symptoms and ventilatory gas exchange. Pacing Clin Electrophysiol 2000;23:32–39.
33. Levine PA, Sholder JA, Young G. Automatic mode switching, is this optimal management of atrial fibrillation? In: Santini M, ed. Proceedings of the International Symposium on Progress in Clinical Pacing 1996, Rome, Italy, December 3–6, 1996. Armonk, NY: Futura Media Services, 1997:331–338.
34. Rawles JM. What is meant by a "controlled" ventricular rate in atrial fibrillation? Br Heart J 1990;63:157–161.
35. Resnekov L, McDonald L. Electroversion of lone atrial fibrillation and flutter including haemodynamic studies at rest and on exercise. Br Heart J 1971;33: 339–350.
36. van Mechelen R, Ruiter J, de Boer H, Hagemeijer F. Pacemaker electrocardiography of rate smoothing during DDD pacing. Pacing Clin Electrophysiol 1985;8: 684–690.
37. Meta DDDR 1250H Multiprogrammable Minute Ventilation, Rate Responsive Pulse Generator with Telemetry Physician's Manual. Englewood, CO: Telectronics Pacing Systems, 1991.
38. Lau CP, Tai YT, Fong PC, Li JP, Chung FL. Atrial arrhythmia management with sensor controlled atrial refractory period and automatic mode switching in patients with minute ventilation sensing dual chamber rate adaptive pacemakers. Pacing Clin Electrophysiol 1992;15:1504–1514.
39. META™ DDDR 1254. User's Guide. Englewood, CO: Telectronics Pacing Systems, 1993.
40. Israel CW, Lemke B (eds.). Modern concepts of automatic mode switching. Herzschrittmacher-therapie & Elektrophysiologie 1999;10 Suppl 1:I/1–I/80.
41. Frohlig G, Helwani Z, Kusch O, Berg M, Schieffer H. Bipolar ventricular far-field signals in the atrium. Pacing Clin Electrophysiol 1999;22:1604–1613.
42. Brandt J, Worzewski W. Far-field QRS complex sensing: prevalence and timing with bipolar atrial leads. Pacing Clin Electrophysiol 2000;23:315–320.
43. Fitts SM, Hill MR, Mehra R, Gillis AM, for the PA Clinical Trial Investigators. High rate atrial tachyarrhythmia detections in implantable pulse generators: low incidence of false-positive detections. Pacing Clin Electrophysiol 2000;23:1080–1086.
44. Barold SS, Sayad D, Gallardo I. Alternating duration of ventricular paced cycles during automatic mode switching of a DDDR pacemaker. J Interv Card Electrophysiol 2002;7:185–187.
45. Israel CW. Mode-switching algorithms: programming and usefulness [German]. Herz 2001;26:2–17.
46. Gelvan D, Crystal E, Dokumaci B, Goldshmid Y, Ovsyshcher IE. Effect of modern pacing algorithms on generator longevity: a predictive analysis. Pacing Clin Electrophysiol 2003;26:1796–1802.
47. Wood MA. Trials of pacing to control ventricular rate during atrial fibrillation. J Interv Card Electrophysiol 2004;10 Suppl 1:63–70.
48. Hayes DL, Higano ST. DDDR pacing: Follow-up and complications. In SS Barold, J Mugica (eds.), New Perspectives in Cardiac Pacing. 2. Mount Kisco, NY: Futura, 1991:473–491.
49. Hayes DL, Higano ST, Eisinger G. Electrocardiographic manifestations of a dual-chamber, rate-modulated (DDDR) pacemaker. Pacing Clin Electrophysiol 1989;12:555–562.

50. Higano ST, Hayes DL, Eisinger G. Sensor-driven rate smoothing in a DDDR pacemaker. Pacing Clin Electrophysiol 1989;12:922–929.
51. Higano ST, Hayes DL. P wave tracking above the maximum tracking rate in a DDDR pacemaker. Pacing Clin Electrophysiol 1989;12:1044–1048.
52. Daubert C, Ritter P, Mabo P, Ollitrault J, Descaves C, Gouffault J. Physiological relationship between AV interval and heart rate in healthy subjects: applications to dual chamber pacing. Pacing Clin Electrophysiol 1986;9:1032–1039.
53. Furman S, Fisher JD. Endless loop tachycardia in an AV universal [DDD] pacemaker. Pacing Clin Electrophysiol 1982;5:486–489.
54. Den Dulk K, Lindemans FW, Bar FW, Wellens HJ. Pacemaker related tachycardias. Pacing Clin Electrophysiol 1982;5:476–485.
55. Hayes DL. Endless-loop tachycardia: The problem has been solved? In: Barold SS, Mugica J, eds. New Perspectives in Cardiac Pacing. Mount Kisco, NY: Futura, 1988:375–386.

Evaluation and Management of Pacing System Malfunctions

Paul A. Levine

7

Given the present reliability and longevity of implanted pacemakers,[1,2] most of the time spent caring for the paced patient will be concerned with evaluating the function of the already implanted pacing system. This chapter will review the differential diagnosis, evaluation, and management of the common malfunctions of single-chamber, dual-chamber, and biventricular pacing systems with respect to the electrical performance of these systems.

THE PACING SYSTEM

The pacemaker, or pulse generator, is a device consisting of a power source and the electronic circuitry that controls the system. Used in this limited context, a diagnosis of "pacemaker malfunction" implies that the device is at fault and that the problem can be corrected by either programming or replacing the unit. Problems can also be the result of a damaged lead, a primary abnormality at the electrode-myocardial interface, or the result of the pulse generator's being programmed inappropriately for the physiologic requirements of the patient. Unexpected behaviors can also be observed due to the interactions of various algorithms, each of which is behaving in a normal manner. While none of these conditions will be solved by replacing the pulse generator, some may be temporarily or permanently managed by reprogramming the pacemaker.

Given that the term *pacemaker* as used in the literature has two meanings, it is strongly recommended that the term *pacemaker* be restricted to the device (*pulse generator*) itself. Thus, when one encounters a malfunction, it should be considered a *pacing system malfunction*. This would promote consideration of all the components of the system, as focusing purely on the pulse generator could overlook the true cause of the problem. Although primary malfunctions of pulse generators do occur, they are the least frequent cause of any of the problems likely to be encountered. A variety of tools are available to facilitate evaluation of pacing system malfunctions, including surface electrocardiogram (ECG), Holter and event monitors, telemetered pacemaker data, pacemaker event counter diagnostics, chest radiograph, and physical examination. Any or all of these sources may be needed to fully evaluate a malfunction.[3] Before proceeding with an operative intervention to replace a device, the manufacturer's technical support services should be contacted when a primary device problem is suspected, because virtually every device has some unique behavioral eccentricities.

BASELINE DATA

It is of paramount importance to gather as much information as possible about the patient and the pacing system (Box 7.1) to make a definitive diagnosis. These data are essential to recognize a variety of malfunctions and pseudomalfunctions. The collection of baseline data concerning the pacing system begins with the implant procedure. This data should include detailed documentation as to the indications for pacing and any studies that impact the specific pacing mode selected. From the implant procedure, the following data should be collected: manufacturer, model, and serial numbers of the pulse generator and lead(s), the acute capture and sensing thresholds, and stimulation impedance measurements.[4] These should be obtained with a pacing system analyzer (PSA) set to the pulse

Box 7.1. Baseline Data Needed for Pacemaker Troubleshooting

Pacemaker System

- Pacemaker generator
  - Manufacturer
  - Model and serial numbers
  - Current programming
  - Date of implant
  - Alerts or recalls
  - Header type
  - Special features
- Lead system
  - Manufacturer
  - Model and serial numbers
  - Polarity and fixation mechanism
  - Pin type
  - Insulation material
  - Date of implant
  - Alerts or recalls

Patient

- Indication for pacemaker
- Implant operative report
- Medical and cardiac diagnoses
- Medications
- History of recent medical procedures (DCC, MRI, electrocautery, etc.)
- History of electrical current exposure, trauma

width of the permanent pacemaker. The actual electrogram (EGM) from the leads should be recorded with a physiologic recorder or ECG machine as this will provide valuable clues to the adequacy of lead position or retrieved from the pulse generator shortly after implantation.[5] At the end of the procedure, the programmed parameters of the pacing system are recorded along with lead function measurements and any other data that can be provided by the telemetric capabilities of the implanted device. Also complete 12-lead ECGs demonstrating full pacing and intrinsic rhythm should be obtained if possible. Following implantation, an *overpenetrated* posteroanterior and lateral chest radiographs should be obtained. A radiograph obtained using the standard technique—which is primarily designed to evaluate the lungs—may not be adequate to document the course and position of the pacing leads within the cardiac silhouette.

Before the patient is discharged from the hospital as well as at each subsequent outpatient pacing system evaluation, a detailed evaluation should be performed. This should include precise measurements of demand and magnet rates, battery and lead status, ECG rhythm strips showing the pacing system function in the demand mode, and a detailed assessment of the capture and sensing thresholds. Where measured data concerning lead and battery function as well as event marker, event counter, and electrogram telemetry are available using the pacemaker–programmer system, these too are obtained and incorporated in the summary of that evaluation.

All data should be thoroughly reviewed before attempting to diagnose a pacing system malfunction. In addition, the physician performing this system evaluation should be familiar with the patient's medical conditions, medications, and device programming as well as any peculiarities or performance alerts related to the pacemaker or leads.[6] One should also inquire about exposure to sources of electrical current (e.g., electrocautery) that may alter device function.

In the case of an intermittent pacing system malfunction or a patient referred for an evaluation of a suspected problem, it is essential to obtain sufficient ECG documentation of the problem. It may be necessary to retrieve these tracings from referring physicians' offices, medical records, and so on. Diligence is required, as "pacemaker malfunctions" are often misinterpretations of normal pacemaker function by persons unfamiliar with pacemaker follow-up evaluations.

DIFFERENTIAL DIAGNOSIS OF SINGLE-CHAMBER PACING SYSTEM MALFUNCTION

Any malfunction that can occur in a single-chamber pacing system can involve either channel of a dual-chamber system. To promote clarity, this section focuses on the common abnormalities associated with single-chamber systems. The next section will concentrate on dual-chamber systems, which require an understanding of both single-channel malfunctions and the complex interaction of the pacemaker's timing cycles with the native rhythm. Where appropriate, features specific to biventricular systems will be discussed.

When presented with a pacemaker problem on an ECG rhythm strip, it is first helpful to determine whether pacing stimuli are present. If present, do they capture the appropriate cardiac chamber? If absent, is there a native depolarization that is properly timed to explain the absence? One also needs to look at the native beats in relation to the paced complexes. Are all the native beats sensed correctly? Do they inhibit or trigger the next paced complex? In essence, these questions define the three major electrocardiographic patterns of single-chamber pacemaker malfunctions: 1) pacing stimuli present with failure to capture, 2) pacing stimuli present with failure to sense, and 3) pacing stimuli absent. Each pattern will be discussed in more detail.

Pacing Stimuli Present with Failure to Capture

To place a malfunction in this group, it is first necessary to be able to identify the pacing stimulus. This is usually obvious in a unipolar pacing system, because the stimuli are physically large (Fig. 7.1), but may become a problem with small bipolar outputs (Fig. 7.2). Pacing stimuli are nonphysiologic electrical transients of very high frequency. Some ECG recording systems, particularly ambulatory and in-hospital monitoring units, use special filters to eliminate high-frequency signals to minimize baseline noise on the recording.[7,8] In these cases, the unipolar signal will be markedly attenuated and the bipolar signal may be effectively erased. Sometimes, the signal is simply isoelectric in a given lead. Thus, if a malfunction of output is suspected, it is essential to record either multiple simultaneous or sequential leads with a system known to accurately reproduce the pacing stimulus artifact. In this case, the technologically older analog recorders are superior to the modern recording systems that digitize the incoming data. Other systems have unique high-frequency detection algorithms intended to identify pacing stimuli. In these systems, detection of a high-frequency signal

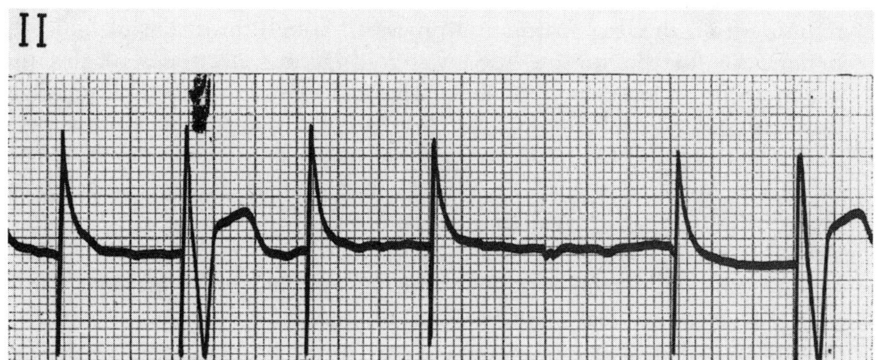

Figure 7.1. Pacing stimuli present with intermittent failure to capture. The large unipolar stimuli are readily identified. The gentle downslope following the ineffective pacing stimulus is an RC decay curve. The pause is due to appropriate sensing of a native QRS, which is virtually isoelectric in this lead. RC = resistance capacitance.

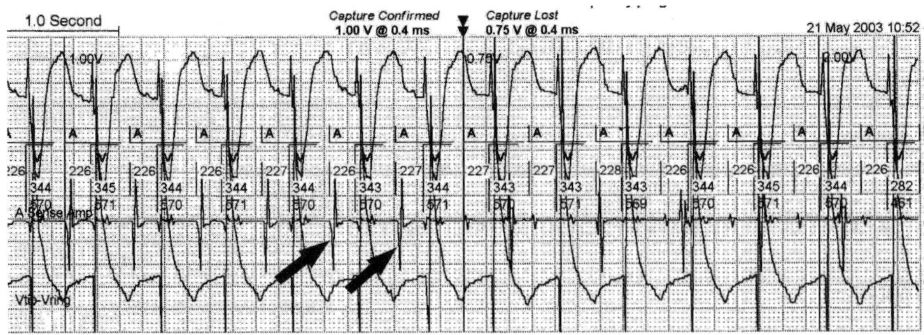

Figure 7.2. Evaluation of the atrial capture threshold while monitoring the surface ECG **(top tracing)**, telemetered event markers and intervals; the atrial electrogram **(middle tracing)** and the ventricular electrogram **(bottom tracing)**. Capture is present at 1.00 volts and 0.4 milliseconds. This is visible on both the surface ECG and the atrial EGM *(arrows)*. With loss of capture at 0.75 volts, there is the loss of the large complex on the atrial EGM and a loss of the visible P wave on the surface ECG. The atrial output is bipolar resulting in a diminutive stimulus artifact that is virtually invisible on the surface ECG. Effective blanking on the intracardiac atrial EGM prevents distortion of the EGM.

results in a uniform, relatively large "pacing artifact" generated by the ECG machine itself. This precludes differentiation of unipolar from bipolar pacing. Even nonpacemaker signals may be displayed as a pacing stimulus with these recording systems.

The differential diagnosis of stimuli present with failure to capture is relatively limited (Table 7.1). A likely etiology can often be established simply by knowing when the problem was encountered with respect to lead implantation. If the loss of capture occurred within hours or days of the implant, the most likely explanation is lead dislodgment. Loss of capture occurring weeks to months after implantation is most likely to be due to high capture thresholds resulting from the lead maturation process although this is less likely in the past decade due to the routine use of steroid-eluting electrodes. If this problem occurs many months to years after implantation, it is usually due to a mechanical or structural problem with the lead (such as damaged insulation or a conductor fracture) or due to an abnormality in the myocardium itself. During this time, it is also appropriate to consider extracardiac causes such as metabolic abnormalities or pharmacologic agents. Failure to program an adequate output safety margin may result in loss of capture due to physiologic variations in the capture threshold. Latency from the pacing stimulus to the onset of the P wave or QRS complex may simulate loss of capture. Eventually, the battery will deplete such that the actual output, despite its programmed value, will fall below the capture threshold, resulting in loss of capture.

Lead Dislodgment: Accompanying the loss of capture with an acute lead dislodgment, there may be changes in the morphology of capture beats, in the

Table 7.1. Differential Diagnosis of Pacing Stimuli Present—Persistent or Intermittent Loss of Capture

Etiology	ECG*	Chest Radiograph[†]	Impedance	Threshold	Management
Lead dislodgment • Early: unstable position • Late: Twiddler's syndrome	Abnormal	Abnormal or Normal	Normal	Elevated	Reposition lead
Lead maturation • Early: inflammatory response • Late: progressive fibrosis	Normal	Normal	Normal	Elevated	Increase output, trial of steroids, or reposition
Late high thresholds • Progressive fibrosis • Myocardial infarction • Cardiomyopathy • Metabolic/drugs • Damaged lead or tissue interface	Normal	Normal	Normal	Elevated	Increase output, correct cause, or replace lead
Insulation failure	Normal[‡]	Normal or conductor abnormality	Decreased	Elevated	Reprogram to unipolar, replace lead
Conductor failure • Lead fracture • Loose set-screw	Normal[§]	Abnormal	Increased	Elevated	Reprogram to unipolar (lead fracture), replace lead, reoperate for set screw
Battery depletion	Normal	Normal	Normal	Elevated[‖]	Replace pulse generator
Functional noncapture • Pseudomalfunction	Normal	Normal	Normal	Normal	Decrease rate, decrease refractory period(s), or increase sensitivity

* In ECG column, *normal* refers to a stable morphology of the evoked potential; *abnormal* refers to a change in the morphology of the evoked potential.
† In the chest radiograph column, *normal* refers to stable lead position and no obvious deformity of the conductor coil; *abnormal* refers to a change in lead position or a deformity of the conductor coil. The insulation is radiolucent and will not be visualized on the x-ray.
‡ The ECG with an insulation failure involving a unipolar lead will show a decrease in the amplitude of the pacing stimulus. An insulation failure involving the outer insulation of a bipolar lead will show an increase in the amplitude of the pacing stimulus. Failure of the internal insulation of a coaxial bipolar lead will show a decrease in stimulus amplitude. This presupposes that all recordings are made with an analog ECG machine.
§ The ECG with an intermittent conductor fracture may show a varying amplitude pacing stimulus if recorded with an analog ECG machine. See Table 7.3 for a total conductor fracture.
‖ Pacing threshold is increased as measured through the depleted generator but is normal through the PSA.
Source: Modified from Levine PA. Pacing system malfunction: Evaluation and management. In: Podrid PJ, Kowey PR, eds. Cardiac Arrhythmia: Mechanisms, Diagnosis, and Management. Philadelphia: Williams & Wilkins, © 1995. By permission of Williams & Wilkins.

dipole of the pacing stimulus, and/or in the lead position identified on a repeat chest radiograph. It is important to obtain the follow-up chest radiograph in an identical projection to that used for the baseline study. Even so, small "microdislodgments" of the lead tip may compromise the electrode contact with the myocardium but not be discernible with radiography. Despite some early reports in the literature to the contrary, neither partial lead dislodgment nor a simple rise in capture threshold due to tissue reaction at the electrode-myocardial interface will result in a significant change in stimulation impedance.[4]

A change in the morphology of the capture beat is often a clue to lead dislodgment, but this is the case only when fusion with the native QRS complex is absent. Fusion can also occur in the atrium. The morphologic changes in the paced P wave when combined with the native atrial depolarization are more difficult to identify because of the smaller size of the atrial complex. In biventricular systems, one has to be concerned with the position of two ventricular leads—one in the right ventricle and the other stimulating the left ventricle.

Correction of a lead dislodgment requires surgical intervention to reposition the lead. Before this is done, the reason for the dislodgment should be investigated. Careful attention should be directed to the original chest radiograph, and an adequate heel on the intracardiac portion of the lead should be sought at the time of lead implantation. Either too little or too much will predispose to dislodgment.[9] One should also review the recorded electrograms from the initial implant, looking for a 2 to 3 mV current of injury pattern ("ST-segment" elevation). The absence of this degree of current of injury has been correlated with an increased incidence of lead dislodgment; the implication is that the electrode is not making good endocardial contact. An examination of the anchoring sleeve for adequate fixation should be done at the time of reoperation.[10]

One should observe several precautions at the time of lead repositioning. When repositioning a dislodged lead, a thrombus may have developed around the lead tip, encasing the passive-fixation tines or fins or active-fixation helix, effectively preventing the lead from being adequately secured at the repeat procedure. Thus, once the lead is thought to be in a good position, the patient should be instructed to take as deep a breath as possible and to cough vigorously so that the electrical and mechanical stability of the lead may be assessed. If the dislodgment is due to Twiddler's syndrome, the most common cause of a late lead dislodgment, the portion of the lead within the pocket should be carefully inspected. If damage to the conductor coil or insulation is noted, the lead should not be reused. If a dislodgment occurs and the reason is not sufficiently apparent that it could be corrected at the second procedure, it would be prudent to remove the dislodged lead and replace it with an active fixation lead. One needs to be aware that use of an active fixation lead does not guarantee chronic stability—dislodgments have been reported years after implantation.[9,11]

High Thresholds; Lead Maturation: When the electrode is first inserted, it is making intimate contact with the endocardium. The presence of foreign material and the pressure of the lead-electrode system against the myocardium induce an inflammatory reaction at the electrode-myocardial interface. This local trauma is responsible for the current of injury pattern on the acute EGM recording. Due to the inflammatory reaction, the electrode is physically displaced from the excitable myocardium. This process increases the capture threshold. In addition, it attenuates the electrogram amplitude and slew rate to compromise sensing. With time, the inflammatory reaction subsides, leaving a thin capsule of fibrous tissue between the electrode and active myocardium. As the distance between the electrode and active myocardium is reduced, the capture and sensing thresholds improve.

Sometimes the inflammatory reaction at the electrode–myocardial interface is excessive, causing the capture threshold to rise above the output of the pacemaker.[11–14] This has been termed *exit block*. If exit block is the reason for loss of capture, there will be no change in the morphology of any capture beats, nor will there be a change in the radiographic position of the lead. Exit block can occur even with steroid-eluting leads and excellent acute capture thresholds; however, if the implanting physician accepts an electrode position with a high threshold (i.e., greater than 1.5 V), there may be an increased likelihood of exit block due to less "reserve" for the threshold to rise. The literature reports the incidence of exit block of less than 5%.[11]

Early experience with systemic steroids to limit acute threshold rises led to the development of the steroid-eluting electrode, which has been effective in attenuating the inflammatory reaction and its associated early rise in capture and sensing thresholds.[15–20] Isolated cases of massive threshold rises have also been encountered with the steroid-eluting leads, although the incidence is probably lower than with non–steroid-eluting leads.[21,22] Acute management of high thresholds, with or without loss of capture, requires increasing the output of the pacemaker. If this is not feasible, one needs to determine the status of the native underlying rhythm. If it is stable and adequate to physiologically support the patient, one might simply wait for the threshold to fall or try a course of high dose systemic steroids. If the underlying rhythm is not stable, one will need to insert a temporary pacemaker lead and consider an urgent intervention to reposition or replace the lead.

If thresholds increase during the early postimplantation period and one elects to use systemic steroids in an attempt to reverse the phenomenon, a regimen of 60 mg of prednisone per day, often administered in divided doses, has been found effective in approximately 50% of patients. In the pediatric population, the dose is 1 mg/kg. Capture thresholds are repeated 4 to 5 days after the initiation of steroids. If there is no change or if there is a further increase in capture thresholds, the steroids are considered ineffective and are simply discontinued. If the threshold, however, has decreased by at least two programming steps (pulse width and/or pulse amplitude), it is likely that the steroids are effective. The steroids are then continued for a month, with biweekly monitoring of capture thresholds. At the end of the month, a slow but progressive tapering schedule is initiated that continues for a minimum of 2 months.

High Thresholds; Chronic Lead: High capture thresholds may develop at any time. Those that are not associated with the acute lead maturation process are not likely to respond to steroids. When this problem is encountered, one should evaluate the patient for transient etiologies, including electrolyte and acid-base abnormalities such as hyperkalemia and acidemia.[15–17,23–26] Also included are pharmacologic agents such as the antiarrhythmic drugs; the 1C agents such as flecainide have developed a particularly poor reputation.[27–30] If a transient cause is identified and it can be corrected, the problem can be managed with a transient increase in output or by use of temporary pacing until the situation has resolved.

Permanent late rises in capture thresholds may also occur with progressive myocardial fibrosis, a primary myopathic process, or myocardial infarction.[31] If the output programmability of the device is not sufficient to overcome these causes, placement of a new lead will be required. Given that the lead is not infected, explantation is *not* mandatory.[32]

One must be very cautious about invoking the diagnosis of a high threshold due to a primary myocardial process in the absence of a change in the morphology of the intrinsic P wave or QRS complex. With a stable native complex on the surface ECG, a more likely explanation is a primary problem developing with the lead itself. If the malfunction were due to a mechanical abnormality developing in the lead, one would expect to see a change in the telemetered or invasively measured stimulation impedance, although this may not always be the case. Normal telemetry values may occur in the presence of an intermittent problem if the lead was functioning properly at the time of the measurements. When the lead impedance is abnormal, a very low impedance value (commonly less than 200 ohms) reflects a failure of the insulation, most commonly the inner insulation in a coaxial bipolar lead. A very high lead impedance (greater than 2000 to 3000 ohms) is consistent with a complete conductor fracture (open circuit). Measurement-to-measurement changes in telemetered lead impedance that are still within the normal range are totally consistent with normal lead function. Changes up to 300 ohms may still be compatible with normal lead function.[33] Further, a change in the measured impedance in the absence of a clinical malfunction, such as a massive rise in capture threshold, noncapture, or a sensing problem, may be a telemetry error. Although this might warrant closer follow-up assessment, an isolated abnormality of a telemetry measurement does not mandate operative intervention.

Lead Insulation Defects: An insulation defect may develop from the intrinsic design and/or a manufacturing limitation as was the case with an early series of 80A polyurethane insulated leads. Most insulation problems, however, are due to extrinsic forces applied to the lead either at or following implant that physically damage the lead. In part, this problem is a direct result of the request by the medical community for thinner leads, both unipolar and bipolar. One method of reducing the lead's diameter is to reduce the thickness of the insulating material. In-line bipolar coaxial leads are the least forgiving of extrinsic stresses for this very reason. Insulation defects have occurred with both silicone rubber and polyurethane insulation material.[34] Industry continues to evaluate new materials having the relative benefits of both polyurethane and silicone rubber while minimizing some of their weaknesses.

Extrinsic stress applied to the lead can result in damage to the insulation and/or a conductor fracture. There are three common mechanical stresses on the lead. The first is the suture sleeve, in which an excessively tight ligature is used to anchor the lead to the underlying fascia. If one sees a visible distortion of the conductor coil either at implant or on a follow-up chest radiograph, the ligature around the suture sleeve and lead is too tight.[35] Although this was originally considered a benign observation, late adverse consequences associated with this area of stress have recently been appreciated.[34] The second source of stress on the lead is the point where the lead traverses the plane between the clavicle and first rib on its way to the subclavian vein.[36,37] The normal motion of the arm causes the space between the clavicle and first rib to widen and narrow, much like the jaws of pliers. This is exacerbated if the course of the lead traverses the costoclavicular ligament or the subclavius muscle in its path to the subclavian vein. The lead located in this position can be repeatedly crushed, pinched, pulled or stretched, resulting in a deformation of the conductor coils, which in turn will predispose to either an insulation failure and/or conductor fracture occurring months to years after implantation (Fig. 7.3). This has been termed the *medial subclavicular musculotendinous complex* and is an increasingly recognized cause of malfunction of both standard pacing and defibrillator leads. A recent recommendation has been to access the axillary or cephalic vein rather than the subclavian vein to avoid both the acute and late complications associated with the implant procedure.[38,39]

A third mechanism involves abrasion of the external insulation. This may occur between overlapping coils of the same or contiguous leads or between the housing of the pulse generator and the lead coiled behind it.

Manifestations of a lead insulation defect are determined, in part, by the location of the defect.[40] In unipolar leads or a defect associated with the proximal conductor of a bipolar lead, there may be extracardiac muscle stimulation due to the electrical current leaking from the defect. Muscle stimulation in the area of a unipolar pacemaker may also be due to an upside-down pacemaker with the anode or indifferent electrode making direct contact with the underlying muscle. The author is also aware of several cases in which the insulating material applied to the pulse generator was damaged, thus allowing for local muscle stimulation with a totally normal lead.

Another manifestation of a lead insulation defect includes changes in the amplitude of the pacing stimulus, although this is difficult to evaluate given the differences in pacemaker stimulus reproduction between different ECG machines. This is best identified with an analog ECG recording system. In a unipolar system, there is a shorter path between the exposed conductor and the pulse generator, resulting in attenuation of the pacemaker stimulus amplitude. When the breach involves the outer insulation covering the anodal conductor

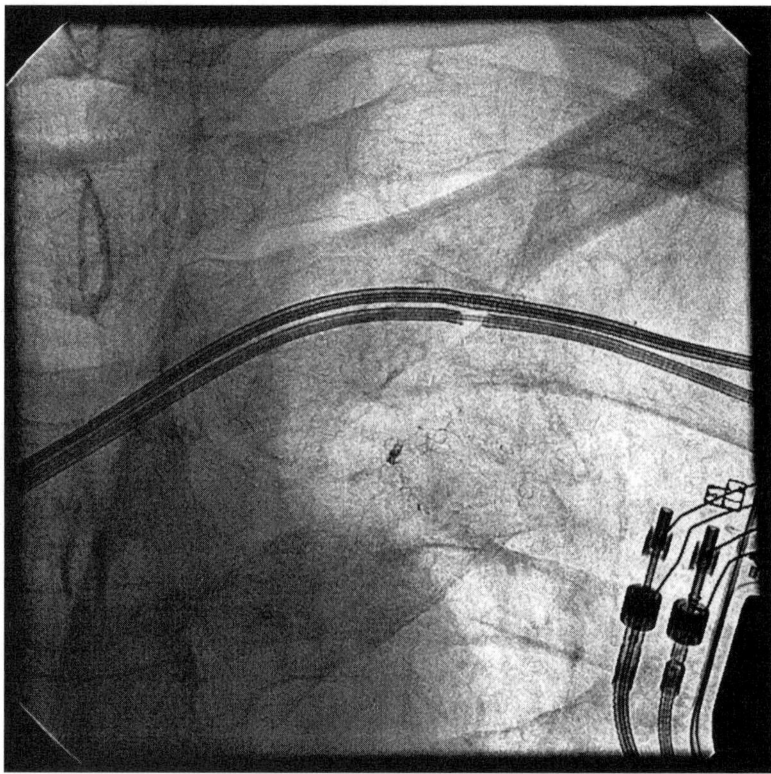

Figure 7.3. Lead fracture diagnosed on chest x-ray. Three years after dual chamber pacemaker implant for sick sinus syndrome this patient was found to have complete loss of ventricular capture and bipolar lead impedance of greater than 2000 ohms. There is a clear fracture of the lead just before it enters the subclavian vein. The fracture may have been due to the subclavian access that passes the lead through the costoclavicular ligament apparatus. There is a slight deformity of the atrial lead at this position suggesting compressive force on this lead as well.

of a bipolar lead, there will then be two pathways for current flow. This will result in a larger "unipolarized" stimulus on the ECG. If the insulation is breached between the distal and proximal conductors of a bipolar lead, the current flow will be short-circuited and little or none of it will ever reach the active electrodes. In this case, the already small bipolar stimulus amplitude will be further attenuated. In any case the shunting of current through the insulation defect and away from the myocardium can result in higher capture thresholds.

Sometimes an intermittent problem is identified on a Holter monitor or is suspected on the basis of symptoms, but when the patient is evaluated in the office, the system is functioning properly. This is particularly likely if the insulation defect occurs between the proximal and distal conductor of a bipolar lead.

When the patient is lying quietly on the examination table, the normal elastic recoil of the conductor coils may separate the two wires even if the insulation between them has been breached. To reveal the problem different maneuvers can be performed while monitoring the ECG, telemetered lead impedance, event markers, and/or electrograms (Fig. 7.4). One technique that is particularly effective in identifying a problem resulting from a ligature that is too tight

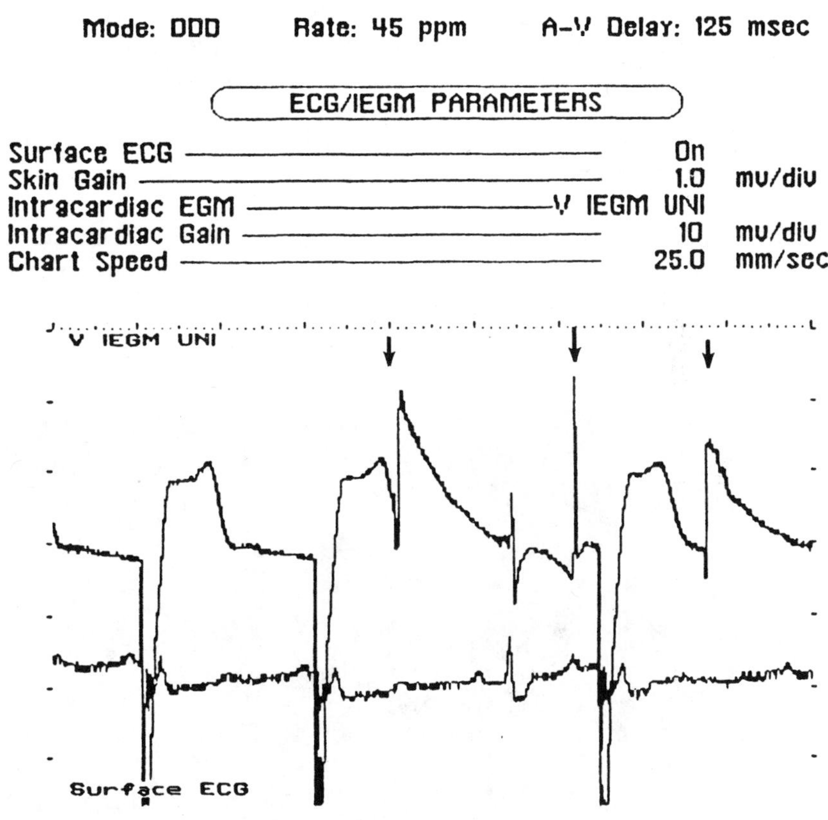

Figure 7.4. Repeated ventricular oversensing with resultant inhibition was demonstrated in this dual bipolar DDD pacing system. Measured data telemetry reported a ventricular lead impedance of less than 250 ohms; the baseline had been 645 ohms. Telemetry of the ventricular electrogram while simultaneously recording a surface ECG demonstrates non-physiologic large electrical transients *(arrows)* occurring at a time when the pacemaker is being inhibited, indicating that the pacemaker is sensing these signals. The ventricular sensitivity had been reduced in an attempt to minimize this oversensing problem. However, the nonphysiologic transients were approximately 20 mV, larger than the least sensitive setting of the pacemaker, and the oversensing continued. However, the reduced sensitivity resulted in undersensing of the native R waves, resulting in competition. The nonphysiologic electrical transients were treated as PVCs by the pacemaker and activated the PVC algorithm, extending the refractory period and resulting in intermittent functional atrial undersensing.

around the anchoring sleeve is for the examiner to trace the course of the subcutaneous portion of the lead with his or her fingers while applying pressure at each point. If there is an insulation defect, the two conductor coils will be pushed together, unmasking the problem. Extending the ipsilateral arm as high as possible, as in reaching toward the ceiling or placing the arm behind the back and rotating the shoulder backward, may unmask a problem caused by the medial subclavian-muscular complex.

Obtaining a chest radiograph may reveal a problem, although the insulation defect alone will not be seen because the insulating material is radiolucent. One might see a deformity of the conductor coil (Fig. 7.5) allowing one to infer the diagnosis when these observations are combined with the clinical and telemetry data. However, a radiographic abnormality in the absence of independent corroboration of a system malfunction would be insufficient grounds to recommend an operative intervention.

Open Circuit: The most common cause of an open circuit is a conductor fracture. The second, but more embarrassing, cause is a failure to adequately tighten the set-screw in the terminal pin connector block of the pulse generator (Fig. 7.6).

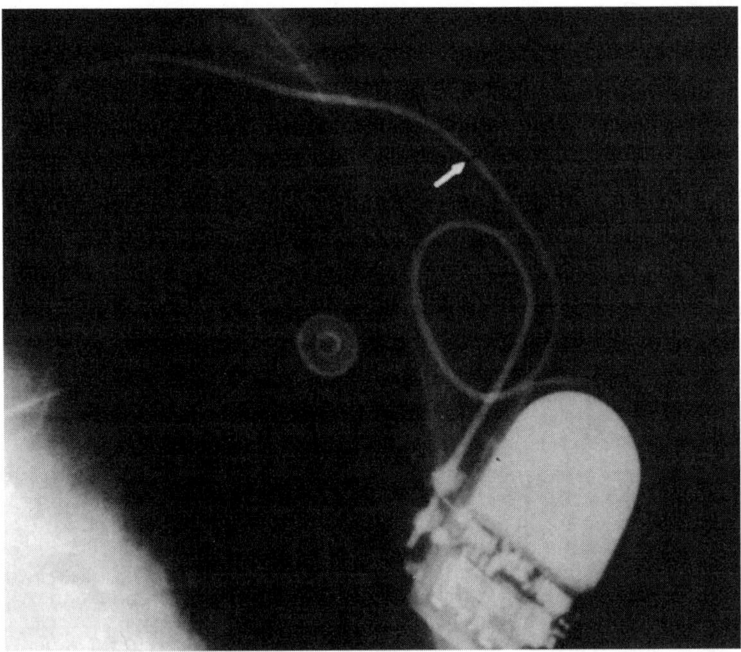

Figure 7.5. In-line bipolar coaxial lead with an indentation *(arrow)* created by a tight ligature around the lead. This has been called a pseudofracture and was previously considered to be of little clinical consequence. It has since been learned that the excessively tight ligature predisposes to both conductor fractures and insulation defects.

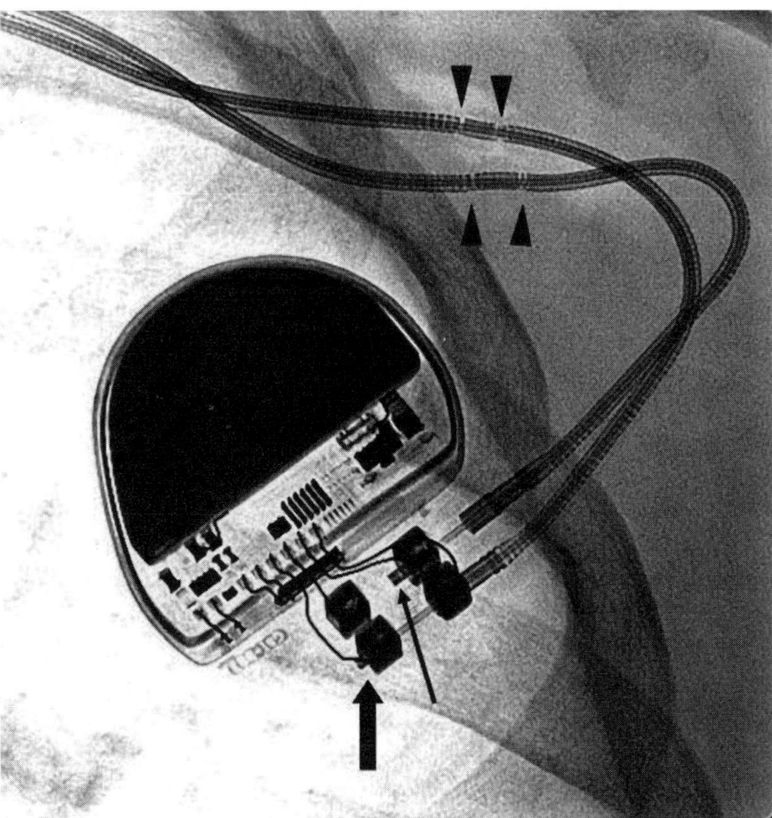

Figure 7.6. Chest radiograph demonstrating displacement of the terminal pin out of the head of a pacemaker. For the atrial lead entering the top of the header (bottom of the figure) the terminal pin is seen extending beyond the header posts for both the ring and tip electrodes *(heavy arrow)*. The ventricular lead, however, does not reach to the header post for the tip electrode *(thin arrow)*. The ventricular lead impedance was unmeasurable. In addition, pseudofractures are seen in both leads due to constriction of the insulation by the tying sleeves *(arrowheads)*.

There are two common clinical manifestations of an open circuit. With a total open circuit, no energy will traverse the gap between the two portions of the lead and there will be an absence of pacing artifacts on the ECG and loss of capture. This is included in the class of malfunction associated with an absent pacing stimulus. If the two ends of the conductor are making any contact at all, the resistance to current flow will be increased to attenuate the amount of current and energy reaching the heart, but a stimulus will be present. If the effective energy reaching the heart is subthreshold, there will be loss of capture. Although a physical break in the conductor is the most common cause of an open circuit and usually does not manifest until months to years after implantation, there are two circumstances when an open circuit can occur at the time of implantation. One is a failure to tighten the set-screw allowing the lead to pull out of the set-screw connector block (see Fig. 7.6). The other involves a small unipolar pacemaker used as a replacement for a larger model pacemaker. If there is air trapped within the pocket, this may serve as an insulator separating the indifferent electrode on the case of the pacemaker from the patient's tissues.[41]

A partially open circuit may also result in pauses due to oversensing. Make-break contact between the ends of the conductor coil or between the terminal pin and an inadequately tightened set-screw within the connector block can cause non-physiologic electrical transients that are detected and reset the pacemaker.

Diagnosis of an open circuit may be facilitated by taking advantage of the diagnostic capabilities incorporated in many present generation pacemakers. Event marker telemetry will confirm an output pulse even if one is not visible on the ECG. Telemetry of lead impedance will demonstrate a significant increase (Fig. 7.7) if the problem is manifested at the time of measurement. A total open circuit will have an infinitely high impedance if the insulation remains intact. However, if there is a concomitant break in the insulation, as may occur when the lead is totally transected, the impedance may be normal or only minimally elevated because the conductor will be exposed to the tissue via the severed insulation.

A radiograph may show the conductor fracture, particularly with unipolar leads. One may have to rotate the patient and take multiple views or use fluoroscopy to eliminate overlapping portions of the lead in a given plane that might obscure the fracture. In-line bipolar coaxial leads are the most difficult with regard to radiographic identification of a conductor fracture. Unless there is total disruption of both conductors at the same place, the intact distal conductor may mask the defect in the proximal conductor.

Recording Artifact: One always needs to be cognizant of recording artifacts. The first-generation digital ECG machines could generate large-amplitude signals even associated with a bipolar stimulus, mimicking the pattern of a unipolar signal and thus suggesting an insulation defect. Because of the digital sampling process some ECG recorders may miss the pacemaker pulse entirely or detect different phases of the pulse, creating dramatic fluctuations in both polarity and amplitude of the pacemaker pulse (Fig. 7.8). To minimize the resultant confusion that occurred in the clinical community, some of the major ECG manufacturers have developed "pacemaker pulse detectors." The newer systems treat any high frequency electrical transient as a pacemaker pulse for which they generate a relatively uniform amplitude signal on the ECG. If there are other causes of infrequent electrical transients, the ECG may look as if there is a pacemaker stimulus when the patient does not even have a pacemaker. In other cases, it may magnify a very low amplitude signal such as that associated with the Vario function or minute ventilation sensor signals of the earlier generation Elema and Telectronics pacemakers, mimicking an unstable runaway situation (Fig. 7.9).

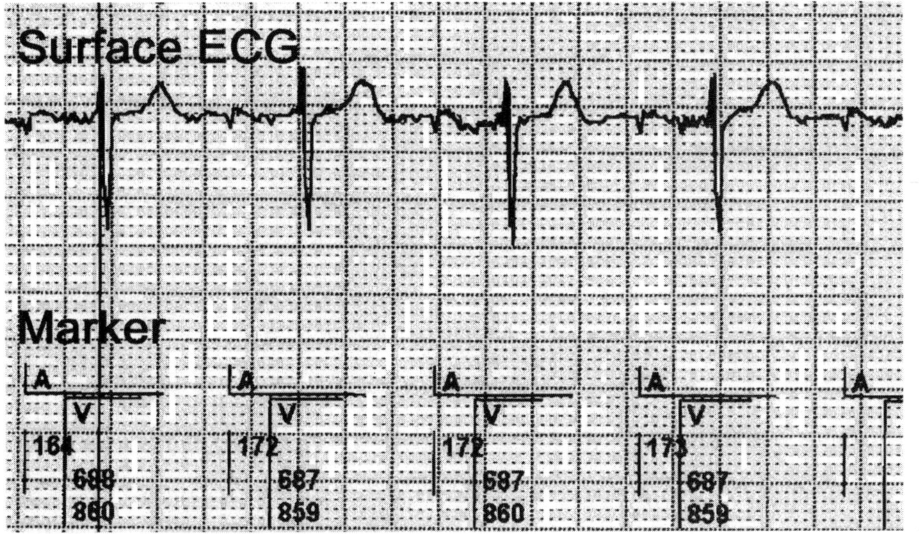

A

Patient/Device Information

Pacemaker Model: Kappa KDR701 PGU427387 Implanted: 12/07/01 3:53 PM

Pacemaker Status: 11/14/02 2:26:17 PM

Estimated remaining longevity: 64-92 months , average: 77 months (Based on Past History)

Battery Status	OK
Voltage	2.77 V
Current	15.75 µA
Impedance	198 ohms

Lead Status: 11/14/02 2:26:17 PM

	Atrial Lead	Ventricular Lead
Output Energy	0.56 µJ	4.59 µJ
Measured Current	0.10 mA	4.60 mA
Measured Impedance	> 9,999 ohms	541 ohms
Pace Polarity	Bipolar	Unipolar

B

Figure 7.7. **A:** This tracing, recorded from a patient with a St. Jude Medical Integrity pacemaker programmed to the DDD mode shows atrial pacing ("A" on marker channel) with intact AV nodal conduction. A ventricular stimulus is not visible on surface ECG. If it weren't for the simultaneously telemetered event markers, one would not know that the pulse generator was releasing a ventricular output pulse ("V" on marker channel). The failure to deliver an effective stimulus to the ventricular channel was due to an open circuit on the ventricular channel with a measured lead impedance of greater than 2500 ohms. **B:** Measured data telemetry indicates that there is an open circuit on the atrial channel of a different patient, implanted with a Medtronic Kappa 700 pacing system. The reported impedance is greater than 9999 ohms, which is the highest impedance that the Medtronic system will report. The pulse current and pulse energy are minimal, which is compatible with an open circuit.

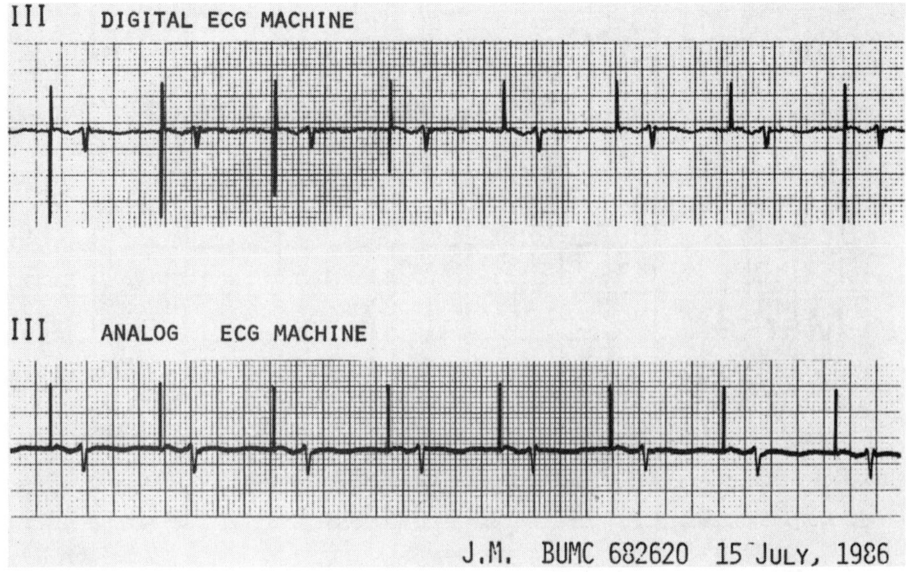

Figure 7.8. A lead III ECG rhythm strip is recorded with both digital **(top)** and analog **(bottom)** ECG machines. The digitizing process causes a marked beat-to-beat fluctuation in the amplitude of the bipolar pacing stimulus. This is an artifact of the recording system. The same surface ECG lead recorded with an analog system has a uniform amplitude pacing stimulus.

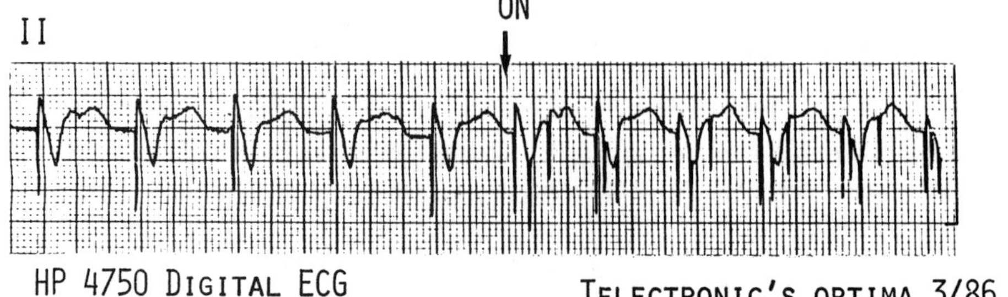

Figure 7.9. To eliminate the marked fluctuation in the amplitude and polarity of the pacing stimulus when it is recorded with the digital ECG system, some manufacturers have introduced additional recording artifacts that may also be misinterpreted. Hewlett-Packard redesigned their Pagewriter II™ model 4750 system to generate a uniform amplitude spike in response to any identified high-frequency transient. In this example, the Vario feature of a Telectronics Optima pacemaker was activated. When Vario is engaged, pacing occurs at 120 ppm for 16 cycles with a progressive decrease in the pulse voltage on each subsequent paced beat until 0 V is reached. To fine-tune each voltage reduction, the pacemaker "dumps" small pulses of energy out of the can. The ECG machine detected each of these small, otherwise invisible, pulses of energy and generated a large stimulus, making it look as though there was a problem. In addition, this particular pacemaker was bipolar and the large stimuli would raise concerns of a lead insulation defect if one did not know about this recording artifact. This design makes ECG interpretation of the impedance-based rate-modulated pacing systems extremely difficult as the entire recording becomes obscured by "stimulus" artifacts.

Functional Noncapture: When a pacing stimulus occurs in the physiologic refractory period of a native depolarization, it will not capture. This is not a primary capture malfunction and should not be classified as such. This may be due to a primary problem of failure to sense or to functional undersensing. Functional undersensing is associated with the basic timing design of the system as with too long a refractory period. It was particularly common in the committed AV sequential (DVI) pacing systems. The atrial stimulus occurs in the refractory period of the native atrial depolarization that conducted to the ventricle. The ventricular output may then coincide with the refractory period of the ventricular depolarization. Thus, in an absolutely normally functioning pacing system, there was functional failure to capture on both the atrial and ventricular channels. A rhythm that will be discussed later, repetitive ventriculo-atrial non-reentrant arrhythmia, is the most common example today where there is both functional loss of capture and functional loss of sensing in the same rhythm. An example of functional loss of capture due to true undersensing is shown in Figure 7.10. The common causes of functional noncapture are listed in Box 7.2.

Pacing Stimuli Present with Failure to Sense

The failure to respond to a physiologically appropriate signal occurring during the alert period of the timing cycle is termed *undersensing*. When undersensing is present, the pacemaker issues pacing stimuli because of the perceived absence of spontaneous cardiac activity. Like failure to capture, undersensing can be a true pacing system malfunction or represent a functional limitation of the system

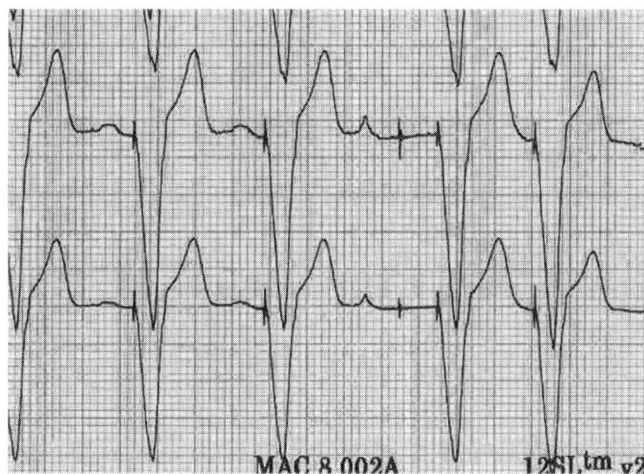

Figure 7.10. The third complex from the left demonstrates primary failure to sense allowing delivery of an output pulse at a time when the tissue in the paced chamber was physiologically refractory. This would be functional loss of capture on the atrial channel due to undersensing of an atrial premature beat.

Box 7.2. Common Causes of Functional Noncapture

Single chamber
- True undersensing
- Long refractory period
- Ectopic activation (PVC, bundle branch block)
- Asynchronous pacing (magnet application, noise reversion)

Dual chamber
- Atrial undersensing
- Atrial asynchronous modes (DDI, DVI)

Blanking period
- Safety pacing
- PVARP extension algorithms post-PVC
- Long PVARP and high base rate
- Mode switching

PVARP = postventricular atrial refractory period; PVC = premature ventricular contraction.

due to the unique algorithms or programmed settings (Fig. 7.11). The differential diagnosis of undersensing along with the diagnostic tests and management options are detailed in Table 7.2. One cause of undersensing is that of inadequate signal amplitude at the time of initial implant. This may result if the patient has no intrinsic rhythm to measure at implant (i.e., temporary ventricular pacing or, on the atrial channel, atrial fibrillation). At implant, device based testing is best but few of the available pacing system analyzers (PSA) use the sensing circuitry of the implanted pacemaker. The filtering characteristics of the PSA may differ significantly from those of the pulse generator and may provide misleading information at implant (Fig. 7.12).[42]

Change in Native Signal: Another etiology of undersensing is that the signal has changed.[43] The change in the signal may be permanent, as with a myocardial infarction or a primary myopathic process. It also may result from a change in the sequence of depolarization, as with development of a bundle branch block. Hyperkalemia results in a widening of the QRS complex and an attenuation of the P wave on the surface ECG. Similar changes will occur with the intracardiac signal or electrogram. Pharmacologic therapy, particularly the antiarrhythmic agents that alter Phase 0 of the cardiac action potential, can change the intrinsic properties of the signal, resulting in undersensing. If possible, these agents should be discontinued before considering an operative intervention to replace or reposition the lead if the primary indication for the procedure is undersensing. One should also check the patient's serum electrolytes and arterial blood gases and correct any identified abnormalities before considering interventions other than programming to a more sensitive setting.

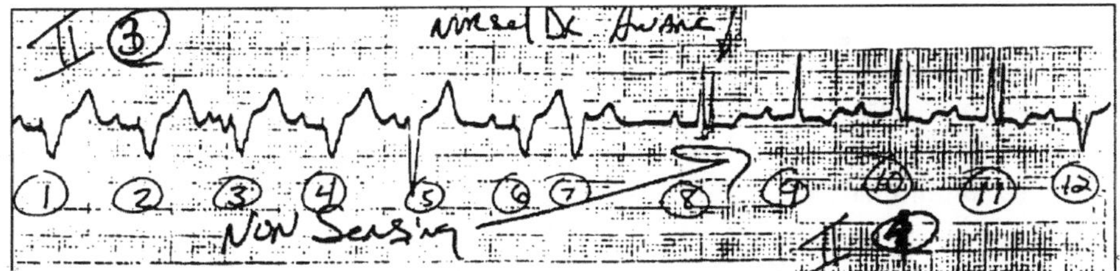

Figure 7.11. A telemetry rhythm strip from a patient with a St. Jude Medical Affinity DR pulse generator with AutoCapture enabled. There is intermittent AV block. When conduction is intact, the low amplitude ventricular output pulse coincides with the native QRS complex resulting in a fusion beat. The resultant evoked response is not detected causing the release of a 4.5-V backup pulse to be delivered in the ST segment. This is shown in complexes 8 and 10 and flagged as "non-sensing" by the clinical staff. This is normal function although it might be labeled functional undersensing.

Inappropriate Programmed Sensitivity: An embarrassing cause of undersensing is an inappropriately programmed sensitivity. Confusion about the terms *high* and *low* sensitivity may result in incorrect programming. When an undersensing problem is encountered, the sensitivity should be *increased* or set to a higher sensitivity so that the system will recognize and respond to smaller amplitude signals. Sensitivity is the amplitude of the signal that can be sensed. A sensitivity of 1 mV would be more sensitive (higher sensitivity) than 2 mV. Similarly, if there is an oversensing problem and one wants to reduce or lower the sensitivity, the incoming signal must be larger than the amplitude chosen for the pacemaker to recognize it as an appropriate signal. Thus, a sensitivity of 4 mV, although a higher number, is really a lower sensitivity than 2 mV. Patients have been inappropriately referred for pulse generator replacement or lead repositioning when the problem was undersensing, which had resulted from a misunderstanding of how to program sensitivity.

Many of the newer pacemakers have incorporated an automatic sensing algorithm.[44] This algorithm monitors the amplitude of the native atrial or ventricular depolarization and either recommends a programmed sensitivity or automatically adjusts the sensitivity to maintain a 2:1 safety margin. The limitation of these automatic algorithms is an inability to respond to isolated premature beats. This may result in the failure to detect isolated ectopic beats resulting in competition or delaying the prompt recognition of a supraventricular or ventricular tachycardia.

Lead Insulation Failure: Lead insulation defects were discussed in the previous section on stimuli present with loss of capture. The breach in the insulation will attenuate the incoming signal. The signal will be an electrical average between the true electrode inside the heart and the false "electrode"—the exposed

Table 7.2. Differential Diagnosis of Pacing Stimuli Present—Intermittent or Persistent Failure to Sense

Etiology	Diagnostic Evaluation*	Management*
Lead dislodgment • Early: unstable position • Late: Twiddler's syndrome	12-lead ECG with pacing; chest radiograph	Reposition lead
Low amplitude electrogram • Small EGM at implant • Ectopic activation (PAC, PVC, bundle branch block, atrial fibrillation) • Medications, electrolytes • Myocardial infarction, cardiomyopathy • Tissue fibrosis, lead maturation	Identification of change in medication, electrolytes, cardiac status	Increase sensitivity, discontinue medication, correct electrolyte or acid–base imbalance, change sensing configuration
Insulation failure	Fall in lead impedance by more than 300 ohms; telemetered EGM	Change sensing configuration until lead can be replaced
Functional undersensing • Magnet application, noise reversion • ERI behavior • PMT interventions • Mode switching • Pacemaker Wenckebach	Careful assessment of pacing intervals, review programmed sensitivity and thresholds	Decrease refractory period(s), increase sensitivity
Inappropriate programming	Review programmed sensitivity and thresholds	Reprogram sensitivity

* Some suggested options may not be available with a given pulse generator. Only definitive management options are listed. In each case, increasing the sensitivity may correct the problem, but, as with a primary lead failure, this may be a temporizing measure only.

Source: Modified from Levine PA. Pacing system malfunction: evaluation and management. In: Podrid PJ, Kowey PR, eds. Cardiac Arrhythmia: Mechanisms, Diagnosis, and Management. Philadelphia: Williams & Wilkins, © 1995. By permission of Williams & Wilkins.

Figure 7.12. To demonstrate the difference between a filtered and unfiltered signal, both of which can be transmitted by telemetry, the standard bipolar ventricular electrogram (VEGM) was recorded when the pacemaker was inhibited. **A:** This is the bipolar VEGM recorded between the tip and ring electrodes. The signal was acquired by the telemetry circuit and transmitted before it was processed by the sensing circuit. The R marker aligns with the intrinsic deflection of the EGM. The visible repolarization artifact representing the T wave demonstrates that the standard telemetry system uses a very broad band-pass filter that does not significantly alter the signal. **B:** The same EGM telemetered after it has been processed by the sensing circuit. This is termed the Sense Amp EGM. Note that the repolarization artifact is virtually eliminated and the signal morphology is markedly altered. The physical amplitude of this signal, as displayed by the programmer, will be directly dependent upon the programmed sensitivity or gain within the pacemaker. (Reprinted by permission from Levine PA. Guidelines to the Routine Evaluation, Programming and Follow-up of the Patient with an Implanted Dual-Chamber Rate-Modulated Pacing System. Sylmar, CA, St. Jude Medical CRMD, 2003.)

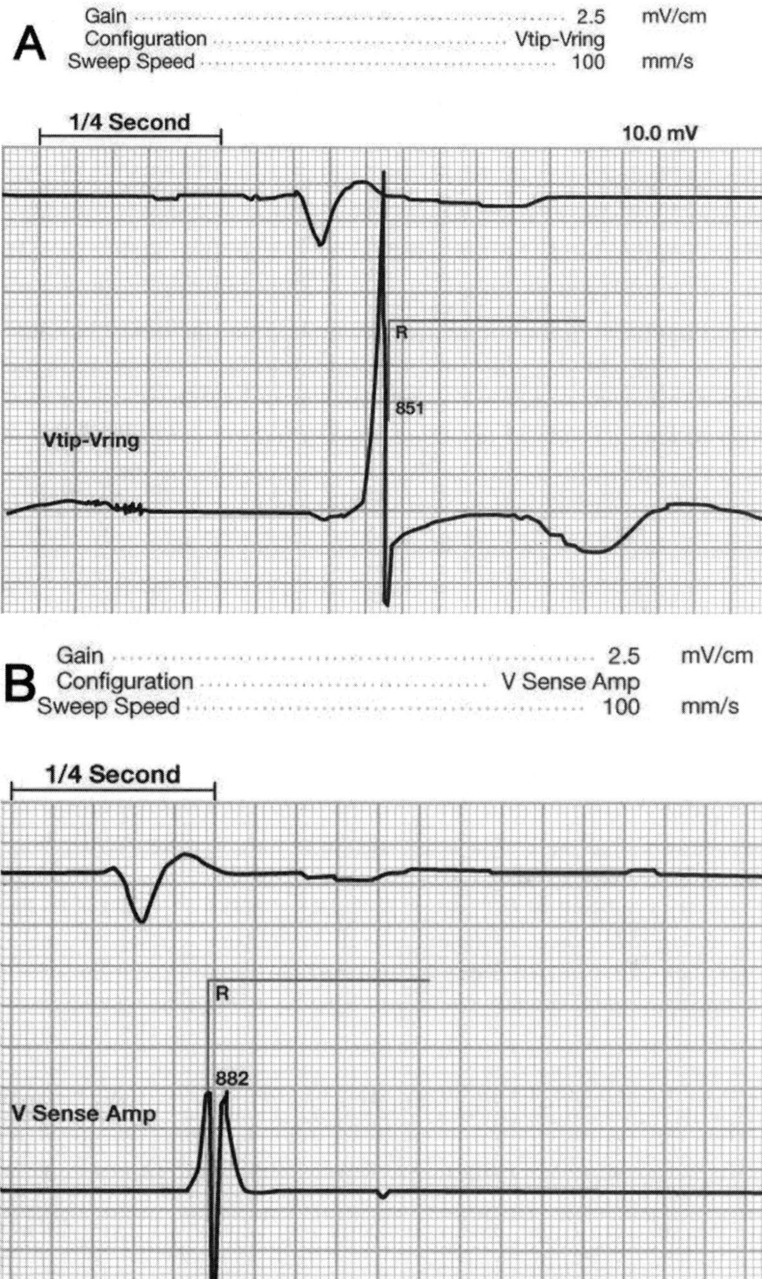
A
Gain 2.5 mV/cm
Configuration Vtip-Vring
Sweep Speed 100 mm/s
1/4 Second
10.0 mV
R
851
Vtip-Vring
B
Gain 2.5 mV/cm
Configuration V Sense Amp
Sweep Speed 100 mm/s
1/4 Second
R
882
V Sense Amp

conductor coil under the insulation defect. If the pacemaker has the ability to telemeter the EGM and there is a baseline recording available, one can compare the two signals. Other suggestive findings include a decrease in stimulation impedance, increase in battery current drain, increase in capture threshold, change in pulse artifact amplitude if recorded with an analog system, and possible extracardiac muscle stimulation. These findings are all corroboratory, supporting the likely cause of the sensing failure being a break in the insulation. One can temporize by increasing the sensitivity of the system, but definitive correction will require repair or replacement of the lead.

Lead Dislodgment: Although lead dislodgment usually results in loss of capture, it is also frequently accompanied by undersensing. The electrode may no longer be in contact with the myocardium, or it may have been totally displaced from the appropriate cardiac chamber. In any case, the incoming signal will be different from and usually smaller than that recorded at implant, resulting in sensing failure. Correction requires repositioning the dislodged lead; however, increasing the sensitivity may restore normal sensing function until the lead can be repositioned.

Electrodes are being introduced to minimize far field sensing. This is accomplished by using a very short interelectrode spacing. While this improves the signal to noise ratio and minimizes oversensing, minor shifts in the orientation of the bipolar dipole between the two closely spaced electrodes may dramatically alter the signal that is being detected.

Lead Maturation: The inflammatory reaction that occurs at the electrode-myocardial interface physically separates the electrode from active functional myocardium. This will attenuate the amplitude of the signal. The signal has been reported to decrease by as much as 20% to 40% when compared to the electrogram amplitude recorded at implantation. It also attenuates the slew rate, which may be the major reason for sensing failure. Treatment requires increasing the sensitivity of the pacemaker while initiating the other suggestions provided earlier for high capture thresholds associated with lead maturation.

Component Malfunction: Problems may occur with the sense amplifier of the pacemaker, resulting in an undersensing problem. There is no good way to assess this noninvasively. Problems with the sense amplifier can certainly be suspected if the telemetered EGM is of large amplitude and good slew rate, given the fact that the telemetry and sensing amplifier of many units are different. Similar observations can be made at the time of operative intervention. If the recorded EGM is large with a good slew rate (>1 V/sec) and the PSA-reported signal amplitude is large, one should suspect that the cause of the problem was intrinsic to the pulse generator. In the differential diagnosis of this problem, this is the least common cause of undersensing.

Functional Undersensing: Functional undersensing is a failure to sense an appropriate physiologic signal but the undersensing is caused by the normal design of the pacemaker (Box 7.3). With respect to single-chamber pacing systems, this most commonly occurs due to native beats falling within the refractory period after a paced or sensed beat, particularly common observation with ventricular pacing in the setting of atrial fibrillation and a rapid ventricular response. Fusion and pseudofusion beats are normal phenomenon. Given that many individuals report these as a "sensing failure," this is another example of functional undersensing. The most common cause of functional undersensing occurs each time a magnet is placed over the pacemaker and induces asynchronous pacing.

If too many signals are sensed by the pacemaker in a very short time, the likelihood is that this is electrical noise rather than true physiologic signals. This is termed *electromagnetic interference* (EMI) or "noise." The presence of EMI precludes the pacemaker's differentiating electrical noise from an intrinsic rhythm. Rather than inhibiting the pacemaker when the patient might be asystolic, the pacemaker reverts to asynchronous function, termed *noise mode operation.*[45]

Pacing Stimuli Absent with Failure to Capture

The next major category of pacing system malfunction occurs when the output stimulus is truly absent (Fig. 7.13). One must be certain that this is not an artifact of a diminutive bipolar pacing stimulus further obscured by being isoelectric in a given lead (Fig. 7.14). Hence, one should record multiple leads simultaneously or sequentially. Indeed, this might be the one indication for using a digital ECG machine that re-creates a uniform amplitude stimulus in response to any high-frequency transient. The differential diagnosis of pacing stimuli absent is summarized in Table 7.3.

Box 7.3. Common Causes of Functional Undersensing

Single chamber
- Long refractory periods
- Noise mode
- Triggered mode

Dual chamber
- Blanking period
- Safety pacing
- Committed DVI pacing
- PVARP extension post-PVC
- Ventricular oversensing
- Long PVARP and high base rate

PVARP = postventricular atrial refractory period; PVC = premature ventricular contraction.

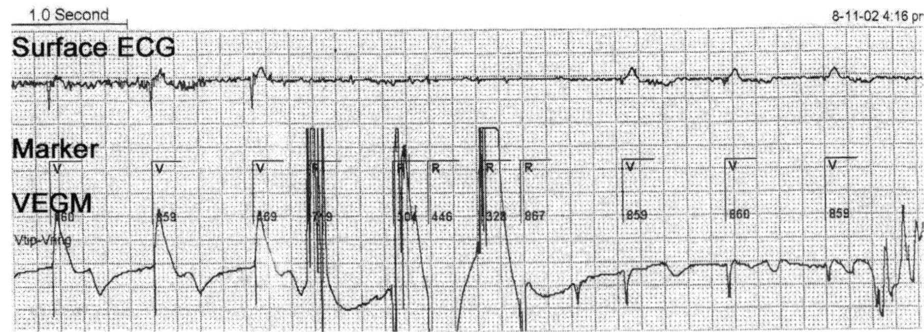

Figure 7.13. Pacing system malfunction, pacing artifact absent. Intermittent pauses occur without a visible pacing artifact. This single chamber VVI pacing system demonstrated repeated pauses due to oversensing. In addition, note the change in amplitude of the pacing stimulus between the three cycles before the pause and the three cycles following the pause. These reflect variations in the delivered energy to the heart as the St. Jude Medical programmer uses an analog circuit for the surface ECG lead. With the lower amount of energy effectively delivered to the heart, the stimulus artifact is smaller and the stimulus distortion of the simultaneously telemetered ventricular (VEGM) is less. In the middle of the tracing corresponding to the pause on the surface ECG, the bipolar ventricular electrogram demonstrates multiple non-physiologic electrical transients and sensing is denoted on the marker channel by the annotation "R." This behavior was subsequently identified as being due to an internal insulation failure of a coaxial bipolar lead. Programming to the unipolar configuration would not eliminate the non-physiologic electrical transients and oversensing. Management required replacement of the lead.

Oversensing: *Oversensing* is the sensing of either a nonphysiologic or a physiologically inappropriate signal. This is particularly common in unipolar pacing systems programmed to a high sensitivity. Sensing skeletal muscle potentials either inhibits the ventricular output if detected on the ventricular channel[46–48] or triggers a ventricular output when sensed on the atrial channel of a DDD system. Bipolar sensing has a greater signal-to-noise ratio, which makes oversensing far less common than with unipolar modes, but oversensing can still occur.[49] Strong electrical fields, as with arc welding equipment or radar installations, can be sensed.[50] Bipolar sensing is relatively immune to the usual myopotential oversensing, but both it and unipolar systems may detect diaphragmatic muscle potentials. Native signals that can be sensed by either bipolar or unipolar sensing configurations are T waves and pacing stimuli afterpotentials.

A cause of oversensing within a normally functioning lead may be found with some active fixation endocardial leads that have both an electrically active collar and helix. If the helix has some side-to-side motion within the collar, the two electrically active metal components may come into contact and a non-physiologic electrical transient is created ("chatter").[51] This signal may be relatively massive, in which case it will not be amenable to programming a reduced

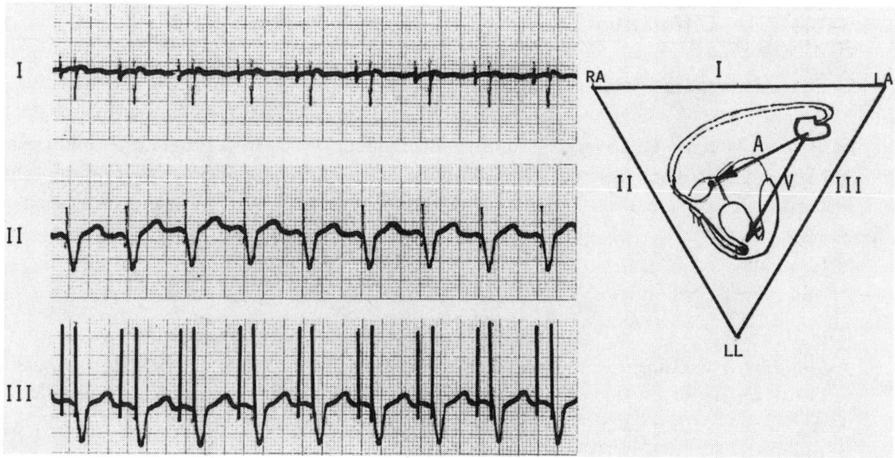

Figure 7.14. In assessing the presence or absence of pacing stimuli and even native complexes, it is imperative to examine multiple leads, recorded either simultaneously or sequentially. Leads I, II, and III are recorded sequentially from a patient with a dual unipolar DDD pacing system. The pulse generator was located in the left pectoral fossa. The basic dipole of the pacing stimuli is parallel to lead III, resulting in the expected large unipolar signals. In lead II, the atrial stimulus is virtually perpendicular to the lead, and thus no stimulus is recorded. In fact, had only lead II been monitored, the rhythm would have been interpreted as P wave synchronous ventricular pacing. In lead I, two pacing stimuli are readily visible, but the ventricular evoked potential is virtually isoelectric. Had this been the only lead monitored, one might have mistakenly made the diagnosis of ventricular noncapture. The multiple leads confirm AV sequential pacing with normal capture. To the right of the rhythm strips, a schematic of the pacing system is diagrammed within Einthoven's triangle. RA is right arm, LA is left arm, and IL is left leg of the standard ECG leads.

sensitivity even though reducing the sensitivity is usually effective management for the physiologic but inappropriate signals such as myopotentials.

Reducing the sensitivity to eliminate oversensing of physiologic but inappropriate signals such as myopotentials or T waves, is recommended only if the native signal for which sensing is desired is sufficiently large to allow it to continue to be appropriately sensed. If reducing the sensitivity will result in undersensing of appropriate signals, one might program the pacemaker to the triggered mode. This will result in a stimulus being triggered rather than being inhibited by oversensing. The "upper rate limit" in the triggered mode will be controlled by the refractory period.

Similar to the generation of nonphysiologic signals in the normally functioning coaxial bipolar leads, a break in the integrity of the inner insulation of an in-line bipolar lead can result in similar nonphysiologic electrical transients that can be sensed. As both conductors are integral to the generation of the false signal, the oversensing will persist in both the bipolar and unipolar sensing configuration. When recorded via telemetered EGMs, these signals are often

Table 7.3. Differential Diagnosis of Pauses—Pacing Stimuli Absent

Etiology	Diagnostic Evaluation	Management
Oversensing • T wave, P wave, R wave • Myopotential/diaphragm • Pacing afterpotential • EMI • Crosstalk • Make-break potentials	Magnet application (pauses eliminated), reduce sensitivity	Reduce sensitivity or program to bipolar sensing configuration, replace with bipolar sensing lead
Open circuit • Conductor fracture • Loose set-screw • Air in pocket (unipolar system) • Lead pin/header mismatch	Lead impedance—high Magnet—pauses persist Chest radiograph—terminal pin not seated properly, lateral may visualize air in pocket, conductor coil discontinuity	Apply pressure dressing (air in pocket), reprogram to unipolar, replace lead, reoperate to tighten set screw
Internal insulation failure	Lead impedance low (<250 ohms) Magnet—pauses persist Chest radiograph—normal or conductor coil deformity	Program to unipolar until lead can be replaced
Component malfunction	Magnet—pauses persist Telemetry—inconsistencies in measured data	Replace pulse generator, operative reassessment of lead function before pulse generator
Pseudomalfunction • Hysteresis • Mode switching • PMT intervention	Native rate slower than paced rate Pauses follow only sensed beats Interrogation of programmed parameters	Reassurance as normal function

Source: Modified from Levine PA. Pacing system malfunction: evaluation and management. In: Podrid PJ, Kowey PR, eds. Cardiac Arrhythmia: Mechanisms, Diagnosis, and Management. Philadelphia: Williams & Wilkins, © 1995. By permission of Williams & Wilkins.

massive (>20 mV), precluding their elimination by a simple reduction in sensitivity (see Fig. 7.4). The only short-term option for a totally pacemaker-dependent patient is to program the pacemaker to the asynchronous or triggered mode. Definitive management requires lead replacement.

When presented with recurrent pauses in the absence of pacing stimuli, one can quickly differentiate oversensing from the other causes of the absence of pacing artifact by applying a magnet to the pacemaker. The magnet will cause the pacemaker to revert to asynchronous function. If the pauses are eliminated, the problem is that of oversensing. To determine the source of the oversensing, it is sometimes necessary to record the surface ECG while the patient is in the environment in which the reported symptoms occur. It may be necessary to have the patient perform provocative maneuvers as were described earlier in the section on lead evaluation. One could also have the patient do upper extremity isometric exercises, tensing the pectoral muscles, or do sit ups to tighten the abdominal muscles in the case of an abdominal implant. The patient should be asked to take very deep breaths if diaphragmatic oversensing is suspected. These maneuvers should be performed while continuously monitoring the rhythm and, if available, in conjunction with telemetered event markers and electrograms.

Open Circuit: This is second to oversensing as a cause of pauses associated with the absence of a pacing stimulus. Event marker telemetry will indicate that the pacemaker released a pulse. A simultaneously recorded ECG will be necessary to demonstrate that this output pulse never reached the heart, as no stimulus artifact is recorded. Measured data telemetry will report an infinitely high stimulation impedance or a dramatic change from the baseline recordings. With an open circuit, there is no current drain associated with the programmed output; thus, the battery current drain will decrease from baseline. Some systems can provide lead impedance measurements on a beat-by-beat basis. Most of the other devices that provide non-invasive lead impedance measurements make individual measurements on a couple of output pulses. Thus, repeated interrogations may be necessary to identify an intermittent problem.

Application of a magnet to the pacemaker will not restore pacing that has failed due to an open circuit because the pacemaker is already generating the output pulse. The problem is that this stimulus is unable to be delivered to the electrode-myocardial interface. An open circuit has a number of possible causes. The most common is a conductor fracture. The second is a failure to tighten the set-screw adequately. Rarely open circuits result from incompatibility between the lead pin and the header connector of the pacemaker or a component problem within the pulse generator.

Pulse Generator Component Malfunction: Pulse generator component malfunction is very rare, and is probably the least frequent cause of a pacing system malfunction. When a systematic design problem predisposes the system to a particular problem, most manufacturers inform physicians by way of a safety alert or technical memorandum. The diagnostic evaluation of a suspected component malfunction includes magnet application, which is unlikely to restore an effective output. Where measured data telemetry is available, it might provide clues, such as the device producing inconsistent measurements or inaccessible information. For example, a high lead impedance suggesting an open circuit but without the expected concomitant decrease in the battery current drain might be obtained. Or a battery current drain that far exceeds that commonly seen at similar output and rate settings might be found. One needs to be aware of what is normal for the implanted pacemaker. If this information is not known, the manufacturer's technical service department should be contacted.

Misinterpretation of Normal Function: Common causes of pauses associated with normal function include the presence of hysteresis or enabling of a sleep or rest rate algorithm, the device being programmed to a lower rate than recalled by the physician, the output being intentionally programmed to zero volts, or the mode being programmed to "off" (ODO, OVO, OAO). In each case, the device would be functioning properly even though the initial rhythms may be misinterpreted as a malfunction. All these causes can be readily identified by interrogating the pacemaker as to its programmed parameters.

Recording Artifacts: Recording artifacts may mimic a pacing system malfunction. Most commonly, this involves a transient disconnection of the monitoring lead, resulting in a loss of the recorded signal. This becomes clear when there is simultaneous failure of the native rhythm as well as the paced rhythm or when there is a depolarization without a repolarization and vice versa. One may have other evidence of continued cardiac function such as the blood pressure or pulse oximetry waveform despite "electrical asystole." Another valuable technique is to assess the patient when the purported rhythm or pacing system failure is occurring. If the problem is real, the patient should be symptomatic. But if the patient is well and simultaneously has a good pulse when the ECG says there is no heartbeat at all, the problem is clearly extrinsic to the patient-pacemaker system.

Intermittent or Persistent Recurrence of Symptoms

When a patient who has a pacemaker calls the physician's office complaining of a recurrence of symptoms or the development of new symptoms, it is both natural and appropriate to be concerned that there may be a problem with the system. All the previously discussed pacing system malfunctions need to be considered. If, on evaluation, the pacing system is shown to be functioning normally, one needs to consider the possibility of intermittent malfunction, programming that is inappropriate for the patient's physiologic needs, or symptoms due to a condition independent of the pacing system. Pacemaker syndrome is particularly common with single-chamber ventricular pacing when the atrium is intact.[52,53] Pacemaker syndrome may also occur in dual-chamber pacing systems (Fig. 7.15) when there is loss of atrial capture or sensing or an inappropriately programmed paced and sensed AV delay. For the evaluation of pacemaker syndrome useful tests include physical examination, ECG, and echo-Doppler techniques.[54,55]

If the concern is that the patient's symptoms are related to chronotropic incompetence and a failure of the pacemaker rate to accelerate appropriately,

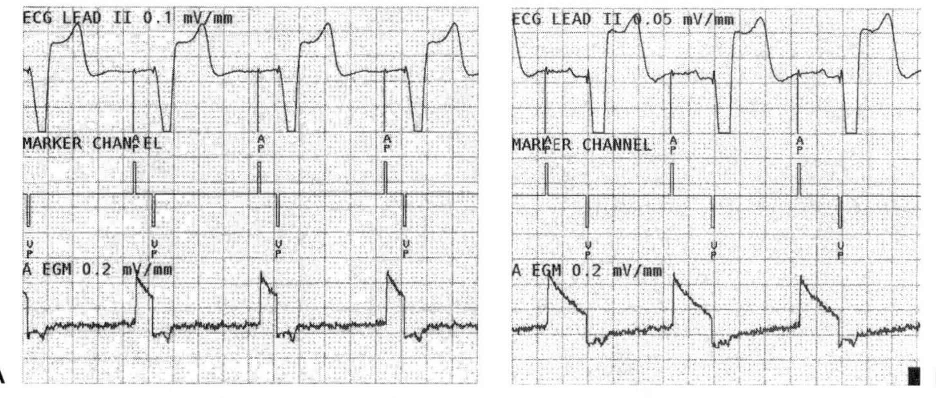

Figure 7.15. A: The patient was complaining of a persistent heaviness in his chest and chronic dyspnea with mild exertion. Atrial and ventricular capture thresholds were stable and low. An atrial-evoked response is not visible in this lead at the programmed AV delay. **B:** Increasing the AV delay unmasked the evoked atrial depolarization. There was marked latency between the atrial stimulus and the resultant P wave. At the original programmed AV delay (shipped value of the manufacturer), the atrial depolarization coincided with the ventricular activation. Markedly lengthening the AV delay allowed for effective atrial transport, a clinical improvement in cardiac output and alleviation of his symptoms of chest heaviness and dyspnea. This is an example of dual-chamber pacemaker syndrome.

enabling rate modulation or re-evaluating the rate modulated parameters would be appropriate.

DUAL-CHAMBER PACING SYSTEM MALFUNCTION

There are five major classes of dual-chamber pacing system malfunction. The first class includes all the abnormalities previously discussed as occurring with single-chamber pacing systems. The abnormalities in this case occur on one or both of the two channels of the dual-chamber system and, in recent years, this has been extended to either lead in a multisite atrial or ventricular system. Although this may sometimes be obvious, there are situations in which the problem will not be readily apparent because of the interaction of the paced rhythm with the native conduction system while the patient remains asymptomatic. The second class consists of the unique rhythms that can occur only with a dual-chamber system, such as crosstalk and endless-loop tachycardia (ELT). The third class of problems occurs when the rate response sensor responds to a physiologically inappropriate signal, which in turn drives the pacemaker. This may also occur in single-chamber pacing systems. The fourth class of problems is primarily due to a lack of understanding of the system and not appreciating the unique behavioral eccentricities of a pacemaker when it is functioning within its design specifications. The fifth group involves a mismatch between the programmed parameters of the pacemaker and the patient's physiology, a prime example being a rhythm termed repetitive non-reentrant ventricular atrial synchrony. Each of these problems is discussed subsequently.

Pacing Stimulus Present with Loss of Capture

Ventricular Loss of Capture: Ventricular loss of capture will sometimes be obvious—as in the patient with high-grade AV block who loses capture on the ventricular channel—but it may be very difficult to identify if there is intact AV nodal conduction. One will then see AV pacing with the ventricular stimulus coinciding with the native QRS such that it appears to capture, particularly if the duration of the native R wave is increased, as with bundle branch block (Fig. 7.16). If the R wave is of normal duration, it will appear as if the patient is having repeated fusion complexes, when actually there is intact native conduction with simultaneous loss of capture. At the time of routine evaluation, one should either increase or decrease the AV interval to confirm that capture is intact. One can also program the pacemaker to a nonsynchronous mode so that the pacing function is dissociated from intrinsic atrial or ventricular activity. All of the causes of loss of capture in single-chamber systems apply to either

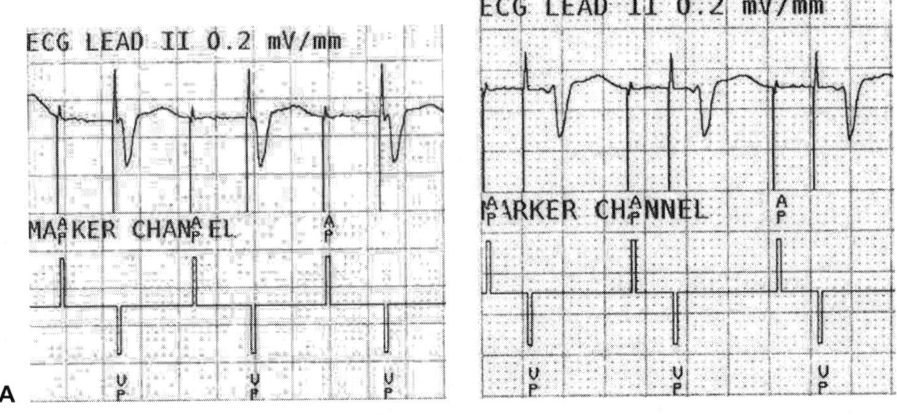

Figure 7.16. **A:** Initial rhythm strip showing AV sequential pacing. As the patient's QRS is mildly widened, it appears as if there is ventricular capture. On the capture threshold test, capture was interpreted as being present down to the lowest output of the pacemaker. This would be unusual for an older generation lead and inconsistent with measurements reported in the prior record. **B:** To further evaluate the system, the AV delay was shortened while the original output settings were maintained. This unmasked loss of capture. At the previous AV delay, the ineffective ventricular output pulses coincided with the conducted QRS complex but did not contribute to ventricular activation. This is termed pseudofusion.

channel of a dual-chamber system. In the case of multisite pacing—as with leads that independently stimulate the right ventricle and the left ventricle, the latter by way of an epicardial or coronary sinus lead—recognition of loss of capture may be a particular challenge. This may be manifested by a widening of the QRS, as the biventricular stimulation results in a narrowing of the paced QRS. However, as one usually associates a wide QRS with a paced ventricular rhythm, unless one had baseline recordings and knew that this was a biventricular system, recognition of loss of capture on one channel may be difficult from the surface ECG alone. Recording a simultaneously telemetered ventricular electrogram may demonstrate "late" activation of the noncaptured chamber, extended event markers showing events sensed within the refractory period as the impulse conducts from one chamber to the other (Fig. 7.17).

Atrial Loss of Capture: All of the causes of loss of capture for single-chamber pacing apply to dual-chamber systems as well. On the atrial channel, particularly with unipolar pacing, even though the atrial-evoked potential is present, it may be obscured by the large atrial stimulus. By the same token, more than one 12-lead ECG has been interpreted as normal AV sequential pacing when there was loss of atrial capture. If ventriculoatrial conduction is present, as reflected by a retrograde P wave in the ST-T wave of the paced ventricular complex, there must have been loss of atrial capture. Sometimes, however, the retrograde P wave is hidden within the T wave or is so small on the surface ECG that it is simply not seen. In this situation, access to atrial electrogram telemetry may prove to be very helpful (see Fig. 7.2).

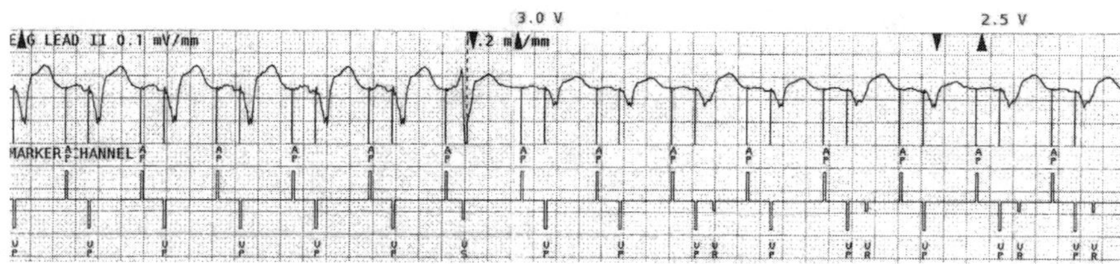

Figure 7.17. This was recorded during a ventricular capture threshold evaluation of a patient with Medtronic InSync model 8040 biventricular pacing system. There is stable biventricular capture at 3.5 volts at the left of the tracing. At 3.0V *(arrowheads)*, there is intermittent loss of LV capture. With the loss of LV capture, there is a slight increase in the QRS duration, which, while apparent when this is specifically sought, would be subtle and difficult to appreciate during routine monitoring. Coincident with the loss of LV capture is a second ventricular marker (VR) indicating left ventricular depolarization is being sensed on the ventricular channel during the pacemaker's refractory period. At 2.5V *(arrowheads)*, there is consistent loss of LV capture.

Programming to the AAI mode or functional AAI mode by reducing the ventricular output to a subthreshold level will readily unmask atrial noncapture. However, this would not be safe to do in the presence of complete heart block even if the atrial capture were intact. In that setting a long PR interval may be programmed. If atrial sensing is present, it is possible to increase the rate to above the native atrial rate. If there is capture, the sinus mechanism will be suppressed and there will be a stable AV sequential paced rhythm (Fig. 7.18). If atrial capture is absent, one will see AV pacing complexes alternating with PV complexes as the sinus P wave occurs during the atrial alert period. The availability of telemetered electrograms in some systems has eliminated the need to use an esophageal lead to record an atrial electrogram to document atrial capture or noncapture. Use of an esophageal lead is still a potential option when the atrial output pulse saturates the electrogram precluding differentiating capture from loss of capture and other techniques prove ineffective.

ASSESSMENT OF ATRIAL CAPTURE THRESHOLD - DDD MODE
(COMPLETE HEART BLOCK)

II 2.5 VOLTS, 0.4 MS PULSE DURATION

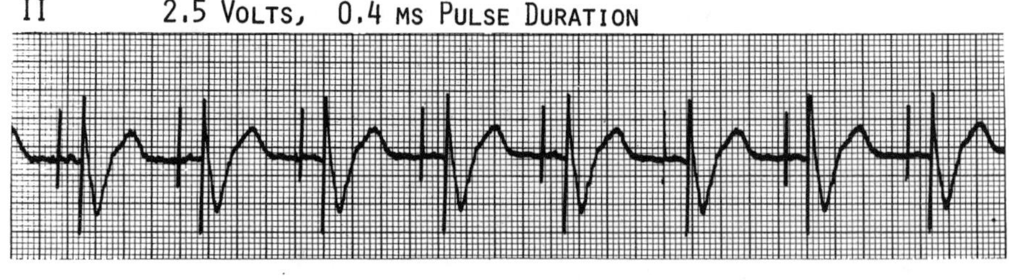

II 2.5 VOLTS, 0.1 MS PULSE DURATION - LOSS OF CAPTURE

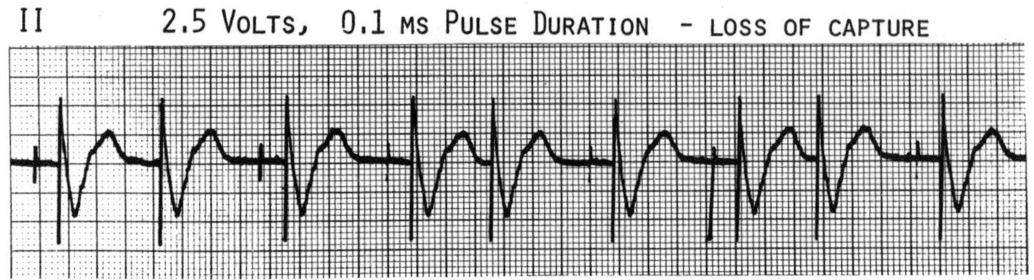

Figure 7.18. To assess atrial capture in the patient with complete heart block, increase the atrial rate above the native sinus rate. This will result in AV sequential pacing **(top)**. As long as atrial capture is intact, the faster paced rate will overdrive–suppress the sinus mechanism. When loss of atrial capture occurs as the atrial output is intentionally reduced, the sinus mechanism will escape; when it falls in an atrial alert period, it will be sensed, triggering a ventricular output resulting in an irregular rhythm. There will be ventricular pacing at all times, thus always protecting the patient. (Reprinted by permission from Levine PA. Confirmation of atrial capture and determination of atrial capture thresholds in DDD pacing systems. Clin Prog Pacing Electrophysiol 1984;2:465–473.)

Dual-Chamber Pacing with Sensing Malfunction

Sensing abnormalities in dual-chamber systems can result in inappropriate triggered pacing or inappropriate suppression of pacing depending on the pacing mode. The causes of sensing abnormalities include all those discussed under single-chamber systems. Functional undersensing is more common in dual-chamber systems due to the refractoriness in both chambers after each paced or sensed event. A well-known historical example is committed DVI pacing with a total lack of atrial sensing and forced functional ventricular undersensing during the AV delay. This occurs because the ventricular channel is rendered refractory following release of the atrial output pulse. A relatively common recent example of both functional undersensing and functional loss of capture is repetitive non-reentrant ventriculoatrial synchronous rhythms.

Undersensing: Loss of atrial sensing when there is an intact sinus rhythm may be more difficult to recognize in the dual-chamber system than in the single-chamber pacing system. For example, in the setting of a sufficiently rapid sinus rate, loss of atrial sensing in the DDD mode when there is intact AV nodal conduction will result in functional DVI pacing with total pacing system inhibition. The potential loss of atrial sensing will not become apparent unless the physician programs the pacemaker to an AV interval that is shorter than the intrinsic conduction.

Atrial undersensing may occur in two settings postimplantation even when a good EGM was obtained at the time of pacemaker implantation. A decrease in the amplitude of the atrial EGM has been demonstrated in both animals and humans during exercise.[56] Thus, atrial undersensing might occur at the higher sinus rates; yet at rest the atrial sensing threshold demonstrates a good margin of safety. Exercise and positional variations in P wave amplitude are also common with single-lead VDD systems using non-contact atrial electrodes. In addition, there may be a transient decrease in the amplitude of the atrial EGM occurring during the early electrode-maturation phase following implantation. Most cases of atrial undersensing occur in the first days or weeks postimplantation and will resolve spontaneously. As such, it would be prudent to observe the patient for weeks to months with the pacemaker programmed to a more sensitive setting before a decision is made to perform a repeat operative procedure.

On the ventricular channel, the ventricular stimulus may repeatedly fall within the native QRS, resulting in either a fusion or a pseudofusion complex. This may be normal because one cannot determine where the intrinsic deflection (ID) that is sensed by the pacemaker occurs within the cardiac depolarization represented by the surface QRS complex. If the ID occurs late within the QRS, then the above behavior is normal. If it occurs before the AV interval timer has completed, the R wave should have been sensed and this behavior represents a malfunction. Unlike atrial undersensing, event marker telemetry will not facilitate this assessment with the pacemaker in the DDD mode. To evaluate ventricular sensing, one can increase the AV interval but only if intrinsic conduction is present and occurs within the lengthened AV delay. If the ventricular stimulus occurs after the QRS complex has ended, there is definitive evidence of ventricular undersensing. One could also program the pacemaker to a single chamber mode (e.g., VVI), at which time ventricular undersensing will become readily apparent.

Oversensing: Oversensing in a dual-chamber system will elicit either inappropriate inhibition or triggering, depending on the channel on which oversensing occurs and the programmed pacing mode. If oversensing occurs on the ventricular channel in the DDD, DDI, or DVI modes, both the atrial and ventricular outputs will be inhibited and the timing cycles reset (Fig. 7.19).

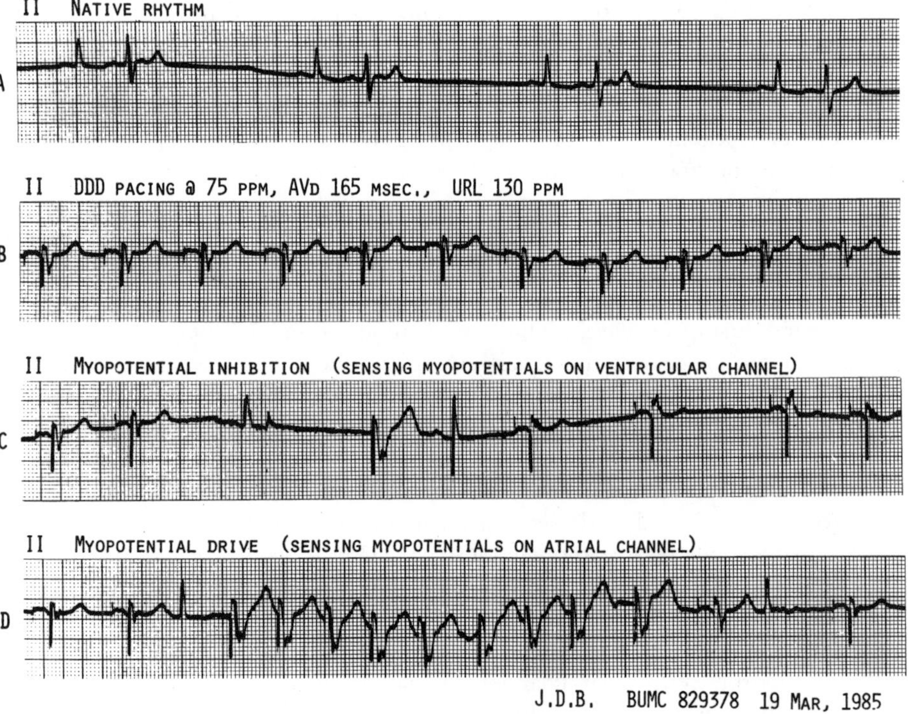

Figure 7.19. In a dual-chamber pacing system, oversensing occurring on the atrial and ventricular channels results in dramatically different rhythms. **A:** The top tracing is the patient's native rhythm prior to implantation of the pacemaker. **B:** The patient's rhythm is totally controlled by the pacemaker. **C:** Ventricular oversensing, in this case of myopotentials, occurs; the pacemaker is inhibited and the rate slows below the programmed lower rate limit. **D:** When there is atrial oversensing, the sensed P triggers a ventricular output. This has been called myopotential drive; it results in brief periods of ventricular pacing at or near the maximum tracking rate or potentially triggering mode switch behavior. (Reprinted by permission from Levine PA. Normal and abnormal rhythms associated with dual-chamber pacemakers. Cardiol Clin 1985;3:595–616.)

Oversensing in a biventricular system will demonstrate similar behaviors to that in a standard DDD system with an occasional exception. Given the instability of the CS lead, dislodgment will result in its withdrawal closer to the coronary sinus placing it in proximity to the left atrium. As such, it may detect a left atrial depolarization causing ventricular inhibition. Left atrial P wave oversensing may result in inhibition of the ventricular output and the loss of CRT.[57]

Unique Dual-Chamber Rhythms

Crosstalk: Crosstalk is the sensing of the far-field signal in the opposite chamber, causing the pacemaker to either inhibit or trigger an output depending on its design. Crosstalk can occur in single-chamber atrial pacing systems in which the far-field QRS is sensed, inhibiting and resetting the basic pacing interval, but crosstalk most commonly refers to ventricular sensing of the far-field atrial stimulus in a DVI, DDI, or DDD pacing system. Sensing this stimulus will result in inhibition of the ventricular output and resetting of the atrial escape interval. In the presence of concomitant AV block, crosstalk can be catastrophic and result in ventricular asystole (Fig. 7.20).[58]

Crosstalk inhibition of ventricular output is most likely to occur in the setting of unipolar pacing leads (atrial and ventricular), high atrial output voltage, high ventricular sensitivity, and short ventricular blanking/refractory periods. Crosstalk is suggested by the failure of ventricular pacing following atrial-paced

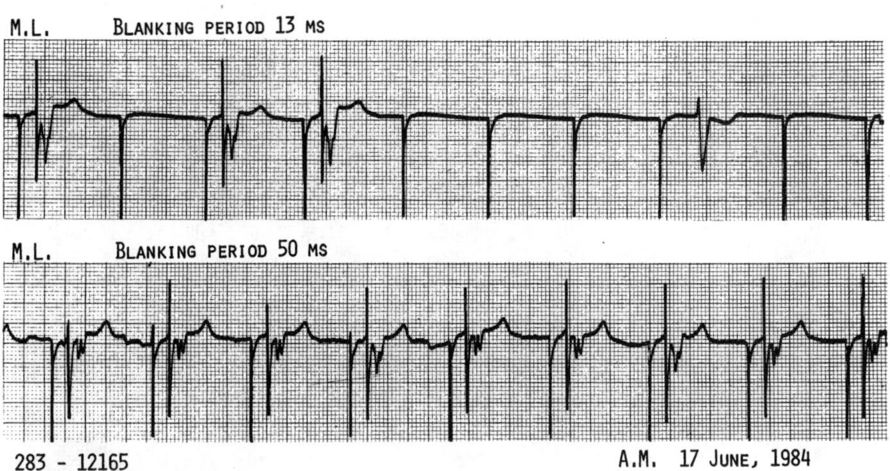

Figure 7.20. **Top:** Classic crosstalk-mediated ventricular output inhibition. This was intentionally induced by programming a short ventricular blanking period, high atrial output, and high ventricular sensitivity. This patient had high-grade AV block, which is the worst setting for crosstalk. The hallmark of crosstalk in a ventricular-based timing system is that the AA interval equals the sum of the atrial escape interval and ventricular blanking period. **Bottom:** In an atrial-based timing system, it may be difficult to differentiate crosstalk from an open circuit. Crosstalk, in this example, was eliminated by increasing the blanking period.

but not atrial-sensed events. Crosstalk is confirmed by telemetered marker channels showing ventricular sensing in the absence of a QRS complex and is corrected by asynchronous pacing (with magnet application or reprogramming), or by extending the ventricular blanking period initiated by the atrial output pulse. As an added insurance against crosstalk-mediated ventricular output inhibition, a special detection or sensing window was added on the ventricular channel. Following the blanking period, this window varies in duration from 51 to 150 milliseconds between manufacturers. A signal sensed during this interval will be treated by the pacemaker as if it were crosstalk, but rather than inhibiting the ventricular output, a ventricular output will be triggered at an abbreviated AV interval (Fig. 7.21).[59]

Another form of crosstalk is far-field R wave (FFRW) oversensing. This has become a significant challenge for mode-switching algorithms that allow the pacemaker to detect rapid atrial rhythms and revert to a nontracking mode (DDI, VVI) from a tracking mode (DDD, VDD). To detect rapid atrial rhythm, these devices can sense atrial events in the Post-Ventricular Atrial Refractory Period (PVARP) and in some cases, within the AV delay. If the far-field paced or native R wave is detected in this period in addition to the native P wave, the system may recognize a falsely high atrial rate and initiate the mode switching (Fig. 7.22).[60] Management requires programming the absolute refractory portion of the PVARP, which is termed the post-ventricular atrial blanking (PVAB) period. In some cases, a far-field R wave associated with a native QRS complex is detected on the atrial channel before it is recognized on the ven-

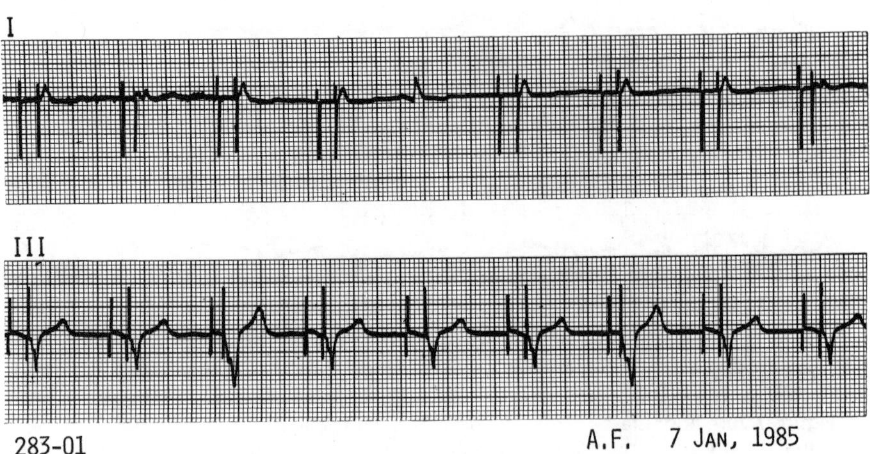

Figure 7.21. Crosstalk that occurs in the presence of a special crosstalk detection window triggers a ventricular output pulse rather than inhibiting it. This usually occurs at a shorter-than-programmed AV interval. Intermittent AV-interval shortening is seen in the two tracings. This reflects episodes of crosstalk triggering a ventricular output pulse. In the top tracing, for example, the second and ninth beats show AV-interval shortening.

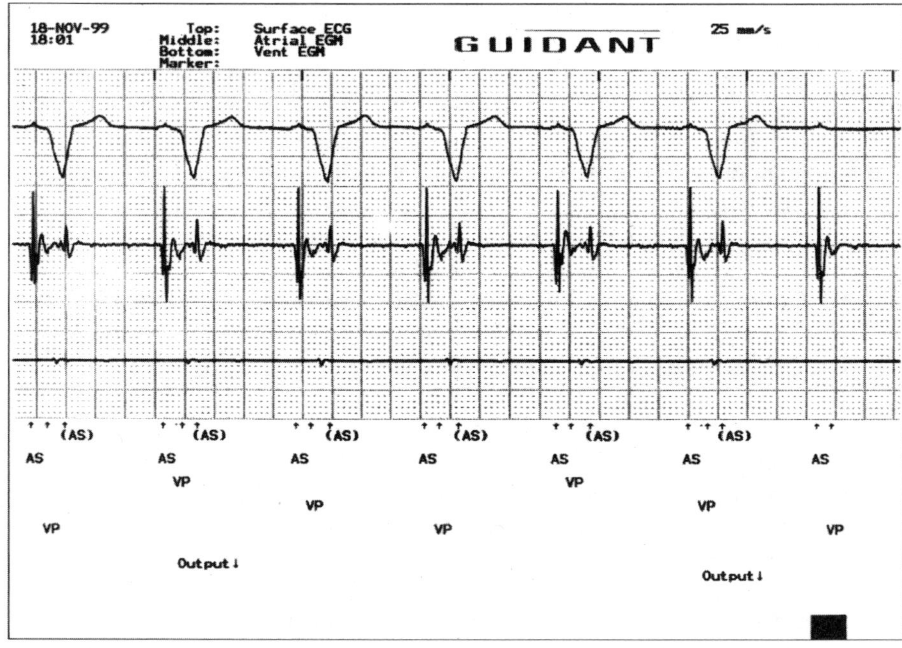

Figure 7.22. Surface ECG, atrial electrogram, ventricular electrogram, and event markers from a patient with a Guidant Discovery that was demonstrating inappropriate mode switching due to far-field R wave oversensing. This recording was obtained during performance of the ventricular capture threshold test as part of the pacing system evaluation. A discrete deflection is visible on the atrial lead coincident with the QRS and identified by the event markers *(AS)*, which means that it is a sensed complex occurring within the refractory period. With loss of capture shown by the last complex on this, there is a disappearance of the second deflection on the AEGM and the marker *(AS)*. Increasing the PVAB eliminated the far-field R wave sensing.

tricular channel. Circuits are being designed to manage this less common situation but it cannot be managed by extending the PVAB.

Pacemaker-Mediated Tachycardias: A pacemaker-mediated tachycardia (PMT) is a tachycardia that is sustained by the continued active participation of the pacemaker in the rhythm. A PMT is not the same as a pacemaker-induced tachycardia, in which the pacemaker induces a tachycardia by intentional or unintentional (undersensing) competition, but once the tachycardia has begun, the pacemaker is inhibited and no longer plays an active role in the rhythm. There are several forms of pacemaker-mediated tachycardias encountered in clinical practice. In the DDD mode, the normally functioning pacemaker is supposed to sense atrial activity and trigger a ventricular output in response to the detected P wave. The DDD pacemaker in a patient in whom atrial fibrillation or flutter develops may track the pathologic atrial signals (e.g., flutter or fibrillatory waves). This will drive the ventricular channel of the pacemaker at or near its maximum tracking rate (MTR).[61]

The first PMTs that became widely recognized in the literature were not due to tracking atrial fibrillation or atrial flutter or oversensing on the atrial channel. Instead, they were due to sensing retrograde atrial activity arising from a premature ventricular contraction (PVC). This set up a repetitive sequence of the sensed retrograde P wave triggering a ventricular output at the end of the maximum tracking rate interval. The delay created by waiting for the MTRI to complete before the ventricular stimulus was released allowed the atrium and AV node to physiologically recover. The depolarization resulting from a ventricular paced beat was again able to conduct in a retrograde direction. This next retrograde P wave would be sensed, triggering another ventricular output and resulting in a sustained PMT.[62,63] Because this resembled the endless loop that can be seen in computers, Furman and associates labeled this rhythm an endless-loop tachycardia (ELT) to differentiate it from the other forms of PMT.[64] The majority of PMTs in the literature are of the endless-loop variety, running either at or below the programmed maximum tracking rate (Fig. 7.23A). The onset of ELT requires at least transient AV dissociation to allow retrograde conduction to occur. Thus, the appearance of ELT should initiate a search for causes of AV dissociation such as atrial undersensing, atrial oversensing, loss of atrial capture, or magnet application to the pacemaker. Once initiated, an endless-loop pacemaker-mediated tachycardia will continue unless there is spontaneous VA block or loss of atrial sensing.

Algorithms to prevent ELT extend the PVARP after a sensed ventricular event that is not preceded by an atrial event (a PVC as defined by the pacemaker) to ensure that any retrograde P wave will fall in the refractory period and not be tracked. A number of adverse rhythms have been associated with automatic extension of the atrial refractory period, leading to sustained pacemaker inhibition with first-degree AV block and a PR interval significantly longer than the programmed PV interval. This situation is created by a P wave coinciding with the PVARP and hence not being sensed. However, the P wave is conducted and the sensed R wave is treated as a PVC by the pacemaker, extending the PVARP and again precluding sensing of the next P wave. Although disconcerting when encountered, it is not dangerous because the patient has an intact native rhythm. To prevent ELT by using a long PVARP yet still allow tracking to high atrial rates some devices employ a rate variable PVARP that automatically shortens at higher rates. Another option is rate responsive AV delay allowing the PVARP to be kept at a longer interval while the sensed AV delay shortens as the rate increases.

ELT may be automatically terminated by specialized algorithms (Fig. 7.24). These algorithms typically extend the PVARP or withhold a ventricular output for one cycle after tracking at the upper rate limit for a number of cycles and intermittently thereafter. If the tachycardia is due to ELT, it is terminated by the failure to track the retrograde P wave. If tachycardia is due to sinus rhythm, the tracking will continue after a single missed beat.[65]

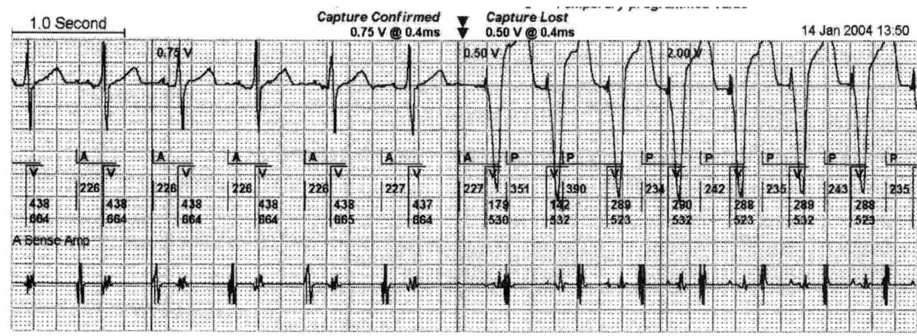

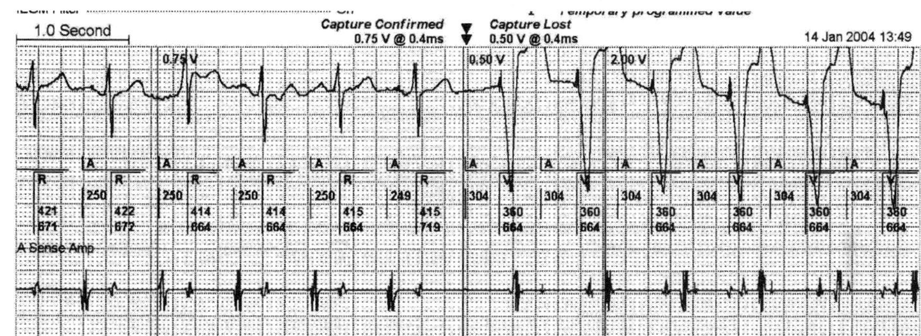

Figure 7.23. This figure shows both a pacemaker endless loop tachycardia (ELT) and a repetitive non-reentrant ventriculoatrial synchronous (RNRVAS) rhythm. These were recorded from the same patient at the time of a follow-up evaluation. Both rhythms were induced by careful programming of the pacemaker. The base rate was increased to 90 ppm during the atrial capture threshold test. **A:** To allow an ELT to occur in this patient with known retrograde conduction, the PVARP was reduced to 125 milliseconds. Upon loss of atrial capture, there was full ventricular capture at the end of the AV delay followed by retrograde conduction. The retrograde P wave was detected by the atrial sensing circuit and triggered the next ventricular output after the sensed AV delay was extended so as to not violate the programmed maximum tracking rate. This rhythm would persist until the pacemaker was reprogrammed or an automatic ELT termination algorithm intervened (see Fig. 7.24). **B:** To demonstrate the RNRVAS rhythm, the AV delay was increased to 300 milliseconds and the PVARP increased to preclude detection of the retrograde P wave. While the long PVARP will prevent an ELT, each subsequent atrial output pulse, even at full output, will be delivered at a time when the atrial myocardium is physiologically refractory as schematically represented by a *heavy solid line* starting with the native (retrograde) P wave as shown on the AEGM. The result is functional loss of capture. The *top horizontal line* within the event markers identifies the duration of the atrial refractory period. As each retrograde P wave coincides with the PVARP, there is also functional undersensing. This alignment is identified by the *thin double arrow*.

A unique ELT has recently been described when a dual-chamber pacemaker is used to provide biventricular pacing where the CS lead is connected to the atrial port and the RV lead is connected to the ventricular port. A PVC arising in the right ventricle will be labeled an R wave. This will trigger the PVARP but if conduction to the LV is delayed such that detection occurs after

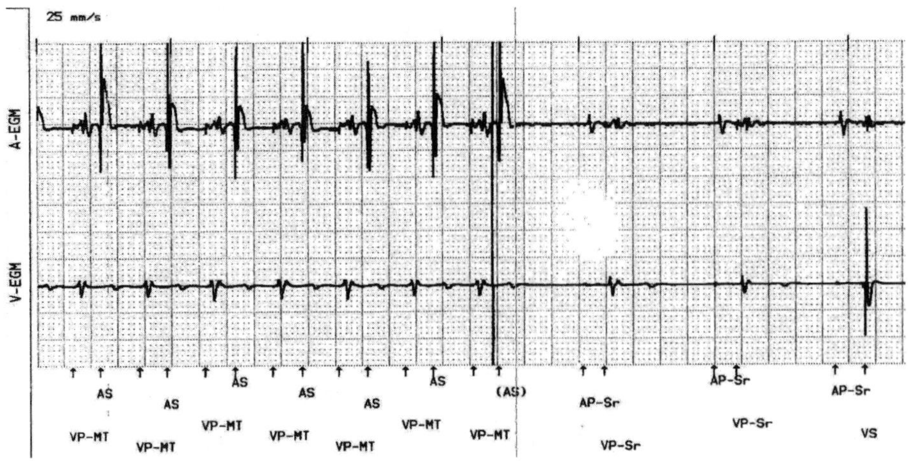

Figure 7.24. Stored EGM from a Guidant Pulsar Max II demonstrating the recognition and automatic termination of an endless loop tachycardia (ELT). **Top tracing:** atrial electrogram (A-EGM). **Middle tracing:** ventricular EGM. **Bottom tracing:** marker channel. Guidant's algorithm extends the PVARP after a number of cycles of atrial sense-ventricle pace (AS-VP) at the maximum tracking (MT) rate. If this rhythm were an ELT, the extended PVARP will preclude responding to the retrograde P wave and prompt termination of the rhythm as occurred. AS denotes atrial event in the refractory period. If the etiology of the atrial events was sinus tachycardia or an intrinsic atrial tachycardia in the setting of high-grade AV block, the extended PVARP would result in a pause due to the lack of tracking of the "blocked" P wave followed by prompt resumption of the rapid rhythm.

the PVARP, the detected LV depolarization will be labeled a P wave and trigger an output in the RV. This is an example of an intraventricular PMT.[66]

Another pacemaker-mediated rhythm resulting from AV dyssynchrony is repetitive non-reentrant ventriculoatrial synchronous rhythm. This rhythm represents a mismatch between the alert and refractory periods of the pacemaker and the heart.[67] It is functionally equivalent to VVI pacing with intact retrograde conduction, but it occurs in the setting of AV pacing. The trigger for this rhythm is identical to the initiating factors for an endless-loop tachycardia (i.e., AV dissociation), that allow retrograde conduction to develop. In this rhythm, the PVARP is programmed to a sufficiently long interval to preclude the retrograde P wave from being detected; hence, a PMT does not begin. If the AV paced rate is sufficiently rapid, whether this is due to a high programmed base rate or sensor-drive, the P wave occurring within the PVARP is not detected (functional undersensing) thus allowing the atrial escape interval to complete, resulting in the delivery of an atrial output pulse. At the high rate, the atrial escape interval is relatively short and may result in the delivery of an atrial output pulse at a time when the atrial myocardium is still refractory on a physiologic basis. This pattern may then be repetitive. A new algorithm called noncompetitive atrial pacing has been introduced in an attempt to preclude such a rhythm by extending atrial output to at least 300 milliseconds after an atrial sensed event (Fig. 7.23B).

UNIQUE BIVENTRICULAR RHYTHMS WITH LOSS OF CAPTURE

When one considers pacing, recognition of a wide QRS is expected, particularly in association with ventricular pacing. In biventricular pacing, the paced complex will be abnormal but usually narrower than the "usual" paced ventricular complex. Unless one has a baseline 12-lead ECG for comparison, this may not be recognized as normal. The LV capture threshold tends to be higher than the RV threshold. LV pacing is usually achieved via a lead placed in the coronary sinus. The fixation mechanisms in this position are not as secure as those associated with endocardial pacing. As such, both lead dislodgment and loss of capture are more common with LV leads than with RV leads. With loss of LV capture, one may see an "obviously" paced ventricular beat. Unless one was aware of the baseline recordings for the patient or that the patient had a biventricular system, loss of capture will not be recognized (see Fig. 7.17). The presentation is also likely to differ from that of the patient with a pacemaker implanted for high grade AV block who develops loss of capture. Patients who are paced for cardiac resynchronization have congestive heart failure. Thus, the loss of CRT may manifest itself as a worsening of their congestive symptoms while the rhythm is intact.

PACEMAKER ECCENTRICITIES AND PSEUDOMALFUNCTION

A pacemaker eccentricity is a unique behavior of the pacemaker that would be unexpected based on a knowledge of the pacing mode but that is normal for that model of pacemaker. A pseudomalfunction is a misdiagnosed problem with pacemaker function that in fact results from normal operation of a pacemaker algorithm or function. The eccentricities of pacemaker function are often not popularized in the literature or the physician's manual for the device. They are frequently brought to the attention of the physician only after consulting with technical support for the manufacturer regarding an unexplained pacemaker behavior. Examples are shown in Figure 7.25. Pseudomalfunctions are a challenge for even the seasoned pacemaker physician given the increasing complexity of the newer devices with less than obvious interactions between available algorithms. A list of common features causing pseudomalfunctions in current pacemaker systems is shown in Box 7.4.

PACEMAKER DIAGNOSTICS

Given the multiplicity of confusing pacemaker rhythms, most manufacturers include various aids within the pacemaker to assist the physician in evaluating the system. These include both real-time diagnostic aids as well as system-overview capabilities. Many real-time diagnostic capabilities have been discussed

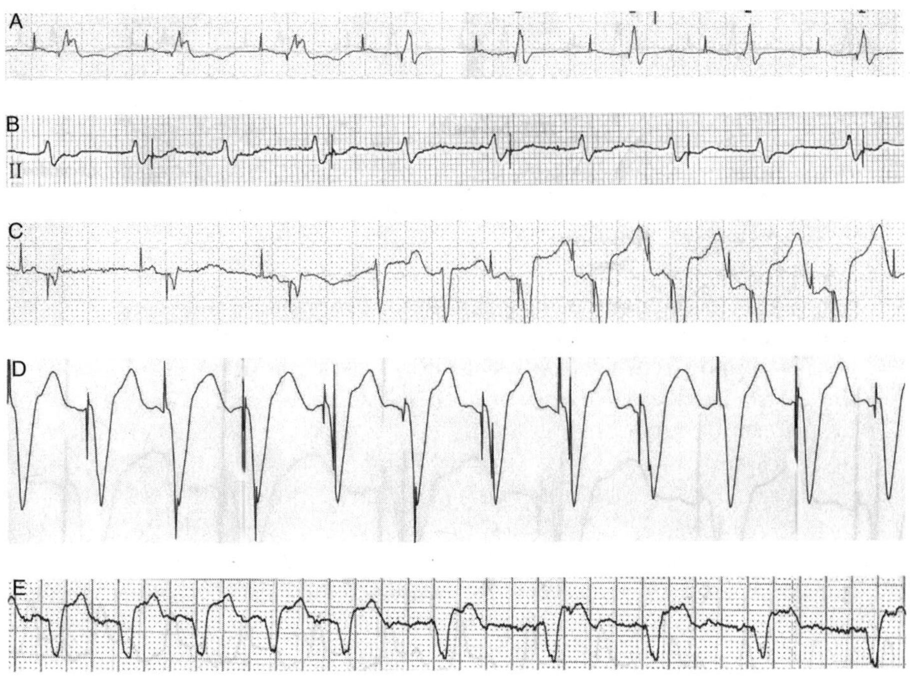

Figure 7.25. Five examples of pseudomalfunctions. **A:** Intrinsic AV search function. After the first three cardiac cycles with atrial pace (Ap)-ventricular pace (Vp) with full ventricular capture, the AV delay is extended to allow for intrinsic conduction. The narrow QRS complexes are pseudofusion complexes that may be mistaken for loss of capture. **B:** Safety pacing during a junctional rhythm simulating ventricular undersensing. With every other cycle the atrial pacing is occurring at the start of the QRS. The QRS is sensed early in the AV delay to trigger safety pacing. **C:** Rate smoothing causing sudden pacing above lower rate limit. The two PVCs after the third AV pacing cycle initiates AV pacing to decrement incrementally from the faster rate established by the ectopy. **D:** St. Jude Medical ventricular autocapture algorithm perfoming threshold determination. After the third QRS complex several complexes occur with two pacing artifacts. The second artifact is the backup pulse that ensures capture while the first pulse is decremented in output. This function can be mistaken for displacement of an atrial lead into the ventricle in a dual chamber pacemaker or pacemaker malfunction. **E:** Medtronic blanked flutter search simulating undersensing. There appears to be tracking of P waves in the first four cardiac cycles. The abrupt rate change is from extension of the PVARP unmasking the flutter from the TARP and initiating mode switching to a slower rate. The flutter waves are poorly seen in this tracing.

in this chapter. The pacemaker physician should make full use of these features to assist in troubleshooting the pacing system.

Measured Data

Measured data is the ability of the pacemaker to provide data regarding battery status, with specific measurements such as battery voltage, current drain, and internal impedance. A decrease in the battery voltage is an appropriate marker

Box 7.4. Pacemaker Functions Associated with Pseudomalfunctions

Pacing When Not Expected	Diagnostic Clue
— Rate smoothing	— Graded rate slowing toward lower rate limit
— Rate drop response	— Abrupt pacing 90–110 bpm after sudden slowing
— Dynamic atrial overdrive	— Atrial pacing after atrial ectopy
— Ventricular rate regularization	— Pacing after shorter V-V intervals in atrial fibrillation
— Ventricular based timing	— Faster ventricular rate during ApVs–ApVp cycle
— Safety pacing	— Ventricular pacing with shortened AV delay
— Separate mode switch rate or post mode switch overdrive rate	— Pacing during or after atrial tachyarrhythmia or oversensing
— Atrial pace for AV resynchronization	— Pacing simultaneous with PVC or delayed after atrial ectopy
— QT sensor check	— QT rate sensor active
— Atrial pacing preference	— Atrial pacing after atrial sensed events
— Automated capture determinations	— Closely coupled stimuli during QRS
No Pacing When Expected	
— Hysteresis	— Pause after sensed events
— Rate smoothing	— Graded rate acceleration toward upper rate limit
— PMT intervention	— Ventricular output absent after As-Vp at upper rate limit
— Mode switching	— Failure to track atrial activity
— Intrinsic AV conduction search	— Periodic extension of AV delay
— Non-competitive atrial pacing	— Delay in atrial output following atrial sense in PVARP
— Separate sleep rate	— Reduced lower rate limit at rest
— Atrial based timing	— Prolongation of V-V interval during ApVs–ApVp cycle
— Automatic sensing check	— Periodic delay in pacing after prolonged pacing
Apparent Undersensing	
— Mode switching	— Failure to track atrial activity
— PMT intervention	— Failure to track single P wave during prolonged AsVp at upper rate limit
— Rate adaptive AV delay	— Evidence of shorter AV delays at faster rates
— Non-tracking modes (DDI, DVI, etc.)	— Typical non-tracking mode behavior
— Blanked flutter search	— Failure to track P wave when atrial tracking at rate <2 times TARP
— Noise mode	— Evidence of EMI

to identify the point at which there is an increase in the frequency of pacemaker surveillance for signs of battery depletion.[68]

Measured data also includes measurements of pulse voltage, charge, current, energy, and stimulation impedance. Lead or stimulation impedance measurements may be particularly helpful in identifying an open circuit, which will be associated with a very high impedance (see Fig. 7.7) or a breach of the internal insulation of a bipolar coaxial lead, in which case, the impedance will be very low.[69,70] One should be cautious with respect to this information. A measurement that is significantly changed from previous results should be reconfirmed to eliminate a telemetry error.

Event Markers

Event markers have been shown in multiple figures in this chapter. These comprise timing information telemetered from the pacemaker to the programmer and are displayed on a screen or printed. Basically, these markers are a report of what the pacemaker is doing. Unique notations or marks are generated for paced and sensed events; in some cases, marks are generated for events occurring during the refractory period as well as an indication of refractory period duration.[71–73]

Event markers are an extremely powerful tool, especially when combined with the simultaneously recorded electrocardiogram. Pauses can be identified as due to oversensing or an open circuit, as shown in Figure 7.7. With diminutive bipolar output pulses that may not be visible on the standard electrocardiogram, telemetered event markers will identify whether the P wave or QRS complex is paced or sensed. The ECG also confirms the response to a pacing stimulus.

Electrograms

The ability to examine the endocardial electrogram (EGM) is very helpful in identifying false signals that are being sensed (oversensing), as shown in Figure 7.4, or in confirming the presence of signals that are not readily identified on the surface ECG, as in Figures 7.2 and 7.17. Some physicians have recommended using the telemetered electrogram as a way of performing a sensing threshold evaluation,[74] but this may be inappropriate. Some systems do not provide a calibration scale; others use a different set of filters in the telemetry amplifier compared with those used in the sense amplifier. In these settings, although there may generally be a close correlation between the amplitude of the telemetered electrogram, there may also be marked discrepancies due to the different filters.

Electrograms may also provide clues as to why there is a sensing problem or why the noninvasively measured sensing threshold is obtained by progressively reducing the sensitivity until intermittent or persistent failure to sense is demonstrated.[75,76] This, however, requires the additional capability of adjusting both the gain and the sweep speed of the signal once it has been frozen. When displayed at a relatively slow recording speed, a complex may look very good with a large amplitude; however, when the signal is displayed at a faster sweep speed, it may be shown to be splintered and/or have segments that are composed of predominantly low-frequency components, with the actual rapid intrinsic deflection being of relatively low amplitude. An example is shown in Figure 7.26. One also needs to be aware that there are two basic electrograms. One reflects the signal after it has been processed by the sense amplifier limiting any morphologic information and may not be calibrated. The other utilizes a relatively broad band-pass filter and although calibrated, the peak-to-peak measurement may not reflect the amplitude of the signal as detected by the sensing circuit because of different filters.

Stored Data

Measured data, event markers, and electrogram telemetry are all considered real-time data. However, if the problem is intermittent, the real-time data may be entirely normal; in such cases, a more extensive evaluation will be required. Further, the real-time diagnostics may identify a developing pacing system problem but one that has not yet resulted in any adverse consequences for the patient. Additional evaluation or even intervention might be warranted, depending on the specific clinical setting. Although stored EGMs triggered by specific events have been a mainstay of ICD diagnostics for almost a decade, they have only been recently introduced to bradycardia devices.[77] EGM storage may be triggered by magnet application by the patient or automatically by the device in response to rapid heart rates.

Event Counters

Event counters provide information about the function of the pacing system over time. This feature may provide an overview of the behavior of the pacing system with respect to specific events or activation of various algorithms, an overview of the general behavior of the system, or a report of the pacing system with respect to time. Each manufacturer has its own set of unique labels for the specific counters in its various products, but, generically, there are three separate capabilities.

Total System Performance Counters: Total system performance counters report the total number of events within each pacing state (atrial sense–ventricular sense, atrial pace–ventricular sense, etc.), sometimes with a further separation as to rate distribution within each pacing state.[78] Many systems will also report the number of premature ventricular sensed events. The potential value to the medical staff caring for the patient is that these counters provide an overview of the behavior of the pacing system since the last evaluation. The interpretation of these counters requires knowledge of the patient's clinical status and the integrity of capture and sensing within the pacing system (Fig. 7.27). For example, if the system reports that all the complexes were paced in the ventricle, either AV or PV, it is a report of the pacemaker's behavior. Loss of atrial or ventricular capture cannot be ascertained from these counters, and a true pacing system problem might go unrecognized if one relies only on the counters.

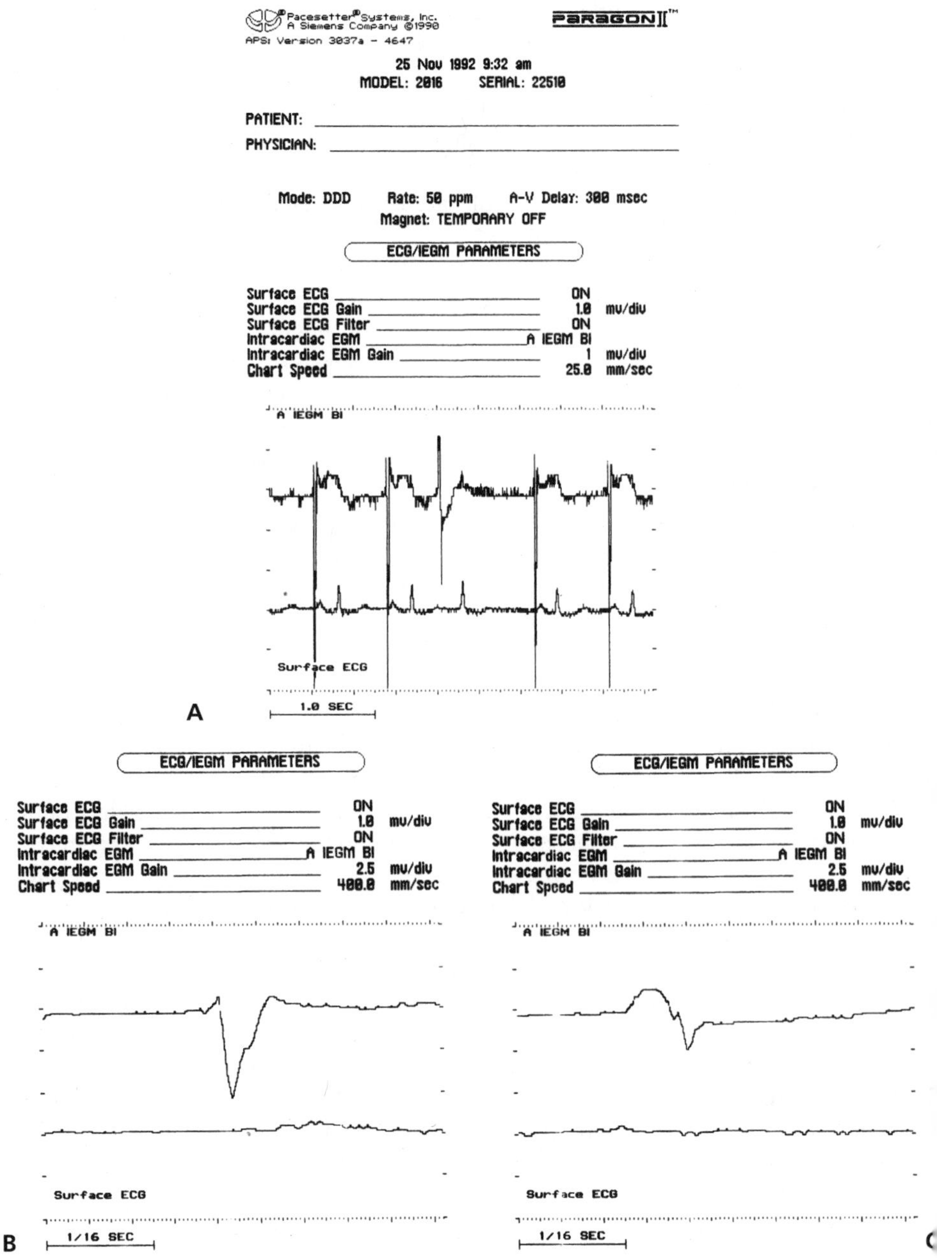

Pacesetter® Systems, Inc.
A Siemens Company ©1990
APS: Version 3037a – 4647

PARAGON II™

25 Nov 1992 9:32 am
MODEL: 2016 SERIAL: 22510

PATIENT: ______________________

PHYSICIAN: ______________________

Mode: DDD Rate: 50 ppm A-V Delay: 300 msec
Magnet: TEMPORARY OFF

ECG/IEGM PARAMETERS

Surface ECG	ON	
Surface ECG Gain	1.0	mv/div
Surface ECG Filter	ON	
Intracardiac EGM	A IEGM BI	
Intracardiac EGM Gain	1	mv/div
Chart Speed	25.0	mm/sec

A IEGM BI

Surface ECG

1.0 SEC

A

ECG/IEGM PARAMETERS

Surface ECG	ON	
Surface ECG Gain	1.0	mv/div
Surface ECG Filter	ON	
Intracardiac EGM	A IEGM BI	
Intracardiac EGM Gain	2.5	mv/div
Chart Speed	400.0	mm/sec

A IEGM BI

Surface ECG

1/16 SEC

B

ECG/IEGM PARAMETERS

Surface ECG	ON	
Surface ECG Gain	1.0	mv/div
Surface ECG Filter	ON	
Intracardiac EGM	A IEGM BI	
Intracardiac EGM Gain	2.5	mv/div
Chart Speed	400.0	mm/sec

A IEGM BI

Surface ECG

1/16 SEC

C

If the pacing system is functioning properly with respect to capture and sensing, the total system performance counters provide insight as to chronotropic function based on the distribution of sensed atrial activity, the response of the sensor, the percentage of time the sensor is controlling the pacemaker, and the status of AV nodal conduction based on the percentage of paced and sensed complexes. Frequent "PVCs" at a low rate may be a marker for intermittent atrial undersensing with intact AV nodal conduction or for accelerated junctional rhythms; a large number of PVCs at a high rate may reflect true ventricular ectopic beats. The data provided by all the event counters need to be correlated with the clinician's knowledge of the patient.

Subsystem Performance Counters: Subsystem performance counters track and report the behavior of specific algorithms or features of the pacing system. These include, but are not limited to, sensor-indicated rates, number of times the PMT algorithm was activated, the amount of time spent at the programmed maximal tracking rate, the number of automatic mode switch episodes, the peak atrial rates that triggered the mode-switch episodes or occurred above a predefined rate, atrial or ventricular high rate episodes, sensor-indicated rates, and a long-term threshold record for those systems with automatic capture assessment algorithms.[79] The value of these counters is that they separate specific events from the overall total system performance counter and provide information with respect to the frequency with which that algorithm or feature was used. These event counters may also provide data that are not obtainable from a standard ECG or Holter monitor.

These counters may be displayed as a summary total, a table of events, a histogram, or a more detailed presentation of each event, depending on the design of the specific counter and the information that is stored. An example of a subsystem performance counter is shown in Figures 7.28 and 7.29.

Time-Based System Performance Counters: A limitation of both the total and subsystem performance counters when the data are displayed in either a cumulative table or histogram format is that specific events will be lost within the overall mass of data. A third counter capability places each of the individual

Figure 7.26. A: Bipolar atrial electrogram with a simultaneously recorded surface ECG. There is an isolated atrial premature beat that appears to be at least 3 mV in amplitude but, when the sensing threshold was assessed, there was intermittent failure to sense at 1 mV. The sensing threshold for the sinus P wave was greater than 5 mV. **B:** Increase in the sweep speed to 400 mm/sec and a reduction in the gain to 2.5 mV/division. This atrial electrogram represents the sinus P wave and it corresponds to the noninvasively measured sensing threshold. **C:** Increase in the sweep speed to 400 mm/sec and a reduction in the gain to 2.5 mV/division. This atrial electrogram represents the atrial premature beat. Much of the amplitude noted when the sweep speed was 25 mm/sec was composed of very low-frequency components. The complex is also splintered with a slew rate significantly lower than the sinus complex, accounting for the intermittent undersensing at a 1-mV sensitivity.

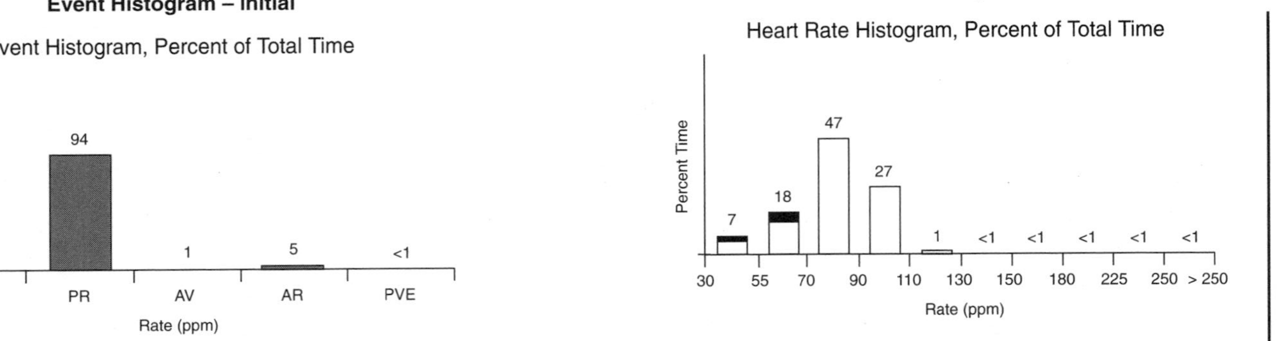

Event Counts – Initial

Rate (ppm)	PV	PR	AV	AR	PVE
30–54	3,699	546,503	28,834	209,108	224
55–69	13,626	2,381,502	70,236	617,575	16
70–89	13,202	10,374,285	242	11	50
90–109	8,650	7,341,430	0	0	478
110–129	70,477	263,498	0	0	4,889
130–149	27	6,001	0	0	2,538
150–179	0	1,689	0	0	770
180–224	0	1,369	0	0	16
225–249	0	1,241	0	0	0
> 250	0	777	0	0	0
Total	**109,681**	**20,918,295**	**99,312**	**821,694**	**8,981**

Total Event Count: 21,957,963

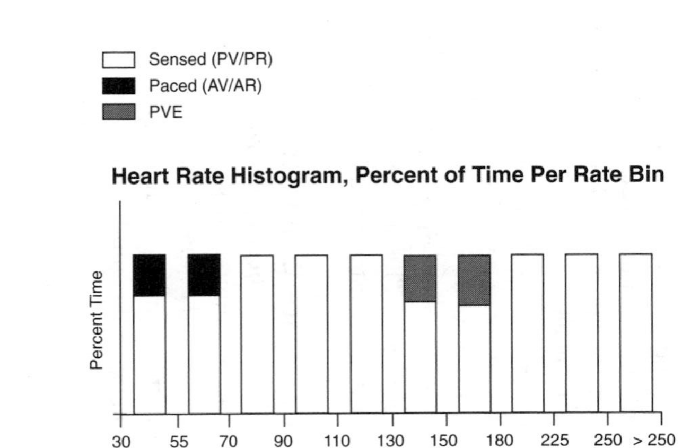

Figure 7.27. Total system performance counter (Event Histogram) from a St. Jude Medical Integrity 5342 pulse generator demonstrating the relative distribution of pacing states, the heart rate based on atrial events (paced or sensed), the absolute number of events in each pacing state at each rate bin over the preceding 192 days, 7 hours, 23 minutes, and 20 seconds. The PVE in this counter reflects events that the pacemaker will treat as PVCs. As these may also be junctional beats, episodes of atrial undersensing with intact conduction, or noise on the ventricular channel and not a true PVC as would be implied to the clinical staff, these are

High Rate Episodes	Page 1

Data Collection Period: 12/13/02 11:04 AM - 04/24/03 4:29 PM (Over Last 4 months)

Atrial High Rate Episodes

Episode Trigger	Mode Switch
Collection Delay	0 sec
Detection Rate	175 bpm
Detection Duration	No Delay

Episode Data

VHR Episodes	0
AHR Episodes	26,524 (23.3 hrs/day - 96.9%)
PVC Singles	407
PVC Runs	83
PAC Runs	7,079,859

Ventricular High Rate Episodes

Detection Rate	180 ppm
Detection Beats	5 beats
Termination Beats	2 beats

Type	Date/Time	Duration hh:mm:ss	Rates (bpm): Max A	Max V	Avg V	Sensor
AHR	12/13/02 11:04 AM	:04:00	254	78	66	72
AHR	12/25/02 10:34 AM	3:18:02	272	135	91	88
AHR	03/20/03 1:23 PM	>96:00:00	254	130	69	61
AHR	04/24/03 1:46 PM	:11	163	126	109	88

A

Atrial High Rate Monitor Detail	Page 1

Atrial High Rate Monitor Detail Zoom - Onset Collected - 04/24/03 3:58 PM

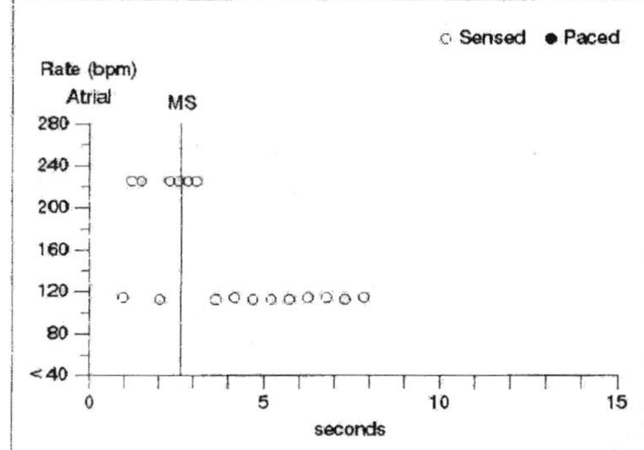

Initial Interrogation

Mode	DDDR
Lower Rate	60 ppm
Upper Tracking Rate	130 ppm
Upper Sensor Rate	130 ppm
Episode Trigger	Mode Switch
Collection Delay	0 sec
Detection Rate	175 bpm
Detection Duration	No Delay

Episode Data

Duration (hh:mm:ss)	00:30:50
Max Atrial Rate	239 bpm
Max Vent. Rate	116 bpm

B

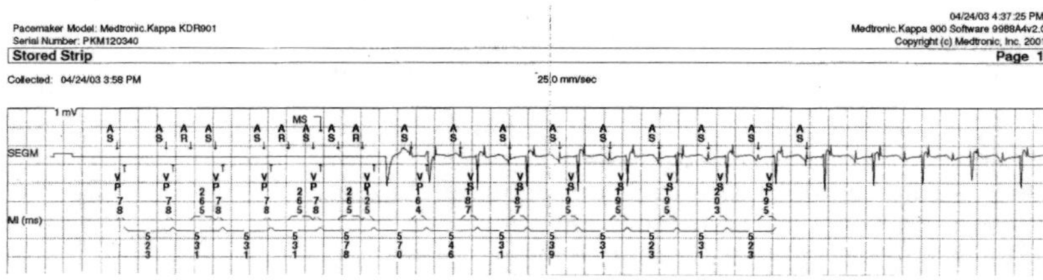

C

Figure 7.28. This is a subsystem performance counter retrieved from a Medtronic Kappa 900 pulse generator. **A:** Page 1 of the High Rate Episode report provides key information on the initial list of episodes with a time and date stamp (AHR = atrial high rate). There is a second page with additional episodes summarized in a similar manner. **B:** This is the High Rate Detail report for one of these episodes. **C:** This is the stored EGM for the episode shown in the High Rate Detail report. The summed EGM (SEGM) records the signal between the atrial and ventricular tip electrodes. Availability of high specific-event diagnostics facilitates the clinician's ability to understand system behavior and episodes that have occurred between scheduled office visits.

events in the specific sequence of their occurrence. These are classified as time-based system performance counters (Fig. 7.30). They have many names, including "rolling trend" and "event record."

There are two subsets to the time-based system performance counter. One is that specific events such as activation of a unique algorithm trigger storage of that event for retrieval at a later date. These are often associated with a time and date stamp (see Fig. 7.28). These, however, will not recognize a symptomatic event that does not also invoke one of the special algorithms in the device.

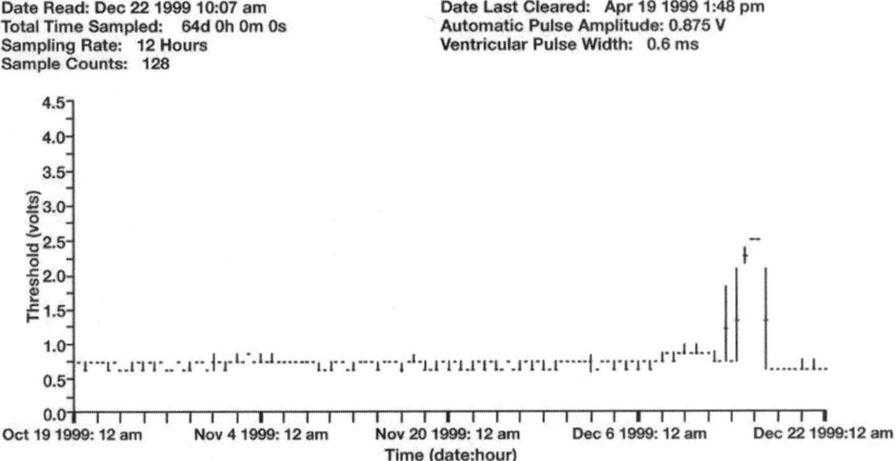

Figure 7.29. Long-term threshold record from a patient with a St. Jude Medical Affinity DR pulse generator with AutoCapture enabled. This is another subsystem performance counter. In this case, it demonstrates a protracted period of a stable low capture threshold in the range of 0.75 V. An abrupt marked increase in the capture threshold occurred 1 week before a scheduled follow-up evaluation. The time course of the threshold rise correlated with an episode of severe acute gastroenteritis resulting in dehydration and marked electrolyte imbalance necessitating hospitalization for a period of 3 days for fluid resuscitation and stabilization. No problems had been suspected with the pacing system and the marked threshold rise was only recognized in retrospect. Had AutoCapture not been enabled and the pacemaker programmed to the standard 2:1 safety margin, there would have been loss of capture. (Reprinted by permission from Levine PA. Guidelines to the Routine Evaluation, Programming and Follow-up of the Patient with an Implanted Dual-Chamber Rate-Modulated Pacing System. Sylmar, CA: St. Jude Medical CRMD, 2003.)

Figure 7.30. A combination of a subsystem and time-based system performance counter from Guidant providing a date stamp for periodic automatic measurements of signal amplitudes and stimulation impedances. This is displayed in both tabular and graphic formats. The total duration of this diagnostic is one year. After that, as new data are added, the oldest data are deleted. Where a signal is not available for measurement because of pacing, the value is reported as NR. When pacing is absent due to continued sensing, the impedance value is reported as NR.

Guidant			Discovery II
			06-AUG-2003 12:53
Institution	CTR.		
Patient		Programmer	037430
Model 1283	Serial 618934	2891 Software	2.7

Daily Measurement - Data Table

Date	Atrial Amplitude (mV)	Atrial Impedance (Ω)	Ventricular Amplitude (mV)	Ventricular Impedance (Ω)
05-AUG-2003	0.6	420	N.R.	370
04-AUG-2003	N.R.	420	N.R.	370
03-AUG-2003	N.R.	420	N.R.	370
02-AUG-2003	N.R.	410	N.R.	370
01-AUG-2003	N.R.	420	N.R.	370
31-JUL-2003	N.R.	410	N.R.	370
30-JUL-2003	N.R.	400	N.R.	370
25-JUL-2003	N.R.	400	N.R.	360
18-JUL-2003	N.R.	410	N.R.	370
11-JUL-2003	N.R.	410	N.R.	370
04-JUL-2003	N.R.	410	N.R.	370
27-JUN-2003	N.R.	410	5.0	380
20-JUN-2003	1.1	410	N.R.	370
13-JUN-2003	N.R.	420	N.R.	380
06-JUN-2003	0.6	420	N.R.	380
30-MAY-2003	N.R.	410	N.R.	380
23-MAY-2003	N.R.	410	N.R.	400
16-MAY-2003	1.4	410	>9.0	380
09-MAY-2003	N.R.	410	N.R.	380
02-MAY-2003	N.R.	410	N.R.	400
25-APR-2003	1.7	410	6.5	400
18-APR-2003	0.7	410	8.9	400
11-APR-2003	N.R.	410	N.R.	400
04-APR-2003	N.R.	410	N.R.	400
28-MAR-2003	N.R.	410	N.R.	400
21-MAR-2003	N.R.	410	>9.0	400
14-MAR-2003	N.R.	410	N.R.	400
07-MAR-2003	N.R.	420	N.R.	400
28-FEB-2003	0.6	410	5.7	400
21-FEB-2003	N.R.	420	>9.0	400
14-FEB-2003	N.R.	420	8.0	410
07-FEB-2003	1.8	410	8.9	400
31-JAN-2003	N.R.	420	>9.0	410
24-JAN-2003	1.6	420	7.2	410
17-JAN-2003	N.R.	430	7.1	410
10-JAN-2003	1.0	420	N.R.	410
03-JAN-2003	1.4	420	7.7	410
27-DEC-2002	1.6	410	N.R.	410
20-DEC-2002	1.6	420	>9.0	410
13-DEC-2002	N.R.	420	>9.0	410
06-DEC-2002	N.R.	420	N.R.	410
29-NOV-2002	N.R.	420	8.5	410
22-NOV-2002	1.7	420	N.R.	420
15-NOV-2002	1.7	420	N.R.	410
08-NOV-2002	1.6	420	8.0	410
01-NOV-2002	2.1	420	>9.0	410
25-OCT-2002	N.R.	420	>9.0	420
18-OCT-2002	N.R.	420	7.7	420
11-OCT-2002	1.8	420	6.4	420
04-OCT-2002	2.0	420	N.R.	420
27-SEP-2002	N.R.	420	N.R.	410
20-SEP-2002	2.6	420	>9.0	410
13-SEP-2002	1.8	420	8.4	410
06-SEP-2002	2.0	420	7.0	410
30-AUG-2002	N.R.	420	7.4	420
23-AUG-2002	N.R.	420	N.R.	420
16-AUG-2002	N.R.	420	8.8	420
09-AUG-2002	1.6	420	8.7	420
02-AUG-2002	1.1	420	>9.0	420

With the continuous recording, the patient may be able to activate a marker to identify the event. The "simple" event counters have been expanded to actual storage of the atrial and/or ventricular electrograms greatly facilitating the diagnosis of infrequent intermittent arrhythmias that either cause symptoms or trigger unique behaviors in the pacemaker.

SUMMARY

As mentioned at the beginning of this chapter, it is important to maintain appropriate records containing all the baseline data and results of the periodic detailed evaluations of the pacing system. These records provide the substrate on which to assess a new observation or information. For biventricular systems, it is helpful to have 12-lead ECGs showing the native depolarization, RV pacing, LV pacing, and biventricular pacing. Depending on the capabilities of the implanted system, it may need to be recorded during the implant procedure. One should also take advantage of the diagnostic capabilities incorporated into many present-generation pacemakers. These features include programmed parameter interrogation, lead and battery function telemetry, event marker and electrogram telemetry, and event counters for native and paced events, including sensor performance and other unique algorithms. Examples of many of these capabilities have been used to illustrate the various conditions described throughout this chapter and a simplified schematic for pacemaker troubleshooting is shown in Figure 7.31.

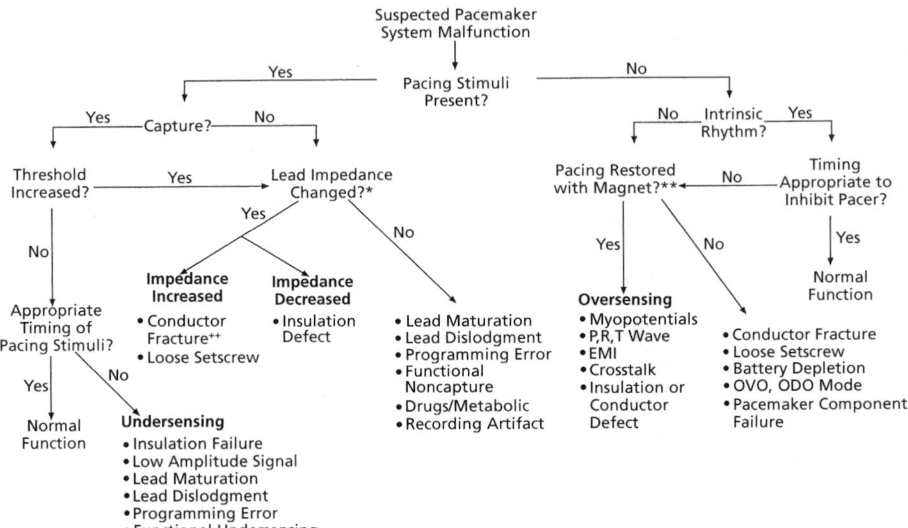

Figure 7.31. Simplified schematic for pacemaker troubleshooting. EMI = electromagnetic interference; *greater than 300 ohm change in impedance as measured at the time of malfunction; **or programmed to asynchronous mode; can have no change in impedance with concomitant insulation failure.

Although these features are helpful, there is no substitute for a thorough understanding of the pacing system, the patient, and the fundamental concepts of pacing.

When a true pacing system malfunction is encountered, the full differential diagnosis should be considered. This includes primary problems arising with the pulse generator, the lead(s), and the patient, as well as the interaction between these three components. It is embarrassing, expensive, and potentially dangerous to subject the patient to an operative procedure to replace a normally functioning pacemaker when the observed "problem" could have been easily corrected by programming the pacemaker or reflected a system eccentricity and was normal. Thus, any prior data that are available should be reviewed, the programmed parameters of the pacing system should be obtained, and all available diagnostic features of the given device should be used before arriving at a final decision and plan. If there are still concerns, each manufacturer provides 24/7 technical support before deciding on an operative intervention. To do less than this may result in an incorrect diagnosis—to the detriment of the patient, the physician, and the overall healthcare economy.

REFERENCES

1. Song SL. The Bilitch report: performance of implantable cardiac rhythm management devices. Pacing Clin Electrophysiol 1994;17:692–704.
2. Furman S, Benedek ZM, Andrews CA, et al. Long-term follow-up of pacemaker lead system. Pacing Clin Electrophysiol 1995;18:271–285.
3. Levine PA. The complementary role of electrogram, event marker and measured data telemetry in the assessment of pacing system function. J Electrophysiol 1987;1: 404–416.
4. Ohm OJ, Breivik K, Hammer EA, et al. Intraoperative electrical measurements during pacemaker implantation. Clin Prog Pacing Electrophysiol 1984;2:1–23.
5. Arnold AG. Predictive value of ST segment elevation in cardiac pacing. Br Heart J 1980;44:416–418.
6. Levine PA, Schuller H, Lindgren A. Pacemaker ECG—an introduction and approach to interpretation. Solna, Sweden: Siemens-Pacesetter, 1986.
7. Sheffield LT, Berson AL, Bragg-Remschel D, et al. AHA special report: recommendation for standards of instrumentation and practice in the use of ambulatory electrocardiography. Circulation 1985;71:626A–636A.
8. Cherry R, Sactuary C, Kennedy HL. The question of frequency response. Amb Electrocardiol 1977;1:13–14.
9. Hecht SR, Berdoff RL. Radiographic recognition of pacemaker lead complications. Clin Prog Electrophysiol Pacing 1986;4:189–198.
10. Veltri EP, Mower MM, Reid PR. Twiddler's syndrome: a new twist. Pacing Clin Electrophysiol 1984;7:1004–1009.
11. Furman S, Pannizzo F, Campo I. Comparison of active and passive adhering leads for endocardial pacing. Pacing Clin Electrophysiol 1979;2:417–427.
12. Trautwein W. Electrophysiological aspects of cardiac stimulation. In: Schaldach M, Furman S, eds. Advances in Pacemaker Technology. New York: Springer-Verlag, 1975:11–23.

13. Furman S, Hurzeler P, Mehra R. Cardiac pacing and pacemakers IV. Threshold of cardiac stimulation. Am Heart J 1977;94:115–124.
14. Irnich W. The chronaxie time and its practical importance. Pacing Clin Electrophysiol 1980;3:292–301.
15. Preston TA, Fletcher RD, Lucchesi BR, et al. Changes in myocardial threshold. Physiologic and pharmacologic factors in patients with implanted pacemakers. Am Heart J 1967;74:235–242.
16. Sowton E, Barr I. Physiologic changes in threshold. Ann NY Acad Sci USA 1969;167:679–685.
17. Preston TA, Judge RD. Alteration of pacemaker threshold by drug and physiologic factors. Ann NY Acad Sci USA 1969;167:686–692.
18. Beanlands DS, Akyurekli Y, Keon WJ. Prednisone in the management of exit block. In: Meere C, ed. Proceedings of the Sixth World Symposium on Cardiac Pacing. Montreal, 1979:Chapter 18–3.
19. Mond H, Stokes K, Helland J, et al. The porous titanium steroid-eluting electrode: a double-blind study assessing the stimulation threshold effects of steroid. Pacing Clin Electrophysiol 1988;11:214–219.
20. Klein HH, Steinberger J, Knake W. Stimulation characteristics of a steroid-eluting electrode compared with three conventional electrodes. Pacing Clin Electrophysiol 1990;13:134–137.
21. Crossley GH, Reynolds D, Kay GN, et al. Treatment of patients with prior exit block using a novel steroid-eluting active fixation lead. Pacing Clin Electrophysiol 1994;17:2042–2046.
22. Ellenbogen KA, Wood MA, Gilligan DM, et al. Steroid eluting high impedance pacing leads decrease short- and long-term current drain: results from a multicenter clinical trial. CapSure Z investigators. Pacing Clin Electrophysiol 1999;22:39–48.
23. O'Reilly MV, Murnaghan DP, Williams MD. Transvenous pacemaker failure induced by hyperkalemia. JAMA 1974;228:336–337.
24. Hughes JC Jr, Tyers GFO, Torman HA. Effects of acid–base imbalance on myocardial pacing thresholds. J Thorac Cardiovasc Surg 1975;69:743–746.
25. Lee D, Greenspan K, Edmands RE, Fisch C. The effect of electrolyte alteration on stimulus requirement of cardiac pacemakers. Circulation 1968;38:VI–124.
26. Gettes LS, Shabetai R, Downs TA, et al. Effect of changes in potassium and calcium concentrations on diastolic threshold and strength–interval relationships of the human heart. Ann NY Acad Sci USA 1969;167:693–705.
27. Fornieles-Perez H, Montoya-Garcia M, Levine PA, Sanz O. Documentation of acute rise in ventricular capture threshold associated with flecainide acetate, PACE 2001;25:871–872.
28. Levick CE, Mizgala HF, Kerr CR. Failure to pace following high dose antiarrhythmic therapy—reversal with isoproterenol. Pacing Clin Electrophysiol 1984;7:252–256.
29. Nielsen AP, Griffin JC, Herre JM, et al. Effect of amiodarone on acute and chronic pacing thresholds. Pacing Clin Electrophysiol 1984;7:462.
30. Hayes DL. Effect of drugs and devices on permanent pacemakers. Cardiology 1991;8:70–75.
31. Szabo Z, Solti F. The significance of the tissue reaction around the electrode on the late myocardial threshold. In: Schaldach M, Furman S, eds. Advances in Pacemaker Technology. New York: Springer-Verlag, 1975:273–287.

32. Love CJ, Wilkoff BL, Byrd CL, et al. Recommendations for extraction of chronically implanted transvenous pacing and defibrillation leads: indications, facilities, training (NASPE Policy Statement). Pacing Clin Electrophysiol 2000;23:544–551.
33. Ben-Zur UM, Platt SB, Gross JN, et al. Direct and telemetered lead impedance. Pacing Clin Electrophysiol 1994;17:2004–2007.
34. Sholder J, Duncan J, Helland J. Clinical and technical considerations of bipolar coaxial pacing leads. Technical Memorandum No. 17. Sylmar, CA: Pacesetter Systems Inc., July 1991.
35. Dunlap TE, Popak KD, Sorkin RP. Radiographic pseudofracture of the Medtronic bipolar polyurethane pacing lead. Am Heart J 1983;106:167–168.
36. Magney JE, Flynn DM, Parsons JA, et al. Anatomical mechanisms explaining damage to pacemaker leads, defibrillator leads and failure of central venous catheters adjacent to the sternoclavicular joint. Pacing Clin Electrophysiol 1993;16:445–457.
37. Jacobs DM, Fink AS, Miller RP, et al. Anatomical and morphologic evaluation of pacemaker lead compression. Pacing Clin Electrophysiol 1993;16:434–444.
38. Magney JE, Staplin DH, Flynn DM, et al. A new approach to percutaneous subclavian venipuncture to avoid lead fracture or central venous catheter occlusion. Pacing Clin Electrophysiol 1993;16:2133–2142.
39. Ong LS, Barold SS, Lederman M, et al. Cephalic vein guidewire technique for implantation of permanent pacemakers. Am Heart J 1987;114:753–756.
40. Levine PA. Clinical manifestations of lead insulation defects. J Electrophysiol 1987;1:144–155.
41. Kreis DJ, LiCalzi L, Shaw RK. Air entrapment as a cause of transient cardiac pacemaker malfunction. Pacing Clin Electrophysiol 1979;2:641–643.
42. Hauser RG, Edwards LN, Giuffree VF. Limitations of pacemaker system analyzers for the evaluation of implantable pulse generators. Pacing Clin Electrophysiol 1981;4:650–657.
43. Ohm OJ. Demand failures occurring during permanent pacing in patients with serious heart disease. Pacing Clin Electrophysiol 1980;3:44–55.
44. Berg M, Frohlig G, Schwerdt H, et al. Reliability of an automatic sensing algorithm. PACE 1992;15:1880–1885.
45. Strathmore NF. Interference in cardiac pacemakers. In: Ellenbogen K, Kay GN, Wilkoff BL, eds. Clinical Cardiac Pacing. Philadelphia: WB Saunders, 1995:770–779.
46. Fetter J, Bobeldyk GL, Engman FJ. The clinical incidence and significance of myopotential sensing with unipolar pacemakers. Pacing Clin Electrophysiol 1984;7: 871–881.
47. Ohm OJ, Morkrid L, Hammer E. Amplitude–frequency characteristics of myopotentials and endocardial potentials as seen by a pacemaker system. Scand J Thorac Cardiovasc Surg Supp 1978;22:41–46.
48. Halperin JL, Camunas JL, Stern EH, et al. Myopotential interference with DDD pacemakers: endocardial electrographic telemetry in the diagnosis of pacemaker-related arrhythmias. Am J Cardiol 1984;54:97–102.
49. Gabry MD, Behrens M, Andrews C, et al. Comparison of myopotential interference in unipolar–bipolar programmable DDD pacemakers. Pacing Clin Electrophysiol 1987;10:1322–1330.
50. Sager DP. Current facts on pacemaker electromagnetic interference and their application to clinical care. Heart Lung 1987;16:211–221.
51. Sarmiento J. Clinical utility of telemetered intracardiac electrograms in diagnosis of design dependent lead malfunction. PACE 1990;13:188–195.

52. Ellenbogen KA, Thames MD, Mohanty PK. New insights into pacemaker syndrome gained from hemodynamic, humoral and vascular responses during ventriculoatrial pacing. Am J Cardiol 1990;65:53–59.
53. Heldman D, Mulvihill D, Nguyen H, et al. True incidence of pacemaker syndrome. Pacing Clin Electrophysiol 1990;13:526.
54. Gee W. Ocular pneumoplethysmography in cardiac pacing. Pacing Clin Electrophysiol 1983;6:1268–1272.
55. Rediker DE, Eagle KA, Homma S, et al. Clinical and hemodynamic comparison of VVI versus DDD pacing in patients with DDD pacemakers. Am J Cardiol 1988;61: 323–329.
56. Frohlig G, Schwerdt H, Schieffer H, et al. Atrial signal variations and pacemaker malsensing during exercise: A study in the time and frequency domain. J Am Coll Cardiol 1988;11:806–813.
57. Lipchenca I, Garrigue S, Glickson M, et al. Inhibition of biventricular pacemaker by oversensing of far field atrial depolarizations. PACE 2000;23:1735–1737.
58. Sweesy MW, Batey RL, Forney RC. Crosstalk during bipolar pacing. Pacing Clin Electrophysiol 1988;11:1512–1516.
59. Barold SS, Belott PH. Behavior of the ventricular triggering period of DDD pacemakers. Pacing Clin Electrophysiol 1987;10:1237–1252.
60. Brandt J, Worzewski W. Far-field QRS complex sensing: prevalence and timing with bipolar atrial leads. Pacing Clin Electrophysiol 2000;23:315–320.
61. Greenspan AJ, Greenberg RM, Frank WS. Tracking of atrial flutter by DDD pacing, another form of pacemaker mediated tachycardia. Pacing Clin Electrophysiol 1984;7:955–960.
62. Den Dulk K, Lindemans FW, Bar FW, et al. Pacemaker-related tachycardias. Pacing Clin Electrophysiol 1982;5:476–485.
63. Levine PA. Postventricular atrial refractory periods and pacemaker mediated tachycardias. Clin Prog Pacing Electrophysiol 1983;1:394–401.
64. Furman S, Fisher JD. Endless-loop tachycardia in an AV universal (DDD) pacemaker. Pacing Clin Electrophysiol 1982;5:486–489.
65. Van Gelder LM, El Gamal MIH, Sanders RS. Tachycardia-termination algorithm: a valuable feature for interruption of pacemaker mediated tachycardia. Pacing Clin Electrophysiol 1984;7:283–287.
66. Barold SS, Byrd CL. Cross-ventricular endless loop tachycardia during biventricular pacing. PACE 2001;24:1821–1823.
67. Levine PA, Love CJ. Pacemaker diagnostics and evaluation of pacing system malfunction. In: Ellenbogen KA, Kay N, Wilkoff BL, eds. Clinical Cardiac Pacing and Defibrillation. 2nd ed. Philadelphia: WB Saunders, 2000:827–875.
68. Freedman RA, Marks ML, Chapman P. Telemetered pacemaker battery voltage preceding generator elective replacement time: use of guide utilization of magnet checks. Pacing Clin Electrophysiol 1995;18:863.
69. Castallenet M, Garza J, Shaners SP, et al. Telemetry of programmed and measured data in pacing system evaluation and follow-up. J Electrophysiol 1987;1:360–375.
70. Winokur P, Falkenberg E, Gerrard G. Lead resistance telemetry: insulation failure prognosticator. Pacing Clin Electrophysiol 1985;8:A–85.
71. Levine PA, Sanders R, Markowitz HT. Pacemaker diagnostics: measured data, event marker, electrogram and event counter telemetry. In: Ellenbogen K, Kay GN, Wilkoff BL, eds. Clinical Cardiac Pacing. Philadelphia: WB Saunders, 1995:639–655.

72. Kruse I, Markowitz HT, Ryden L. Timing markers showing pacemaker behavior to aid in the follow-up of a physiologic pacemaker. Pacing Clin Electrophysiol 1983;6:801–805.
73. Olson W, Goldreyer BA, Goldreyer BN. Computer-generated diagnostic diagrams for pacemaker rhythm analysis and pacing system evaluation. J Electrophysiol 1987;1:367–387.
74. Goldschalger N. After the implant: principles of follow-up, intel reports. Cardiac Pacing Electrophysiol 1991;10:1–4.
75. Levine PA, Sholder J, Duncan JL. Clinical benefits of telemetered electrograms in the assessment of DDD function. Pacing Clin Electrophysiol 1984;7:1170–1177.
76. Sarmiento JJ. Clinical utility of telemetered intracardiac electrograms in diagnosing a design-dependent lead malfunction. Pacing Clin Electrophysiol 1990;13:188–195.
77. Newman D, Dorian P, Downar E, et al. Use of telemetry functions in the assessment of implanted antitachycardia device efficiency. Am J Cardiol 1992;70:616–621.
78. Hayes DL, Higano ST, Eisinger G. Utility of rate histograms in programming and follow-up of a DDDR pacemaker. Mayo Clin Proc 1989;64:495–502.
79. Lascault GR, Frank R, Himbert C, et al. Pacemaker Holter function and monitoring atrial arrhythmias. Eur JCPE 1992;2:285–293.

The Implantable Cardioverter Defibrillator

Michael R. Gold

8

The implantable cardioverter-defibrillator (ICD) has undergone a remarkable transformation over the past 20 years. The early devices were large, requiring thoracotomy for epicardial patch placement, and were implanted in the abdomen. This complex surgery resulted in postoperative hospitalization averaging approximately 1 week. The pulse generators had a longevity of less than 2 years, had almost no diagnostic capabilities, and had pacing capabilities that were limited to only backup ventricular pacing. Modern devices provide detailed information about the morphology and rates of arrhythmias, and store electrocardiographic signals before, during, and after therapy. Heart rate variability and rates are catalogued independent of arrhythmias and lead impedance and sensed electrogram amplitudes (i.e., R-waves and P-waves) are measured regularly and stored in memory. The downsizing of pulse generators, in combination with improvements of lead design and shock waveforms, allows the simplicity of defibrillator implantation to approach that of pacemakers, with outpatient placement now feasible. Despite the marked reduction in size and increase in diagnostic capabilities, device longevity is now over 6 years. Devices have the capabilities to treat multiple problems, not only life-threatening ventricular arrhythmias but also bradyarrhythmias with dual-chamber devices, atrial arrhythmias, and congestive heart failure with biventricular pacing.

INDICATIONS

The indications for ICD implantation remained unchanged for many years. Initially, the devices were only implanted in patients who had survived an aborted cardiac arrest or an episode of sustained ventricular tachycardia that was refractory to antiarrhythmic drug therapy. The use of ICDs for the secondary prevention of sudden cardiac death was the standard for more than a decade. However, several landmark studies established the role of ICD therapy for primary prevention of sudden death in high-risk subjects, and today a majority of new implants in the United States are performed for this indication. A summary of the current indications for ICD therapy is shown in Box 8.1.[1]

Box 8.1. Indications for Implantable Cardioverter-Defibrillator Therapy

Class I

1. Cardiac arrest due to ventricular tachycardia or ventricular fibrillation not due to a transient or reversible cause.
2. Spontaneous sustained ventricular tachycardia in association with structural heart disease.
3. Unexplained syncope with clinically relevant and hemodynamically significant sustained ventricular tachycardia, or ventricular tachycardia induced at electrophysiology study, when drug therapy is ineffective, not tolerated, or not preferred.
4. Nonsustained ventricular tachycardia with coronary artery disease, prior myocardial infarction, left ventricular dysfunction, and inducible sustained ventricular tachycardia or fibrillation at electrophysiology study that is not suppressible by a Class I antiarrhythmic drug.
5. Spontaneous sustained VT in patients who do not have structural heart disease that is not amenable to other treatments.

Class IIa

1. Patients with LV ejection fraction ≤ 30%, at least 1 month post myocardial infarction and 3 months post coronary artery revascularization surgery.

Class IIb

1. Cardiac arrest presumed to be due to ventricular fibrillation when electrophysiology testing is precluded by other medical conditions.
2. Severe symptoms (e.g., syncope) attributable to sustained ventricular tachyarrhythmias while awaiting cardiac transplantation.
3. Familial or inherited conditions with a high risk for life-threatening ventricular tachyarrhythmias such as long QT syndrome or hypertrophic cardiomyopathy.
4. Nonsustained ventricular tachycardia with coronary artery disease, prior myocardial infarction, left ventricular dysfunction, and inducible sustained ventricular tachycardia or fibrillation at electrophysiology study.
5. Recurrent syncope of undetermined etiology in the presence of ventricular dysfunction and inducible ventricular arrhythmias at electrophysiology study when other causes of syncope have been excluded.
6. Syncope of unexplained etiology or family history of unexplained sudden cardiac death in association with typical or atypical right bundle-branch block and ST-segment elevations (Brugada syndrome)
7. Syncope in patients with advanced structural heart disease in which thorough invasive and noninvasive investigation has failed to define a cause.

The AVID study compared ICD implantation with antiarrhythmic drug use (primarily amiodarone) in patients with aborted cardiac arrest or poorly tolerated ventricular tachycardia (VT).[2] Patients were randomized to initial therapy with an ICD or to class III antiarrhythmic drugs. There was a significant reduction in mortality in the groups randomized to ICD implantation. The benefit of the ICD was most marked in the patients with a reduced left ventricular ejection fraction (≤0.35). In the Canadian Implantable Defibrillator

Study (CIDS), 659 patients with ventricular tachycardia, ventricular fibrillation, or syncope were randomized to antiarrhythmic therapy with amiodarone or ICD implantation. A 20% reduction in mortality was observed in the ICD group, although it did not reach statistical significance.[3] However, subsequent analyses showed that a left ventricular ejection fraction less than 0.35, age over 70 years, and advanced congestive heart failure were characteristics of the patients who were most likely to benefit from ICD implantation.[4] In the CASH study, 288 patients with a history of cardiac arrest were randomized to receive metoprolol, amiodarone, propafenone, or to undergo ICD implantation. There was an increased mortality in the group treated with propafenone, and a 28% decreased mortality at the 4-year follow-up evaluation in the patients who received ICDs.[5] These studies established the benefit of ICD therapy as first-line treatment among patients with a history of life-threatening arrhythmias (i.e., secondary prevention), particularly in individuals with left ventricular dysfunction; thus, antiarrhythmic drugs have been relegated to adjunctive therapy to reduce arrhythmia recurrence rates. The AVID II study will address the issue directly of the role of ICD therapy for secondary prevention among patients with preserved left ventricular systolic function.

Once the relative safety of ICD implantation became apparent, the use of this therapy for primary prevention of sudden death was studied. The MADIT and MUSTT trials evaluated patients with coronary artery disease, left ventricular systolic dysfunction, nonsustained ventricular tachycardia, and inducible sustained monomorphic ventricular tachycardia. In the MADIT study, patients were randomized to either receive an ICD or "conventional" medical therapy, which was most commonly amiodarone.[6] In the MUSTT study, patients were randomized to either no antiarrhythmic therapy or electrophysiologically guided drug therapy. In 46% of the latter group, ICD implantation was performed because of the failure of antiarrhythmic drugs to suppress inducible arrhythmias.[7] Despite these differences in study design, the results of the two trials were remarkably similar; ICD use decreased mortality more than 50% in these cohorts with ischemic cardiomyopathy.[8]

It is interesting that the magnitude of mortality reduction in these primary prevention trials appears even larger than in the studies of patients with a history of aborted cardiac arrest or sustained ventricular tachycardia. One possible explanation for this apparent paradox is that the groups who were evaluated in primary prevention studies had lower mean ejection fractions and higher incidences of congestive heart failure, two potent predictors of mortality.

Expanding the indications for ICD use is an area of intense investigation. The analysis of the MUSTT registry of patients with coronary artery disease, reduced ejection fraction, and no inducible sustained ventricular tachycardia demonstrated a disturbingly high mortality rate, even though it was significantly lower than that among patients with inducible ventricular tachycardia.[9] This indicates that methods of risk stratification, other than by electrophysiology testing, are necessary. The MADIT II study was a prospective randomized trial of 1232 subjects with previous myocardial infarction and ejection fraction of

0.30 or less.[10] Spontaneous nonsustained VT or electrophysiology testing were not required for enrollment in this trial. The ICD and control groups had similar clinical characteristics with a mean age of approximately 65 years, 67% with congestive heart failure (NYHA II–IV) and mean left ventricular ejection fraction of 0.23. In addition, beta blocker and angiotensin converting-enzyme inhibitor use was approximately 70% among each group. During a mean follow-up of 20 months, the mortality rates were 14.2% in the ICD group and 19.8% in the control group (Hazard ratio 0.69, 95% confidence interval, 0.51–0.93, $P = .016$). In a controversial decision, reimbursement for ICD implantation among Medicare patients was approved only for those patients who met MADIT II criteria and had intraventricular conduction delay, as evidenced by a QRS duration of 120 milliseconds or greater.

Several other primary prevention studies evaluated patients with a reduced left ventricular ejection fraction without requiring the presence of coronary artery disease. The SCD HeFT study evaluated more than 2500 subjects with congestive heart failure (NYHA II and III) and left ventricular systolic dysfunction (ejection fraction ≤ 35%), irrespective of etiology (i.e., ischemic or nonischemic cardiomyopathies). ICD implantation, but not amiodarone, was shown to reduce all-cause mortality. Similar mortality reductions were observed among the subgroups with ischemic and nonischemic cardiomyopathies. The DEFINITE study randomized 458 subjects with dilated, nonischemic cardiomyopathy and frequent ventricular ectopy to receive an ICD or optimal medical therapy. There was a strong trend toward a mortality reduction in the ICD cohort, and a significant reduction in the incidence of sudden cardiac deaths ($P = .006$).[11]

Not all high-risk groups benefit from ICD implantation, as shown by the CABG Patch trial. In this study, patients with ischemic cardiomyopathy and an abnormal signal-averaged electrocardiogram were randomized to receive an ICD or no antiarrhythmic treatment at the time of coronary artery bypass surgery. No effect on mortality was observed with ICD use in this cohort.[12] The DINAMIT study evaluated patients with acute myocardial infarction, left ventricular systolic dysfunction and reduced heart rate variability. No mortality benefit was observed with ICD implantation. The reasons for the failure of these studies to show a benefit of ICD therapy are unclear. The use of noninvasive risk modifiers, such as signal-averaged ECG or heart rate variability, may be insufficient to identify a high-risk cohort. Also, the competing mortality risks early post-MI or post bypass surgery may offset any benefit of ICD therapy. However, these studies clearly demonstrate that clinical trials and not "common sense" needs to guide the decision to implant devices.

One cohort that is particularly difficult to manage is those patients with structural heart disease and a history of syncope. These patients have been excluded from most prospective, randomized studies because, on one hand, they do not have documented arrhythmias to be included in secondary prevention studies, and, on the other hand, they cannot be classified as asymptomatic to be included in primary prevention trials. Present guidelines recommend ICD implantation in patients with inducible ventricular tachycardia and syncope (see Box 8.1). However, initial treatment with an ICD in patients with syncope and dilated cardiomyopathy, regardless of the results of electrophysiology testing, is rapidly becoming standard clinical practice,[13,14] despite the lack of randomized studies to support this strategy. The retrospective analyses that have been performed consistently indicate high rates of appropriate ICD therapy in this population, comparable to patients with documented sustained ventricular arrhythmias. Many of these patients now meet other indications for ICD implantation (e.g., MADIT II or SCD HeFT), so their management is less controversial. Patients with primary electrical disease, such as the Brugada syndrome and long QT syndrome, are another cohort in whom ICD use is becoming more common, particularly in those patients with a history of syncope or ventricular arrhythmias.[15]

PULSE GENERATORS AND LEAD SYSTEMS

Early ICD pulse generators were large and bulky. The size (115 to 145 cm^3) and weight (195 to 235 g) of these devices mandated abdominal implantation, typically in the left upper quadrant either subcutaneously or most often under the rectus muscle. The surgical procedure for abdominal ICD implantation is more extensive than for endocardial pacemakers, in part because it requires tunneling leads from the chest. The abdominal location of the pulse generator and the surgical procedure required were likely responsible for the higher complication rates observed with early ICD implantation, particularly infection and lead fractures.

Modern pulse generator size has decreased significantly. With the downsizing of these devices (30 to 39 cm^3, 70 to 84 g), routine subcutaneous pectoral implantation is possible,[16] although these pulse generators are still significantly larger than pacemakers. This implantation approach is not associated with any increased risk of complications.[17] Despite the large size of the early pulse generators, their battery life was only approximately 2 years. With improvement in battery design and reduction of monitoring current drain, the expected life span of many ICD pulse generators is now more than 6 years. This has obvious and important implications for the cost effectiveness of this therapy.[18]

Modern ICD pulse generators have very sophisticated programmability and internal circuitry. All pulse generators have noninvasive pacing induction, with the capabilities for programmed ventricular stimulation. With real-time telemetry of intracardiac electrograms, the pacing, shocking impedances, and pacing thresholds of the ICD lead systems can be monitored noninvasively as well, to aid in the assessment of lead function. Detailed data logging is present, including precise measurements of arrhythmia rates, time of occurrence, and response to therapy. In addition, stored electrograms provide a recording of the arrhythmia at the time of device activity. This is most useful in assessing the appropriateness of therapy (i.e., shocks for atrial fibrillation versus ventricular tachycardia) and any malfunctions of the system. Finally, the capacitors in the pulse generator need to be charged periodically to avoid very prolonged charging during spontaneous arrhythmia; such capacitor reformation would mandate office visits every 2 to 3 months for patients, but now it is performed automatically by the pulse generator.

The lead systems for sensing, pacing, and the delivery of shocks have also changed significantly over the past decade. The evolution of ICD lead systems is shown in Figure 8.1. Although transvenous defibrillation was developed by

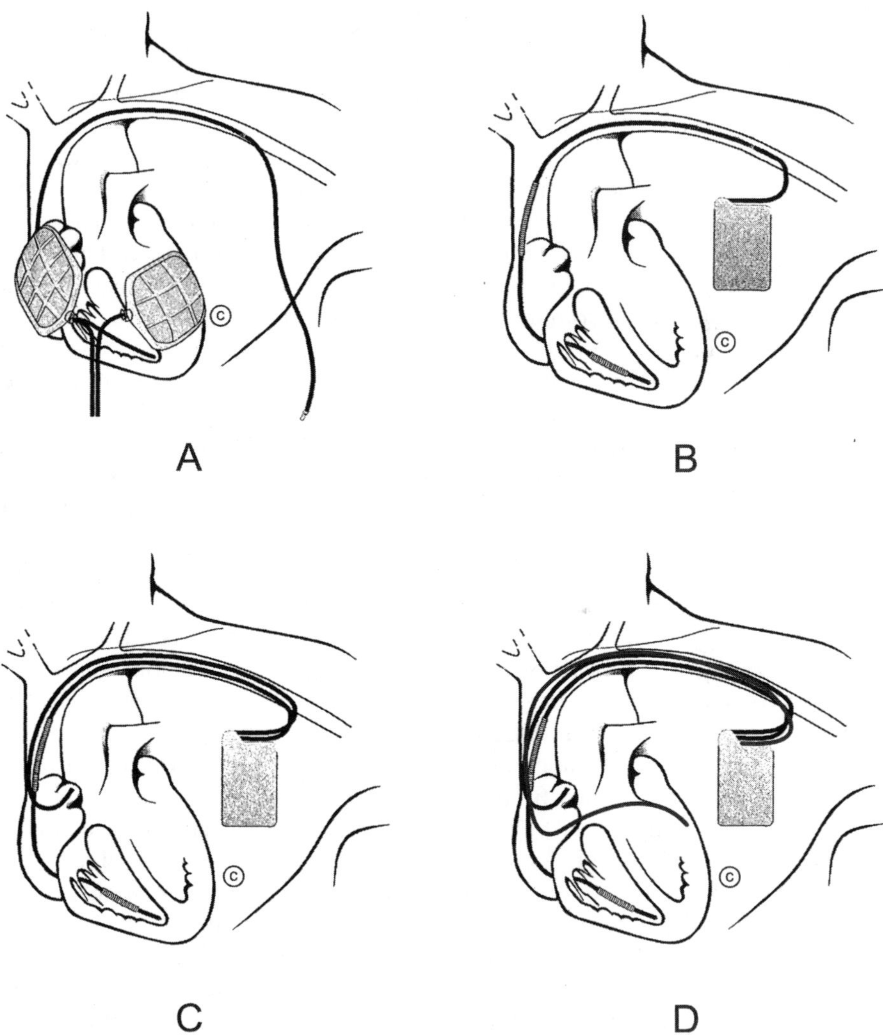

Figure 8.1. Schematic drawings of defibrillation lead systems. **A:** Epicardial system with two sensing leads on the left ventricle and patches on the left and right ventricles. **B:** Active pectoral pulse generator with dual coil lead system. **C:** Dual-chamber pectoral lead system. **D:** Biventricular ICD system (CRT-D).

Mirowski in his pioneering studies of the ICD,[19] the initial commercial systems used epicardial sensing leads and patches placed on the heart. Subsequently, the development of integrated leads incorporating both rate-sensing electrodes and defibrillation coils that led to the routine use of nonthoracotomy lead systems. The pectoral placement of pulse generators allowed further improvement in lead technology, because the pulse generator shell can serve as an extrathoracic electrode and actually become part of the lead system. These active pulse generator systems further simplify the implantation procedure while enhancing defibrillation efficacy.[20]

ICD leads can be coaxial or multilumen, with insulation of silicone, polyurethane, or fluoropolymers. Both single-coil and dual-coil defibrillation leads are available, with active or passive fixation. Coaxial lead design was dominant until the mid-1990s. This is characterized by a coiled conductor with an outside insulation layer, both surrounded by another conductor. Typically the tip conductor would be central with the ring conductor and then the defibrillation conductor more peripheral. Multilumen leads are preferred today, with conductors running in parallel through a single insulating lead body. The advantages of this design include greater space efficiency resulting in smaller leads, and greater resistance to compressive forces by including extra lumens within the lead body.

Lead insulation can have an important impact on long-term stability and function. Silicone is inert, biostable, and biocompatible, but has a high coefficient friction. It is soft, making it prone to damage during implantation and can swell over time. Polyurethane is biocompatible, has a high tensile strength making small lead diameters possible, and a low coefficient of friction, but is prone to environmental stress cracking and metal ion oxidation. Recent reports highlight the high failure rate of polyurethane leads,[21] so they should be avoided given the superiority of alternative insulators. Fluoropolymers (e.g., PTFE and ETFE) are the most biocompatible, have high tensile strength allowing small lead size, but are stiff, susceptible to damage from traction when the lead migrates, and they are prone to insulation micro defects and have a difficult manufacturing process. Today's lead systems have an insulating body of silicone, and in some instances supplemented by an outside polyurethane layer (not used for insulation) to reduce friction, abrasion, and scar formation. Metal ion oxidation is avoided as polyurethane is not in direct contact with the conductors. The conductors are often insulated with an extra thin layer of fluoropolymer.

Dual-chamber ICDs are now used more frequently than single chamber devices. For dual-chamber systems, a separate atrial lead is used. These are typically simple bipolar pacemaker leads, with no unique design for being part of an ICD. Radiographs of a dual-chamber lead system, including a dual-coil integrated defibrillation lead and an active left pectoral pulse generator, are shown in Figure 8.2. Despite the rapid acceptance of this technology, all of the early large studies establishing ICD indications evaluated only single-chamber systems. The first large study to evaluate directly the impact of dual chamber pacing

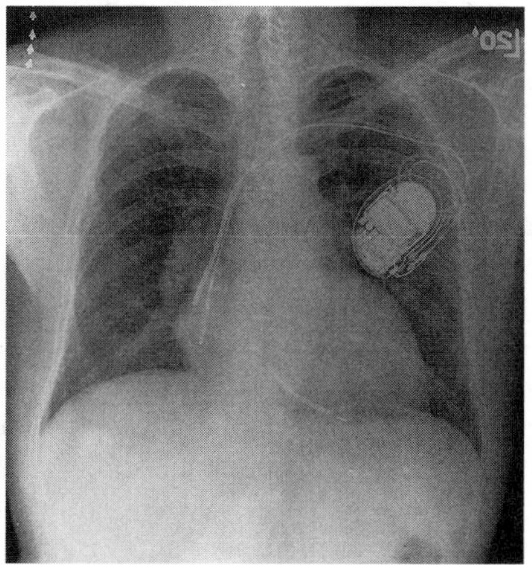

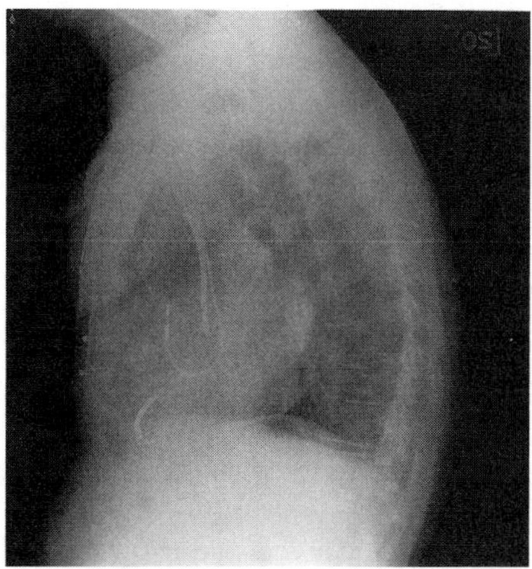

Figure 8.2. Radiographs of a dual-chamber ICD lead system. **Left:** Posterior-anterior view. **Right:** Lateral view. Note the integrated, dual-coil lead with the tip in right ventricular apex. There is a separate right atrial bipolar pacing lead and a left pectoral pulse generator.

among ICD patients was DAVID.[22] This was a single blind, randomized trial of 506 subjects with standard indications for ICDs. Patients underwent implantation with a dual chamber ICD and were randomized to ventricular backup pacing (VVI at 40 bpm) or dual chamber rate responsive pacing (DDDR at 70 bpm). Surprisingly, dual-chamber pacing was associated with worse clinical outcomes. The 1-year survival free of the primary endpoint of mortality or CHF hospitalization was 83.9% for patients randomized to VVI pacing and 73.3% for those patients randomized to DDDR pacing (Hazard ratio 1.61, $P \leq .03$). The results of this study have challenged the approach of indiscriminate use of dual chamber pacing among ICD patients.

IMPLANTABLE CARDIOVERTER-DEFIBRILLATOR IMPLANTATION

ICD systems are implanted by electrophysiologists in nearly 90% of patients, often without the use of an operating room or general anesthesia.[23] The downsizing of ICD pulse generators allowing for routine pectoral implantation simplified the operative procedure and costs,[24] so that the implantation technique now approaches that of a permanent pacemaker; however, the acute testing and management of these devices still requires electrophysiology expertise. It is for this reason that current guidelines require the presence of an electrophysiologist for the implantation procedure.[25]

Whether implanted in an operating room, a multipurpose procedure room, or an electrophysiology laboratory, and whether general anesthesia or conscious sedation are employed, the basic concepts of ICD surgery are the same. Meticulous sterile technique must be used and patients should receive perioperative intravenous antibiotics. The antibiotics chosen should provide adequate activity against staphylococcal species, as these are the most common bacteria associated with early device infections. Typically, vancomycin or a cephalosporin are used. Local irrigation of the pulse generator pocket with antibiotic solution is often performed, although controlled data establishing the efficacy of this additional step are lacking. A physiologic recorder is necessary for evaluating electrophysiologic signals, and heart rhythm, blood pressure, and respiration must be monitored. This can either be performed invasively with an arterial line and endotracheal intubation or more commonly with electrocardiographic monitoring, a brachial cuff, and pulse oximetry. Finally, the patient should be connected to a transthoracic defibrillator with skin pads for backup defibrillation therapy if needed during defibrillation testing. Two functional external defibrillators (preferably with a biphasic waveform) should always be available during defibrillation testing.

The sites of venous access and methods of obtaining access are similar to that for permanent pacemakers. Unless contraindicated by an atrioventricular (AV) fistula, venous anomaly, previous chest surgery (i.e., mastectomy), severe dermatologic conditions, or scarring, a left-sided approach is preferred. Cutdown to the cephalic vein or percutaneous axillary vein access may be preferable to subclavian puncture to reduce the incidence of subclavian crush observed with these large leads.[26] Leads need to be well secured to the pectoral fascia, because dislodgment of defibrillation leads remains the most common perioperative complication.[27] The transvenous defibrillator leads are implanted in the same fashion as pacemaker leads. The preferred location is the right ventricular apex with the distal coil entirely within the right ventricular cavity. Adequate sensing (R waves > 5 mV) and pacing (threshold < 1.0 V) of the right ventricular lead need to be established. If a dual-chamber ICD is implanted, then a separate atrial lead is placed, again with adequate sensing and pacing parameters required. Only bipolar leads are used in ICD systems. For dual-chamber devices, atrial leads with closely spaced electrodes are used to reduce the risk of far-field sensing of ventricular electrograms. For biventricular pacing ICDs (CRT-D), a third lead is implanted, typically in a lateral branch of the coronary sinus venous system. These leads are passive fixation and may be unipolar or bipolar.

Acute defibrillation testing is performed to ensure an adequate safety margin for the treatment of spontaneous arrhythmias. In common usage, the defibrillation threshold (DFT) is defined as the lowest energy that successfully terminates ventricular fibrillation. Unlike the pacing threshold, however, the DFT is *not* an absolute value above which defibrillation will always be successful and below which it will always fail. Instead, the likelihood of defibrillation at any energy level is a probability of success. The relationship between probability of successful defibrillation versus the energy delivered yields a sigmoidal shaped curve (Fig. 8.3). The goal of defibrillation testing is to ensure that the maximal energy output of the device has an extremely high (>99%) probability of terminating ventricular fibrillation in a given patient. There are different methods to determine the DFT, and each method provides a value with different significance.

The DFT value derived from each testing method establishes different positions on the defibrillation success curve for a given patient. For example, a single termination of fibrillation with a given energy level (DFT, Table 8.1) identifies an energy that may terminate fibrillation in as few as 25% of repeated attempts due to the probabilistic nature of defibrillation. By demonstrating that this same shock energy terminates ventricular fibrillation three times without failure; however, it may be concluded that that energy level is high on the probability curve for success and in fact has at least a 75% chance of terminating fibrillation on further attempts.[28]

Understanding precisely what a given DFT value represents allows the physician to program an appropriate safety margin of energy output above the DFT to ensure termination of all ventricular fibrillation episodes. In practice, the simple convention of programming output to 10J greater than the DFT is widely accepted and usually provides reliable defibrillation. This method is expedient at implant; but through careful DFT testing, lesser energy margins may be satisfactory as well[29] (Table 8.1).

There are many testing algorithms to assess defibrillation efficacy and determine a value for DFT (Fig. 8.4), but two methods predominate: the single-energy success and step-down protocols. For both methods, the first shock is typically set at least 10J less than the maximal output of the device. Ventricular fibrillation is induced by pacing through the right ventricular electrode or with a low-energy shock on the T wave. The pulse generator will then automatically sense the arrhythmia, charge, and deliver a shock. If the first shock is successful, then this energy level can be repeated once or twice more (single-energy success method). This technique allows for minimal testing to establish adequate acute defibrillation efficacy. Alternatively, in the "step-down method" the shock energy is decreased on each trial until a shock energy is reached that fails to defibrillate. The lowest energy level to successfully defibrillate is the DFT.[28] This energy level may be tested an additional one or two times if desired to further ensure the likelihood of success. Other algorithms that can be used to determine DFT are the binary search method, in which shock energy is decreased or increased depending on the results of the preceding defibrillation trial,[30] or the Bayesian search method (Fig. 8.4). When ICD shocks fail, a high-output internal or transthoracic shock should be given immediately for arrhythmia termination. There is increasing interest in minimizing defibrillation testing. Consequently, the practice of testing only one episode of ventricular fibrillation and then programming devices to maximum output is gaining in popularity. This strategy probably works because of the very high efficacy of modern lead system and shock waveforms.[31] There is even a growing practice of performing no defibrillation testing at the time of implantation, although the prospective data to support this strategy are lacking.

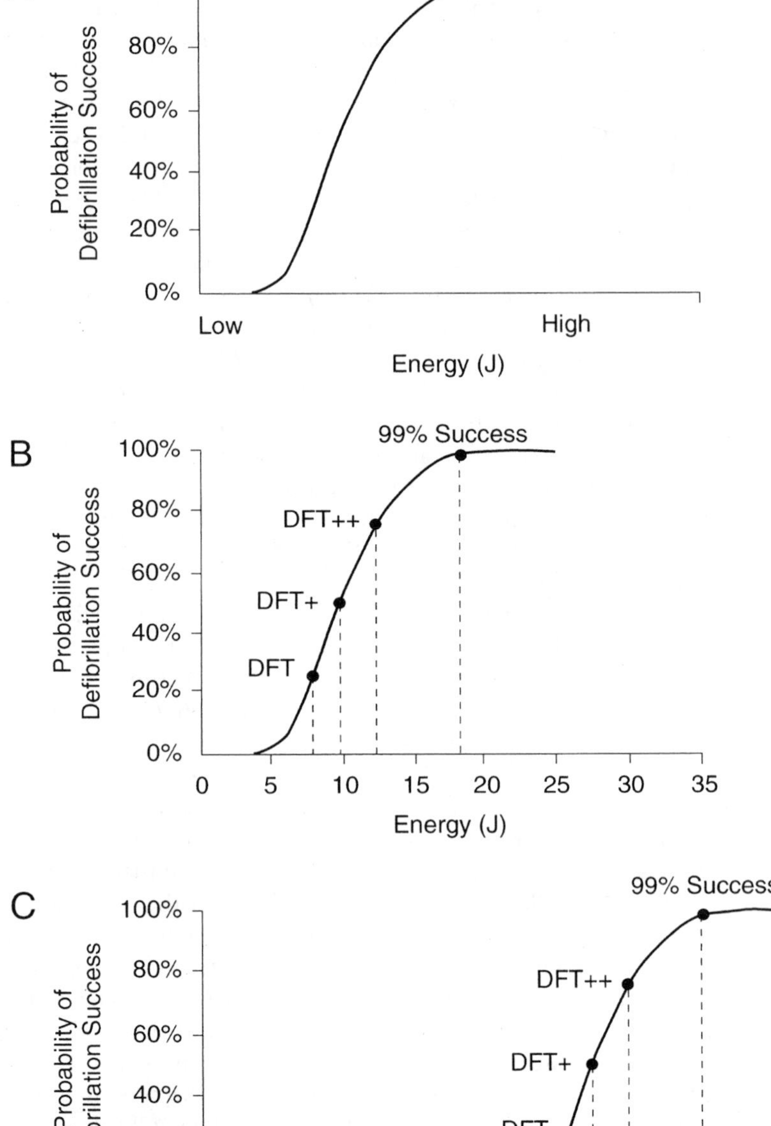
A
100%
80%
60%
40%
20%
0%
Probability of Defibrillation Success
Low
High
Energy (J)
B
99% Success
DFT++
DFT+
DFT
100%
80%
60%
40%
20%
0%
Probability of Defibrillation Success
0
5
10
15
20
25
30
35
Energy (J)
C
99% Success
DFT++
DFT+
DFT
100%
80%
60%
40%
20%
0%
Probability of Defibrillation Success
0
5
10
15
20
25
30
35
Energy (J)

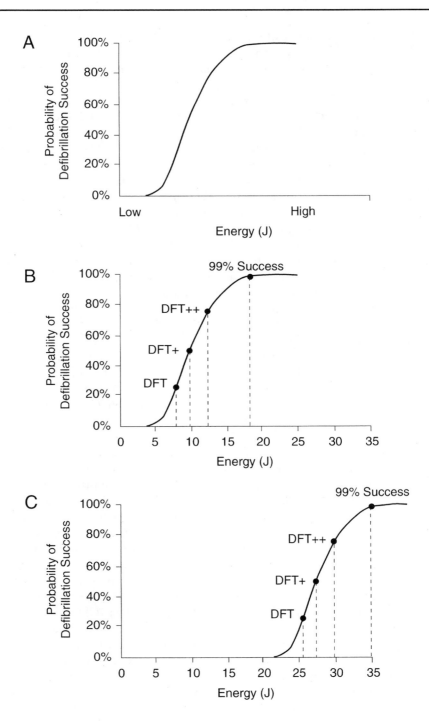

Table 8.1. Safety Margins for ICDs Based on DFT Method

Method	Technique	Definition	Estimated Minimal Energy for 99% Success
DFT	Step-down to failure	Lowest energy level yielding a single successful defibrillation	2 × DFT
DFT+	Step-down to failure and repeat last successful energy	Lowest energy level yielding two successful defibrillations without a failure	1.5 × DFT
DFT++	Step-down to failure and repeat last successful energy twice	Lowest energy level yielding three successful defibrillations without a failure	1.2 × DFT or + 5J
Bayesian	Testing in up or down increments based on response to previous attempt	Completion of a four-shock algorithm	Bayesian DFT 100V
Single energy, two successes	Single energy level tested twice	Two successful defibrillations without failure at the same energy level	2 × DFT
Single energy, three successes	Single energy level tested three times	Three successful defibrillations without failure at the same energy level	1.7 × DFT

Note: Recommendations are based on extensive animal studies and mathematical modeling, *appropriate testing in each patient is mandatory*. (See Singer I, Lang D. The defibrillation threshold. In: Kroll MW, Lehmann MH, eds. Implantable Cardioverter Defibrillator Therapy. The Engineering Clinical Interface. Norwell: Kluwer Academic, 1996:89–129.)

◀

Figure 8.3. Graphical representation of the relationship between probability of successful defibrillation versus energy level of shock. **A:** The generalized defibrillation success curve is sigmoidal in shape. **B:** Defibrillation success curve for a hypothetical patient. If the DFT is measured as a single successful defibrillation at a given energy level (DFT), the confidence for repeated success is lower than if an energy level is tested that defibrillates two (DFT) or three times (DFT) without failure. The safety margin for programming is the difference between the measured value of DFT and the energy needed for greater than 99% successful defibrillation. In this case the safety margins are approximately 10, 8, and 6 J for DFT, DFT^+, and DFT^{++}, respectively (see Table 8.2). The energy level for 99% success is never really known for any patient, however. The safety margins for any measure of DFT are estimated empirically based on the assumption that the shape of the DFT curve is relatively consistent between patients. **C:** In this hypothetical patient, all measures of DFT are high. Using a safety margin of 10 joules added to the DFT^+ or DFT^{++} would require a device with at least 37-J output to ensure greater than 99% successful defibrillation. This patient would require revision of the lead system to reduce the DFTs or the implantation of a high-output device.

Alternatively, determination of the upper limit of vulnerability (ULV) has been used to estimate the DFT while minimizing or even eliminating the need for ventricular fibrillation inductions.[32] By delivering shocks of decreasing energy synchronized to the T wave, a minimal energy level is found that does not induce ventricular fibrillation while lower energies induce fibrillation. The lowest energy value that does not induce fibrilla-

Step Down Protocols

Start
DFT > 20J ← F — 20J — S → Repeat 20J — S×1 → DFT + = 20J; S×2 → DFT ++ = 20J
DFT ≤ 20J
S
DFT = 20J ← F — 15J — S → Repeat 15J — S×1 → DFT + = 15J; S×2 → DFT ++ = 15J
DFT ≤ 15J
S
DFT = 15J ← F — 10J — S → Repeat 10J — S×1 → DFT + = 10J; S×2 → DFT ++ = 10J
DFT ≤ 10J
S
DFT = 10J ← F — 5J — S → Repeat 5J — S×1 → DFT + = 5J; S×2 → DFT ++ = 5J
DFT ≤ 5J

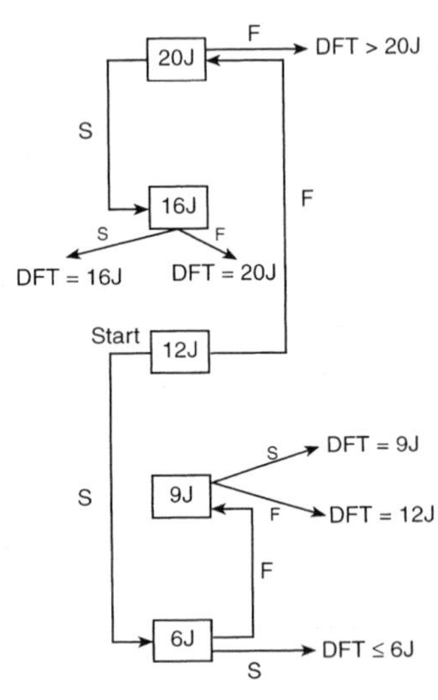

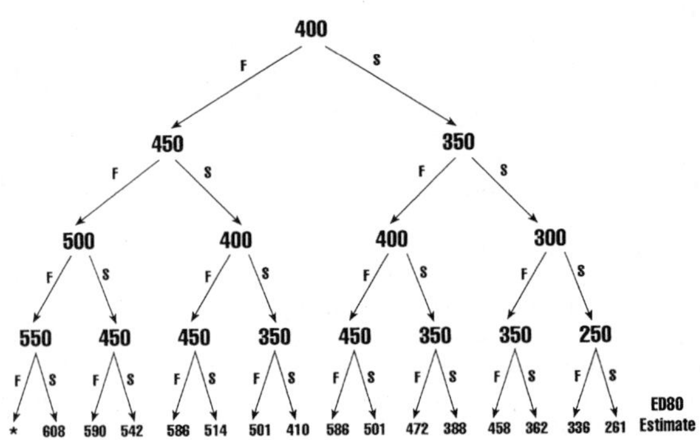

tion is the ULV. The ULV is probabilistic as is the actual DFT. The ULV is highly correlated with the DFT, and may obviate inductions of ventricular fibrillation although multiple shocks in sinus rhythm are required.[32]

At least 2 minutes, and more typically 3 to 5 minutes, should be allowed between defibrillation episodes to ensure full hemodynamic recovery and minimize any cumulative effects of multiple shocks. The appropriate sensing of each episode of induced arrhythmia should be confirmed after each induction. The sensitivity is typically decreased at implant testing (e.g., from 0.3 to 1.2 mV) as an additional safety measure to assure that there will be adequate sensing of spontaneous ventricular arrhythmias. Although acute defibrillation testing is typically performed using the implanted pulse generator, an external defibrillator that delivers identical shocks as the pulse generator can also be used.

The postoperative management of the patient includes monitoring of vital signs and heart rhythm during the recovery from anesthesia or conscious sedation, as well as the completion of a course of perioperative antibiotics. A chest radiograph is performed to document lead position and to rule out complications from the implantation such as a pneumothorax. Typically, the lead function is assessed noninvasively before the patient is discharged from the hospital. Repeat predischarge defibrillation testing is no longer recommended. The duration of postoperative hospitalization has decreased remarkably with modern ICD technology. Often patients are discharged less than 24 hours after surgery, and some implants can be performed on an outpatient basis for primary prevention indications.

The follow-up of patients after ICD implantation usually consists of an early evaluation of wound healing and lead integrity. This is often performed approximately 2 to 4 weeks after implantation. At that visit, chronic pacing outputs can be programmed and lead function can be assessed noninvasively.

Figure 8.4. DFT testing algorithms. The step-down protocol is most commonly used clinically. Starting at 10 J less than the maximal output of the device (20 J in this example), a successful defibrillation may either be repeated at this energy (single-energy success protocol) or stepped down incrementally until failure. The lowest energy level to successfully defibrillate is the DFT. By repeating this energy once or twice without failure, the DFT and DFT are defined. J = joules, S = successful defibrillation, F = failed defibrillation. The binary search protocol starts at intermediate energy levels and again the lowest energy level to defibrillate is the DFT. This energy may be repeated for verification.

The Bayesian search protocol shown here was developed for use with St. Jude Medical defibrillators. The numerical values represent the voltage output for defibrillation testing using Ventritex devices. The algorithm was constructed mathematically and verified in clinical testing. The voltage output specified by the algorithm after completing the series of four inductions of ventricular fibrillation identifies the ED 80 or energy that terminates 80% of fibrillation episodes (* = DFT > 550 V). (Bayesian protocol reproduced by permission from Malkin RA, Herre JM, McGowen L, et al. A four-shock Bayesian up-down estimator of the 80% effective defibrillation dose. J Cardiovasc Electrophysiol 1999;10: 973–980.)

Traditionally ICD patients are evaluated with device interrogation and threshold testing every 3 months. However, given the reliability of modern pulse generators and leads, follow-up every 6 months among clinically stable patients is rapidly becoming the norm. Transtelephonic monitoring of ICDs is growing in popularity, and this approach can further reduce the frequency of office visits.

RATE SENSING

Sensing of ventricular tachyarrhythmias is a critically important function of an ICD system. The ability to sense small amplitude signals rapidly during ventricular fibrillation, while not oversensing T waves or noise in the absence of tachyarrhythmias, is mandatory for proper ICD function. This goal was difficult to achieve with fixed gain sensing,[33] as is used in pacemaker systems. An example of undersensing of ventricular fibrillation by such a fixed gain sensing circuit is shown in Figure 8.5. All contemporary pulse generators use automatic adjustment of amplifier gain or sensing threshold to ensure appropriate detection of ventricular arrhythmias. These algorithms effectively increase the amplifier sensitivity over time between sensed or paced ventricular events to search for

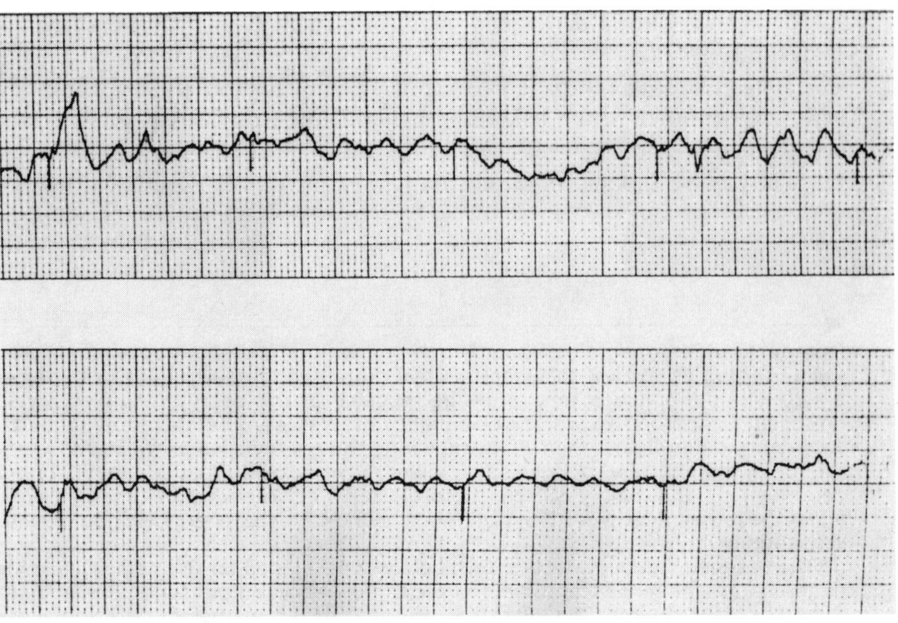

Figure 8.5. Undersensing of ventricular fibrillation. The patient had an ICD without automatic sensing adjustment and ventricular fibrillation developed while on telemetry monitor. The lower rate VVI pacing artifacts are noted indicative of undersensing of ventricular fibrillation.

low-amplitude fibrillatory electrograms that may be missed at lower sensitivities. One such algorithm is shown in Figure 8.6. In addition to these sophisticated sensing algorithms, the need for stable lead performance is mandatory to ensure normal detection of tachyarrhythmias.

Undersensing of ventricular fibrillation was rarely noted with early epicardial or bipolar transvenous leads after automatic gain or sensitivity was employed. However, with the development of integrated nonthoracotomy leads, undersensing of ventricular tachyarrhythmias was reported.[34] These leads initially used extended bipolar sensing, in which the right ventricular coil serves both for sensing and as an electrode for high-energy shocks. Undersensing was most commonly observed with the redetection of ventricular fibrillation following failed shocks. The most likely mechanism of this phenomenon is stunning of local myocardium following shocks, resulting in the diminution of the electrogram near the tip of the lead. With positioning of the right ventricular shocking coil farther from the rate sensing electrode tip, post-shock undersensing is minimized.[35] Data from large clinical trials of integrated transvenous leads have demonstrated excellent detection of ventricular tachycardia and fibrillation, indicating that clinically important undersensing is very rare.[36] However, the optimal spacing between the lead tip and the right ventricular shocking coil is unknown. As the coil is moved farther from the tip, and thus farther from the myocardium, local stunning is reduced but defibrillation thresholds increase. At present, both true bipolar sensing, with a dedicated tip and ring, and integrated sensing, where the distal coil is used for both sensing and shocks, are available.

Another area of potential difficulty with sensing occurs when ICDs are used in conjunction with separate pacemakers. The proximity of the endocardial pacemaker and ICD leads within the ventricle can lead to several problems, including double counting during pacing, which can cause inappropriate shocks,

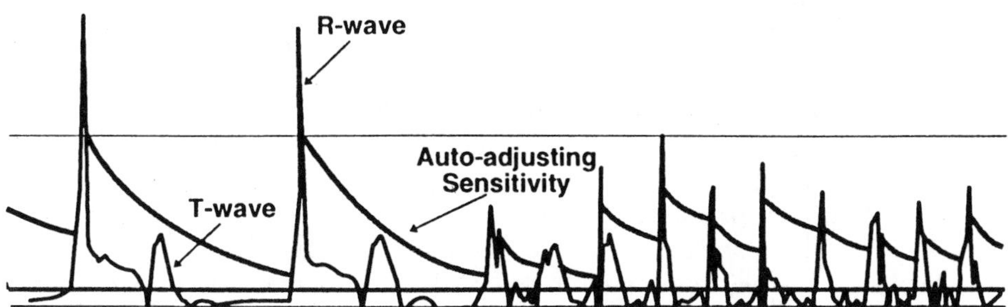

Figure 8.6. A schematic representation of automatic sensitivity during sinus rhythm and ventricular fibrillation. In sinus rhythm, sensitivity increases slowly to avoid oversensing T waves. However, with the onset of ventricular fibrillation, high sensitivity is maintained to minimize undersensing. (Reproduced with permission from Medtronic Inc., Minneapolis, MN.)

and sensing of pacemaker pulses during ventricular fibrillation, which can inhibit therapy. The problems of pacemaker–ICD interactions are largely of historical interest with the development of dual-chamber, rate-responsive ICD systems. Such systems provide all of the basic capabilities of permanent pacemakers, obviating implanting or retaining separate devices.

Although undersensing of ventricular tachyarrhythmias is very unusual with modern lead systems and pulse generators, oversensing of other biologic signals is now more common.[37] The maximum sensitivity of pulse generators is increased (up to 0.15 mV) with contemporary low noise amplifiers. At maximal sensitivity, myopotentials arising from the diaphragm or pectoral muscles can cause inappropriate ICD discharges. This problem is more likely to occur during periods of ventricular pacing, when the amplifier sensitivity is maximized. Often a history of coughing or straining preceding ICD discharges can be elicited from the patient, suggesting that myopotential oversensing is present. Such oversensing can be confirmed by monitoring ventricular electrograms during provocative maneuvers such as handgrip, Valsalva, or deep inspiration. Several strategies have been used to prevent further ICD oversensing, including decreasing the maximum sensitivity of the pulse generator, decreasing the bradycardic pacing rate, or increasing the AV delay to minimize ventricular pacing, prolonging the detection intervals to prevent shocks from transient oversensing, and implanting a separate rate sensing lead in the right ventricular outflow tract more distant from the diaphragmatic surface.[38] Oversensing of T-waves with double counting is another problem observed more frequently with modern pulse generators because of increased maximum sensitivity and aggressive sensing algorithms. Again, this can often be avoided with device reprogramming including reducing the maximum sensitivity, prolonging the refractory period or reducing the aggressiveness of the autosensitivity algorithm.

Extensive data logging capabilities are present in pulse generators. All systems provide beat-to-beat interval data for detected tachyarrhythmias. This is helpful for identifying the arrhythmias associated with shocks. For instance, very irregular intervals are suggestive of atrial fibrillation, whereas the sudden onset of a regular tachycardia is indicative of either monomorphic ventricular tachycardia or paroxysmal supraventricular tachycardia. A very rapid rhythm with nonphysiologic intervals (<130 msec) is indicative of a sensing malfunction, typically due to either a lead insulation defect or a loose set-screw in the pulse generator header.[39]

A further diagnostic tool in devices is stored electrograms. This significantly improves the physician's ability to interpret the appropriateness of defibrillation shocks.[40] The electrodes used to record the electrogram may or may not be the same electrodes used for the detection of arrhythmias. "Near-field" electrograms are recordings of the local bipolar ventricular electrogram, which is also used for arrhythmia detection. This can either be a true bipolar sensing, with recording from the electrode tip to a more proximal ring, or extended bipolar sensing from the tip to a right ventricular shocking coil. For "far-field" electrograms, recordings are made between shocking electrodes, which for a typical transve-

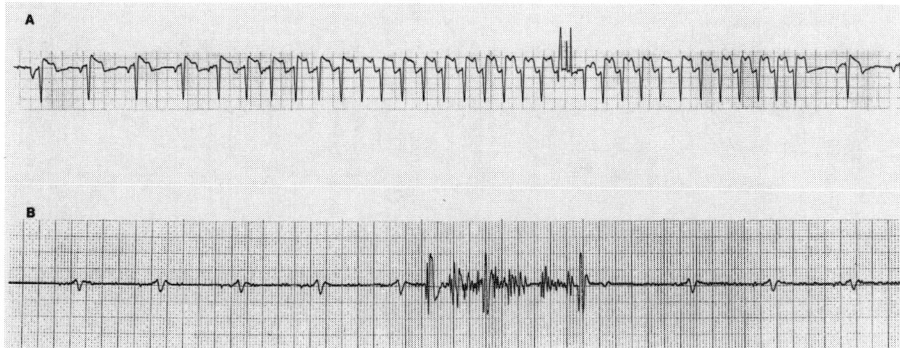

Figure 8.7. Stored electrograms during ICD activity. **A:** "Far-field" electrograms during a short episode of atrial flutter are shown. The arrhythmia was detected but no shock was delivered because the pulse generator was programmed to the noncommitted mode. The patient had received multiple other shocks for longer episodes of atrial fibrillation and flutter. Note the unchanged electrogram morphology (QRS complex) indicative of a supraventricular arrhythmia and the atrial activity in both sinus rhythm and atrial flutter that can be observed with "far-field" electrograms that are recording signals between the shocking coils in the ventricle and superior vena cava. **B:** Noise due to an insulation break is shown from an electrogram from the rate sensing bipolar lead ("near field"). The patient experienced multiple shocks without preceding symptoms, and a shock in sinus rhythm was documented.

nous lead system includes a right ventricular coil, a left pectoral active pulse generator, and often a more proximal coil in the right atrium or superior vena cava. Far-field recordings potentially allow for the identification of atrial activity to aid in arrhythmia classification. In addition, the change in morphology of ventricular arrhythmias is often more obvious in the far-field electrograms. The source of stored electrograms is important for interpreting arrhythmia episodes, particularly inappropriate therapy. For example, if the far-field electrogram recorded from the shocking electrodes is being monitored, then this is not the same signal that is being sensed by the amplifier for the determination of tachyarrhythmias. Thus, if no tachycardia is noted at the time of therapy for a rapid rate, then oversensing of the rate-sensing lead can be deduced, but extraneous "noise" will not be demonstrated. Examples of stored electrograms are shown in Figure 8.7. With dual-chamber ICDs, direct atrial recordings further simplify the interpretation of arrhythmias (Fig. 8.8).

ARRHYTHMIA DETECTION

Arrhythmia detection requires effective sensing of the intrinsic cardiac activity and the fulfillment of the programmed detection algorithm. For ventricular tachycardia, most ICDs require that a certain number of consecutive R-R intervals be shorter than the tachycardia detection interval for the VT zone (Fig.

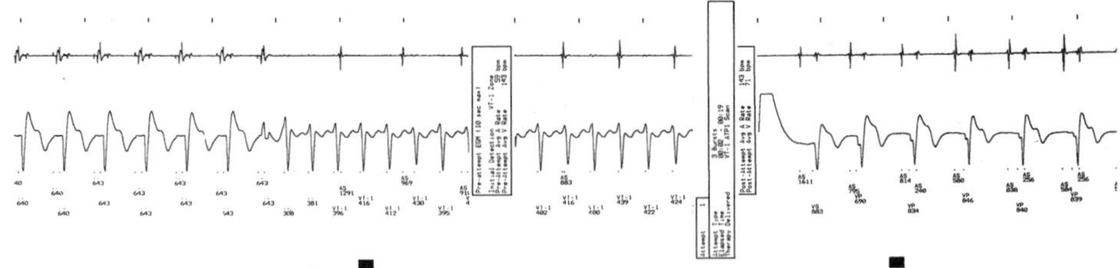

Figure 8.8. Stored electrogram from a dual-chamber ICD. The bipolar atrial electrogram is shown on the **top panel**. Below is the far-field electrogram in the triad configuration (sensing from right ventricle to right atrium and left pectoral pulse generator). Initially the patient is in sinus rhythm but ventricular tachycardia with clear AV dissociation develops. Following a burst of antitachycardia pacing (not shown), sinus rhythm is restored on the **far right panel** of the electrogram. Note how the atrial electrogram simplifies the interpretation of rhythms.

8.9). Because the ventricular fibrillation (VF) electrograms may transiently be very low in amplitude and undersensed, the ventricular fibrillation detection algorithms require that a certain percentage (typically 75%) of R-R intervals in a rolling window of cardiac cycles be shorter than the ventricular fibrillation detection interval (see Fig. 8.9). After each delivered therapy, the ICD must determine whether the tachycardia was terminated. The redetection criteria after therapies are usually somewhat less demanding than the initial detection criteria for each zone. The detection criteria in the VT zone may be modified by algorithms to prevent inappropriate therapy for supraventricular tachycardias.

IMPLANTABLE CARDIOVERTER-DEFIBRILLATOR THERAPIES

Pacing

All ICD pulse generators have pacing capabilities. This can be simple backup bradycardia support (VVI mode), more physiologic pacing modes with or without rate responsiveness (e.g., DDDR), or high-rate pacing for the termination of ventricular tachycardia or supraventricular tachyarrhythmias (SVT or atrial flutter). Ventricular pacing prevents long pauses that occur spontaneously or following shocks for ventricular tachyarrhythmias. Such post-shock pauses can contribute to the hemodynamic compromise associated with these arrhythmias. In fact, in some patients syncopal episodes associated with appropriate ICD therapy are due to the post-shock pause and not to the primary tachyarrhythmia.

The use of dual-chamber ICD systems has increased dramatically since they were first approved in 1997. It is estimated that approximately 70% of new ICD systems (not including biventricular pacing devices) implanted in the United States are dual-chamber devices. This is a much greater percentage than the 5% to 10% of patients who received both pacemakers and ICDs previously, suggesting that this usage is not due solely to the need for atrial pacing for stan-

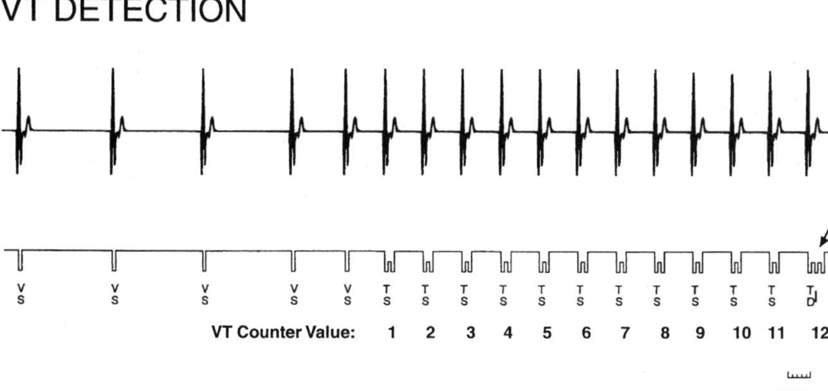

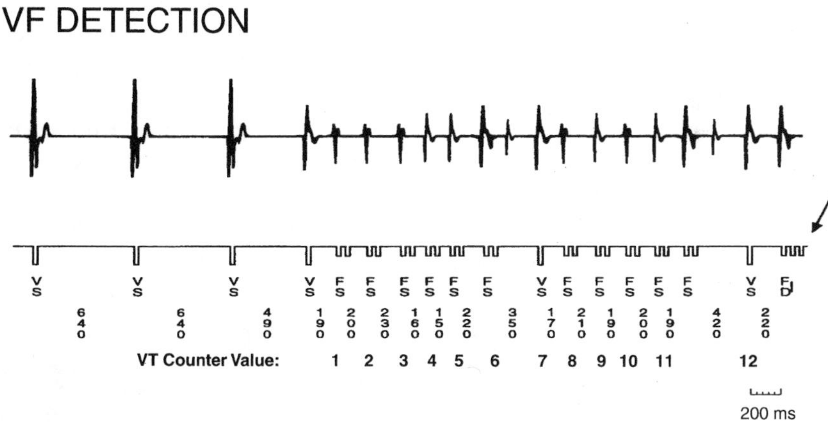

Figure 8.9. Basic ventricular tachycardia (VT) and fibrillation (VF) detection algorithms. In both panels, the tracings are from top to bottom: ventricular electrogram, marker channel, and counter value (labeled) for detection. VS = ventricular sensing below tachycardia detection rate, TS = sensing in the VT zone, TDI = tachycardia detection completed *(arrow)*; FS = sensing in the VF zone, FDI = fibrillation detection completed *(arrow)*. **Top:** For ventricular tachycardia detection in this example, the criteria are 12 consecutive intervals shorter than the tachycardia detection interval of 400 milliseconds. If an interval longer than 400 milliseconds had occurred in this episode, the counter would have been reset to zero at that point. **Bottom:** For ventricular fibrillation detection, occasional undersensing is anticipated. The detection criteria in this example are 12 out of 16 consecutive intervals shorter than the fibrillation detection interval of 320 milliseconds. Here two long intervals of 350 and 420 milliseconds are recorded due to signal drop out; however, fibrillation is still detected. (Courtesy of Medtronic, Inc.)

dard indications. Many factors are likely responsible for this discrepancy. Dual-chamber ICDs are likely being implanted in an "anticipatory" manner, such as in patients who may receive negative chronotropic drugs or those with conduction system abnormalities (e.g., first-degree AV block or QRS prolongation), when permanent pacemakers would not have been used. Also, dual-chamber ICDs are being implanted for reasons other than to provide atrial-based bradycardia pacing, such as to improve arrhythmia discrimination[41] or to provide therapy for atrial tachyarrhythmias. However, the DAVID study has demonstrated the potential adverse effects of dual chamber pacing.[22] Moreover, the results of dual chamber discrimination algorithms to prevent inappropriate shocks has been disappointing.[42] Hopefully, newer algorithms will prove more useful.[43] These observations and the results of the DAVID study suggest that right ventricular pacing should be minimized in ICD patients who do not have pacemaker indications. This can be achieved in single-chamber systems by programming a low rate (e.g., VVI 40 bpm). For dual-chamber ICD systems, prolonging the AV delay, or activating features such as AV search hysteresis can serve to reduce the percentage of ventricular pacing. In contrast to avoiding ventricular pacing with single and dual-chamber devices, biventricular ICDs (CRT-D) are designed specifically to pace the right and left ventricles. These systems are indicated for patients with severe CHF (NYHA III-IV), left ventricular systolic dysfunction and QRS prolongation, typically left bundle branch block.

Antitachycardia Pacing

High-rate, overdrive pacing is very effective for terminating ventricular tachycardia. Adaptive algorithms are used, in which the pacing rate is set based upon the tachycardia cycle length of each episode of tachycardia (Fig. 8.10). Randomized studies have shown similar efficacy of burst (constant cycle length in the train) and ramp (decremental cycle lengths) pacing in this setting (Fig. 8.11).[44] Interestingly, the success rates for pace termination of spontaneous episodes of ventricular tachycardia are higher than for induced episodes, typically approximately 90%, whereas arrhythmia acceleration rates are low (1% to 3%).[44,45] Presumably, the high efficacy of terminating spontaneous ventricular tachycardias is due to the slower rates of these episodes compared with induced tachycardias. These observations support a strategy of empiric programming of antitachycardia pacing in patients with the underlying substrate for monomorphic ventricular tachycardia.[45] There is a relative paucity of data concerning the clinical predictors of unsuccessful pace termination of ventricular tachycardia, other than rapid tachycardia rates (>200 bpm) and very poor left ventricular function.[44,45] However, even very rapid tachycardias can be pace terminated in a sufficient proportion of episodes to justify programming pacing at rates above 200 bpm to reduce the number of shocks.[46] In a randomized study comparing antitachycardia pacing with low-energy cardioversion (Fig. 8.12), similar termination and acceleration rates were observed,[47] indicating no advantage to low-energy shocks for the initial treatment of monomorphic ventricular tachycardia.

Defibrillation

Defibrillation is achieved when a critical mass of myocardium is depolarized by establishing a critical voltage gradient throughout the ventricular tissue.[48] The dispersion of the voltage gradient and current flow depends on the positioning

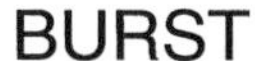

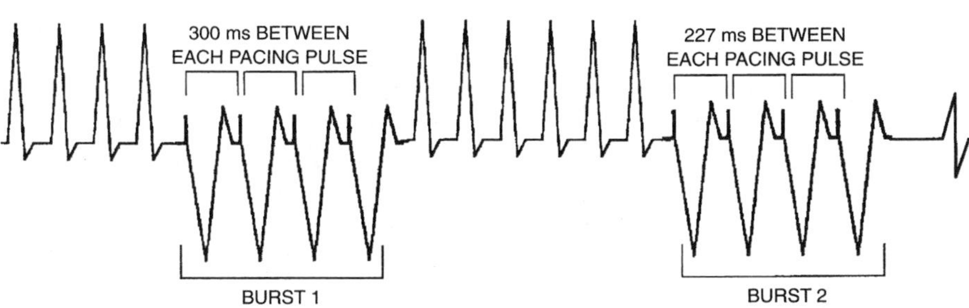

RAMP

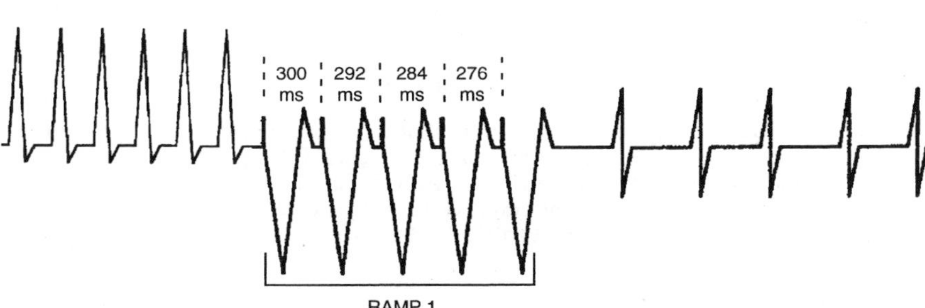

Figure 8.10. Schematic representation of burst and ramp antitachycardia pacing (ATP). **Top:** Four beats of ventricular tachycardia are followed by the first burst of ATP at 300 milliseconds for four beats. The rate for this burst is determined as a programmable percentage of the tachycardia cycle length. Tachycardia continues after Burst 1, so after redetection Burst 2 is delivered at a programmable rate faster than Burst 1 (227 milliseconds in this example). The pacing interval for subsequent bursts will decrement further until a minimum pacing cycle length is reached, all ATP attempts are delivered, or the tachycardia terminates. **Bottom:** In ramp ATP there is decrement in the pacing interval between consecutive stimuli. The initial pacing rate starts as a percentage of the tachycardia cycle length. Multiple ramp attempts can be programmed with shorter intervals in each subsequent attempt. (Courtesy of Guidant Corp.)

of the high-voltage lead electrodes in and/or around the heart. Failure to defibrillate may be due to a residual mass of fibrillating tissue or immediate reinduction of fibrillation in areas of low electrical gradient. All ICD pulse generators achieve defibrillation by applying voltage to a capacitor, which is then discharged through the lead system. The resulting waveform is an exponentially declining voltage, which is prematurely terminated or truncated before full capacitor discharge. Thus, the maximal *delivered* energy for an ICD is always less than the *stored* energy necessary to fully charge the capacitor. In the early ICD systems, monophasic waveforms were used that were truncated at about 35% of

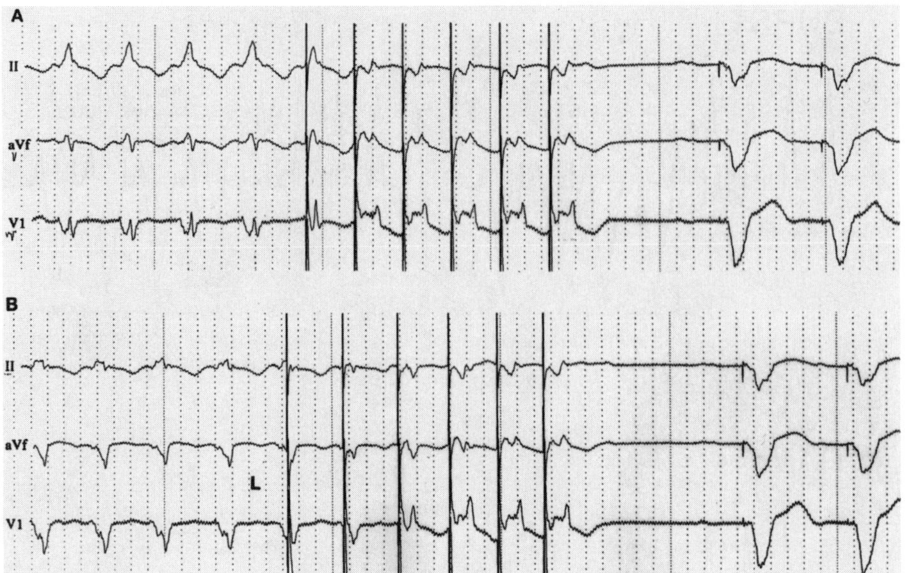

Figure 8.11. Antitachycardia pacing termination of ventricular tachycardia. Examples of **(A)** burst and **(B)** ramp pacing to terminate tachycardia in a patient are shown. Note that the morphology and rate of ventricular tachycardia differ in two episodes in the same patient, illustrating the utility of adaptive rate pacing from the ICD. Bradycardia pacing is present at the termination of ventricular tachycardia.

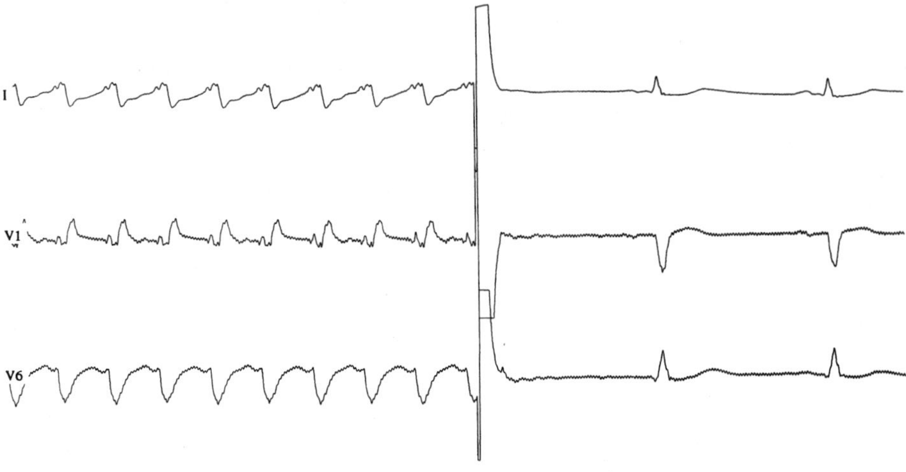

Figure 8.12. An example of low-energy cardioversion (0.5 J) for the termination of ventricular tachycardia. The shock is shown by the high-voltage artifact on the electrocardiographic recordings, which was followed by the restoration of sinus rhythm.

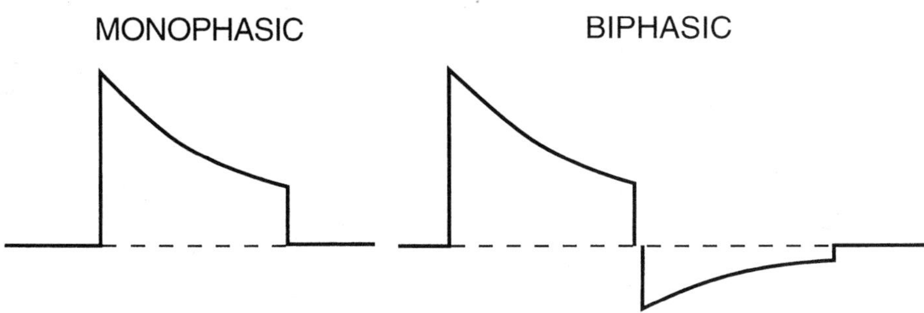

Figure 8.13. Schematic representation of defibrillation waveforms. The time course of the delivered voltage for monophasic and biphasic shocks are shown. Note that shock waveforms are truncated exponentially declining pulses.

the leading edge voltage; this is referred to as a 65% *tilt* monophasic shock (Fig. 8.13). This waveform was chosen because animal studies have shown a lower defibrillation efficacy with shorter or longer duration pulses. However, human studies have now demonstrated that defibrillation thresholds are not affected by pulse duration over a wide range of pulse widths, including tilts up to 95%.[49] Accordingly, adjusting pulse width is unlikely to have significant effects on defibrillation efficacy. The truncation of shocks from ICD pulse generators allowed the development of more complex waveforms, because the undelivered voltage remaining on the capacitors at the end of the pulse is still available. Biphasic waveforms were shown consistently to reduce defibrillation energy requirements compared with monophasic shocks.[50,51] For biphasic shocks, the polarity of the voltage pulse is reversed after the termination of the initial positive phase and a second negative phase is delivered. Biphasic waveforms have become the standard waveform for all ICD pulse generators. More complicated ascending ramp waveforms are presently under investigation, but it is unclear if there will be a sufficient reduction of defibrillation thresholds to merit changing waveforms in implantable devices.

Another factor that can affect defibrillation thresholds is the polarity of the defibrillation shock. Initially, studies of transvenous lead systems used the right ventricular coil as the cathode for shocks. However, reverse polarity, or anodal shocks, result in significantly lower defibrillation thresholds.[52,53] Shock polarity has much less effect on biphasic defibrillation thresholds than on monophasic thresholds.[54,55] Reversing the shock polarity may only improve defibrillation efficacy when high thresholds are present.[53,54] In this case, the first phase of the biphasic waveform is similar to a monophasic shock—that is, making the right ventricular coil the anode (positive) for the first phase of the shock is optimal. The polarity of the shock is programmable, but to minimize defibrillation testing the initial configuration to evaluate should be the right ventricular coil as the anode. In some devices different high voltage electrodes may be reprogrammed in or out of the circuit as well.

Capacitance is another factor that may affect defibrillation efficacy. Capacitors are important components of pulse generator size, so if defibrillation thresholds are decreased with lower capacitance, then pulse generator size could be reduced. Decreasing capacitance to 60 or 90 μF reduces defibrillation thresholds modestly in some studies,[56,57] but had no effect on stored energy requirements and increased peak voltage in other studies.[58,59] The defibrillation safety margin is reduced with lower capacitance because of the higher peak voltages required, so the strategy of marked reductions of pulse generator capacitance is unlikely to be pursued in the future.

Once biphasic waveforms became ubiquitous, the most important advance for lowering defibrillation thresholds was the development of active pulse generators. With the downsizing of pulse generator size to allow for pectoral placement, the pulse generator shell can become part of the lead system. Such active pulse generators are also known as "hot cans" or "active cans." The active can was first evaluated in humans by Bardy and colleagues using a shocking configuration from a right ventricular coil to a left pectoral pulse generator.[60] This lead system was termed the unipolar configuration because only a single endocardial electrode is used, analogous to unipolar pacing where the pacemaker pulse generator serves as the return pathway for current from the right ventricular electrode. These investigators showed that adequate defibrillation thresholds (<20 J) could be achieved in approximately 90% of patients with this simple single coil lead system. Subsequently, it was confirmed that defibrillation thresholds were lower in the unipolar configuration than in a dual-coil, transvenous configuration (where current is delivered between two coils, one in the right ventricle and the other in the superior vena cava).[61] Defibrillation thresholds are relatively insensitive to pulse generator size,[62] indicating that defibrillation efficacy will not be affected adversely as pulse generators get progressively smaller.

The effect of combining an active pectoral pulse generator with a dual-coil lead was evaluated independent of the development of the unipolar lead configuration. This was called the "triad" configuration because of the presence of three shocking electrodes, the active can and two transvenous coils. In the initial study of this lead system, it was shown that the mean defibrillation threshold decreased 36% compared with a dual-coil shocking vector.[63] This benefit was due more to the lowering of impedance with the active can than to an improvement in the shocking vector. Subsequent studies compared the defibrillation efficacy of multiple lead configurations.[64] Defibrillation thresholds in the triad lead configuration were again much lower than in the dual-coil transvenous lead configuration, as well as 23% lower than in the single-coil unipolar configuration. In the largest study comparing active can defibrillation configurations, the unipolar and triad configurations were measured in 50 patients.[65] Both the mean and the variability of defibrillation thresholds were lower in the triad configuration. In this study, 98% of patients had a threshold less than 15 J. Of particular clinical relevance is the reduction of the number of patients with high thresholds, because such patients have an inadequate safety margin and often require complicated implantation procedures to test multiple lead positions or shocking vectors. The uniformly low thresholds with dual-coil, active can lead systems have simplified implantation testing of these systems.

The effect of proximal coil position has also been evaluated. When shocking between two coils and no active can, positioning a second lead in the left subclavian vein is optimal because it directs current more toward the left side of the heart compared with a more proximal position in the superior vena cava.[66] However, no such benefit of the proximal coil position is observed when an active can is part of the shocking circuit,[67] indicating that single-pass dual-coil leads with fixed intercoil spacing should minimize defibrillation thresholds without the need for additional leads. This has become the standard lead system for implants. Single-coil leads are still used in pediatric patients because complications from the proximal coil are more common as a result of continued growth of the child.

The anatomic position of an active pulse generator is important for determining its effect on defibrillation thresholds. In the right pectoral region, there is no significant change in thresholds with the use of an active can compared with a dual-coil transvenous lead.[68] This is because an active can increases defibrillation current requirements due to a worsened shock vector, which is directed away from the left ventricle and toward the right shoulder. The reduction in impedance with the active can offsets the increased current resulting in no net effect on threshold. In the left abdominal position, defibrillation thresholds decreased with an active can in one study and were unchanged in another study.[69] In either case, these observations imply that active devices can be used when replacing older abdominal pulse generators.

Despite the marked reduction of defibrillation thresholds with active pectoral pulse generators, there are still some patients with unacceptably high thresholds. Unfortunately, identifying these patients prospectively is difficult. Raitt and colleagues evaluated the clinical predictors of defibrillation efficacy in 101 patients with a unipolar defibrillation system.[70] The only independent predictors of the biphasic defibrillation threshold were left ventricular mass and resting heart rate. However, all correlations with defibrillation thresholds were weak. Similarly, no routine clinical factors reliably predict high thresholds in the triad configuration.[71] The possible causes of high DFTs at implant and potential corrective measures are listed in Table 8.2.

Fortunately, the proportion of patients with high defibrillation thresholds is small with left pectoral active can lead systems. If an adequate safety margin cannot be demonstrated at implantation, then further testing is necessary. The simplest change is to reverse the polarity of the shocks. Other changes that can be made include repositioning leads, placing a second coil, implanting a subcutaneous patch or array,[72] or adding a type III antiarrhythmic drug such a dofetilide or sotalol which can reduce thresholds. Although most popular ICDs have maximal energy outputs of about 30J, most manufacturers also produce high-energy units with delivered energy up to 36J. These high output devices

Table 8.2. Causes and Corrections for High DFTs at Implant

Cause of Elevated DFT	Diagnosis	Correction
Poor lead position	On fluoroscopy distal coil out of RV, proximal coil low in atrium	Reposition lead
Increased high-voltage impedance	Data from defibrillation attempt, commanded determination of impedance	Check header connections, reposition lead and/or coils, add SVC to single-coil system, add SQ array, relieve pneumothorax
Pneumothorax	High-shock impedance, fluoroscopy, dyspnea	Relieve pneumothorax
Hypoxia	Low oxygen saturation	Lighten sedation, assist ventilation
Ischemia	Chest pain, ECG changes, hypotension	Anti-ischemic therapy
Multiple defibrillations	Numerous previous defibrillation attempts	Implant device in best configuration and retest
Antiarrhythmic drugs or anesthetics	Exclude other etiologies	Retest after stopping drugs, stop inhaled anesthetics
Poor current distributions	High or low shocking impedance, poor lead positions	Reposition coil, add SVC coil to single-coil system, add SQ array
Shunting current through guidewires or retained leads	Retained guidewires, temporary or permanent pacing leads	Retest after removing wires or leads
Suboptimal waveform or tilt	Exclusion of other causes, failure of multiple lead configurations	Confirm, shocking impedance, use biphasic waveform, reprogram tilt, pulse width, polarity
Poor myocardial substrate	Exclusion of other causes, failure of multiple plead configuration	Add coils, SQ array, epicardial patches to circuit, use high output device

RV = right ventricle; SVC = superior vena cava; SQ = subcutaneous.

are useful in patients with elevated DFTs despite testing different lead configurations.

Traditionally an implantation safety margin of at least 10J between the measured defibrillation thresholds and the maximal output of the pulse generator is considered adequate. This is because such safety margins are associated with very low arrhythmic death rates in patients with first-generation devices and epicardial patch lead systems.[73] This has led to the common practice of programming shock strengths to at least 10J greater than the defibrillation thresholds measured at implantation. Results from the Low Energy Safety Study (LESS) suggest that a safety margin of approximately 5J may be adequate with modern ICD systems employing biphasic waveforms, transvenous leads, and active pectoral pulse generators when rigorous DFT testing (DFT++) is used.[29]

Traditionally, defibrillation thresholds were measured only at implantation. This strategy was supported by studies that showed no significant change of defibrillation thresholds chronically with epicardial lead systems.[74] However, mean defibrillation thresholds with transvenous leads and monophasic waveforms increase over time, and this can lead to an inadequate safety margin that may require operative revision of the lead system.[75] However, more recent studies indicate that defibrillation thresholds are stable with biphasic waveforms. In a study evaluating chronic changes of monophasic and biphasic defibrillation thresholds in the same patients, monophasic thresholds increased 23% during a mean follow-up time of 8 months, while biphasic thresholds were essentially unchanged.[76] More long-term follow-up evaluations confirmed the overall stability of biphasic defibrillation thresholds, although a small minority of patients may show an increase.[29,77] Thus, routine reevaluation of defibrillation function is not commonly performed anymore. Such testing is still necessary among patients treated with antiarrhythmic drugs, particularly amiodarone, those patients with marginal defibrillation efficacy at implantation and among patients in whom the initial shock failed to terminate a spontaneous episode of ventricular tachycardia or fibrillation.

ATRIAL DEFIBRILLATORS

In the 1990s, a dedicated atrial-only defibrillator was developed and tested in a multinational clinical trial (Metrix Atrial ICD, InControl, Inc., Redmond WA). The study showed this device to be successful in terminating atrial fibrillation automatically or on patient or physician command in a group of highly selected patients. This device is no longer in production largely due to poor patient acceptance of painful shock therapy for atrial fibrillation and the concern for ventricular fibrillation induction by an improperly timed shock in the absence of backup ventricular defibrillation capabilities. At present there are several devices that provide automated or commanded atrial defibrillation therapy. These devices are also a fully functional ventricular defibrillator and are capable of delivering a variety of atrial antitachycardia pacing therapies.[78,79] The atrial antitachycardia pacing has been reported to terminate more than half of atrial tachyarrhythmias.[79,80] Moreover, the use of atrial therapies (both shocks and pacing) can significantly reduce atrial fibrillation burden[81] and it is associated with an improvement of quality of life.[82] Despite these data supporting the role of atrial defibrillators, the adoption of this technology into clinical practice has been disappointing. At present, combined atrial and ventricular ICDs are typically used in patients with a history of atrial fibrillation who are receiving ICDs for standard clinical indications. They are also employed in patients with congestive heart failure, where clinical deterioration is often more pronounced during atrial arrhythmias.

FUTURE DIRECTIONS

It is very likely that the rapid growth of ICD implants will continue given the results of recent primary prevention studies such as SCD HeFT and COMPANION, and as the implantation and management of devices are further simplified. Currently, there are over 2 million people in the United States with heart failure, including about 400,000 new cases annually, who could benefit from ICD implantation based on the results of randomized clinical trials.

It is unlikely that there will be major changes in the primary functions of ICD pulse generators in the near future. Bradycardia pacing, antitachycardia pacing, and shocks from active pectoral pulse generators are ubiquitous features of devices that will be maintained. The most rapidly growing segment of the ICD market is the biventricular pacing devices (CRT-D). This trend is likely to continue, given the functional and mortality benefit demonstrated with this therapy and as placement of left ventricular leads becomes more routine. The biphasic waveform of a capacitive discharge is also unlikely to be abandoned, unless dramatic reductions of defibrillation thresholds are observed with alternative waveforms such as ascending ramps. Pulse generator size will continue to decrease with improvement of battery and capacitor technology. However, at some point this may compromise device longevity, which is a potential disadvantage given the improvement in survival in patients with a reduced ejection fraction with contemporary medical therapy. With first-generation devices in the 1980s, the annual mortality of patients with congestive heart failure was 20% to 40%, so devices with a 3-year longevity were often sufficient and the only device that many patients needed. The annual mortality today is less than 7% in patients receiving angiotensin-converting enzyme inhibitors, aldosterone antagonists and beta blockers, even for those patients with NYHA class III symptoms; thus, device longevity is important even for the sickest group of patients with ventricular arrhythmias.

Arrhythmia discrimination continues to be a problem for ICD therapy. Even with dual-chamber devices, the delivery of shocks for atrial arrhythmias or extraneous noise remains a major problem. Such inappropriate shocks may be decreased with algorithms incorporating aspects of the frequency content of signals, electrogram morphology, or by comparing signals from multiple leads.

Strategies to prevent ventricular arrhythmias are not well developed. Ventricular arrhythmias are often preceded by ectopy or more prolonged changes in heart rate or repolarization variability. Decreases of heart rate variability or increases of the magnitude of T-wave alternans could be a trigger for preventative therapy. Therapies could include overdrive pacing, local release of antiarrhythmic agents by a drug pump, or stimulation of cardiac afferent nerves to initiate neurally mediated changes of autonomic function.

Intravascular hemodynamic monitors could also be combined with such systems, either to allow early detection of heart failure exacerbations or to trigger therapy such as pacing or drug pumps. Similarly, hemodynamic or electrocardiographic monitors could be used to diagnose myocardial ischemia and initiate therapy such as intravascular infusion of beta blockers or antiplatelet agents. These would also likely be effective antiarrhythmic strategies, as ischemia and hemodynamic deterioration are potent triggers of ventricular arrhythmias.

Finally, the follow-up assessment of patients with ICDs continues to evolve. Remote monitoring of ICDs has been developed; either through a telephone or Internet link, and both interrogation and programming of devices are possible, which would aid in the management of patients who have received shocks or for more routine evaluations.

SUMMARY

ICD therapy has undergone a remarkable transformation in the 20 years since the devices were first approved for human use. The early devices were "shock boxes" with almost no diagnostic capabilities, and they required sternotomy or thoracotomy for epicardial patch implantation with typical postoperative hospitalizations of approximately 1 week. Pulse generator longevity was less than 2 years. Modern devices provide detailed information about the rate and morphology of electrocardiographic signals before, during, and after therapy. The simplicity of defibrillator implantation now approaches that of pacemakers, because of the downsizing of pulse generators and improvements of lead design and shock waveforms. Despite the increase in diagnostic capabilities and the marked reduction in size, device longevity is now over 6 years. Routine outpatient ICD implantation is feasible and will certainly increase. Further advances in lead technology and arrhythmia discrimination algorithms should increase the efficacy and reliability of therapy. Finally, devices have the capabilities to treat multiple problems in addition to life-threatening ventricular arrhythmias, such as atrial arrhythmias and congestive heart failure.

REFERENCES

1. Gregoratos G, Abrams J, Epstein AE, et al. ACC/AHA/NASPE 20002 guidelines update for implantation of cardiac pacemakers and antiarrhythmia devices: executive summary article. Circulation 2002;106:2145–2161.
2. The Antiarrhythmic Versus Implantable Defibrillator (AVID) Investigators. A comparison of antiarrhythmic-drug therapy with implantable defibrillators in patients resuscitated from near-fatal ventricular arrhythmias. N Engl J Med 1997;337: 1576–1583.
3. Connolly SJ, Gent M, Roberts RS, et al. Canadian Implantable Defibrillator Study (CIDS). A randomized trial of the implantable cardioverter defibrillator against amiodarone. Circulation 2000;101:1297–1302.
4. Sheldon R, Connolly S, Krahn A, et al. Identification of patients most likely to benefit from implantable cardioverter-defibrillator therapy: the Canadian Implantable Defibrillator Study. Circulation 2000;101:1660–1664.
5. Kuck K-H, Cappato R, Siebels J, et al. Randomized comparison of antiarrhythmic drug therapy with implantable defibrillators in patients resuscitated from cardiac arrest: the Cardiac Arrest Study Hamburg (CASH). Circulation 2000;102:748–754.

6. Moss A, Hall J, Cannom D, et al. Improved survival with an implanted defibrillator in patients with coronary disease at high risk of ventricular arrhythmias. N Engl J Med 1997;335:1933–1940.
7. Buxton AE, Lee DL, Fisher JD, et al. A randomized study of the prevention of sudden death in patients with coronary artery disease. N Engl J Med 1999;341: 1882–1890.
8. Gold MR, Nisam S. Primary prevention of sudden cardiac death with implantable cardioverter defibrillators: lessons learned from MADIT and MUSTT. Pacing Clin Electrophysiol 2000;23:1981–1985.
9. Bigger JT. Prophylactic use of implanted cardiac defibrillators in patients at high risk for ventricular arrhythmias after coronary-artery bypass graft surgery. Coronary Artery Bypass Graft (CABG) Patch Trial Investigators. N Engl J Med 1997;337:1569–1575.
10. Buxton AE, Lee KL, DiCarlo L, et al. Electrophysiologic testing to identify patients with coronary artery disease who are at risk for sudden death. N Engl J Med 2000;342:1937–1945.
11. Kadish A, Dyer A, Daubert JP, et al. Prophylactic defibrillator implantation in patients with nonischemic dilated cardiomyopathy. N Engl J Med 2004;350:2151–2158.
12. Moss AJ, Zareba W, Hall WJ, et al: Prophylactic implantation of a defibrillator in patients with myocardial infarction and reduced ejection fraction. N Engl J Med 2002;346:877–883.
13. Knight BP, Goyal R, Pelosi F, et al. Outcome of patients with nonischemic dilated cardiomyopathy and unexplained syncope treated with an implantable defibrillator. J Am Coll Cardiol 1999;33:1964–1970.
14. Andrews NP, Fogel RI, Pelargonio G, et al. Implantable defibrillator event rates in patients with unexplained syncope and inducible sustained ventricular tachyarrhythmias: a comparison with patients known to have sustained ventricular tachycardia. J Am Coll Cardiol 1999;34:2023–2030.
15. Nademanee K, Veerakul G, Mower M, et al. Defibrillator versus β-blockers for unexplained death in Thailand (DEBUT): A randomized clinical trial. Circulation 2003;107:2221–2226.
16. Pacifico A, Wheelan KR, Nasir N, et al. Long-term follow-up of cardioverter-defibrillator implanted under conscious sedation in the prepectoral subfascial position. Circulation 1997;95:946–950.
17. Gold MR, Peters RW, Johnson JW, et al. Complications associated with pectoral cardioverter-defibrillator implantation: comparison of subcutaneous and submuscular approaches. J Am Coll Cardiol 1996;28:1278–1282.
18. Larsen GC, Manolis AS, Sonnenberg FA, et al. Cost-effectiveness of the implantable cardioverter-defibrillator: effect of improved battery life and comparison with amiodarone therapy. J Am Coll Cardiol 1992;19:1323–1334.
19. Mirowski M, Mower MM, Gott VL, et al. Feasibility and effectiveness of low-energy catheter defibrillation in man. Circulation 1973;47:79–85.
20. Bardy GH, Johnson G, Poole JE, et al. A simplified, single-lead unipolar transvenous cardioversion-defibrillation system. Circulation 1993;88:543–547.
21. Ellenbogen KA, Wook MA, Shepard RK, et al. Detection and management of an implantable cardioverter defibrillator lead failure: incidence and clinical implications. J Am Coll Cardiol 2003;41:73–80.
22. The DAVID Investigators. Dual-chamber pacing or ventricular backup pacing in patients with an implantable defibrillator: the dual chamber and VVI implantable defibrillator (DAVID) trial. JAMA 2002;288:3115–3123.

23. Fitzpatrick AP, Lesh MD, Epstein LM, et al. Electrophysiological laboratory, electrophysiologist-implanted, nonthoracotomy-implantable cardioverter/defibrillators. Circulation 1994;89:2503–2508.
24. Gold MR, Froman D, Kavesh NG, et al. A comparison of pectoral and abdominal transvenous defibrillator implantation: analysis of costs and outcomes. J Interven Cardiac Eletrophysiol 1998;2:345–349.
25. Hayes DL, Naccarelli GV, Furman S, et al. NASPE training requirements for cardiac implantable electronic devices: selection, implantation, and follow-up. PACE 2003; 26:1556–1562.
26. Roelke M, O'Nunain SS, Osswald S, et al. Subclavian crush syndrome complicating transvenous cardioverter defibrillator systems. Pacing Clin Electrophysiol 1995;18:973–979.
27. Gold MR, Peters RW, Johnson JW, Shorofsky SR. Complications associated with pectoral implantation of cardioverter-defibrillators. Pacing Clin Electrophysiol 1997;20:208–211.
28. Singer I, Lang D. Defibrillation threshold: clinical utility and therapeutic implications. Pacing Clin Electrophysiol 1992;15:932–949.
29. Gold MR, Higgins S, Klein R, et al. Efficacy and temporal stability of reduced safety margins for ventricular defibrillation. Primary results from the Low Energy Safety Study (LESS). Circulation 2002;105:2043–2048.
30. Shorofsky SR, Peters RW, Rashba EJ, Gold MR. Comparison of step-down and binary search algorithms for determination of defibrillation threshold in humans. PACE 2004;27:218–220.
31. Gold MR, Breiter D, Leman R, et al. Safety of a single successful conversion of ventricular fibrillation before the implantation of cardioverter defibrillators. PACE 2003;26:483–486.
32. Swerdlow CD. Implantation of cardioverter defibrillators without induction of ventricular fibrillation. Circulation 2001;103:2159–2164.
33. Singer I, Adams L, Austin E. Potential hazards of fixed gain sensing and arrhythmia reconfirmation for implantable cardioverter defibrillators. Pacing Clin Electrophysiol 1993;16:1070–1079.
34. Berul CI, Callans DJ, Schwartzman DS, et al. Comparison of initial detection and redetection of ventricular fibrillation in a transvenous defibrillator system with automatic gain control. J Am Coll Cardiol 1995;25:431–436.
35. Cooklin M, Tummala RV, Peters RW, et al. Comparison of bipolar and integrated sensing for redetection of ventricular fibrillation. Am Heart J 1999;138:133–136.
36. Gold MR, Shorofsky SR. Transvenous defibrillation lead systems. J Cardiovasc Electrophysiol 1996;7:570–580.
37. Reiter MJ, Mann DE. Sensing and tachyarrhythmia detection problems in implantable cardioverter defibrillators. J Cardiovasc Electrophysiol 1996;7:542–558.
38. Peters RW, Cooklin M, Brockman R, et al. Inappropriate shocks from implanted cardioverter defibrillators caused by sensing of diaphragmatic myopotentials. J Intervent Cardiac Electrophysiol 1998;2:367–370.
39. Peters RW, Foster AH, Shorofsky SR, et al. Spurious discharges due to late insulation break in endocardial sensing leads for cardioverter defibrillators. Pacing Clin Electrophysiol 1995;18:478–481.
40. Marchlinski FE, Callans DJ, Gottlieb CD, et al. Benefits and lessons learned from stored electrogram information in implantable defibrillators. J Cardiovasc Electrophysiol 1995;6:832–1851.

41. Dijkman B, Wellens HJJ. Dual chamber arrhythmia discrimination in the implantable cardioverter defibrillator. J Cardiovasc Electrophysiol 2000;11:1105–1115.
42. Deisenhofer I, Kolb C, Ndrepepa G, et al. Do current dual chamber cardioverter defibrillators have advantages over conventional single chamber cardioverter defibrillators in reducing inappropriate therapies? A randomized, prospective study. J Cardiovasc Electrophysiol 2001;12:134–142.
43. Gold MR, Shorofsky SR, Thompson JA, et al. Advanced rhythm discrimination for implantable cardioverter defibrillators using electrogram vector timing and correlation. J Cardiovasc Electrophysiol 2002;13:1092–1097.
44. Newman D, Dorian P, Hardy J. Randomized controlled comparison of antitachycardia pacing algorithms for termination of ventricular tachycardia. J Am Coll Cardiol 1993;21:1413–1418.
45. Schaumann A, Muhlen FVZ, Herse B, et al. Empirical versus tested antitachycardia pacing in implanted cardioverter defibrillators: a prospective study including 200 patients. Circulation 1998;97:66–74.
46. Wathen MS, Sweeney MO, DeGroot PJ, et al. Shock reduction using antitachycardia pacing for spontaneous rapid ventricular tachycardia in patients with coronary artery disease. Circulation 2001;104:796–801.
47. Bardy GH, Poole JE, Kudenchuk PJ, et al. A prospective randomized repeat-crossover comparison of antitachycardia pacing with low-energy cardioversion. Circulation. 1993 Jun;87(6):1889–1896.
48. Dillon SM. The electrophysiologic effects of defibrillation shocks. In: Kroll MW, Lehmann MH, eds. Implantable Cardioverter Defibrillator Therapy. The Engineering Clinical Interface. Norwell: Kluwer Academic, 1996:31–61.
49. Gold MR, Shorofsky SR. Strength-duration relationship for human transvenous defibrillation. Circulation 1997;96:3517–3520.
50. Saksena S, An H, Mehra R, et al. Prospective comparison of biphasic and monophasic shocks for implantable cardioverter-defibrillators using endocardial leads. Am J Cardiol 1992;70:304–310.
51. Block M, Hammel D, Bocker D, et al. A prospective randomized cross-over comparison of mono- and biphasic defibrillation using nonthoracotomy lead configurations in humans. J Cardiovasc Electrophysiol 1994;5:581–590.
52. Strickberger SA, Hummel JD, Horwood LE, et al. Effect of shock polarity on ventricular defibrillation threshold using a transvenous lead system. J Am Coll Cardiol 1994;24:1069–1072.
53. Shorofsky SR, Gold MR. Effects of waveform and polarity on defibrillation thresholds in humans using a transvenous lead system. Am J Cardiol 1996;78:313–316.
54. Olsovsky MR, Shorofsky SR, Gold MR. Effect of shock polarity on biphasic defibrillation thresholds using an active pectoral lead system. J Cardiovasc Electrophysiol 1998;9:350–354.
55. Strickberger SA, Man KC, Daoud E, et al. Effect of first-phase polarity of biphasic shocks on defibrillation threshold with a single transvenous lead system. J Am Coll Cardiol 1995;25:1605–1608.
56. Bardy GH, Poole JE, Kudenchuk PJ, et al. A prospective randomized comparison in humans of biphasic waveform 60-μF and 120-μF capacitance pulses using a unipolar defibrillation system. Circulation 1995;91:91–95.
57. Swerdlow CD, Kass RM, Davie S, et al. Short biphasic pulses from 90 microfarad capacitors lower defibrillation threshold. Pacing Clin Electrophysiol 1996;19:1053–1060.

58. Poole J, Kudenchuk P, Dolack G, et al. A prospective randomized comparison in humans of 90μF and 120μF biphasic pulse defibrillation using a unipolar pectoral transvenous defibrillation system. J Cardiovasc Electrophysiol 1995;6:1097–1100.
59. Block M, Hammel D, Bocker D, et al. Internal defibrillation with smaller capacitors: a prospective randomized cross-over comparison of defibrillation efficacy obtained with 90-μF and 125-μF capacitors in humans. J Cardiovasc Electrophysiol 1995;6:333–342.
60. Bardy GH, Johnson G, Poole JE, et al. A simplified, single-lead unipolar transvenous cardioversion-defibrillation system. Circulation 1993;88:543–547.
61. Haffajee C, Martin D, Bhandari A, et al. A multicenter, randomized trial comparing an active can implantable defibrillator with a passive can system. Pacing Clin Electrophysiol 1997;20:215–219.
62. Poole JE, Bardy GH, Dolack GL, et al. A prospective randomized evaluation of implantable cardioverter-defibrillator size on unipolar defibrillation system efficacy. Circulation 1995;92:2940–2943.
63. Gold MR, Foster AH, Shorofsky SR. Effects of an active pectoral-pulse generator shell on defibrillation efficacy with a transvenous lead system. Am J Cardiol 1996;78:540–543.
64. Gold MR, Foster AH, Shorofsky SR. Lead system optimization for transvenous defibrillation. Am J Cardiol 1997;80:1163–1167.
65. Gold MR, Olsovsky MR, Pelini MA, et al. Comparison of single- and dual-coil active pectoral defibrillation lead systems. J Am Coll Cardiol 1998;31:1391–1394.
66. Stajduhar KC, Ott GY, Kron F, et al. Optimal electrode configuration for pectoral transvenous implantable defibrillation: a prospective randomized study. J Am Coll Cardiol 1996;27:90–94.
67. Gold MR, Olsovsky MR, DeGroot PJ, et al. Optimization of transvenous coil position for active can defibrillation thresholds. J Cardiovasc Electrophysiol 2000;11: 25–29.
68. Kirk MM, Shorofsky SR, Gold MR. Right sided active pectoral pulse generators do not reduce defibrillation thresholds. Pacing Clin Electrophysiol 1999;22:747.
69. Neuzner J, Schwarz T, Strasser R, et al. Effect of the addition of an abdominal hot can cardioverter/defibrillator pulse generator on the defibrillation energy requirements in a single-lead endocardial defibrillation system. Eur Heart J 1997;18: 1655–1658.
70. Raitt MH, Johnson G, Dolack GL, et al. Clinical predictors of the defibrillation threshold with the unipolar implantable defibrillation system. J Am Coll Cardiol 1995;25:1576–1583.
71. Hodgson DM, Olsovsky MR, Shorofsky SR, et al. Clinical predictors of defibrillation thresholds with an active pectoral pulse generator lead system. PACE 2002;25: 408–413.
72. Higgins SL, Alexander DC, Kuypers CJ, et al. The subcutaneous array: a new lead adjunct for the transvenous ICD to lower defibrillation thresholds. Pacing Clin Electrophysiol 1995;18:1540–1548.
73. Epstein AE, Ellenbogen KA, Kirk KA, et al. Clinical characteristics and outcome of patients with high defibrillation thresholds: a multicenter study. Circulation 1992;86: 1206–1216.
74. Wetherbee JN, Chapman PD, Troup PJ, et al. Long term internal cardiac defibrillation threshold stability. Pacing Clin Electrophysiol 1989;12:443–450.

75. Venditti FJ, Martin DT, Vassolas G, et al. Rise in chronic defibrillation thresholds in nonthoracotomy implantable defibrillator. Circulation 1994;89:216–223.
76. Gold MR, Kavesh NG, Peters RW, et al. Biphasic waveforms prevent the chronic rise of defibrillation thresholds with a transvenous lead system. J Am Coll Cardiol 1997;30:233–236.
77. Tokano T, Pelosi F, Flemming M, et al. Long-term evaluation of the ventricular defibrillation energy requirement. J Cardiovasc Electrophysiol 1998;9:916–920.
78. Dijkman B, Wellens HJ. Diagnosis and therapy of atrial tachyarrhythmias in the dual chamber implantable cardioverter defibrillator. J Cardiovasc Electrophysiol 2000;11:1196–1205.
79. Gold MR, Sulke N, Schwartzman DS, et al. Clinical experience with a dual-chamber implantable cardioverter defibrillator to treat atrial tachyarrhythmias. J Cardiovasc Electrophysiol 2001;12:1247–1253.
80. Adler SW, Wolpert C, Warman E, et al. Efficacy of pacing therapies for treating atrail tachyarrhythmias in patients with ventricular arrhythmias receiving a dual-chamber implantable cardioverter defibrillator. Circulation 2001;104:887–892.
81. Friedman PA, Kijkman B, Warman EN, et al. Atrial therapies reduce atrial arrhythmia burden in defibrillator patients. Circulation 2001;104:1023–1028.
82. Newman DM, Dorain P, Paquette M, et al. The effect of an implantable cardioverter defibrillator with atrial detection and shock therapies on patient perceived health-related quality of life. Am Heart J 2002;145:841–846.

Cardiac Resynchronization Therapy

Michael O. Sweeney

9

A HEART FAILURE EPIDEMIC

There are 4 to 5 million people living with chronic heart failure and an additional 400,000 newly diagnosed yearly.[1–3] The incidence of heart failure is 10 per 1000 for individuals who are older than 65 years of age. The increasing incidence of heart failure is due primarily to the advancing age of the population with coronary artery disease, which is now the principal cause of heart failure associated with reduced ventricular function (dilated cardiomyopathy, DCM).[4] Mortality due to progressive heart failure associated with DCM has declined. In the Framingham study, total mortality was 24% and 55% within 4 years of developing symptomatic heart failure for women and men, respectively.[4] These statistics approximate well the natural history of heart failure as the subject population was untreated by contemporary standards. Recognition of the beneficial effects of ACE inhibitors, diuretics, digoxin, and beta-blockade has yielded substantial reductions in mortality due to progressive pump failure. However, despite these improvements in medical therapy, symptomatic heart failure still confers a 20% to 25% risk of premature death in the first 2½ years after diagnosis.

Almost all heart failure patients will have at least one acute episode with symptoms requiring hospitalization and treatment with intravenous medications to stabilize their condition. Hospital discharges for heart failure totaled approximately 1,000,000 in 2001 and have increased more than 150% from 1979. Hospitalization for management of heart failure imposes the highest cost by diagnosis-related grouping (DRG) to the US healthcare system.

ABNORMAL ELECTRICAL TIMING IN HEART FAILURE ASSOCIATED WITH DILATED CARDIOMYOPATHY

Disordered electrical timing frequently accompanies heart failure associated with DCM. Disordered electrical timing alters critical mechanical relationships that further impair left ventricular (LV) performance. It is now recognized that there are four levels of electromechanical abnormalities associated with heart failure associated with DCM.[5,6] These are prolonged atrioventricular (AV) delay, interventricular delay, intraventricular delay, and intramural delay.

Prolonged Atrioventricular Delay

Optimal AV coupling is necessary for maximum ventricular pumping performance. The normal AV interval results in atrial contraction just before the pre-ejection (isovolumic) period of ventricular contraction that maximizes ventricular filling (LV end diastolic pressure, or pre-load) and cardiac output by the Starling mechanisms. This optimal timing relationship also results in diastolic filling throughout the entire diastolic filling period, prevents diastolic mitral regurgitation (MR) and maintains mean left atrial pressure at low levels (Fig. 9.1).

Alterations in the AV coupling can be understood by analysis of Doppler mitral inflow patterns (Fig. 9.2). Prolonged AV conduction disrupts these relationships and may degrade ventricular performance. Significantly prolonged AV conduction results in displacement of atrial contraction earlier in diastole such that atrial contraction may occur immediately after or even within the preceding ventricular contraction. This may result in atrial contraction before venous return is completed, thereby reducing the atrial contribution to pre-load and diminishing ventricular volume and contractile force. It may also initiate early mitral valve closure, limiting diastolic filling time. Diastolic MR may also occur with prolonged AV conduction because once closed, valve cusps may separate again before ventricular contraction as a result of the development of a left ventricular-left atrial gradient in diastole induced by atrial contraction with premature and incomplete mitral valve closure (Fig. 9.3).

Interventricular Delay

Optimal inter- and intraventricular coupling is more important than AV coupling for maximum ventricular pumping function. Normal ventricular electrical activation is rapid and homogeneous with minimal temporal dispersion throughout the wall. This elicits a synchronous mechanical activation and ventricular contraction. Exploration of the link between the sequence of cardiac electrical activation and mechanical function is one of the most exciting contemporary areas of research in heart failure but recognition of the importance of normal ventricular activation patterns for optimal pumping function dates back 75 years. Wiggers observed that asynchronous delayed activation of the ventricular musculature induced by electrical stimulation had adverse hemodynamic consequences in mammals and proposed that the more muscle activated before excitation of the Purkinje system, the greater the asynchrony and the weaker the resulting contraction.[7] Forty years later, Schlant reached similar conclusions and concluded that asynchronous ventricular activation imposed by significant interventricular conduction delay (LBBB) was hemodynamically disadvantageous due to loss of the "idioventricular kick."[8] This is a term applied to improved systolic function resulting from coordinated myocardial segment activation. This was attributed to the greater stretch and increased contractility

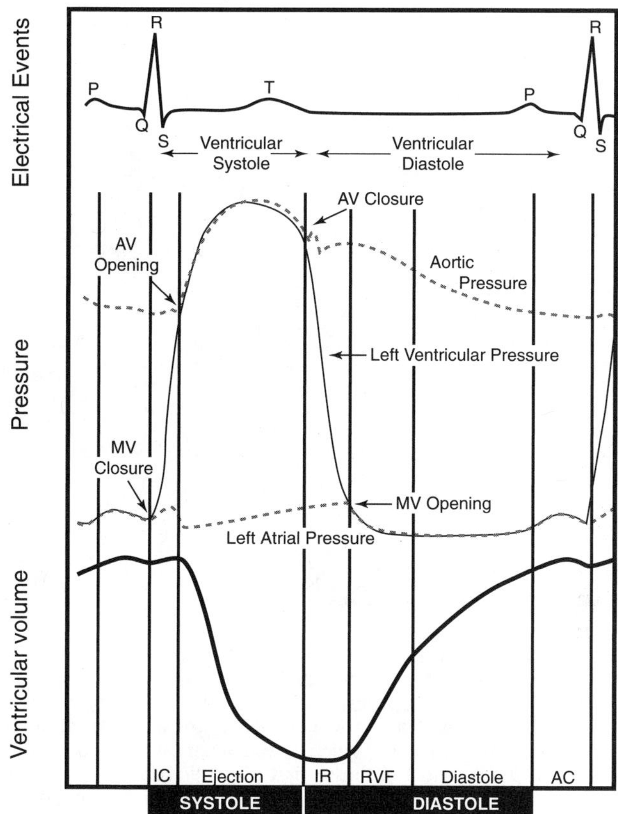

Figure 9.1. Events of the cardiac electrical cycle. Atrial contraction followed by relaxation produces a negative pressure gradient, causing a surge of blood in the LV at end diastole. Reversal of the atrioventricular pressure gradient initiates mitral valve (MV) closure because of a rapid decrease in pressure between the MV cusps pulling them into apposition. A brief period of isovolumetric contraction exists after MV closure and before AV opening during which the maximal rate of pressure change (peak + dP/dt) occurs. Rapid ejection occurs during ventricular systole and is terminated when ventricular pressure falls below aortic pressure, closing the aortic valve (AV). A brief period of isovolumic relaxation follows during which the maximal rate of pressure decline (peak – dP/dt) occurs. As the left ventricular (LV) pressure continues to decline and fall below atrial pressure, the MV opens and diastolic ventricular filling begins. Normal diastolic filling is characterized by an initial rapid increase in ventricular filling during early diastole followed by a slow phase of filling during mid-diastole. A second rapid increase in ventricular filling occurs in late diastole as a result of atrial contraction.

(by Starling's law) of later contracting areas that is imparted by earlier contraction of other areas.

Chronic DCM is often accompanied by delayed ventricular electrical activation manifest as prolonged QRS duration (QRSd), most commonly in the form of left bundle branch block (LBBB). The prevalence of prolonged QRSd in heart failure associated with DCM varies between studies but appears to be

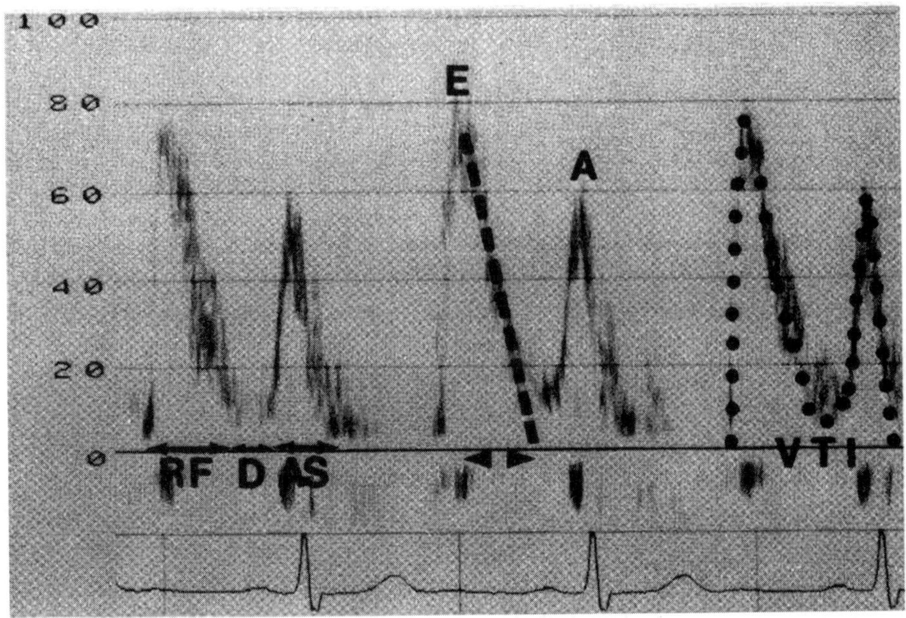

Figure 9.2. Doppler mitral inflow patterns. This figure shows left ventricular (LV) filling velocities from a normal subject, recorded at the level of the mitral leaflet tips (apical window) with pulsed-wave Doppler. The mitral flow velocity curve is composed of the peak initial velocity (E wave) and the velocity at atrial contraction (A wave). This comprises the diastolic filling period, which is the interval from the onset of the E velocity to the cessation of the A velocity. In the first diastolic complex, the periods of rapid filling (RF), diastasis (D), and atrial systole (AS) are labeled. In the second complex, early diastolic (E) and atrial systolic (A) maximum velocities are indicated. The dashed line denotes the slope of decay of the peak early diastolic velocity and the arrowheads mark the deceleration time. The third complex shows how planimetry of the diastolic velocity curve as a function of time yields the velocity-time integral (VTI), which indicates diastolic "stroke distance."

in the range of 25% to 50%. Prolonged QRSd is a potent predictor of mortality in heart failure associated with DCM. In the VEST study, which assessed the efficacy of vesnarinone in patients with DCM and class II-IV heart failure, age, creatinine, ejection fraction, heart rate, and QRSd were found to be independent predictors of mortality. Cumulative survival from all-cause mortality decreased proportionally with QRSd. The relative risk of the widest QRSd group was five times greater than the narrowest.[9] The association between LBBB in DCM and increased risk of sudden death and total mortality in DCM has subsequently been demonstrated in large population studies.[10]

Interventricular coupling refers to coordinated contraction of the right ventricle (RV) and LV. *Interventricular delay* refers to a relative delay in mechanical activation of each ventricle, most commonly LBBB where the RV begins its contraction before the LV. The delay in onset of left ventricular activation results in reversal of the normal sequence between right and left ventricular

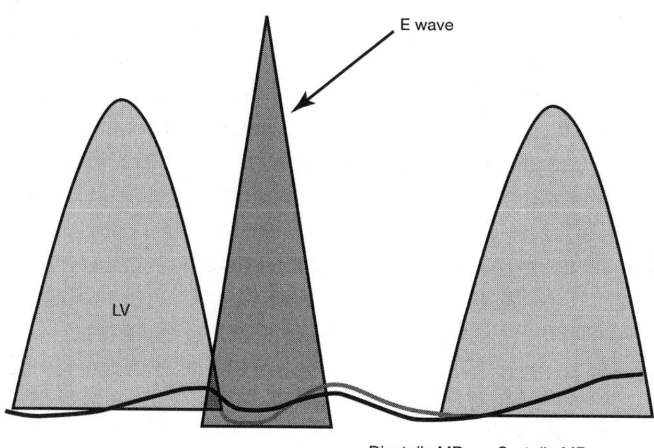

Figure 9.3. Schematic representation of hemodynamic effects of prolonged native AV conduction on left ventricular performance. The absence of the "a" wave before ventricular contraction may result in suboptimal ventricular filling and diastolic mitral regurgitation.

mechanical events that persists throughout the cardiac cycle.[11] Asynchronous ventricular contraction and relaxation results in dynamic changes in ventricular pressures and volumes throughout the cardiac cycle. This results in abnormal septal deflections that alter the regional contribution to global ejection fraction. Earliest ventricular depolarization is recorded over the anterior surface of the RV and latest at the basal-lateral LV.[12] In canine models with induced LBBB, increasing the delay between RV and LV contraction increases the delay between the upslope of LV and RV systolic pressure. The increase in interventricular delay was associated with decreased LV + dP/dt and decreased stroke work, presumably the result of ventricular interdependence and impairment of the septal contribution to LV ejection due to displacement after onset of RV ejection.[13]

Pacing models can be used to induce asynchronous ventricular activation, with early activation occurring at the pacing site.[14,15] Regions of late activation are subject to greater wall stress and develop local myocyte hypertrophy accompanied by reductions in sarcoplasmic reticulum calcium-ATPase and phospholamban.[16] Chronic asynchronous ventricular activation redistributes the mechanical load within the ventricular wall and leads to reduction of blood flow and myocardial wall thickness over the site of early activation.[15,17] This ventricular remodeling may contribute to progression of heart failure. In addition to these effects, delayed, sequential activation of papillary muscles may aggravate mitral regurgitation.[18]

Intraventricular Delay

The third level of synchrony exists within each ventricle. Normally, the rapid spread of contraction from the LV septum endocardially to the base of the heart creates coordinated, efficient contraction. With LBBB, and delayed propagation of the electrical impulse across the LV, the septum begins contraction substantially earlier than the lateral wall. When one segment of the ventricle, such as the septum, contracts earlier than another segment, such as the lateral wall, the lateral wall stretches, absorbing some of the initial force, then begins its late contraction, stretching the septum. Shortening of earlier activated regions is wasted work because pressure is low and no ejection is occurring. Delayed shortening of late activated regions occurs at higher wall stress because the early regions have already developed tension, yet it is also characterized by wasted work because the early regions may now undergo paradoxical stretch. The resulting contraction is mechanically inefficient, with diminished ejection at an increased metabolic cost. This is accompanied by increased end systolic volume and wall stress and reduced LV + dP/dt and diastolic filling time. The net result is an acute decline in systolic function of approximately 20%.

Intramural Delay

Studies of activation maps have shown different activation timing and sequence between endocardial and transmural activation. This suggests the possibility of intramural activation delay between the endocardial and myocardial layer.[19] The negative effects, if any, of intramural delay on ventricular pumping function, are uncertain.

CARDIAC RESYNCHRONIZATION THERAPY

Recognition of the contribution of disordered electrical timing to reduced ventricular performance suggested the possibility that pacing techniques could favorably modulate contractile dyssynchrony and delayed AV timing. The fundamental premise of this therapeutic strategy is that left ventricular preexcitation may correct inter- and intraventricular conduction delays and permit optimization of left-sided AV delay, thereby improving ventricular pumping function.

The first report of the potential hemodynamic benefit of left univentricular pacing used epicardial leads placed on the high right atrium and lateral left ventricular (LV) free wall during surgery for aortic valve replacement in patients with LBBB.[20] de Teresa and colleagues[20] noted that left ventricular ejection fraction was maximal when septal motion was simultaneous with free wall contraction and diminished when septal and free wall motion were dyssynchronous, such as during spontaneous activation with LBBB or during right ventricular (RV) apical pacing. The term "cardiac resynchronization" was first used 10 years later when Cazeau and colleagues[21] used epicardial leads on all four cardiac chambers to modify the ventricular activation sequence and improve hemodynamic performance in heart failure due to dilated cardiomyopathy accompanied by LBBB.

Mechanisms of Cardiac Resynchronization Therapy

Improved Pumping Function: Atrioventricular Optimization and Ventricular Resynchronization: Correction of physiologically disadvantageous prolonged AV conduction (*AV optimization*) can be achieved with left ventricular preexcitation. Optimization of the AV interval during CRT can be conceptualized by examining mitral flow velocity curves using two-dimensional echocardiography.

When left ventricular preexcitation is inadequate, the result is similar to a prolonged AV interval as shown in Figure 9.3. Note atrial contraction occurs too early and does not contribute to increased LVEDP (absence of A wave on mitral inflow velocity). Atrial contraction occurs before venous return is completed causing reduced ventricular volume and contractile force. It may also initiate early mitral valve closure, thereby limiting diastolic filling time. Diastolic MR may also occur because once closed, the mitral valve may drift open again before ventricular contraction.

When the programmed AV interval is too short, LV preexcitation occurs too early relative to atrial systole (Fig. 9.4). Note that diastolic filling occurs throughout all of diastole. Atrial contraction now occurs simultaneously with LV contraction resulting in increased left atrial pressure and loss of atrial contribution to ventricular systole, reducing cardiac output. A shorter AV interval lengthens the diastolic filling period by abolishing premature mitral valve closure due to the LV-left atrial pressure gradient seen with long AV delays. This also eliminates diastolic MR. However, the diastolic filling period should not be used as the only guideline to optimize the AV interval. Despite optimization of the diastolic filling period, hemodynamic deterioration will occur at too short an AV interval if atrial contraction occurs against a closed mitral valve. This could

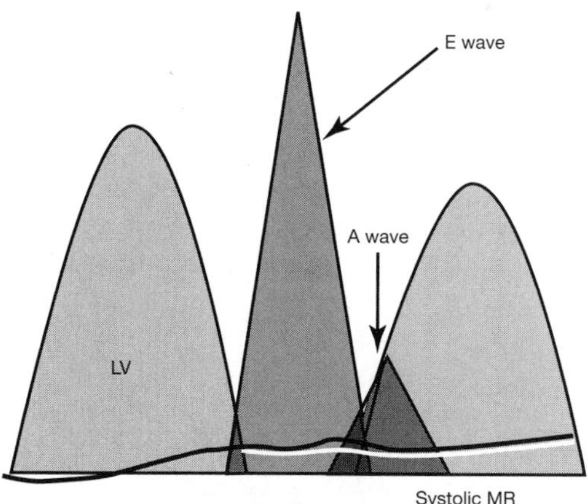

Figure 9.4. Schematic representation of hemodynamic effects of too short an AV interval on left ventricular performance. The atrial contraction is incomplete at the time of ventricular systole. This leads to ventricular under-filling, systolic mitral regurgitation, and atrial contraction against closed AV valves.

result in a decrease in cardiac output and increase in mean left atrial pressure despite optimization of the diastolic filling period.

LV preexcitation at the optimal AV interval is shown in Figure 9.5. The relation of atrial contraction to the onset of ventricular contraction is now optimal, resulting in diastolic filling throughout the entire diastolic filling period. An appropriate relation now exists between mechanical left atrial and left ventricular contraction so that mean left atrial pressure is maintained at a low level with left atrial contraction occurring just before left ventricular contraction. This causes an increase in LVEDP (preload) and cardiac output. Note diastolic MR is eliminated and systolic MR is reduced.

Acute hemodynamic studies have shown that AV delay is a significant determinant of changes in all LV systolic parameters (+ dP/dt, aortic systolic pressure, aortic pulse pressure).[22] For CRT "responders" (see below). LV + dP/dt and aortic pulse pressure AV delay functions are positive and unimodal, with a peak effect at approximately 50% of the native PR interval. The optimal AV delays for the same pacing chamber and parameter varied widely among patients and often differed for pulse pressure and LV + dP/dt within an individual.[22] The acute increase in LV + dP/dt with optimal AV delay may be in the range of 15% to 45%.[22,23]

The hemodynamic benefit of LV preexcitation is primarily due to *ventricular resynchronization* rather than AV optimization, however. The decreased LV + dP/dt and decreased stroke work associated with interventricular delay can be eliminated by CRT[13] and improvements in RV to LV delay correlate with improvements in EF.[24] Furthermore, CRT improves pumping function while decreasing myocardial energy consumption.[25]

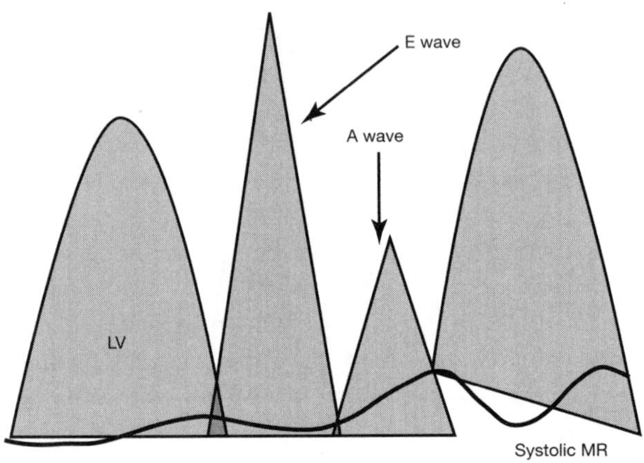

Figure 9.5. Schematic representation of hemodynamic effects of optimal AV interval on left ventricular performance. The optimal AV interval prevents mitral regurgitation, maximizes ventricular filling and reduces mean atrial pressure.

Reverse Left Ventricular Remodeling: In addition to improvement in acute hemodynamic performance, it has now been clearly demonstrated that CRT improves chronic left ventricular pumping function. This improvement is accompanied by Doppler echocardiographic (conventional two-dimensional and tissue imaging) evidence of reverse left ventricular remodeling.[26–28] These remodeling effects include reduction in left ventricular volume, redistribution of cardiac mass, reduced mitral orifice size and reduced mitral regurgitation.

Other Effects of Cardiac Resynchronization Therapy: Reduction in Functional Mitral Regurgitation

Functional MR frequently accompanies DCM and results from an imbalance between the closing and tethering forces that act on the mitral leaflets and has been elegantly described by Breithardt and colleagues.[18] This is strongly dependent on alterations in ventricular shape as the tethering forces that act on the mitral leaflets are higher in dilated, more spherical ventricles. These geometric changes alter the balance between tethering and closing forces and impede effective mitral closure. Ventricular dilatation and increased chamber sphericity increase the distance between the papillary muscles to the enlarged mitral annulus as well as to each other, restricting leaflet motion and increasing the force needed for effective mitral valve closure. This mitral valve closing force is determined by the systolic left ventricular pressure-left atrial pressure difference, which is called the transmitral pressure gradient. Under these conditions, the mitral regurgitant orifice area will be largely determined by the phasic changes in transmitral pressure. Increasing the transmitral pressure can reduce the effective regurgitant orifice area. CRT acutely reduces the severity of functional MR and this reduction is quantitatively related to an increase in LV + D*P*/dt max and transmitral pressure.[18] This is distinct from the reduction in MR due to reduced LV dimensions from remodeling associated with chronic CRT.

Functional mitral regurgitation may also occur due to delayed sequential activation of the papillary muscles due to intraventricular delay.[18] This accounts for the acute hemodynamic deterioration reported in some patients after ablation of the AV junction and institution of RV apical pacing, which mimics LBBB.[29,30] This can be ameliorated by CRT.[31]

Implementation of Cardiac Resynchronization Therapy

There are currently three approaches to achieving left ventricular pacing. The transvenous approach uses specially designed delivery sheaths and tools for cannulating the coronary sinus to permit delivery of pacing leads into the epicardial venous circulation serving the left ventricular free wall. Left ventricular pacing lead placement can also be achieved under direct visualization using a cardiac surgical approach. Finally, transvenous left ventricular endocardial pacing via transseptal puncture has been described in the rare circumstance where neither the transvenous epicardial nor surgical options are viable.[32,33]

Approach to Transvenous Left Ventricular Lead Placement

Early attempts at epicardial LV pacing via the coronary veins utilized standard endocardial pacing leads designed for right ventricular pacing or coronary sinus leads designed for left atrial pacing.[34] This approach was met with predictable difficulties, including lead dislodgment, high pacing thresholds and inability to reach the target coronary venous branch. Currently available tools and techniques achieve a greater than 90% transvenous LV lead placement success rate.

Typically, the coronary sinus is cannulated with a specially designed sheath that serves as a workstation for LV lead placement. Such sheaths are available in a variety of diameters and shapes intended to overcome unpredictable anatomic variation in right heart anatomy. Although directional sheaths permit unassisted cannulation of the coronary sinus ostium in some cases, most implanters cannulate the coronary sinus with a deflectable electrophysiology catheter or a coronary angiography catheter. The sheath is then advanced into the coronary sinus body using the catheter as a railing system (Fig. 9.6).

Once the coronary sinus is successfully cannulated, retrograde venography is performed to delineate the coronary venous anatomy (Fig. 9.7). This is done with a standard balloon occlusion catheter and hand injections of contrast material. Care must be taken to achieve a good seal within the main body of the coronary sinus in order to obtain maximal opacification of the distal vasculature. Underfilling the coronary venous system is a common mistake that may result in failure to identify potentially suitable targets for LV pacing lead place-

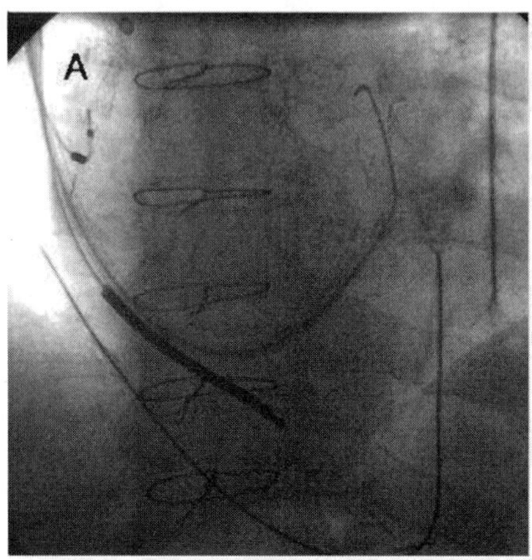

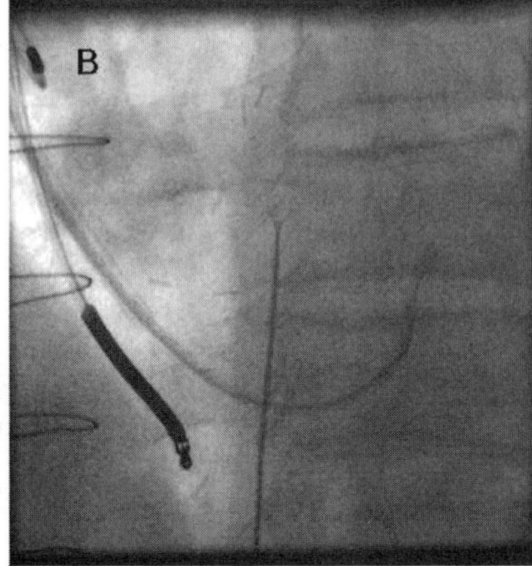

Figure 9.6. Cannulation of the coronary sinus using a coronary guide catheter and an over-the-wire technique. **A:** The guidewire has been directed into the coronary sinus by the sheath in the right atrium. The sheath is advanced over the wire. Note LV lead delivery sheath within main body of coronary sinus. **B:** The guidewire is withdrawn into the sheath.

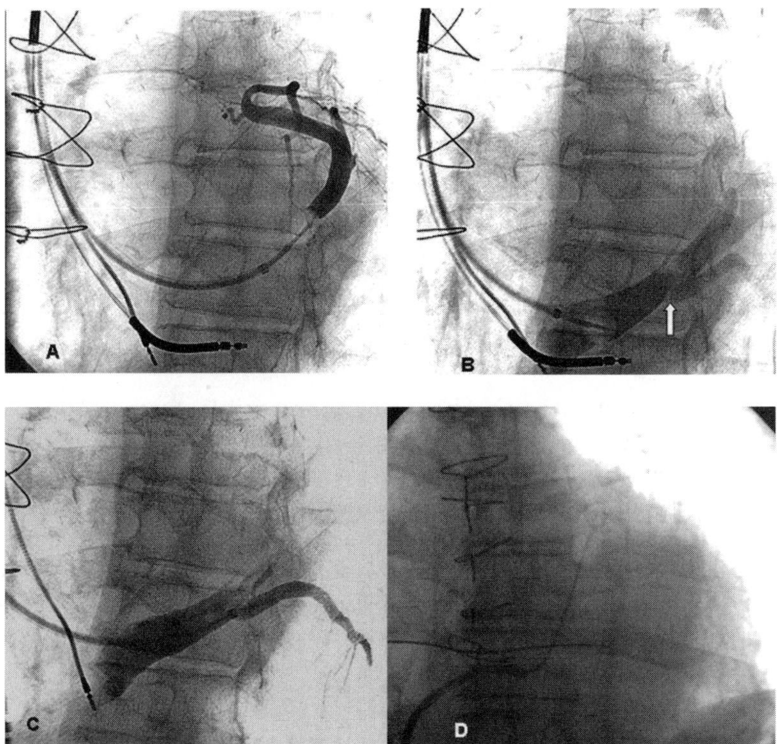

Figure 9.7. Retrograde coronary venogram. **Panel A:** With the balloon occlusive catheter in the distal coronary sinus there appear to be no satisfactory lateral veins for lead placement. **Panel B:** Repeat venogram with the balloon proximal in the coronary sinus partially fills a more proximal branch missed on the distal injection. **Panel C:** Subselection of the proximal branch with the inner sheath of the guide system depicts this branch well. **Panel D:** Retrograde coronary sinus venogram by the femoral approach in another patient.

ment. Occasionally the inflated balloon will occlude the ostium of a suitable branch vessel for LV lead placement, therefore occlusive venography at multiple levels within the main CS are advisable (see Fig. 9.7).

Currently available transvenous LV pacing leads may be either stylet driven or use over-the-wire delivery similar to percutaneous coronary intervention. Fixation relies primarily on "wedging" the lead tip into a distal site within the target vein such that the outer diameter of the lead closely approximates the inner luminal diameter of the vein. Some current LV lead designs incorporate one or more tines, which may assist with fixation by catching on a valve or promoting thrombosis, but are probably otherwise irrelevant. Active fixation technologies are in development and will likely incorporate various self-retaining bends or cants that compress the distal segment of the lead against the outer wall of the vein and the epicardial surface of the heart.

Factors Limiting Successful Transvenous Left Ventricular Lead Placement

Complex and unpredictable anatomic and technical considerations may preclude successful delivery of the LV lead to an optimal pacing site.

Inability to Cannulate the Coronary Sinus: It is difficult to estimate the true percentage of cases in which the coronary sinus cannot be cannulated because this is clearly influenced by operator experience. It is probably in the range of 1% to 5%. When the coronary sinus cannot be located by the superior approach, an adaptation of the inferior approach described for complex electrophysiology procedures is often successful in localizing the CS ostium (see Fig. 9.7).

Coronary Venous Anatomy: Absent or Inaccessible Target Veins: The coronary venous circulation demonstrates considerably more variability than the parallel arterial circulation (Fig. 9.8). Careful studies of retrograde coronary venography have revealed that the anterior interventricular vein is present in 99% of patients and the middle cardiac vein is present in 100%. These veins are generally undesirable for LV preexcitation because they do not reach the late activated portion of the LV free wall. Unfortunately, approximately 50% patients have only a single vein serving the LV free wall. Anatomically, this is a lateral

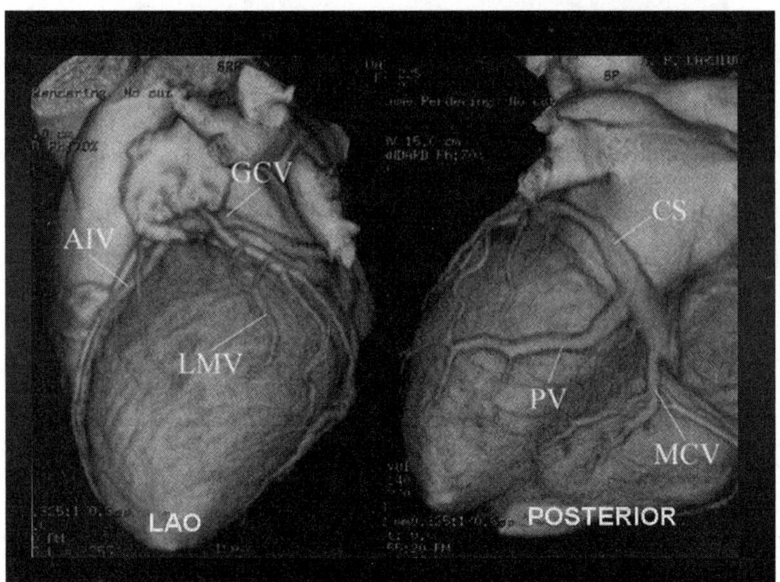

Figure 9.8. Three-dimensional reconstruction of epicardial coronary venous anatomy using computed tomography. (Reproduced with permission from Tada H, et al. Three-dimensional computed tomography of the coronary venous system. J Cardiovasc Electrophysiol 2003;14:1385.)

marginal vein in slightly more than 75% and a true posterior vein that ascends the free wall in approximately 50% of patients.[35] Thus, as many as 20% of patients may not have a vein that reaches the optimal LV free wall site for delivery of CRT. In some instances target veins are present but too small for cannulation with existing lead systems, or paradoxically too large to achieve mechanical fixation (Figs. 9.9 and 9.10).

Coronary Venous Tortuousity: Another commonly encountered difficulty in transvenous LV lead placement is tortuousity of the target vessel take-off or main segment. These anatomic constraints can be extremely difficult to overcome and often require the use of multiple LV lead designs and delivery systems (Fig. 9.11).

High Left Ventricular Stimulation Thresholds and Phrenic Nerve Stimulation: The principal limitation of the transvenous approach is that the selection

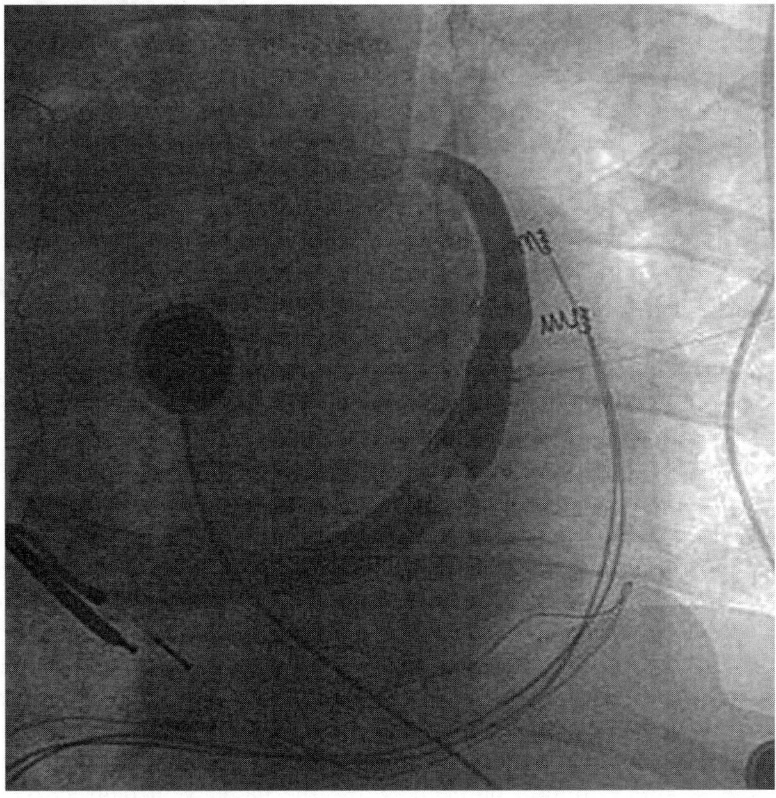

Figure 9.9. Absence of lateral marginal or posterior cardiac veins serving the LV free wall revealed by retrograde coronary venography.

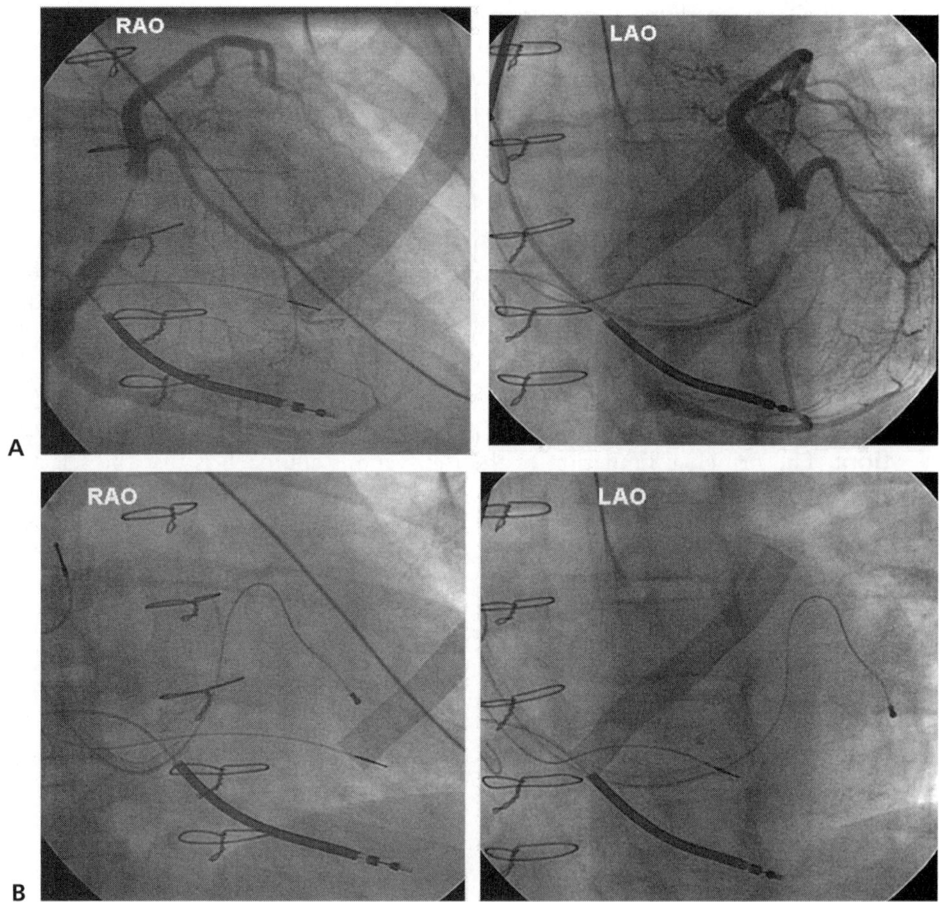

Figure 9.10. Panel A: RAO and LAO retrograde coronary venograms demonstrating very large lateral marginal vein descending toward the left ventricular apex. This patient has a unipolar ventricular pacing lead that was abandoned with the new ICD system. **Panel B:** LV lead descended to terminus of lateral marginal vein.

of sites for pacing is entirely dictated by navigable coronary venous anatomy. A commonly encountered problem is that an apparently suitable target vein delivers the lead to a site where ventricular capture can be achieved at only very high output voltages or not at all. This presumably relates to the presence of scar on the epicardial surface of the heart underlying the target vein and cannot be anticipated by fluoroscopic examination *a priori* (Fig. 9.12). If this is not successful, surgical placement of LV leads permits more detailed mapping of viable sites in the anatomic region of interest (see Fig. 9.12).

A second common problem is that the target vein delivers the lead to a site that results in phrenic nerve stimulation and diaphragmatic pacing. This can be difficult to demonstrate during implantation when the patient is supine and

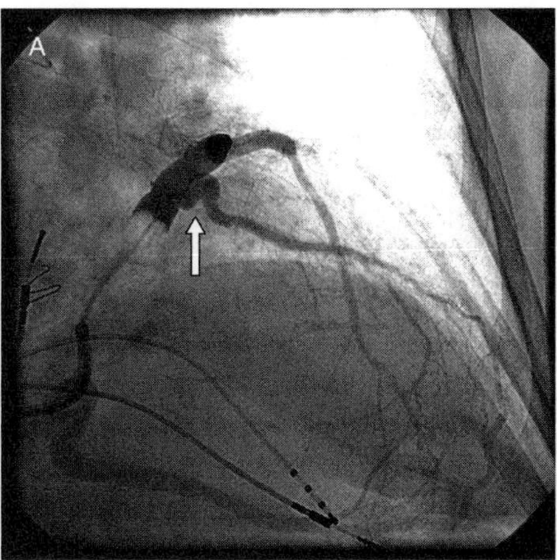

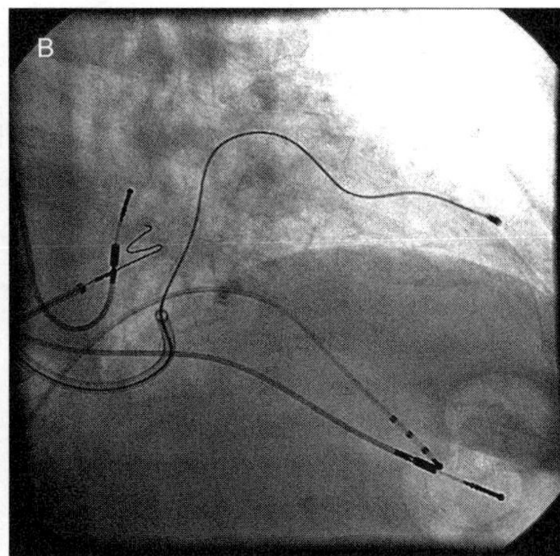

Figure 9.11. Panel A: "Shepherd's Crook" take-off of lateral marginal vein, with kink just beyond take off *(arrow)*. **Panel B:** A 6-Fr over-the-wire LV lead could not navigate the venous kinking but a 4-Fr over-the-wire lead successfully navigated the kinked portion of vein.

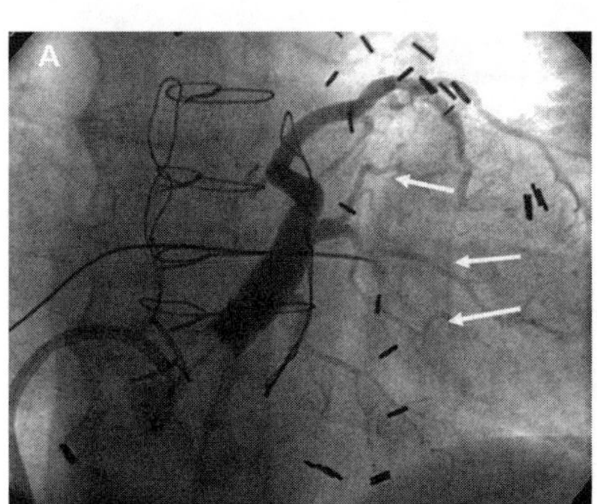

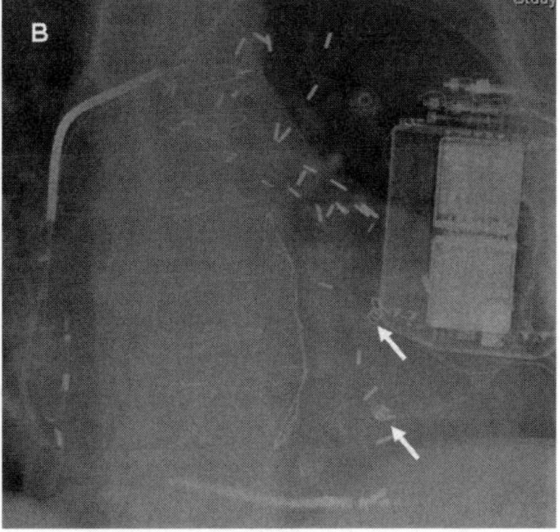

Figure 9.12. Panel A: Multiple diminutive lateral marginal veins. LV pacing threshold exceeded 6 V in all locations *(arrows)* in this vein system due to epicardial scar due to prior infarct (note surgical clips associated with prior coronary revascularization). **Panel B:** PA chest radiograph of surgically placed epicardial LV pacing leads *(arrows)* in same patient. Note LV free wall position of leads approximates obtuse marginal artery location in circumflex territory, where epicardial mapping identified viable sites for LV pacing. The second lead is a "back-up" that can be accessed if needed without repeat thoracotomy.

sedated but may be immediately evident when the patient is later active and changes body positions, even in the absence of lead dislodgment. Occasionally, if there is a significant differential in the capture thresholds for phrenic nerve stimulation versus LV capture, this can be overcome by manipulation of LV voltage output. However, many experienced implanters recognize that once phrenic nerve stimulation is observed acutely (during implantation), it is almost invariably encountered during follow-up despite manipulation of output voltages and therefore alternative site LV pacing is sought (Fig. 9.13). As with high LV capture thresholds, occasionally phrenic nerve stimulation can be overcome by repositioning the LV lead more proximally within the target vein (Fig. 9.14).

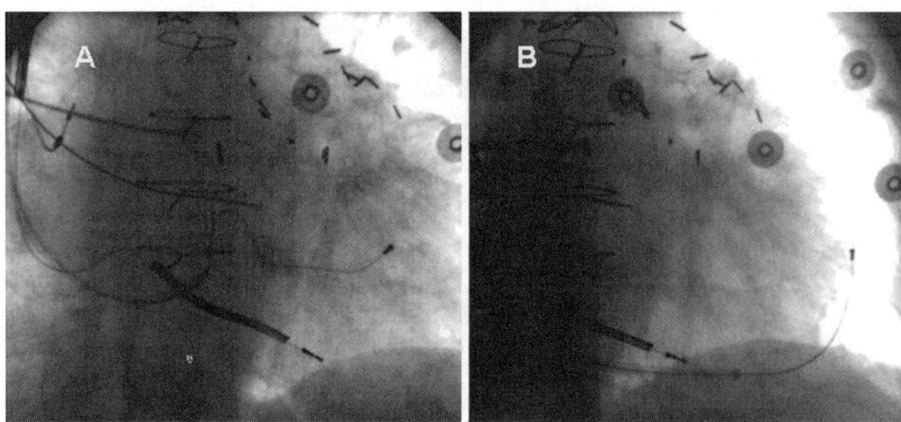

Figure 9.13. Panel A: LV lead is positioned in a lateral marginal vein but this site was rejected due to insuperable phrenic nerve stimulation. **Panel B:** Repositioning of the LV lead in a large posterior vein that was ascending the LV free wall eliminated phrenic nerve stimulation.

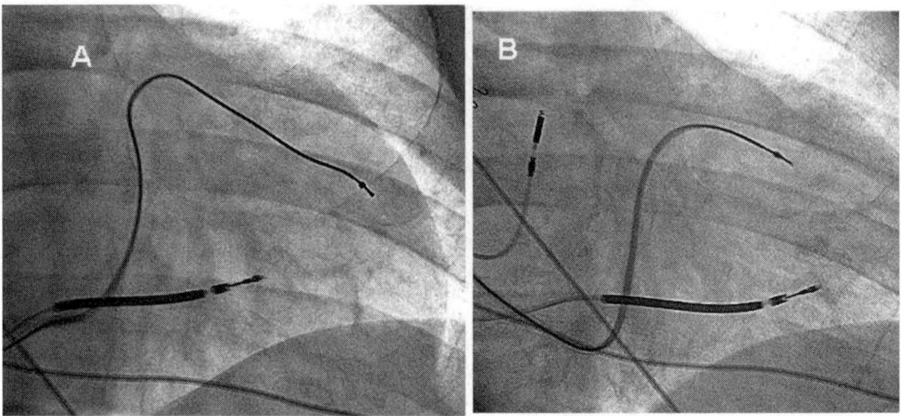

Figure 9.14. Panel A: LV lead positioned in lateral marginal vein. This site was rejected due to phrenic nerve stimulation. **Panel B:** Repositioning of a larger diameter LV lead more proximally in the same vein eliminated phrenic nerve stimulation.

Surgical Approach to Left Ventricular Lead Placement

The first clinical trial of CRT used a hybrid epicardial LV, endocardial RV pacing lead configuration for multisite ventricular stimulation simply because the technique for transvenous epicardial LV pacing had not been developed.[36]

There are several current approaches to surgical placement of LV pacing leads. Many surgeons still use a full left lateral thoracotomy, which permits full visualization of the LV free wall, but results in significant postoperative pain and an extended recovery period. More recently, a minimally invasive approach has been developed. In this approach, the patient is prepared lying on his or her right side with the left arm suspended overhead. Two or three "porthole" incisions are made in the left axillary space for access to the LV free wall (Fig. 9.15). Two epicardial LV leads are placed typically placed using the obtuse marginal branches of the circumflex coronary artery as regional landmarks, approximately 1 cm apical to the mitral annulus. After the leads are placed, the capped terminal pins are tunneled to a provisional pocket on the chest wall. The patient is then re-prepared and draped on his or her back; the provisional pocket is opened and terminal pins are tunneled to the pectoral pocket. One critical difference in patient preparation for surgical versus transvenous LV lead placement is that it is better to have the patient a little "dry" (well diuresed) in the former and a little "wet" (diuretics withheld) in the latter. In the case of the transvenous approach, adequate hydration may minimize the risk of contrast-induced renal failure. In contrast during the surgical approach volume overload may increase lung volume. This increases the hemodynamic consequences of single lung ventilation, particularly on right heart function and may limit LV visualization if complete left lung deflation cannot be achieved.

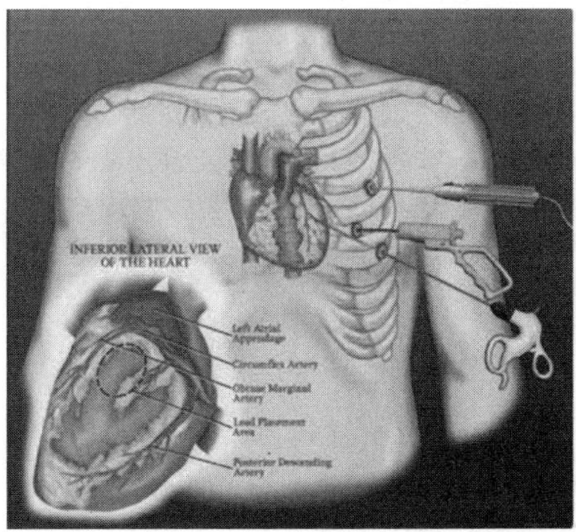

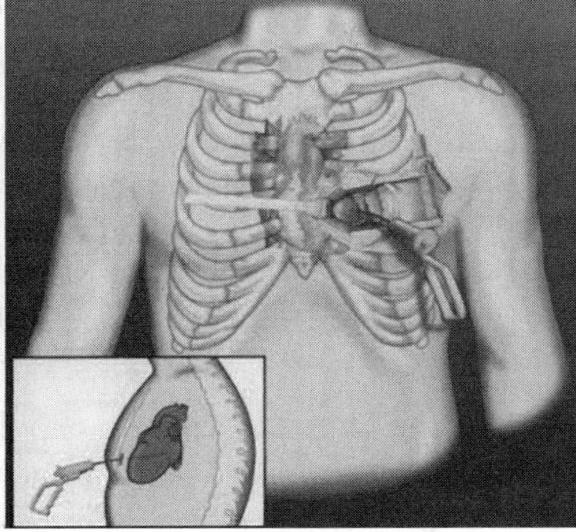

Figure 9.15. Surgical approach to minimally invasive placement of epicardial left ventricular pacing leads via "port hole" approach **(left)** or limited left lateral thoracotomy **(right)**. (Courtesy of Medtronic, Inc.)

Optimal Left Ventricular Lead Placement

The optimal site for LV pacing is a complex and unsettled consideration. It is probably true that the optimal site varies between patients and is likely to be modified by venous anatomy, regional and global LV mechanical function, myocardial substrate, characterization of electrical delay, and other factors. The success of resynchronization is dependent on pacing from a site that causes a change in the sequence of ventricular activation that translates to an improvement in cardiac performance. Such systolic improvement and mechanical resynchronization does not require electrical synchrony[12] and explains the lack of correlation between change in QRSd and clinical response to CRT. Ideally the pacing site or sites that produce the greatest hemodynamic effect would be selected.

However, current clinical evidence permits some generalizations LV pacing site selection for optimal acute hemodynamic response. At least three different independent investigations comparing the acute effects of different pacing sites in similar DCM populations have reported parallel evidence that stimulation site is a primary determinant of CRT hemodynamic benefit.

Auricchio and colleagues[36,37] showed a positive correlation between the magnitude of pulse pressure and LV + dP/dT increases and left ventricular pacing site. The percent increases in pulse pressure and LV + dP/dT averaged over all AV delays were significantly larger at mid-lateral free wall LV epicardial pacing sites compared to any other sample left ventricular region. Furthermore, increases at the mid-anterior sites were smaller than all other sites.

These observations were extended in an analysis of 30 patients enrolled in the PATCH-CHF II trial (Fig. 9.16).[38] Left ventricular stimulation was delivered at the lateral free wall or mid-anterior wall. Free wall sites yielded significantly larger improvements in LV + dP/dT and pulse pressure than anterior sites. Furthermore, in one third of patients, stimulation at anterior sites worsened acute LV hemodynamic performance, whereas free wall stimulation improved it, and the opposite pattern was never observed. This difference in acute hemodynamic response correlated with intrinsic conduction delays (Fig. 9.17). This may be interpreted as evidence that stimulating a later activated LV region produces a larger response because it more effectively restores regional activation synchrony. Thus, the negative effect of anterior wall stimulation at all AV delays in some patients may be due to preexcitation of an already relatively early activated site thereby exaggerating intraventricular dyssynchrony.[39]

Interestingly, in PATH-CHF a small number of patients with heart failure and LBBB achieved optimal hemodynamic improvement with RV versus LV or biventricular pacing.[40] Electroanatomic mapping has demonstrated that the RV apex is frequently delayed in LBBB and in select patients, left ventricular preexcitation can be achieved by RV apical pacing due to early

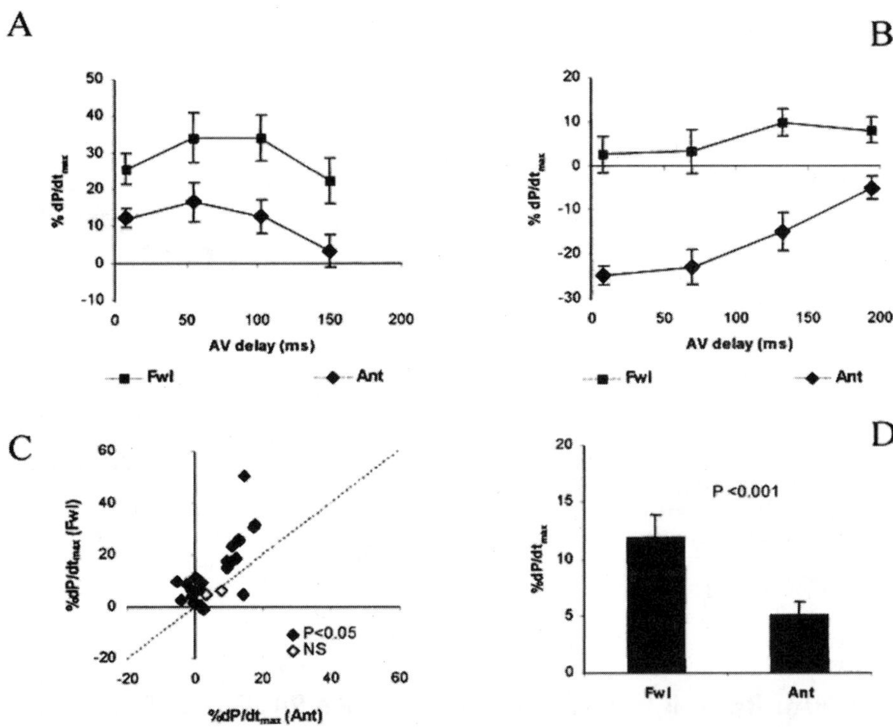

Figure 9.16. Effect of CRT stimulation site on acute hemodynamic response in 30 patients enrolled in PATCH-CHF-II trial. Left ventricular stimulation was delivered at free wall (FWL) or anterior wall (ANT) sites. FWL sites yielded significantly larger LV + dP/dT and pulse pressure than ANT sites. In one-third of patients stimulation at ANT sites worsened hemodynamic function, whereas FWL stimulation improved it. The opposite pattern was never observed. See text for details.

breakthrough into the left ventricle at this site (Angelo Auricchio, MD, personal communication).

Methods for identifying the best site during implantation are not yet of proven clinical benefit. Furthermore, even if optimal LV pacing sites could be identified *a priori*, access to such sites is potentially constrained by variations in coronary venous anatomy. Despite rapid evolution of implantation techniques including guiding sheaths and catheters and over-the-wire delivery systems, a suitable pacing site on the LV free wall cannot be achieved in 5–10% of patients. Even when the coronary venous anatomy is suitable and navigable, some free wall sites are rejected due to unacceptably high pacing thresholds related to epicardial scar or unavoidable phrenic nerve stimulation. Surgical placement of epicardial LV pacing leads or endocardial LV stimulation[41] are options when the coronary venous approach fails.

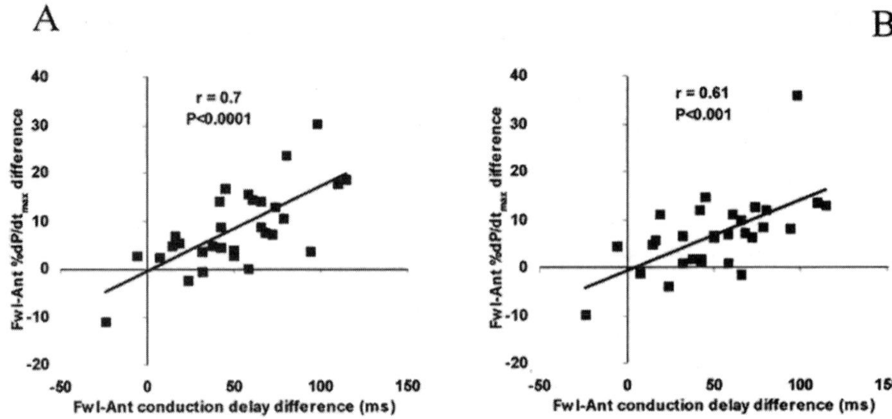

Figure 9.17. Correlation between free wall (FWL) and anterior wall (ANT) intrinsic conduction delay differences and the LV + dP/dt_{max} response differences during FWL and ANT stimulation for left ventricular pacing **(A)** and biventricular pacing **(B)**. Positive conduction delay differences correspond to more delayed FWL activation. Positive LV + dP/dt_{max} differences correspond to a larger FWL stimulation response (percentage change from baseline).

CARDIAC RESYNCHRONIZATION THERAPY PACING SYSTEMS

Leads and Electrodes

Non-independently Programmable Ventricular Polarity Configurations: Transvenous and epicardial LV pacing leads may be either unipolar or bipolar, though the former dominates current applications. Multiple ventricular pacing polarity configurations are therefore possible. Since programmed polarity settings are common to both ventricular leads and since the type (bipolar or unipolar) of these leads may not be the same, the following considerations apply.

In a dual bipolar polarity configuration, both lead tips are the active electrodes (cathodes) and the ring(s) are the common (non-stimulating) anode. However, the type of ventricular leads implanted define the pacing/sensing vector (Fig. 9.18). With two unipolar leads, the bipolar setting results in no pacing or sensing. If both leads are bipolar, both rings act as the common electrode. If one lead is bipolar (RV) and the other lead is unipolar (typically LV), the ring on the bipolar lead acts as the common electrode (non-stimulating anode). This configuration results in "shared-ring" bipolar pacing and sensing. This hybrid bipolar/unipolar stimulation configuration is used in most contemporary CRT pacing systems.

In a dual unipolar polarity configuration, the lead tips are the active electrodes; the noninsulated device case is the common electrode (see Fig. 9.18). This configuration is uncommonly used in CRT pacing systems and is not feasible in CRT ICD systems due to the concerns regarding ventricular oversensing.

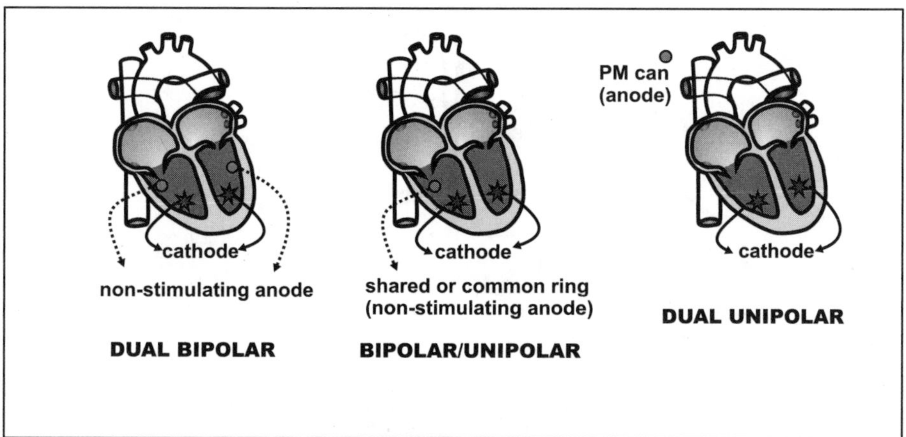

Figure 9.18. Various combinations of lead polarities for biventricular pacing. (Reproduced by permission from Barold SS, Stroobandt RX, Sinnaeve AF, eds. Cardiac Pacemakers Step by Step, An Illustrated Guide. Boston: Blackwell Science, 2003.)

Pulse Generators: Conventional dual chamber pulse generators or specially designed multisite pacing pulse generators may be used for CRT applications (Fig. 9.19). A conventional dual chamber pulse generator is well suited for CRT in patients with permanent AF. In this situation, the ventricular port is used for the RV lead and the atrial port is used for the LV lead. This permits programming of independent outputs and ventricular-ventricular timing by manipulation of the AV delay. The programming mode can be either DDD/R or DVI/R (see subsequent discussion). A conventional dual chamber pulse generator can also be used for atrial-synchronous biventricular pacing. The single ventricular output must be divided to provide simultaneous stimulation of the RV and LV (dual cathodal system with parallel outputs). This is achieved with a Y-adapter and results in simultaneous RV and LV sensing, which may result in ventricular double-counting and loss of CRT (see later sections) or pacemaker inhibition in the case of LV lead dislodgment into the coronary sinus with sensing of atrial activity.

First-generation multisite pacing pulse generators similarly provide a single ventricular output for simultaneous RV and LV stimulation; however, two separate ventricular channels internally connect in parallel. This connection is made for both the lead tip and ring connections and eliminates the need for a Y-adapter. However, this configuration still provides simultaneous RV and LV sensing with associated limitations.

Second generation multisite pacing pulse generators have independent ventricular ports. Each ventricular lead therefore has separate sensing and output

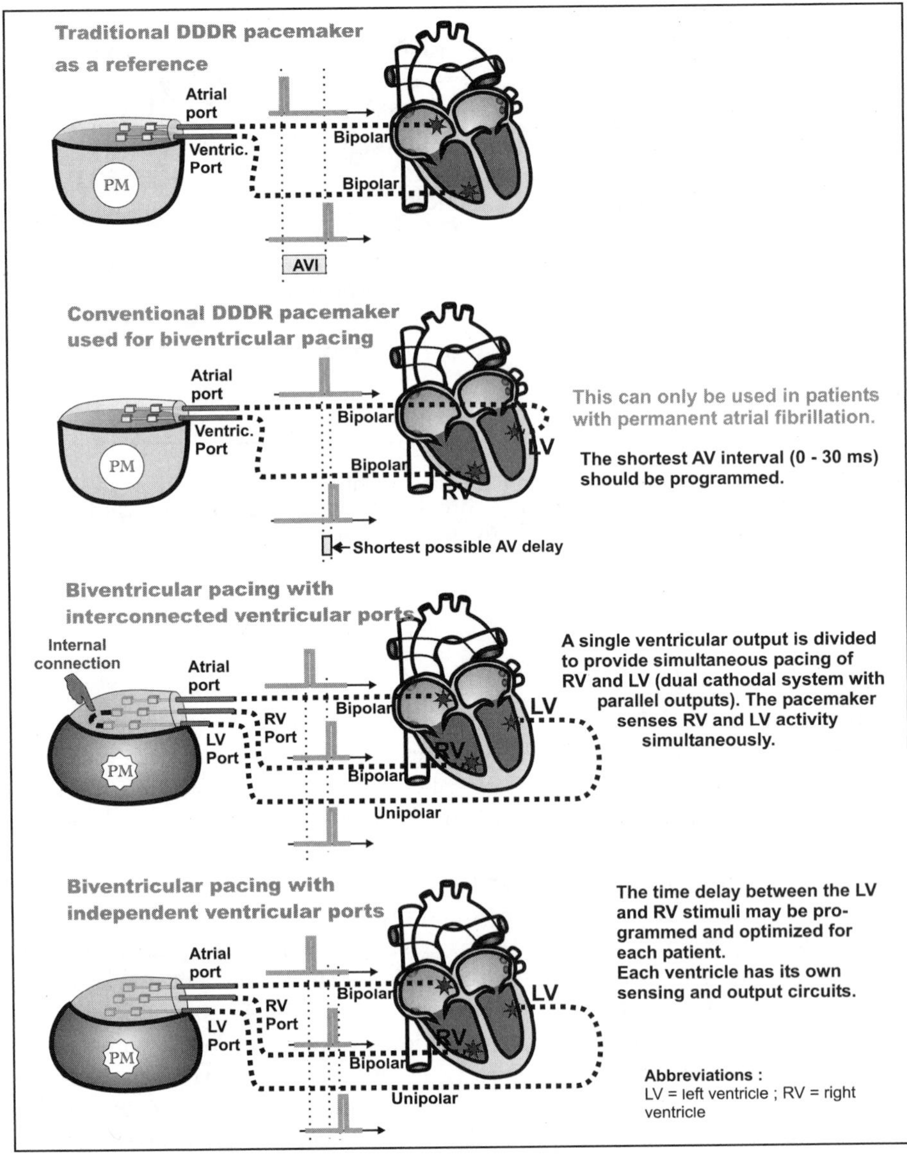

Figure 9.19. Various pulse generator configurations for biventricular pacing. (Reproduced by permission from Barold SS, Stroobandt RX, Sinnaeve AF, eds. Cardiac Pacemakers Step by Step, An Illustrated Guide. Boston: Blackwell Science, 2003.)

circuits. This arrangement permits optimal programming of outputs and time delay between RV and LV stimulation for each patient. It also eliminates the potential complications of biventricular sensing.

Biventricular or Univentricular Stimulation for Cardiac Resynchronization Therapy

It is important to note that uncertainty about the requirement of RV stimulation during CRT, uneasiness about long-term LV lead performance, and unavailability of pacing systems with separately programmable ventricular outputs influenced the use of biventricular pacing, as opposed to left univentricular pacing, in large scale randomized clinical trials. A particular concern is LV lead dislodgment which risks for potentially lethal bradycardia and has a reported incidence of 5% to 10% in larger studies.[42–44] However, there is some scientific evidence that right ventricular stimulation might not be necessary for optimal CRT response. Left univentricular pacing alone has acute hemodynamic effects that are similar or superior to those achieved with biventricular pacing in some patients.[27,45–47] Blanc and co-workers recently extended these observations.[48] Functional capacity (6 minute walk and maximal O_2 uptake), ventricular size and function, and blood norepinephrine levels before and after 12 months of left univentricular pacing were evaluated in 22 patients with dilated cardiomyopathy, LBBB NYHA class III or IV heart failure. The LV lead was placed in a lateral coronary vein when possible and all patients had sinus rhythm to allow atrial synchronous left univentricular pacing with an AV delay initially programmed to 100 milliseconds. Significant improvements in functional capacity, echocardiographic mitral regurgitation, and LV end-diastolic diameter were observed with favorable trend toward improvement in LVEF. Thus these results are encouraging and support persistent benefit (at least to 1 year) of left univentricular pacing in some patients.

At present, it is not possible to identify patients who will respond better to LV alone compared to biventricular pacing, or neither; and it is not clear how to identify the optimal pacing site. Other factors will warrant RV lead placement in many patients. Patients with reduced LV ejection fraction and at least moderately symptomatic heart failure are at risk for sudden cardiac death due to ventricular arrhythmias and this risk can be reduced by ICD therapy.[49–52] Current ICD systems require RV lead for tachyarrhythmia sensing and high voltage therapies and have a long record of safety and reliability in this regard. Further data on the safety and reliability of LV leads for tachyarrhythmia sensing and possibly defibrillation[53] are essential before RV leads are abandoned in CRT pacing and CRT defibrillation systems. It is likely that systems incorporating an RV lead will continue to predominate. If LV pacing systems can become as reliable as RV pacing systems, the paradigm could shift.

PROGRAMMING CONSIDERATIONS IN CARDIAC RESYNCHRONIZATION THERAPY

Pacing Modes

It is axiomatic that for maximal delivery of CRT, ventricular pacing must be continuous.

DDD mode guarantees AV synchrony and ventricular pacing with all atrial events in the physiologic heart rate range. However, DDD mode increases the probability of atrial pacing (depending upon programmed lower rate limit) that may alter the left sided AV timing relationship due to interatrial conduction time and atrial pacing latency.

VDD mode guarantees the absence of atrial pacing and synchronizes all atrial events to ventricular pacing at the programmed AV delay. However, if the sinus rate is below the lower programmed rate limit, AV synchrony is lost because the VDD mode is operationally VVI.

Although conventional dual-chamber pacemakers are not designed for biventricular pacing and generally do not allow programming of an AV delay of zero, or near zero, they are being increasingly used with their shortest AV delay (0 to 30 milliseconds) for CRT in patients with permanent AF. The advantages include programming flexibility, elimination of the Y-adapter (required for conventional VVIR devices), protection against far-field sensing of atrial activity (an inherent risk of dual cathodal devices with simultaneous sensing from both ventricles), and cost. When a conventional dual-chamber PM is used for CRT, the LV lead is usually connected to the atrial port and the RV lead to the ventricular port. This provides for (1) LV stimulation before RV activation (LV preexcitation), and (2) protection against ventricular asystole related to oversensing of far-field atrial activity when the LV lead is dislodged toward the AV groove. The DVIR mode is ideally suited for this application. The DVIR mode behaves like the VVIR mode except that there are always two closely coupled independent ventricular stimuli thereby facilitating comprehensive evaluation of RV and LV pacing and sensing performance. The DVIR mode also provides absolute protection against far-field sensing of atrial activity in case of LV lead dislodgment because no sensing occurs on the "atrial" (LV) lead in the DVIR mode.

Ventricular Double-Counting Causing Loss of Cardiac Resynchronization Therapy and Spurious Ventricular Therapies

In first generation CRT and CRTD systems, pacing and sensing occurs from RV and LV simultaneously. Double counting involves the spontaneous wide QRS complex of LBBB (Fig. 9.20). This produces temporal separation of RV and LV electrograms (EGM). The degree of separation depends on the severity of the interventricular conduction delay and the location of the electrodes. The LV EGM may be sensed sometime after detection of the RV EGM if the LV signal extends beyond the relatively short ventricular blanking period initiated by RV sensing. This is more likely to occur when a long post-ventricular atrial

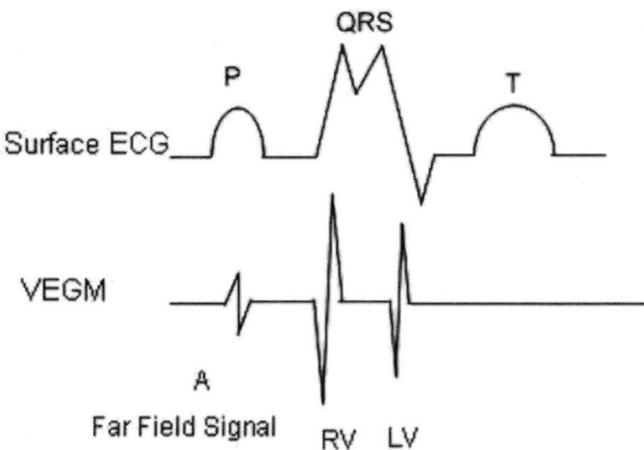

Figure 9.20. Origin of temporally dispersed RV and LV electrograms during biventricular sensing in left bundle branch block.

refractory period (PVARP) is programmed. In this circumstance, sinus P waves, particularly during sinus tachycardia and first-degree AV block (which are common in heart failure patients) that displace the P wave into the PVARP where it cannot be tracked. This results in loss of ventricular pacing and CRT. This situation is commonly triggered by PVARP extensions after a premature ventricular contraction (PVC). Spontaneous AV conduction occurs in the form of a preempted upper rate Wenckebach response with loss of ventricular pacing and CRT (Fig. 9.21). In CRTD systems, this may result in ventricular double counting and misclassification of sinus tachycardia or rapidly conducted AF as ventricular tachycardia resulting in spurious therapies. During true ventricular episodes, such as ventricular tachycardia, the LV EGM may precede the RV EGM and may result in spurious shocks because the rate is misclassified as VF.

Failure to deliver CRT at high sinus rates can be minimized by shortening the PVARP, increasing the upper tracking limit and deactivating the PVC response in the DDD/R mode. Additionally, atrial fibrillation should be aggressively treated to prevent rapid ventricular response and emergence of spontaneous QRS complexes. New CRT systems prevent ventricular double-counting by using an IVRP (interventricular ventricular refractory period). Ventricular sensed events (i.e., LV sensing) during the IVRP do not restart PVARP (Fig. 9.22).

Atrioventricular Optimization

AV optimization is important for maximal hemodynamic response to CRT but not essential, because ventricular pumping function can be improved by CRT even in the presence of permanent AF. Nonetheless, acute hemodynamic studies have consistently demonstrated that AV optimization "re-times" the left atrial-left ventricular relationship and can result in 15% to 40% improvement in indices

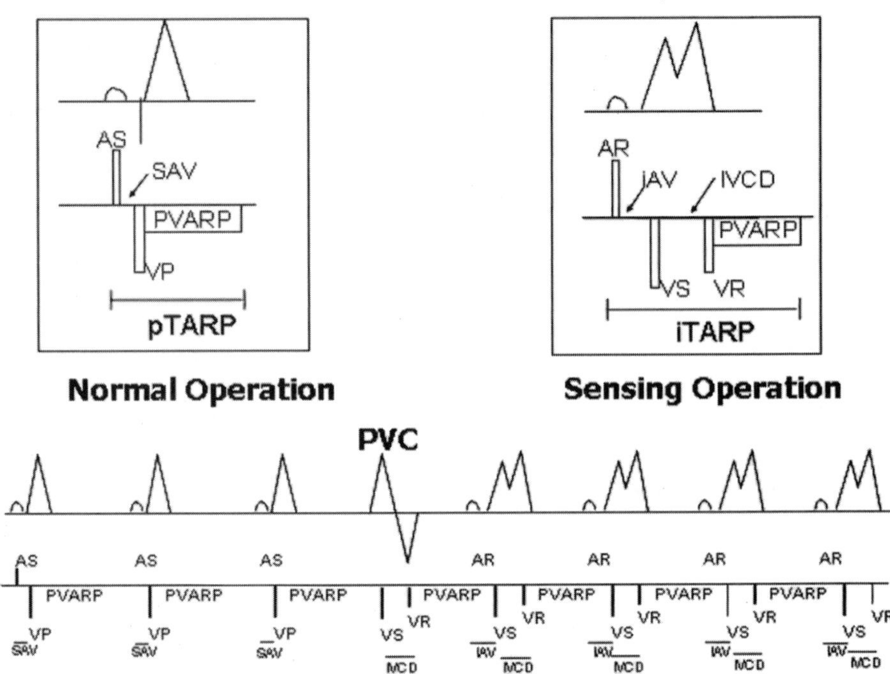

Figure 9.21. Onset of ventricular double-counting and failure to deliver CRT due to loss of atrial tracking during CRT. See text for details.

of left ventricular systolic performance acutely. Furthermore, small changes in AV delay may nullify hemodynamic benefit of CRT.

Presently, two methods of AV optimization are commonly applied. One method uses an echo-guided Doppler analysis of transmitral blood flow velocities to approximate an optimal timing relationship between atrial systole and ventricular filling. This is a rather tedious process and may be physiologically unsound because the basis for the technique was derived from studies of patients with permanent AV block and conventional dual chamber pacing with right ventricular apical stimulation. Nonetheless, this was the technique for AV optimization used in the MIRACLE study.[42] Empiric observation suggested that most optimized AV delays derived using this technique were in the range of 80 to 100 milliseconds regardless of other considerations. The process of AV optimization using this technique is shown in Figures 9.23 to 9.25.

A second approach to AV optimization for maximal positive change in LV + dP/dt is derived from the intrinsic AV interval measured from the local right atrial and RV endocardial EGMs using two linear equations.[54] If the native QRSd is greater than 150 milliseconds, then estimated optimal AV delay (EOAVD) = AxiAVI + B (milliseconds) and EOAVD = CxiAVI + D (millisec-

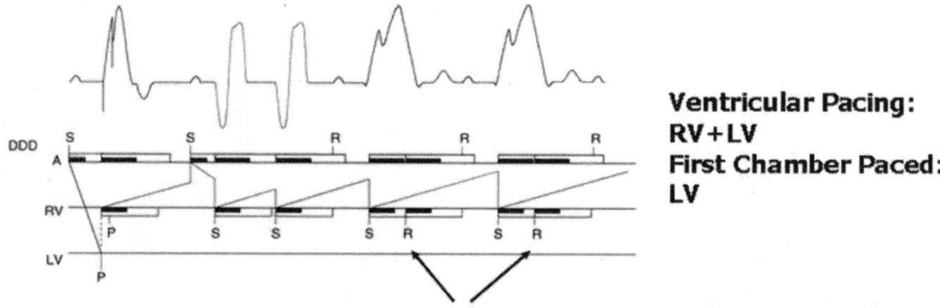

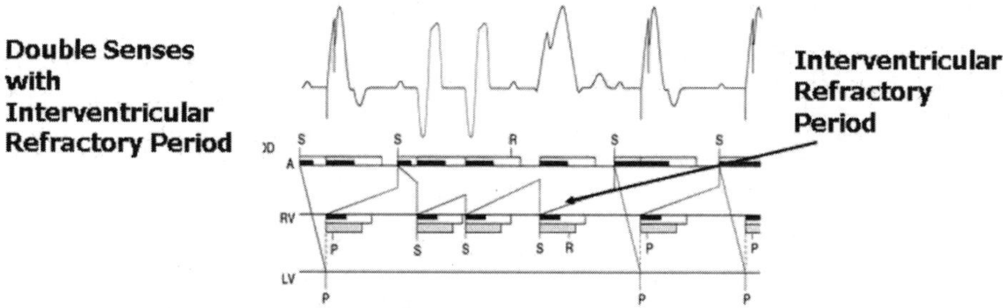

Figure 9.22. Prevention of ventricular double-counting with an interventricular refractory period. A = atrium; RV = right ventricle; LV = left ventricle; R = refractory event; S = sensed event; P = paced event. See text for details.

onds), where iAVI = intrinsic AV interval, A = 0.7, B = −55 milliseconds, and D = 0 milliseconds. These regression formulas can be very closely approximate by the following simple rules: the estimated optimal programmed AV delay for patients with QRSd greater than 150 milliseconds is 50% of the intrinsic AV interval and 75% for QRSd of 120 to 150 milliseconds. This strategy was used in the study design of the Comparison of Medical Therapy, Pacing, and Defibrillation in Heart Failure (COMPANION) trial[44] that showed significant reductions in mortality and heart failure hospitalizations with CRT at 1 year.

It is almost certainly true that the optimal AV delay will likely differ as heart rate and cardiac loading conditions change, such that the optimal AV delay at one point in time may not predict optimal AV timing under other conditions. Furthermore, the importance of AV delay optimization at rest for chronic clinical and hemodynamic effect remains to be shown.

Pacing Outputs

It is critically important that voltage output be adjusted to exceed ventricular capture threshold for LV and RV in common cathodal devices. Since there are

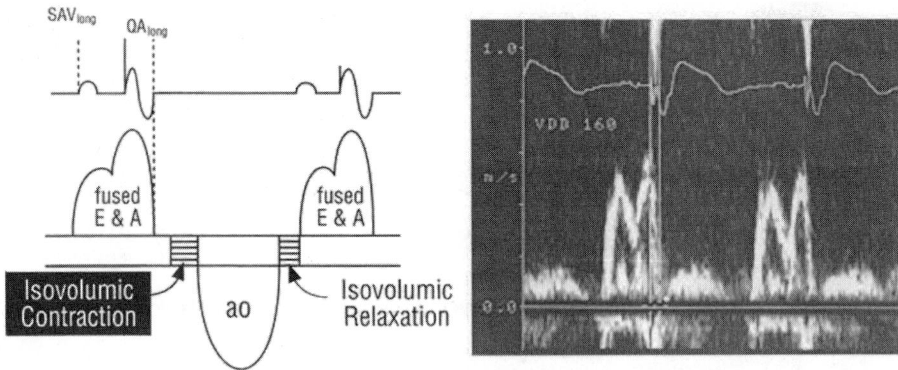

Figure 9.23. Doppler echo of transmitral blood flow with long AV delay. When the AV delay is too long, mitral valve closure may not be complete, since atrial contraction is not followed by a properly time ventricular systole. Left ventricular pressure increases above the left atrial pressure at the end of the diastolic filling period and results in diastolic, or "pre-systolic" mitral regurgitation.

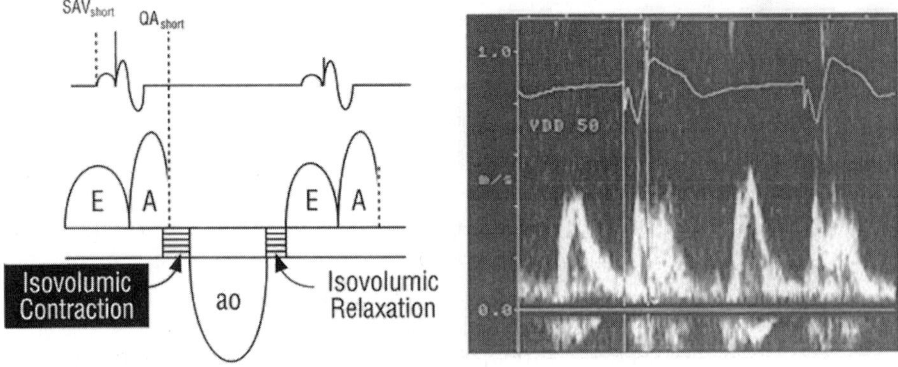

Figure 9.24. Doppler echo of transmitral blood flow with short AV delay. Note truncation of diastolic filling period due to premature closure of mitral valve (atrial and ventricular contraction occur simultaneously).

commonly differences in capture thresholds between ventricular chambers, this means that the voltage output must exceed capture threshold in chamber with highest threshold (usually the LV) (Fig. 9.26). Newer pulse generators that permit independent programming of ventricular outputs provide greater flexibility in this regard. Similarly, RV and LV voltage outputs may be separately programmable in the situation where a standard DDD device is used to provide RV and LV stimulation in the DVI mode for CRT in permanent AF (see previous discussion). Extending the pulse width to 1 msec or greater may produce

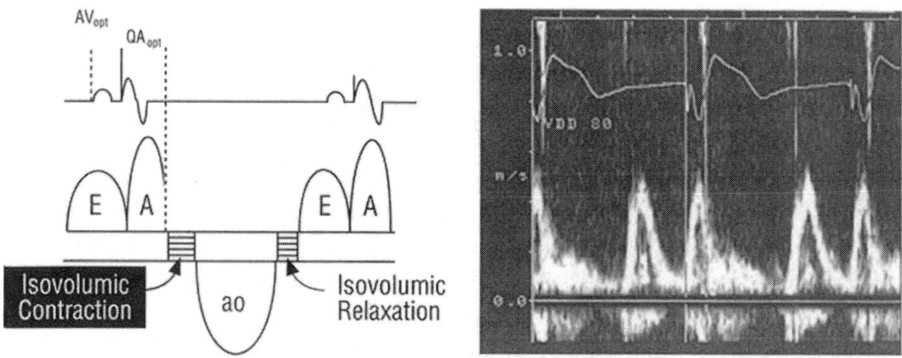

Figure 9.25. Doppler echo transmitral blood flow at optimal AV delay. The relation of atrial contraction to the onset of ventricular contraction is now optimal, resulting in diastolic filling throughout the entire diastolic filling period. An appropriate relation now exists between mechanical left atrial and left ventricular contraction so that mean left atrial pressure is maintained at a low level with left atrial contraction occurring just before left ventricular contraction. AV optimization is noted by return of the normal E-A separation. Transmitral flood and LV diastolic filling time are increased, which improves to increased cardiac output. If a large amount of diastolic MR can be abolished, a beneficial effect is obtained because of lower left atrial and higher left ventricular preload at the onset of ventricular contraction.

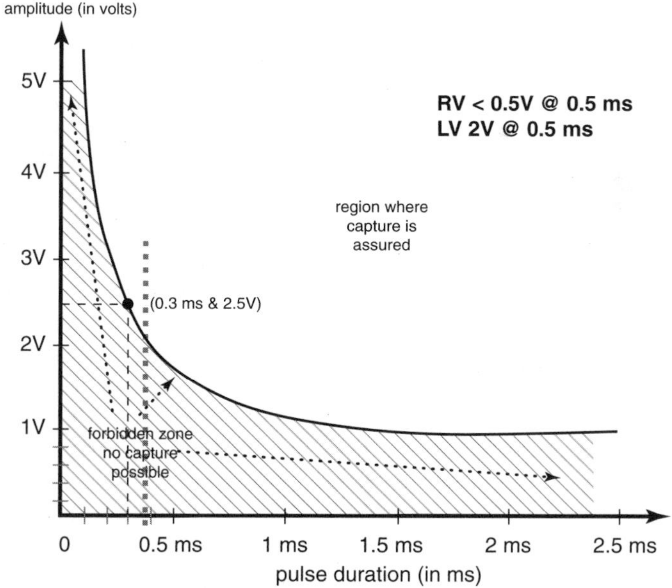

Figure 9.26. Strength-duration curve considerations for biventricular pacing. In common cathodal systems, the ventricular output must exceed the capture threshold for the chamber with the highest threshold, typically the LV.

consistent capture at sites that have unacceptable thresholds at standard pulse widths.

Interventricular Timing

Implantation of a biventricular pacing system with separately programmable LV and RV stimulation outputs and timing delay would allow adjustments to be made during follow-up. It is presently unclear what benefit, if any, manipulation of interventricular timing would provide during biventricular pacing.[27] This is highlighted by the emerging evidence (see earlier) that univentricular left ventricular pacing is probably either equivalent or superior to biventricular pacing acutely and chronically.

CARDIAC RESYNCHRONIZATION THERAPY PACEMAKER ELECTROCARDIOGRAPHY/DETERMINING LEFT VENTRICULAR AND RIGHT VENTRICULAR CAPTURE

The 12-lead ECG is essential to ascertain RV and LV capture during follow-up of CRT systems without separately programmable ventricular outputs. It is recognized that five distinct 12-lead ventricular activation patterns may be seen during threshold determination. These are (1) intrinsic rhythm during loss of RV and LV capture or pacing inhibition (native QRS), (2) isolated RV stimulation, (3) isolated LV stimulation, (4) biventricular stimulation, and (5) biventricular stimulation with anodal capture (Figs. 9.27 to 9.32).

Ventricular pacing thresholds should ideally be performed independently and in the VVI mode at a rate superseding the prevailing ventricular rate to obtain continuous ventricular capture without fusion. Alternately, thresholds can be performed in the VDD or DDD mode at very short AV delays to ensure full ventricular capture without fusion. In general, it is advisable to initiate threshold determinations at maximum output (voltage and pulse duration) because there is often a significant differential in capture thresholds between RV and LV.

In devices without separately programmable ventricular outputs RV and LV capture can only be determined by ECG analysis during common ventricular voltage decrement. This requires inspection of a 12-lead ECG to demonstrate a change in electrical axis that confirms independent LV and RV capture.

Pacing from the RV apex produces a negative paced QRS complex in the inferior leads simply because the activation starts in the inferior part of the heart and travels superiorly away from the inferior leads. The mean QRS frontal plan axis is superior either in the left or right superior quadrant. Pacing from the RVOT produces a frontal plane axis that is "normal," meaning, inferiorly directed (positive QRS in inferior leads). Isolated LV pacing produces a rightward axis, similar to maximal ventricular preexcitation over a left-sided accessory pathway. Biventricular pacing (RV + LV) produces a right superior axis as a result of

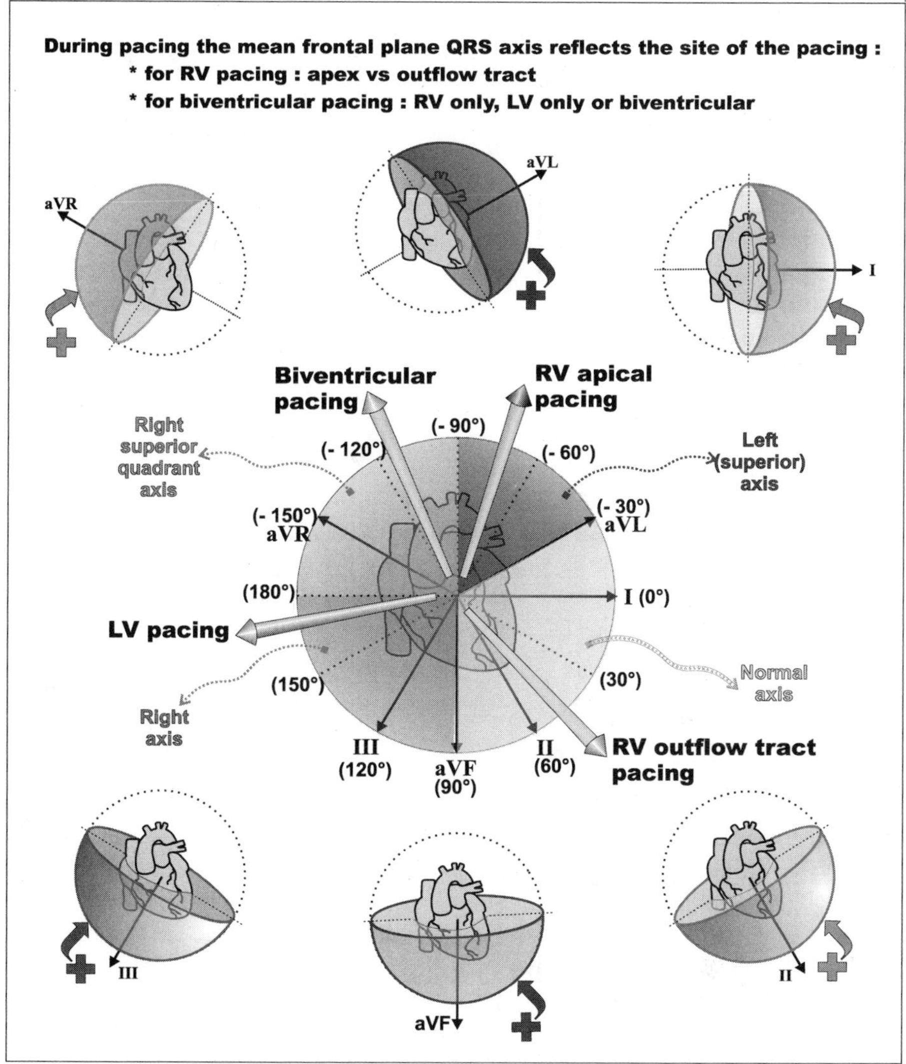

Figure 9.27. Mean QRS axis in the frontal plane during ventricular pacing at different sites and configurations. (Reproduced by permission from Barold SS, Stroobandt RX, Sinnaeve AF, eds. Cardiac Pacemakers Step by Step, An Illustrated Guide. Boston: Blackwell Science, 2003.)

fusion of RV and LV electrical axes. A qR or Qr complex in lead I is rare in uncomplicated RV apical pacing. It is present in 90% of cases of biventricular pacing. In biventricular pacing, loss of the q or Q wave in lead I is 100% predictive of loss of LV capture.

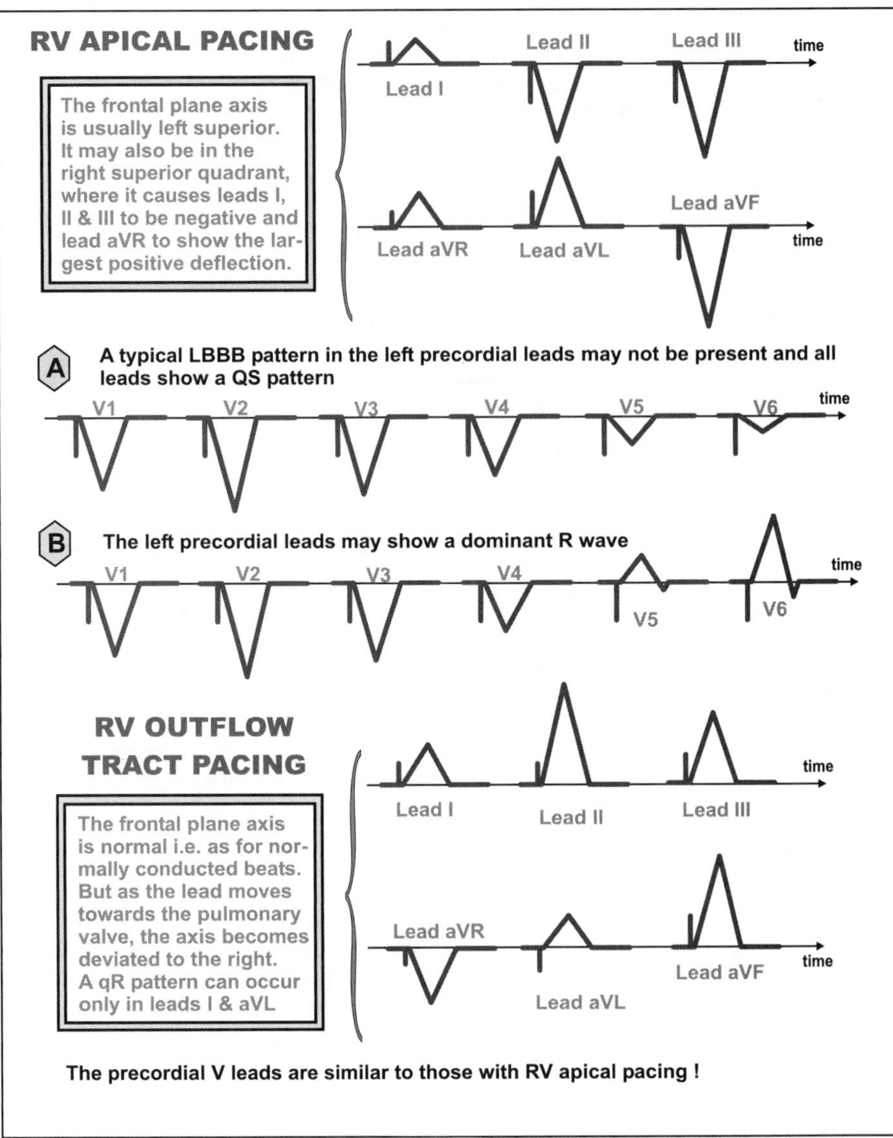

Figure 9.28. EKG QRS patterns during RV pacing from different sites. (Reproduced by permission from Barold SS, Stroobandt RX, Sinnaeve AF, eds. Cardiac Pacemakers Step by Step, An Illustrated Guide. Boston: Blackwell Science, 2003.)

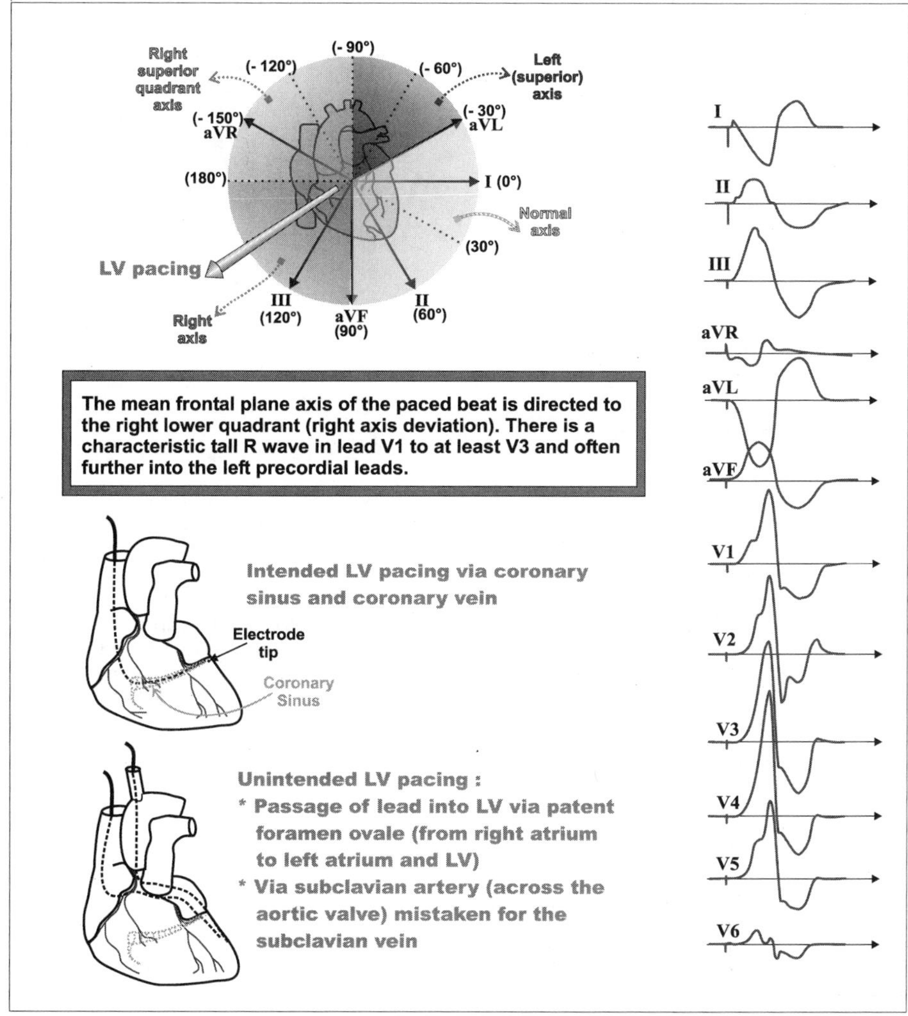

Figure 9.29. EKG QRS patterns during LV free wall pacing. (Reproduced by permission from Barold SS, Stroobandt RX, Sinnaeve AF, eds. Cardiac Pacemakers Step by Step, An Illustrated Guide. Boston: Blackwell Science, 2003.)

CARDIAC RESYNCHRONIZATION THERAPY RESPONDERS AND NONRESPONDERS

Despite the technical limitations for achieving reliable, long-term transvenous LV stimulation, the majority of appropriately selected patients respond to CRT. Nonetheless, approximately 18% to 30% of patients fail to respond clinically to CRT.[42,55,56] In some cases, failure to respond may simply indicate that despite

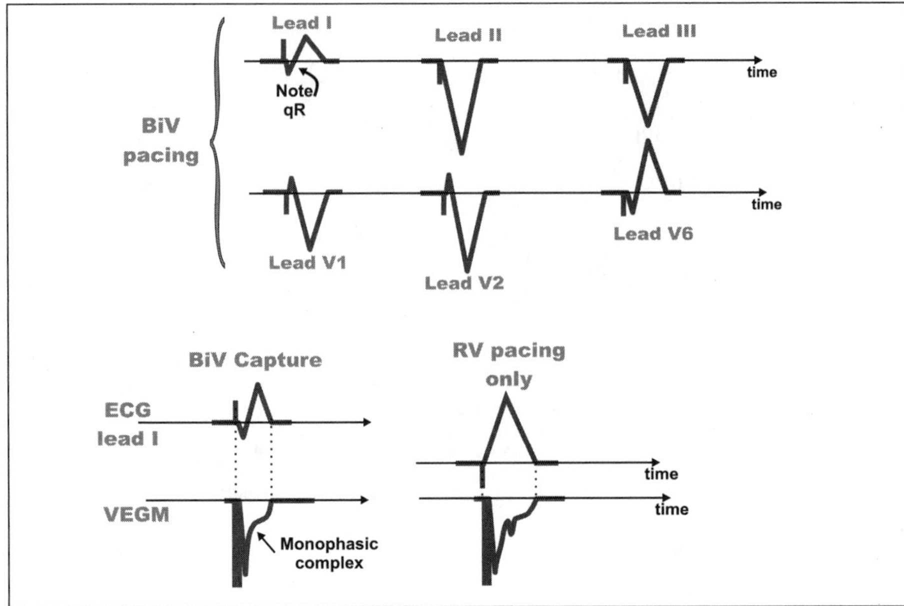

Figure 9.30. Analysis of EKG QRS patterns to ascertain RV and LV capture in CRT systems without separately programmable ventricular outputs. (Reproduced by permission from Barold SS, Stroobandt RX, Sinnaeve AF, eds. Cardiac Pacemakers Step by Step, An Illustrated Guide. Boston: Blackwell Science, 2003.)

delayed ventricular activation, mechanical activation is not dyssynchronous.[57,58] It is likely, however, that technical limitations are a major factor. In the MIRACLE study a lateral marginal vein site serving the LV free wall was obtained in only 43% of patients. This number is probably an overestimate because the larger diameter stylet driven leads used during MIRACLE typically traverse the "Shepherd's Crook" curve of the anterior interventricular vein before they descend the LV. Many of the "lateral" sites were probably really anterolateral rather than true lateral marginal vein sites. Thus, at least 57% of patients in MIRACLE may have had suboptimal LV lead positions. It is conceivable that some of these patients were actually made worse by CRT due to LV pacing at suboptimal sites, particularly among the patients with relatively narrow QRSd (less than 150 milliseconds).[38] As reviewed previously, CRT with stimulation at a LV free wall site consistently improves short-term systolic function more than stimulation at an anterior site does (Figs. 9.33 and 9.34). These differences may account for the varied results and large individual difference observed among clinical studies.

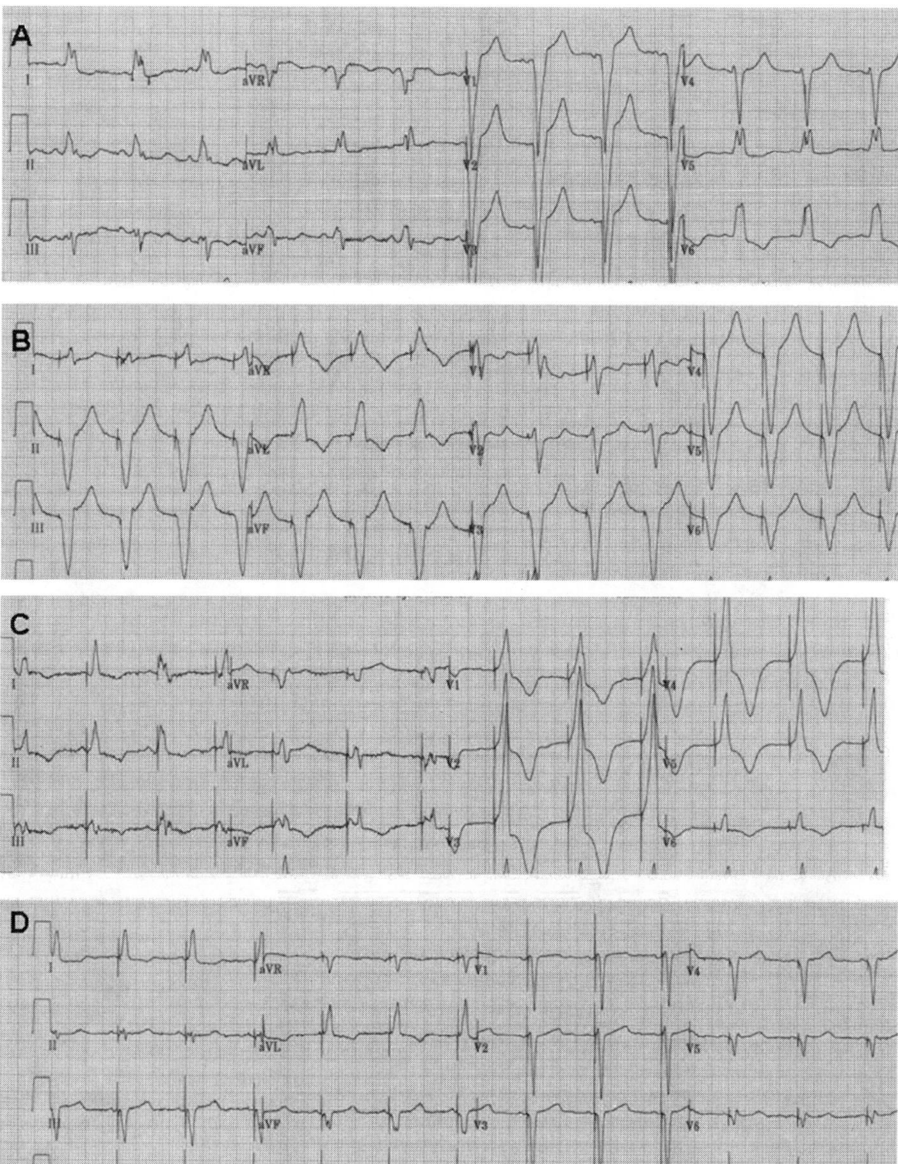

Figure 9.31. Twelve lead ECGs of uni- and biventricular pacing. **Panel A:** Non-paced intrinsic ventricular activation with LBBB. **Panel B:** RV only pacing. **Panel C:** LV only pacing. **Panel D:** Biventricular pacing. Note the markedly shortened QRS duration.

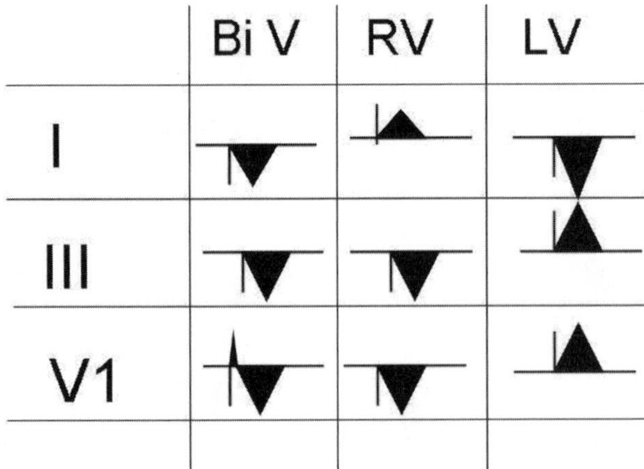

Figure 9.32. Clues for assessing LV capture by assessing ECG leads I, III, and V1. Bi V = biventricular pacing; RV = right ventricular pacing; LV = left ventricular pacing.

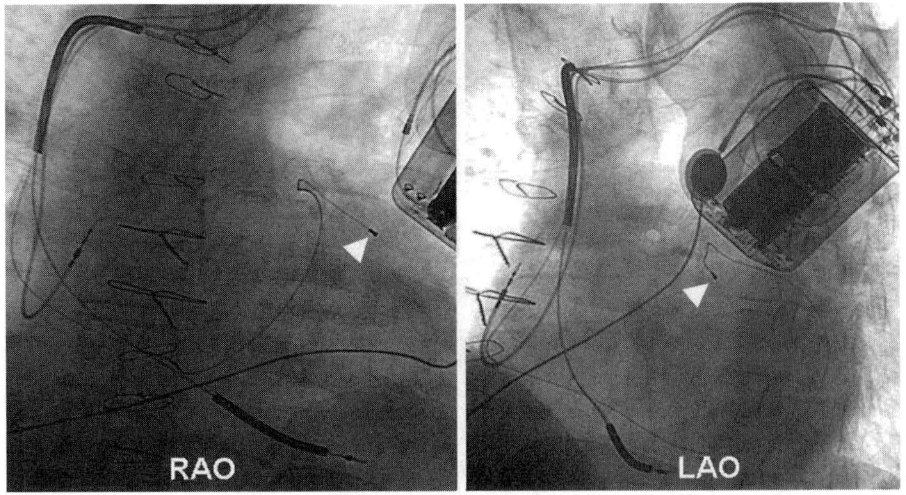

Figure 9.33. CRT nonresponder. Note position of left ventricular (LV) electrode in the proximal anterior interventricular vein. The LV lead tip is designated by the *arrowhead*. Note lack of spatial separation of right ventricular and LV leads in lateral view. This patient suffered progressive heart failure until his demise.

PATIENT SELECTION FOR CARDIAC RESYNCHRONIZATION THERAPY

Ventricular dyssynchrony is the pathophysiologic target of CRT. Techniques for selecting patients with significant ventricular dyssynchrony likely to benefit from CRT are rapidly evolving. The optimal criteria would identify all patients with a high probability of response and reject all patients with a low probability of response. To date, QRSd determined from the surface ECG has been most

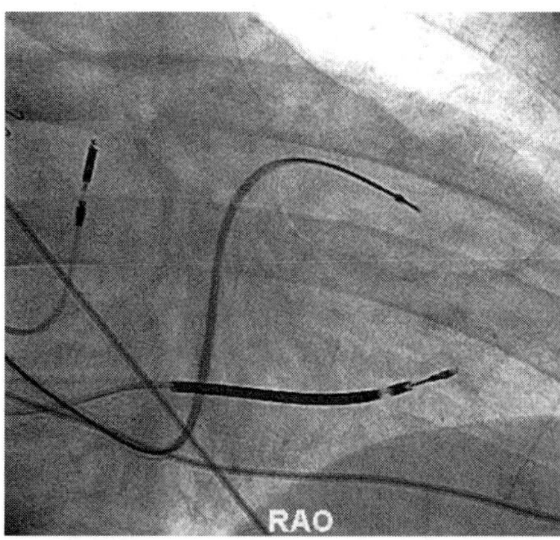

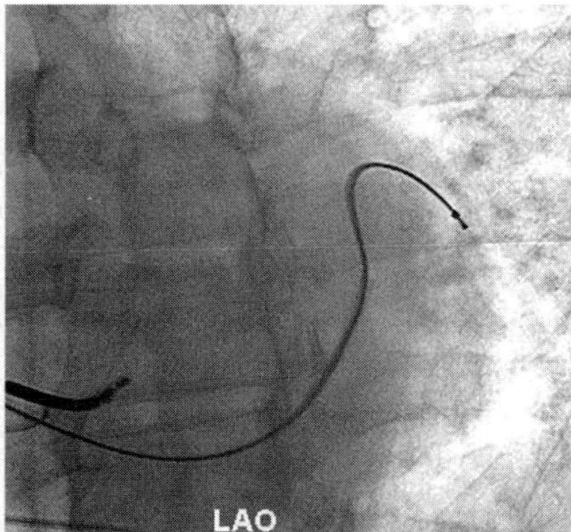

Figure 9.34. CRT responder. Note position of left ventricular (LV) lead in lateral marginal vein on LV free wall. Note the wide spatial separation of right ventricular and LV leads in lateral view. This patient had a marked improvement in heart failure symptoms.

Box 9.1. ACC/AHA/NASPE Guidelines for Cardiac Resynchronization Therapy in Patients with Congestive Heart Failure and Dilated Cardiomyopathy

- Advanced symptomatic heart failure (NYHA III–IV) refractory to optimal medical therapy
- LVEF ≤ 35%
- QRS duration > 130 × ms

NYHA = New York Heart Association; LVEF = left ventricular ejection fraction.

extensively evaluated as a selection criteria for CRT on the premise that electrical delay is a reliable marker for spatially dispersed mechanical activation (Box 9.1). Numerous studies have reproducibly demonstrated that baseline QRSd is an important predictive favor of acute hemodynamic improvement with CRT. Auricchio et al. (22) showed that there was a positive correlation between the surface QRS duration and the percentage of change in LV + dP/dt and pulse pressure during CRT. This observation was corroborated by Nelson and colleagues.[23] Baseline QRS duration modestly predicted systolic response, as assessed by maximal rate of pressure defined as percent change in LV + $dP/dt_{max} = 0.61 \times QRS_d - 70.2$. Combining baseline QRSd and LV + dP/dt_{max} improved the predictive accuracy for identifying CRT clinical responders. Patients with baseline QRSd of 155 milliseconds or greater and baseline LV + dP/dt_{max} of 700 mm Hg/sec or less consistently yielded the greatest acute hemodynamic response to CRT (percent change LV + $dP/dt_{max} \geq 25\%$).

Prediction curves for contractile function response using baseline QRSd derived from the PATH-CHF and PATH-CHF II studies are shown in Figure 9.35.[59] The specificity curve indicates that 80% of CRT nonresponders had a QRSd less than 150 milliseconds. The sensitivity curve indicates that 80% of CRT responders had a QRSd greater than 150 milliseconds. The overlap between these QRSd ranges was populated with CRT responders and nonresponders. The predictive accuracy of QRSd to separate responders from nonresponders is fairly constant around 80% with a threshold cut-off between 120 and 150 milliseconds. If the QRSd is greater than 150 milliseconds, the likelihood of CRT response is greater. An important qualification is that this analysis is based on acute hemodynamic response to CRT. It is possible that acute hemodynamic response does not correlate precisely with chronic clinical improvement. However, these observations appear to be corroborated by the COMPANION Trial, where little or no benefit of CRT or CRTD on death or heart failure hospitalization was observed among patients with baseline QRSd less than 150 milliseconds.[44]

QRSd may not reliably predict CRT response for several reasons. It is important to remember that QRSd reflects both right and left ventricular activation. In many patients with LBBB, the delay in ventricular activation resides entirely within the left ventricle, as anticipated. However, in some patients with LBBB, delayed right ventricular activation accounts for a significant proportion of electrical delay manifest on the surface ECG (Fig. 9.36). Another reason is

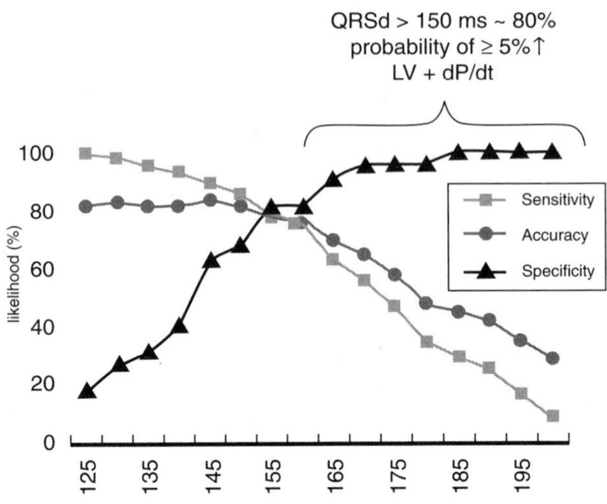

Figure 9.35. Sensitivity, specificity, and accuracy likelihoods are plotted for different QRS thresholds between 120 and 200 milliseconds using acute hemodynamic data from PATH-CHF and PATH-CHF II. Specificity curve indicates that 80% of nonresponders have QRSd less than 150 milliseconds. Sensitivity curve indicates that 80% of responders have QRSd greater than 150 milliseconds. CRT response is defined as greater than 5% acute increase in LV + dP/dt.

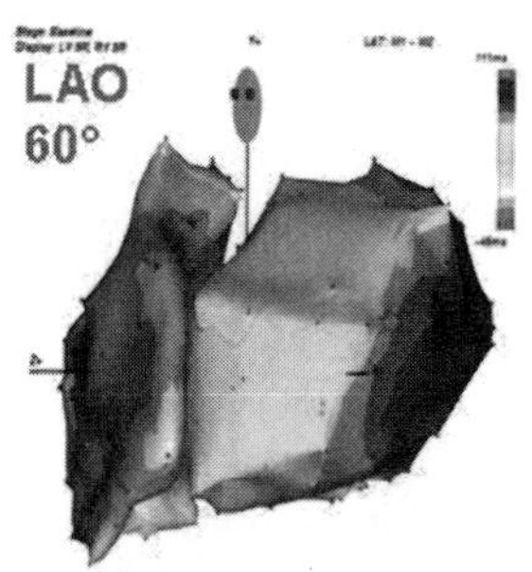

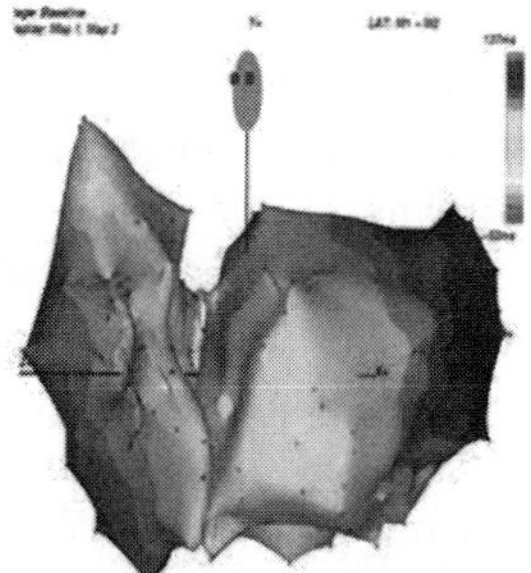

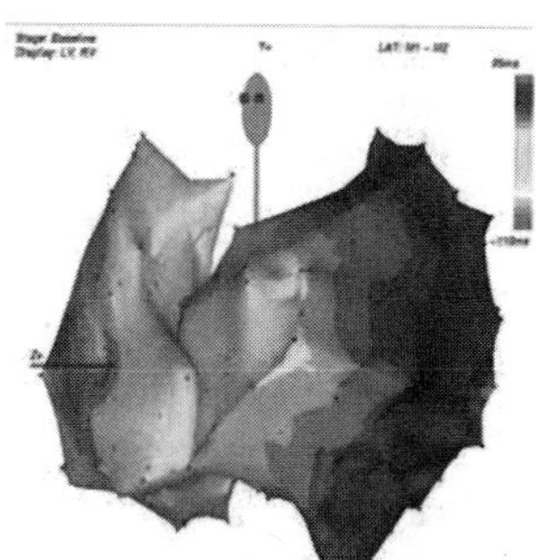

Total Ventricular Activation Time: 157 ms

RV Activation Time: 57 ms LV Activation Time: 100 ms

Total Ventricular Activation Time: 189 ms

RV Activation Time: 85 ms LV Activation Time: 104 ms

Total Ventricular Activation Time: 205 ms

RV Activation Time: 130 ms LV Activation Time: 75 ms

Figure 9.36. Electroanatomic endocardial activation maps showing heterogeneity of electrical delay in LBBB. See text for details. (Reproduced with permission from Auricchio et al., Pacing Clin Electrophysiol 2001;24, No. 4, Part II, Page 736, abstract # 791.)

the intriguing observation that a prolonged QRSd may not be accompanied by dyssynchronous, mechanical activation.[57,58] In this situation, despite electrically delayed ventricular activation CRT would not be anticipated to modify mechanical performance.

Recognition of the potential limitations of QRSd for predicting CRT response has stimulated interest in techniques for directly measuring baseline ventricular dyssynchrony. Intraventricular synchrony can be assessed echocardiographically from the delay between the maximal posterior displacement of the septum and the maximal displacement of the LV posterior wall measured from an M-mode short axis view of the LV. Pitzalis and colleagues[57] found that the delay between septal and posterior wall LV motion improved from a mean of 192 milliseconds to a mean of 14 milliseconds after 1 month of CRT, and was the only echocardiographic marker (including interventricular delay, ejection fraction, mitral regurgitant duration, and mitral regurgitant area) associated with a favorable response to CRT, defined as a greater than 15% improvement in LV systolic volume index.

Another promising echocardiographic technique to identify dyssynchrony and target patients for CRT is Doppler strain rate imaging. This uses tissue Doppler signals to quantify the rate of regional myocardial deformation, providing a sensitive estimate of regional myocardial shortening and lengthening that correlates with LV + dP/dt and systolic function in healthy and diseased hearts.[60] In LBBB, Doppler strain imaging demonstrates maximal septal contraction occurring before aortic valve opening and accompanied by lateral wall lengthening, consistent with studies in animal model.[14] The septum then lengthens after aortic valve opening and does not contribute to ejection. Peak lateral wall contraction is observed very late in systole and persists into the postsystolic period. During CRT, systolic contraction can be demonstrated to occur simultaneously in both septal and lateral walls, contributing equally to ejection.[61] The use of this technique in patient selection for CRT remains to be defined in clinical trials but preliminary results appear encouraging. Ventricular dyssynchrony detected by tissue Doppler imaging has been shown to predict acute and chronic response (including remodeling) to CRT in several studies.[62–65]

Numerous clinical variables have also been evaluated for predicting likelihood of CRT responsiveness. Baseline contractile function indexed by LV + dP/dt_{max} has been shown to inversely correlate with its subsequent change during LV pacing. Heart failure functional class is positively correlated with CRT response. In several studies, equivalent benefit was observed with CRT in NYHA class III-IV patients but no significant benefit in class II.[42,43] Left ventricular ejection fraction has not been shown to correlate with likelihood of CRT response in any study. Some studies have suggested that ischemic cardiomyopathy is less likely to respond to CRT than non-ischemic cardiomyopathy,[55] but not others.[42,44] Sinus rhythm does not appear to be necessary for CRT response. Patients in permanent AF had a similar acute hemodynamic response as sinus rhythm in PATH-CHF and similar long-term function improvements in other trials.[42,66–68] There is very limited data on CRT in RBBB that suggests the possibility of similar intermediate term response as LBBB in one trial[69] but not another.[44]

Further complicating the matter of patient selection for CRT is the fascinating observation that some patients with DCM and significant mechanical dyssynchrony have a normal or near-normal QRSd.[70–73]

In summary, 80% of patients with QRSd greater than 150 milliseconds will have a hemodynamic improvement with CRT and the probability of response is positively correlated with QRS duration. Patients with QRSd less than 150 milliseconds are less likely to respond to CRT though this is not uniformly true. Improvements in asynchrony seem to be the determinant of the improvements obtained with CRT, and this may be independent of QRS duration. Patients with more advanced heart failure symptoms are more likely to respond to CRT than patients with less severe symptoms. There is limited data suggesting that patients with non-ischemic cardiomyopathy respond more consistently than ischemic CMP and LBBB more consistently than RBBB. Permanent atrial fibrillation does not preclude CRT response.

Finally, RV apical pacing alone may cause prolonged QRSd and ventricular desynchronization. Ventricular desynchronization imposed by ventricular pacing even when AV synchrony is preserved causes increased left atrial diameters and reduced LV fractional shortening and is associated with increased risks of atrial fibrillation, heart failure and death among patients with normal baseline QRSd.[74,75] Therefore, it is logical to speculate that multisite (RV + LV) or alternate single site (LV) pacing may be more physiologic among patients in whom ventricular dyssynchrony is due to unavoidable ventricular pacing (i.e., persistent heart block). Intriguing studies suggest that pacing at the LV septum or apex maintains ventricular pumping function at sinus rhythm levels despite pacing-induced QRSd prolongation, possibly because of early engagement of the specialized conduction system resulting in a more physiologic propagation of electrical conduction.[76]

CLINICAL TRIALS OF CARDIAC RESYNCHRONIZATION THERAPY

CRT is an effective adjunctive treatment for moderately-severely symptomatic heart failure associated with depressed left ventricular function and ventricular dyssynchrony.[42,66,77] The aggregate experience with CRT among clinical trials involving more than 3500 patients demonstrates a consistent clinical benefit (Table 9.1). The magnitude of the benefits is modest and concordant. These include about a 1-step improvement in NYHA class, a 10-point improvement in quality of life measures, a 1 to 2 mL/kg/min improvement in peak VO_2, a 50 to 70 meter improvement in 6-minute hall walk, and a trend toward reduced heart failure hospitalizations. A meta-analysis of randomized trials of CRT using these first-generation pacing systems in 1634 patients found that heart failure deaths were reduced by 51% (from 3.5% to 1.7%) and heart failure hospitalizations were reduced by 29%.[78]

CLINICAL TRIALS OF CARDIAC RESYNCHRONIZATION THERAPY WITH IMPLANTABLE CARDIOVERTER-DEFIBRILLATORS

Sudden cardiac death is the leading cause of mortality in the United States. It is estimated that 200,000 to 400,000 sudden deaths occur annually.[79] The vast majority of these deaths occur among patients with symptomatic heart failure associated with reduced left ventricular function.

Survival from out-of-hospital cardiac arrest remains abysmal; it is estimated that less than 20% of victims will leave the hospital alive.[80] The principal reason for this dismal statistic is unavailability, or delayed time to, successful defibrillation. Prevention, or at least effective treatment, of the first episode of cardiac arrest is thus critically important. These realities have focused attention on identification and treatment of patients at risk for sudden death due to ventricular arrhythmias.

The results of large scale randomized treatment trials in patients with reduced left ventricular function and VF or hemodynamically unstable sustained uniform VT that occurs spontaneously or can be induced consistently demonstrate a survival advantage associated with ICD therapy compared to antiarrhythmic drugs.[49,51,81–83] Accordingly, ICD therapy can be recommended as first-line treatment for primary and secondary prevention of sudden cardiac death in these settings.

A similar mortality benefit for ICD therapy was subsequently demonstrated in MADIT II among patients with ischemic cardiomyopathy and left ventricular ejection fraction less than 30% without prior electrophysiology study.[50] These findings were extended in SCD-HeFT, which demonstrated a 23% mortality reduction among patients with ischemic or non-ischemic cardiomyopathy,

Table 9.1. Randomized Trials of CRT: Enrollment Criteria

Study	Design	N	NYHA	QRSd	LVEF	LVEDD
PATH-CHF	Randomized, single blind, controlled	42	II-IV	>120	<35	NA
VIGOR-CHF	Randomized, controlled	53	II-IV	>120	<30	NA
PATH-CHF II	Acute hemodynamic	43	II-IV	>120	<30	NA
InSync OUS	Uncontrolled	81	III-IV	>150	<35	>60
MUSTIC	Uncontrolled	67	III-IV	>150	<35	>60
MIRACLE	Randomized, double-blind, controlled	266	III-IV	>130	<35	>55

Study	Baseline NYHA	3-month NYHA	Baseline QRSd	3-month QRSd	Baseline LVEF	3-month LVEF
PATH-CHF	3.0 ± 0.3	2.0 ± 0.7	NA	NA	NA	NA
InSync OUS	3.37	2.15	179	143	20.9	23.9
MUSTIC	NA	NA	176 ± 19	NA	23.0 ± 7	NA
MIRACLE	3.0 ± 0.3	2.0 ± 0.3*	160	150	23.3	26.5

Results

Study	Baseline Peak VO_2	3-month Peak VO_2	Baseline QOL	3-month QOL	Baseline 6-min Walk	3-month 6-min Walk
PATH-CHF	13.9 ± 0.8	17.0 ± 1.1	49.0 ± 4	21.0 ± 4	362 ± 18	443 ± 13
InSync OUS	NA	NA	55	34	299	418
MUSTIC	13.7 ± 3.9	16.2 ± 4.7	51.0 ± 20	29.0 ± 21	320 ± 97	399.2 ± 100
MIRACLE	13.9	15.1	59.2 ± 19	39.6 ± 24*	314 ± 84	339 ± 127*

* 6-month comparison.

CRT = cardiac resynchronization therapy; LVEF = left ventricular ejection fraction; LVEDD = left ventricular end-diastolic dimension; NYHA = New York Heart Association; QOL = Minnesota Living with Heart Failure Quality of Life; VO_2 = oxygen uptake determination; OUS = outside United States.

NYHA class II-III heart failure and left ventricular ejection fraction 35% or less.[52] The mortality reduction among patients with ischemic cardiomyopathy approximated that observed in MADIT II and validates the findings of that study. More importantly, the equivalent mortality reduction among patients with NDCMP definitively demonstrates that the primary prevention mortality benefits of ICD therapy seen in ischemic CMP are transferable to NDCMP. Accordingly, ICD therapy can be recommended as first-line treatment for primary prevention of sudden cardiac death in either of these settings as well.

The incidence of ventricular dyssynchrony (usually LBBB or other interventricular conduction delay) as designated by prolonged QRS duration greater than 120 milliseconds among patients with chronic congestive heart failure and reduced systolic function is in the range of 35% to 40%.[84,85] It is not surprising therefore, that intense interest has focused on CRT combined with ICD therapy for prevention of sudden death and treatment of congestive heart failure. Despite impressive technical hurdles, CRT has been successfully hybridized with conventional ICD therapy delivery systems and implanted successfully in humans.

CONTAK Cardioverter-Defibrillator, MIRACLE Implantable Cardioverter-Defibrillator, and COMPANION

Three studies of CRT ICDs involving more than 2500 patients have been reported (Table 9.2). The study populations were similar to trials of CRT (without defibrillation capability) except there was a conventional indication for ICD therapy. CONTAK CD showed a significant improvement in NYHA class, 6-minute hall walk, peak V02 and standardized quality of life.[86] Post-hoc analysis showed that the greatest benefit was observed in the patients with the most advanced heart failure. However, the primary goal of a 25% reduction in heart failure, as measured by a composite outcome of death, heart failure hospitalization, worsening heart failure requiring other interventions, and ventricular arrhythmias, was not met. Patients receiving CRT ICDs had a 21% reduction in this composite endpoint ($P = .17$). However, the study was probably underpowered to detect significant differences in this composite endpoint, particularly because 80% of the patients were NYHA I or II after 6 months of CRT. MIRACLE ICD showed a reduction in NYHA class and improvement in quality of life but not 6-minute hall walk.[43] Importantly, neither of these studies provided data on the effect of CRT ICDs on mortality and limited data on whether the clinical benefits of CRT or CRT ICDs are sustainable for more than 12 months.

The COMPANION trial compared CRT, CRT ICDs, and optimal medical therapy among 1602 patients with ischemic and nonischemic cardiomyopathy, left ventricular ejection fraction less than 35%, QRS duration greater than 120 milliseconds, and PR interval greater than 150 milliseconds. Compared to medical therapy, mortality was reduced by CRT ICDs (36%) and CRT (24%), although only the reduction associated with CRT ICDs was statistically significant.[44]

Table 9.2. Randomized Trials of CRTD for Primary and Secondary Prevention of Sudden Death and Treatment of Congestive Heart Failure

	MIRACLE ICD	CONTAK CD	COMPANION
Target population	CHF + QRSd prolongation + ICD	CHF + QRSd prolongation + ICD	CHF + QRSd prolongation + ICD
Treatment	ICD vs. CRTD	ICD vs. CRTD	CRT vs. CRTD vs. medical management
Patients enrolled	364	581	1602
Arrhythmia qualifier	ICD indication	ICD indication	ICD indication
LVEF (%) qualifier	≤35	<35	≤35 + LVEDD ≥ 60 mm*
CHF qualifier (NYHA Class)	II–IV	II–IV	III–IV
QRS duration qualifier (ms)	>120	>130	>120
Improvement in NYHA Class	65% decreased 1 class vs. 50% control	23% decreased 1 class, 11.6% decreased 2 classes vs. control	Not reported
Improvement in 6-minute hall walk (m)	No difference	35 overall; 47 class IV	Not reported
Improvement in QOL	7.2 ± 2.0	6	Not reported
Improvement in VO_2 (mL/kg/min)	1.1	0.9 overall; 1.8 class IV	Not reported
Death or CHF hospitalization	Not reported	Not reported	40% ↓ CRTD, 35% ↓ CRT
Death	Not reported	Not reported	36% ↓ CRTD, 24% ↓ CRT
Comments	Single blind	Double blind	PR > 150 ms; single blind; mortality reduction with CRT not stat. significant

CRTD = cardiac resynchronization therapy + defibrillation; LVEF = left ventricular ejection fraction; LVEDD = left ventricular end-diastolic dimension; NYHA = New York Heart Association; QOL = Minnesota Living with Heart Failure Quality of Life; VO_2 = oxygen uptake determination; Not reported = indicates data have not been published.

Retrospective analysis of these and other ICD trials clearly demonstrates that the mortality benefit of ICD therapy is almost entirely confined to older patients with the most severely depressed left ventricular systolic function and more advanced symptomatic heart failure. However, it is crucial to recognize that none of the ICD trials cited previously specified heart failure as a requisite for entry, and even though the majority of patients had mild to moderate heart failure symptoms (NYHA class II or III), many were not receiving optimal medical therapy. Although post-hoc analysis has consistently demonstrated a mortality benefit among the "sickest" patients *in ICD trials*,[87] none of these trials before SCD-HeFT and COMPANION specifically enrolled patients with heart failure. Patients with severely reduced LVEF and highly symptomatic heart failure may pose unique problems for mortality reduction using ICD therapy. These patients are at equivalently high risk for lethal ventricular arrhythmias and death due to progressive heart failure. Mortality generally increases with increasing NYHA functional class; however, the proportion of sudden deaths

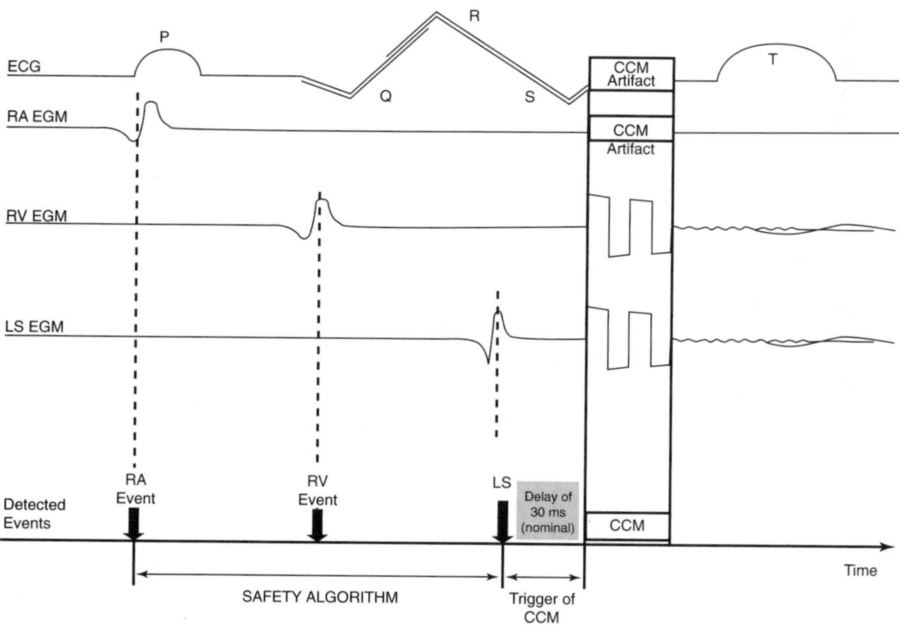

Figure 9.37. Schematic timing of electrical events in a device for cardiac contractility modulation (CCM). Surface ECG, right atrial electrogram (RA EGM), right ventricular (RV) EGM, and local sensed (LS) ventricular EGM are represented. The CCM pulse is delivered 30 to 60 milliseconds after the sensed local ventricular EGM to correspond to the plateau of the local action potential. The pulse is visible on surface ECG as stimulus artifact in the terminal portion of the QRS complex. (Reproduced by permission from Pappone C, et al. First human chronic experience with cardiac contractility modulation by nonexcitatory electrical currents for treating systolic heart failure: mid-term safety and efficacy results from a multicenter study. J Cardiovasc Electrophysiol 2004;15:418–427.)

declines from 50% to 80% among patients with class II symptoms to 5% to 30% among patients with class IV symptoms.[88,89] Furthermore, sudden bradyarrhythmic death in advanced heart failure[90] may occur spontaneously or after successful termination of VT/VF "storms" in ICD patients ("cardiac annihilation")[91] and further diminish the mortality benefit of ICD therapy.

NON-EXCITATORY CARDIAC CONTRACTILITY MODULATION

Cardiac contractility modulation is an evolving device based therapy for heart failure that does not rely upon the presence of ventricular dyssynchrony for a therapeutic effect. Using standard pacing leads and an implantable pulse generator, *non-excitatory* electrical stimuli are delivered to the right ventricular myocardium 30 to 60 milliseconds after the sensed local electrogram (Fig. 9.37). The pulse is biphasic with a duration of 20 to 40 milliseconds and amplitude up to 10 V. Because this stimulus is delivered during ventricular refractoriness it does not participate in the electrical excitation of the ventricle. Instead, this stimulus prolongs the local action potential duration thereby enhancing the sarcolemmal calcium transient. This in turn increases cardiac contractility. A significant inotropic effect has been demonstrated in animal and human studies.[92,93] In patients with the device implanted for 32 weeks, significant improvements in ejection fraction, exercise time, and quality of life were demonstrated.[93] At the time of this writing, this therapy is beginning clinical trials in the United States. The benefits of this therapy as an alternative or adjunct to cardiac resynchronization therapy are unknown.

REFERENCES

1. Schocken DD, Arrieta MI, leaverton PE, Ross EA. Prevalence and mortality of congestive heart failure in the United States. J Am Coll Cardiol 1992;20:301–306.
2. Ho KKL, Anderson KM, Kannel WB, et al. Survival after the onset of congestive heart failure in the Framingham Heart Study subjects. Circulation 1993;88:107–115.
3. Massie BM, Shah NB. Evolving trends in the epidemiologic factors of heart failure. Am Heart J 1997;133:703–712.
4. Kannel WB, Plehn JF, Cupples A. Cardiac failure and sudden death in the Framingham study. Am Heart J 1988;115:869–875.
5. Auricchio A, Abraham WT. Cardiac resynchronization therapy: current state of the art. Cost versus benefit. Circulation 2004;109:300–307.
6. Leclerc C, Kass DA. Retiming the failing heart: principles and current clinical status of cardiac resynchronization. J Am Coll Cardiol 2002;39:194–201.
7. Wiggers C. The muscular reactions of the mammalian ventricles to artificial surface stimuli. Am J Physiol 1925;73:346–378.
8. Schlant RC. Idioventricular kick. Circulation 1966;33 (Suppl III):III–209.
9. Gottipaty VK, Krelis SP, Lu F, et al. The resting electrocardiogram provides a sensitive and inexpensive marker of prognosis in patients with chronic congestive heart failure. J Am Coll Cardiol 1999;33:145A. Abstract.

10. Baldasseroni S, Opasich C, Gorinii M, et al. Left bundle branch block is associated with increased 1-year sudden death and total mortality rate in 5517 outpatients with congestive heart failure: a report from the Italian Network on Congestive Heart Failure. Am Heart J 2002;143:398–405.
11. Grines CL, Boshore TW, Boudoulas H, et al. Functional abnormalities in isolated left bundle branch block: the effect of interventricular asynchrony. Circulation 1989;79:845–853.
12. Leclerq C, Faris O, Runin R, et al. Systolic improvement and mechanical resynchronization does not require electrical synchrony in the dilated failing heart with left bundle–branch block. Circulation 2002;106:1760–1763.
13. Verbeek XA, Vernooy K, Peschar M. Intra-ventricular resynchronization for optimal left ventricular function during pacing in experimental left bundle branch block. J Am Coll Cardiol 2003;42:558–567.
14. Prinzen FW, Hunter WC, Wyman BT, et al. Mapping of regional myocardial strain and work during ventricular pacing: experimental study using magnetic resonance imaging tagging. J Am Coll Cardiol 1999;33:1735–1742.
15. Prinzen FW, Augustijn CH, Arts T, Allessi MA, Reneman RS. Redistribution of myocardial fiber strain and blood flow by asynchronous activation. Am J Physiol 1990(259):H300–308.
16. Spragg DD, Leclercq C, Loghmani M, et al. Regional alterations in protein expression in the dyssynchronous failing heart. Circulation 2003;108:929–932.
17. Prinzen FW, Cheriex EC, Delhaas T, et al. Asymmetric thickness of the left ventricular wall resulting from asynchronous electric activation: a study in dogs with ventricular pacing and in patients with left bundle branch block. Am Heart J 1995;130:1045–1053.
18. Breithardt OA, Sinha AM, Schwammenthal E, et al. Acute effects of cardiac resynchronization therapy on functional mitral regurgitation in advanced systolic heart failure. J Am Coll Cardiol 2003;203:765–770.
19. Auricchio A, Fantoni C, Regoli F, et al. Characterization of left ventricular activation in patients with heart failure and left bundle branch block. Circulation (in press).
20. de Teresa E, Chamorro JL, Pulpon LA, et al. An even more physiologic pacing. Changing the sequence of activation. In: Steinbech K GD, Laskovics A, et al., eds. Cardiac Pacing. Proceedings of the VIIth World Symposium on Cardiac Pacing, 1984. Darmstadt, Germany: Steinkoopff Verlag; 1984:395–400.
21. Cazeau S, Ritter P, Bakdach S, et al. Four chamber pacing in dilated cardiomyopathy. Pacing Clin Electrophysiol 1994;17:1974–1979.
22. Auricchio A, Stellbrink C, Block M, et al. Effect of pacing chamber and atrioventricular delay on acute systolic function of paced patients with congestive heart failure. The Pacing Therapies for Congestive Heart Failure Study Group. The Guidant Congestive Heart Failure Research Group. Circulation 1999;99(23):2993–3001.
23. Nelson GS, Curry CW, Wyman BT, et al. Predictors of systolic augmentation from left ventricular preexcitation in patients with dilated cardiomyopathy and intraventricular conduction delay. Circulation 2000;101(23):2703–2709.
24. Kerwin WF, Botvinick EH, O'Connell JW, et al. Ventricular contraction abnormalities in dilated cardiomyopathy: effect of biventricular pacing to correct interventricular dyssynchrony. J Am Coll Cardiol 2000;35:1221–1227.

25. Nelson GS, Berger RD, Fetics BJ, et al. Left ventricular or biventricular pacing improves cardiac function at diminished energy cost in patients with dilated cardiomyopathy and left bundle branch block. Circulation 2000;105:3053–3059.
26. St John Sutton MG, Plappert T, Abraham WT, et al, for the MIRACLE Study Group. Effect of cardiac resynchronization therapy on left ventricular size and function in chronic heart failure. Circulation 2003;105(1985–1990).
27. Sogaard P, Egeblad H, Pedersen AK, et al. Sequential versus simultaneous biventricular resynchronization for severe heart failure: evaluation by tissue Doppler imaging. Circulation 2002;106:2078–2084.
28. Lau CP, Yu CM, Chau E, et al. Reversal of left ventricular remodeling by synchronous biventricular pacing in heart failure. Pacing Clin Electrophysiol 2000;23: 1722–1725.
29. Van Oosterhout MFM, Prinzen FW, Arts T, et al. Asynchronous electrical activation induces asymmetrical hypertrophy of the left ventricular wall. Circulation 1998;98: 588–595.
30. Cannan CR, Higano ST, Holmes DR. Pacemaker induced mitral regurgitation: an alternative form of pacemaker syndrome. Pacing Clin Electrophysiol 1997;20: 735–738.
31. Nunez A, Alberga MT, Cosio FG, et al. Severe mitral regurgitation with right ventricular pacing successfully treated with left ventricular pacing. Pacing Clin Electrophysiol 2002;25:226–230.
32. Garrigue S, Jais P, Espil G, et al. Comparison of chronic biventricular pacing between epicardial and endocardial left ventricular stimulation using Doppler tissue imaging in patients with heart failure. Am J Cardiol 2001;88(8):858–862.
33. Jais P, Takahashi A, Garrigue S, et al. Mid-term follow-up of endocardial biventricular pacing. Pacing Clin Electrophysiol 2000;23:1744–1747.
34. Daubert CJ, Ritter P, LeBreton H, et al. Permanent left ventricular pacing with transvenous leads inserted into the coronary veins. Pacing Clin Electrophysiol 1998;21:239–345.
35. Meisel E, Pfeiffer D, Engelmann L, et al. Investigation of coronary venous anatomy by retrograde venography in patients with malignant ventricular tachycardia. Circulation 2001;104:442–447.
36. Auricchio A, Stellbrink C, Sack S, et al. The Pacing Therapies for Congestive Heart Failure (PATH-CHF) study: rationale, design, and endpoints of a prospective randomized multicenter study. Am J Cardiol 1999;83(5B):130D–135D.
37. Auricchio A, Klein H, Tockman B, et al. Transvenous biventricular pacing for heart failure: can the obstacles be overcome? American Journal of Cardiology 1999;83(5B): 136D–142D.
38. Butter C, Auricchio A, Stellbrink C, et al. Effect of resynchronization therapy stimulation site on the systolic function of heart failure patients. Circulation 2001; 104(25):3026–3029.
39. Fauchier L, Marie O, Casset-Senon D, et al. Interventricular and intraventricular dyssynchrony in idiopathic dilated cardiomyopathy: a prognostic study with fourier phase analysis of radionuclide angioscintigraphy. J Am Coll Cardiol 2002;40(11): 2031–2033.
40. Auricchio A, Stellbrink C, Sack S, et al. Long-term clinical effect of hemodynamically optimized cardiac resynchronization therapy in patients with heart failure and ventricular conduction delay. J Am Coll Cardiol 2002;39(12):2026–2033.

41. Garrigue S, Jais P, Espil G, et al. Comparison of chronic biventricular pacing between epicardial and endocardial left ventricular stimulation using doppler tissue imaging in patients with heart failure. Am J Cardiol 2001;88:858–862.
42. Abraham WT, Fisher WG, Smith AL, et al. Cardiac resynchronization in chronic heart failure. N Engl J Med 2002;346(24):1845–1853.
43. Young JB, Abraham WT, Smith AL, et al. Combined cardiac resynchronization and implantable cardioversion defibrillation in advanced chronic heart failure: the MIRACLE ICD Trial. JAMA 2003;289:2685–2694.
44. Bristow MR, Feldman AM, Saxon LA, et al. COMPANION. In: Heart Failure Society of America, Late Breaking Clinical Trial Presentation; 2003.
45. Blanc JJ, Etienne Y, Gilard M, et al. Evaluation of different ventricular pacing sites in patients with severe heart failure: results of an acute hemodynamic study. Circulation 1997;96:3273–3277.
46. Kass DA, Chen CH, Curry C, et al. Improved left ventricular mechanics from acute VDD pacing in patients with dilated cardiomyopathy and ventricular conduction delay. Circulation 1999;99(12):1567–1573.
47. Touiza A, Etienne Y, Gilard M, et al. Long-term left ventricular pacing: assessment and comparison with biventricular pacing in patients with severe congestive heart failure. J Am Coll Cardiol 2001;38:1966–1970.
48. Blanc JJ, Bertault–Valls V, Fatemi M, et al. Long-term benefits of left univentricular pacing in patients with congestive heart failure. Circulation 2004; In press.
49. Moss AJ, Hall WJ, Cannom DS, et al. Improved survival with an implanted defibrillator in patients with coronary disease at high risk for ventricular arrhythmia. N Engl J Med 1996;335:1993–1940.
50. Moss AJ, Zareba W, Hall WJ, et al. Prophylactic implantation of a defibrillator in patients with myocardial infarction and reduced ejection fraction. N Engl J Med 2002;346(12):877–883.
51. Buxton AE, Lee KL, Fisher JD, et al. A randomized study of the prevention of sudden death among patients with coronary artery disease. N Engl J Med 1999;341:1882–1890.
52. Bardy GH. The Sudden Cardiac Death in Heart Failure Trial (SCD-HeFT). In: Late–Breaking Clinical Trials, American College of Cardiology; 2004.
53. Butter C, Meisel E, Engelmann L, et al. Human experience with transvenous biventricular defibrillation using an electrode in a left ventricular vein. Pacing and Clin Electrophysiol 2002;25(3):324–331.
54. Auricchio A, Kramer A, Spinelli J, et al. Can the optimum dosage of resynchronization therapy be derived from the intracardiac electrogram? J Am Coll Cardiol 2002;39:124. Abstract.
55. Reuter R, Garrigue S, Barold SS, et al. Comparisons of characteristics in responders versus nonresponders with biventricular pacing for drug-resistant congestive heart failure. Am J Cardiol 2002;89:346–350.
56. Bax JJ, Mohoek SG, Marwick TJ, et al. Left ventricular dyssynchrony predicts benefit of cardiac resynchronization therapy in patients with end-stage heart failure before pacemaker implantation. Am J Cardiol 2003;92:1238–1240.
57. Pitzalis MV, Iacoviello M, Romito R, et al. Cardiac resynchronization therapy tailored by echocardiographic evaluation of ventricular asynchrony. J Am Coll Cardiol 2002;40:1615–1622.
58. Kerckhoffs RC, Bovendeerd PH, Kotte JC, et al. Homogeneity of cardiac contraction despite physiological asynchrony of depolarization: a model study. Ann Biomed Eng 2003;31:536–547.

59. Kadhiresan V, Vogt J, Auricchio A, et al. Sensitivity and specificity of QRS duration to predict acute benefit in heart failure patients with cardiac resynchronization. Pacing Clin Electrophysiol 2000;23(II):555. Abstract.
60. D'Hooge J, Heimdal A, Jamal F, et al. Regional strain and strain rate measurements by cardiac ultrasound: principles, implementation and limitations. Eur J Echocardiography 2000;1:154–170.
61. Breithardt OA, Stellbrink C, Herbots L, et al. Cardiac resynchronization therapy can reverse abnormal myocardial strain distribution in patients with heart failure and left bundle branch block. J Am Coll Cardiol 2003;42:486–494.
62. Sogaard P, Egeblad H, Kim W, et al. Tissue Doppler imaging predicts improved systolic performance and reversed left ventricular remodeling during cardiac resynchronization therapy. J Am Coll Cardiol 2002;40:723–730.
63. Baxx JJ, Yu C-M, Lin H, et al. Comparison of acute changes in left ventricular volume, systolic and diastolic functions, and intraventricular synchronicity after biventricular pacing and right ventricular pacing for congestive heart failure. Am Heart J 2003;145:G1–G7.
64. Bax JJ, Molhoek SG, Marwick TH, et al. Usefulness of myocardial tissue Doppler echocardiography to evaluate left ventricular dyssynchrony before and after biventricular pacing in patients with idiopathic dilated cardiomyopathy. Am J Cardiol 2003;91:94–97.
65. Yu C-M, Fung W-H, Lin H, et al. Predictors of left ventricular reverse remodeling after cardiac resynchronization therapy for heart failure secondary to idiopathic dilated or ischemic cardiomyopathy. Am J Cardiol 2002;91:684–688.
66. Auricchio A, Stellbrink C, Sack S, et al. Long-term benefit as a result of pacing resynchronization in congestive heart failure: results of the PATH-CHF Trial. Circulation 2000;102:II–693A.
67. Linde C, Leclerc C, Rex S, et al. Long-term benefits of biventricular pacing in congestive heart failure: Results from the Multisite Stimulation in Cardiomyopathy (MUSTIC) Study. J Am Coll Cardiol 2002;40:111–118.
68. Linde C, Braunschweig F, Gadler F, Bailleul C, Daubert JC. Long-term improvement in quality of life by biventricular pacing in patients with chronic heart failure: results from the MUSTIC Study. Am J Cardiol 2003;91:1090–1095.
69. Aranda JM, Curtis AB, Conti JB, Stejskal-Peterson S. Do heart failure patients with right bundle branch block benefit from cardiac resynchronization therapy? Analysis of the MIRACLE Study. J Am Coll Cardiol 2002;39:96A. Abstract.
70. Yu C-M, Yang H, Lau C-P, et al. Regional left ventricular mechanical asynchrony in patients with heart disease and normal QRS duration. Pacing Clin Electrophysiol 2003;26:562–570.
71. Achilli A, Sassara M, Ficili S, et al. Long term effectiveness of cardiac resynchronization therapy in patients with refractory heart failure and "narrow" QRS duration. J Am Coll Cardiol 2003;42:2117–2124.
72. Kass DM. Predicting cardiac resynchronization response by QRS duration. J Am Coll Cardiol 2003;42:2125–2127.
73. Gaspirini M, Mantica M, Galimberti P, et al. Beneficial effects of biventricular pacing in patients with a "narrow" QRS duration. Pacing Clin Electrophysiol 2003; 26:169–174.
74. Sweeney MO, Hellkamp AS, Ellenbogen KA, et al. Adverse effect of ventricular pacing on heart failure and atrial fibrillation among patients with normal baseline

QRS duration in a clinical trial of pacemaker therapy for sinus node dysfunction. Circulation 2003;23:2932–2937.

75. The DAVID Trial Investigators. Dual-chamber pacing or ventricular backup pacing in patients with an implantable defibrillator: the Dual Chamber and VVI Implantable Defibrillator (DAVID) Trial. JAMA 2002;288(24):3115–3123.
76. Peschar M, de Swart H, Michels KJ, Reneman RS, Prinzen FW. Left ventricular septal and apex pacing for optimal pump function in canine hearts. J Am Coll Cardiol 2003;41(7):1218–1226.
77. Cazeau S, Leclerlq C, Lavergne T, et al. Effects of multisite biventricular pacing in patients with heart failure and intraventricular conduction delay. N Engl J Med 2001;344:873–880.
78. Bradley DJ, Bradley EA, Baughman KL, et al. Cardiac resynchronization and death from progressive heart failure: a meta-analysis of randomized controlled trials. JAMA 2003;289:730–740.
79. Gillum RF. Sudden coronary death in the United States. Circulation 1989;79: 756–765.
80. Moss AJ. Sudden cardiac death and national health. Pacing Clin Electrophysiol 1993;16:2190–2191.
81. The Antiarrhythmics versus Implantable Defibrillator (AVID) Investigators. A comparison of antiarrhythmic-drug therapy with implantable defibrillators in patients resuscitated from near-fatal ventricular arrhythmias. N Engl J Med 1997;337: 1576–1583.
82. Kuck KH, Cappato R, Siebels J, Ruppel F, for the CASH Investigators. Randomized comparison of antiarrhythmia drug therapy with implantable defibrillators in patients resuscitated from cardiac arrest: the Cardiac Arrest Study Hamburg (CASH). Circulation 2000;102:748–754.
83. Connolly SJ, Gent M, Roberts RS, et al. Canadian implantable defibrillator study (CIDS): a randomized trial of the implantable cardioverter defibrillator against amiodarone. Circulation 2000;101:1297–1302.
84. Shamim W, Francis DP, Yousufuddin M, et al. Intra-ventricular conduction delay: a prognostic marker in congestive heart failure. Int J Cardiol 1999;70:171–178.
85. Gerber TC, Nishimura R, Holmes DR, et al. Left ventricular and biventricular pacing in congestive heart failure. Mayo Clin Proc 2001;706:803–812.
86. Higgins SL, Hummel JD, Niazi IK, et al. Cardiac resynchronization therapy for the treatment of heart failure and intraventricular conduction delay and malignant ventricular tachyarrhythmia. J Am Coll Cardiol 2003;42:1454–1459.
87. Moss AJ. Implantable cardioverter defibrillator therapy: the sickest patients benefit the most. Circulation 2000;101:1638–1640.
88. MERIT-HF Study Group. Effect of metoprolol CR/XL in chronic heart failure: metoprolol CR/XL randomized intervention trial in congestive heart failure (MERIT-HF). Lancet 1999;353:2001–2007.
89. Uretsky B, Sheahan G. Primary prevention of sudden cardiac death in heart failure: will the result be shocking? J Am Coll Cardiol 1997;30:1589–1597.
90. Luu M, Stevenson WG, Saxon LA, Stevenson LW. Diverse mechanisms of unexpected cardiac arrest in heart failure. Circulation 1989;80:1675–1680.
91. Mitchell LB, Pineda EA, Titus JL, Bartosch PM, Benditt DG. Sudden death in patients with implantable cardioverter defibrillators: importance of post-shock electromechanical dissociation. J Am Coll Cardiol 2002;39(8):1323–1328.

92. Mohri S, He KL, Dickstein M, et al. Cardiac contractility modulation by electrical currents applied during the refractory period. Am J Physiol Heart Circ Physiol 2002;282:H1642–H1647.
93. Pappone C, Augello G, Rosanio S, et al. First human chronic experience with cardiac contractility modulation by nonexcitatory electrical currents for treating systolic heart failure: mid-term safety and efficacy results from a multicenter study. J Cardiovasc Electrophysiol 2004;15:418–427.

ICD Follow-up and Troubleshooting

Henry F. Clemo and Mark A. Wood

10

The implantable cardioverter-defibrillator (ICD) is the treatment of choice for aborted sudden cardiac death and sustained ventricular arrhythmias in the absence of acute myocardial infarction or reversible causes. Patients with these devices need regular follow-up by a physician knowledgeable of ICDs to ensure appropriate functioning and avoid potential problems. Further, the physician must be able to investigate and solve any problems that may arise with the ICD.

FOLLOW-UP AFTER IMPLANTABLE CARDIOVERTER-DEFIBRILLATOR PLACEMENT

After implanting the device and before discharging the patient from the hospital, the implanting physician should observe the following procedures:

1. Inspect the ICD site for evidence of hematoma or infection.
2. Counsel the patient about keeping the ICD site clean and dry for 1 week as well as avoiding raising the arm ipsilateral to the ICD above the shoulder or reaching for the horizon for 2 to 4 weeks.
3. Interrogate the ICD and perform a noninvasive check of lead resistances as well as lead sensing and pacing thresholds.
4. Obtain chest radiographs in the anteroposterior and lateral views to ascertain appropriate lead positions.
5. Discuss driving, activity, and occupational restrictions appropriate for the patient's condition. Most states have mandatory driving restrictions for 6 to 12 months following a syncopal event due to ventricular arrhythmias.[1]

In addition, some devices emit audible alert tones to indicate battery depletion, high lead impedances or prolonged charge times. These tones should be demonstrated to the patient and their importance emphasized.

The ICD patient should be seen again at 2 to 4 weeks after the implantation surgery to ascertain whether the wound is healing appropriately. The ICD pocket should be carefully examined for evidence of infection. The ICD system should be checked as outlined below to ensure that the lead is stable and the device is functioning. Patients should be seen every 3 to 6 months thereafter until the device approaches elective replacement indicators, at which time more frequent follow-up assessments are warranted.

ROUTINE FOLLOW-UP

The purpose of subsequent follow-up visits is to assess the patient's condition, check the stability and performance of the ICD system and the adequacy of programmed therapies, provide patient education, and investigate potential device malfunctions.

History and Physical Examination

The history and physical examination can be invaluable for understanding the performance of a patient's ICD. The patient should be asked about the occurrence of shocks or syncope. In particular, conditions such as congestive heart failure and cardiac ischemia, which may precipitate ventricular tachyarrhythmias, should be evaluated. Conditions such as chronic obstructive pulmonary disease, infection, anemia, and dehydration that can precipitate supraventricular tachyarrhythmias and inappropriate shocks should be investigated. The patient should be questioned as to whether particular body positions have triggered ICD therapy. A drug history should be obtained at each visit, because some medications could change pacing, sensing, and defibrillation thresholds; others could cause electrolyte imbalances that may interfere with appropriate ICD function.[2] Furthermore, patients who have congestive heart failure or recurrent cardiac ischemia should be placed on effective doses of beta blockers, angiotensin-converting enzyme inhibitors, and "statins," all of which reduce the incidence of sudden cardiac death and possibly the frequency of delivered ICD therapy.[3–5] The patient should also be examined for ICD infection or erosion. Early detection of impending device erosion can prevent the possibility of catastrophic ICD system infection.

Device Interrogation

At each visit, information retrieved from the device using an ICD programmer should be examined carefully in a systematic fashion.

Programmed Parameters: Programmed parameters include detection and treatment algorithms for ventricular tachyarrhythmias, therapies for bradyarrhythmias, and various alert settings. Review of these parameters may reveal erroneous programming that can potentially result in inappropriate or suppressed ICD therapy. For example, failure to program a VT zone could prevent delivery of effective therapy for undetected ventricular tachycardia. On the other hand, failure to use supraventricular tachyarrhythmia (SVT) discrimination schemes could allow SVTs such as atrial fibrillation to trigger inappropriate ICD therapy.

Occasionally, patients who have ICD therapies suspended when they undergo surgery are left unprotected when these therapies are not reactivated after completion of their procedures.

System Data: System data include lead impedances, battery voltage, capacitor charge time, and defibrillation circuit resistance. Initial examination of this data can quickly reveal potential problems with the ICD system including battery depletion (low battery voltage or prolonged charge time), faulty capacitor function (prolonged charge time), lead insulation failure (low impedance), or lead conductor fracture (high impedance). These values should be compared to information recorded from previous visits and to the guidelines for the specific ICD model. In particular, lithium–silver–vanadium oxide batteries are used in ICDs. These batteries have unusual voltage discharge characteristics and approach end-of-life voltage in a less predictable fashion than pacemaker batteries.

Elective replacement indicators for ICDs are based on battery voltage with or without charge time criteria specific for each model of ICD. The charge times reflect the time required to charge the capacitor to high voltages. Prolonged charge times may indicate battery depletion, capacitor or component malfunction, or excessive times between capacitor reformation. The reformation process restores the insulating dielectric between the capacitor plates needed for optimal capacitor function. This is usually performed automatically by the device at 3- to 6-month intervals. When the ICD battery voltage is approaching elective replacement status, the patient should be observed on a more frequent basis (i.e., monthly or bimonthly) to allow for timely ICD generator replacement.

Event Logs: Event logs include ventricular and supraventricular tachyarrhythmia episodes/electrograms and therapies, bradyarrhythmia information, and system component alerts. Obviously, each episode of ventricular tachycardia (VT), ventricular fibrillation (VF), and SVT should be reviewed carefully to ensure that detection was appropriate and that the therapy was effective. Several companies have introduced the ability to remotely interrogate ICDs using monitoring stations based in the patient's home. The retrieved data from the ICD are transmitted by telephone line to a secure server that may be accessed by authorized healthcare providers over the Internet (Fig. 10.1). This information may allow physicians to assess the device programming, activity, and performance without the patient leaving home.

System Component Testing

The system components that require intermittent testing include the sensing and pacing thresholds. These should be determined at each visit. Occasionally, defibrillation threshold testing may need to be done.

Sensing: Sensing of intrinsic intracardiac signals by atrial and ventricular leads must be determined to make sure that atrial and ventricular tachyarrhythmias are being reliably detected. Some ICDs include a semiautomated check of sensing,

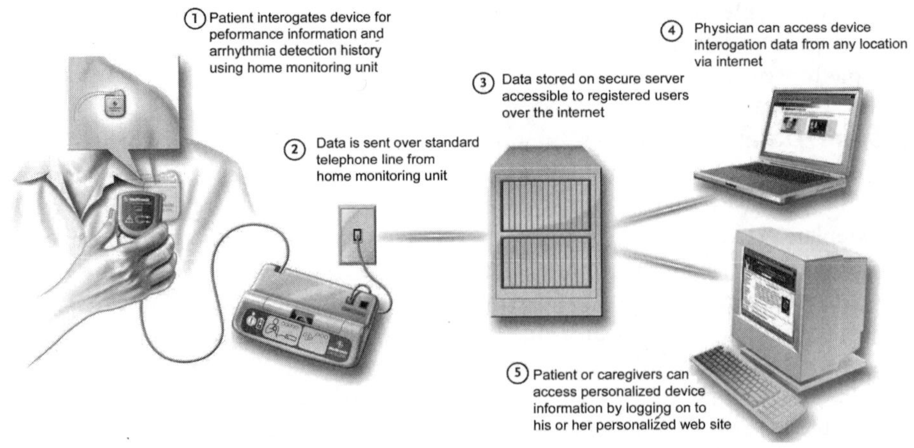

Figure 10.1. Schematic of home based remote ICD monitoring system. (Figure courtesy of Medtronic, Inc.)

whereas others require that bradycardia pacing be temporarily inhibited while a telemetered calibrated intracardiac electrogram strip is printed. Myocardial infarction, congestive heart failure, cardiac surgery, and lead dislodgment, maturation, fracture, or perforation can all cause significant decreases in sensed intracardiac electrogram amplitude.

The intracardiac electrogram should be observed while the patient is performing arm movements, deep breathing, coughing, and other maneuvers. If either high-frequency signals or a failure to sense surface electrocardiographic events are seen, lead conductor fracture, insulation failure or lead/header problems should be suspected. The intracardiac electrogram should also be examined for diaphragmatic myopotentials, T wave sensing, or far-field sensing.

In biventricular devices, sensing of both left and right ventricular leads should be ascertained. Potential double counting of sensed ventricular events should be checked in those devices that sense between right and left ventricular tip electrodes to right ventricular ring or defibrillation electrodes.

Pacing Thresholds: Pacing thresholds for atrial and ventricular leads should be checked to ensure reliable pacing for bradyarrhythmias. Significant changes in pacing thresholds could be caused by lead fracture, perforation, or dislodgment; congestive heart failure or ischemia; and medications or serum electrolyte abnormality. Because bradycardia pacing can shorten the longevity of the ICD battery by months or years, every attempt should be made to minimize unnecessary pacing (e.g., ventricular fusion, and elevated lower rate limit) and excessive outputs.

Both right and left ventricular pacing thresholds should be checked in biventricular devices to ascertain effective biventricular pacing. Additionally, diaphragmatic and chest wall pacing should be checked at maximal left ventricular voltage and pulse duration.

Defibrillation Threshold Testing: Defibrillation threshold (DFT) testing may have to be repeated using the noninvasive electrophysiology study capability of the ICD. Situations in which repeat DFT testing should be done include addition of a new antiarrhythmic drug to the patient's treatment program or cardiac events such as myocardial infarction or cardiac surgery. All of these conditions may potentially change the rate and morphology of ventricular tachyarrhythmias or the minimal energy required for defibrillation (DFT). Testing is also warranted to evaluate failed therapies or to assess sensing during ventricular tachycardia or ventricular fibrillation. Routine yearly defibrillation testing has been advocated by some, but the yield for significant problems has been low.[6,7]

Implantable Cardioverter-Defibrillator Programming

Programming of ICDs can be complex and frustrating. The successful programming of an ICD depends on a good understanding of a particular patient's arrhythmias and the symptoms from those arrhythmias, as well as the underlying cardiac pathophysiology and the patient's medications. In addition, a thorough knowledge of the capabilities of the patient's ICD is essential. The various parameters that may be programmed are shown in Table 10.1.

Ventricular Tachyarrhythmia Detection: Most devices allow for multiple zones of ventricular tachyarrhythmia detection based on heart rate. Often, a zone is programmed for slower, relatively well-tolerated ventricular tachycardia (VT zone), and another zone is programmed for faster, hemodynamically unstable ventricular tachycardia or fibrillation (VF zone). For example, a VT zone may be set for rates of 160 to 200 beats per minute (bpm) with the VF zone for rates over 200 bpm. The rate limits for these zones are usually set 10 bpm slower than the documented ventricular arrhythmia rate to ensure reliable detection. Ventricular tachycardia induced by electrophysiologic testing is often much faster than the patient's spontaneous arrhythmia and is not usually an accurate guide to setting the rate limits.

The ventricular sensitivity must allow for the detection of very low amplitude ventricular fibrillation signals and is typically set to 0.3 mV, or more sensitive settings. Criteria for the number of beats or the time duration above the tachycardia rate in each zone must also be programmed to complete the detection algorithm. An example of a ventricular tachyarrhythmia detection scheme as programmed in a dual-chamber ICD is shown in Figure 10.2.

In the VT zone, various enhancements are available to decrease the risk of supraventricular tachyarrhythmias triggering therapy. In single-chamber ICDs, stability, suddenness of onset, and duration of arrhythmia may be used to increase the specificity for ventricular arrhythmias. These features are described further in Table 10.2. Some defibrillators offer the option of using electrogram duration or morphology to aid in discriminating between supraventricular

Table 10.1. Basic Parameters for ICD Programming

Parameter	Function	Programming*	Comments	Cautions
VF zone	Detection rate for fastest VF zone: rate of VF zone must be on at all VT/VF in multizone hemodynamically programming or rate for single zone	VF zone; rate of hemodynamically unstable VT Single zone: 10 bpm < spontaneous VT	VF zone must be on at all times, only shock RX available	Programmed rate > spontaneous VT rate causes failure to detect
VT zone	Detection rate for slower VTs in multizone programming	On or off; usually 10 bpm < spontaneous VT	ATP and cardioversion RX available	Programmed rate > spontaneous VT rate causes detection failure
Initial detection (no. of intervals and/or duration)	Number of intervals or time above rate limit to diagnose VT/VF	VF zone: 75% intervals > VF rate VT zones: Number of consecutive intervals or time (seconds) above rate limit	VF typically 12 of 16, or 18 of 24 beats > VF rate or 1–2 seconds VT typically 8–20 beats > VT rate or 2–5 seconds	Short criteria may treat criteria delay RX
Redetection	Number of intervals or time after RX to assess RX success or failure	Similar to initial detection but shorter criteria	Similar to initial detection but shorter criteria	Same as initial detection
Ventricular sensitivity	Amplitude of EGM that can be detected	Usually 0.18–0.3 mV	High sensitivity needed to detect small EGM in VF	Failure to detect VF if not sensitive enough; oversensing if too sensitive

SVT discriminators	Differentiates SVT from VTs	See Table 9.2	See Table 9.2	See Table 9.2
ATP	Painless pace termination of VT	On or off	Often initial RX for VTs <200 bpm	May prolong time to shock RX; may accelerate VT to shock RX
Type of sequence (burst or ramp)	Burst: all paced intervals the same Ramp: decrements between paced intervals in sequence	Burst or ramp	Ramp therapy considered more aggressive but equal efficacy for spontaneous VTs	May prolong time to shock RX; may accelerate VT to shock RX
Coupling interval	Interval from VT beat fulfilling detection to first beat of ATP	Typically 80–90% of VT cycle length	May be same as R-R%	Too long or short an interval prevents capture
R-R%	Sets rate for first sequence of ATP	Typically 80–90% of VT cycle length	Consider number of sequences to deliver	Values <80% VT cycle length likely to accelerate VT
# Pulses	Number of paced beats delivered within each ATP sequence	Typically 5–15 beats	Some algorithms add 1 pulse to each sequence	Short trains may fail to penetrate VT circuit; long trains may reinitiate VT
Decrement	Amount the intervals shorten between (burst) and/or within sequence (ramp)	Typically 10–30 msec	Value should consider number of sequences to be delivered	Large decrements may rapidly reach minimal ATP interval value
# Sequences	Maximal number of ATP sequences attempted	Typically 3–6 sequences	Most VT terminated with ≤3 sequences	Large number of sequences prolongs time to shock RX
Sustained high rate	Overrides SVT discriminators to initiate RX after programmed duration	Highly individualized for each patient, typically 1–5 min	Only requires programming when discriminator algorithms active	Excessively long duration will delay therapy for misdiagnosed VT

Table 10.1. Basic Parameters for ICD Programming (*Continued*)

Parameter	Function	Programming*	Comments	Cautions
Minimum ATP interval	Limits maximal rate of ATP pacing	Typically 240–300 msec	VT > 200 bpm less likely to terminate with ATP	Short intervals may accelerate VT
Cardioversion/ Defibrillation	Shock therapy	Always on in all zones (rarely is disabled in a very slow VT zone)	Only RX in VF or single zone; initial RX or follows ATP in VT zones	Painful at all energy levels
Energy	Magnitude of shock in joules or as voltage	VF: DFT + 5–10 J VT: at or above smallest successful energy	VT often terminated with 2–10 J	Failed first shocks prolong time to effective RX and are painful
Pathway/Polarity	Path of current flow between electrodes	Typically RV coil negative (cathodal) and can ± proximal coil positive (anodal)	Most devices can reprogram polarity; new devices can program coils in or out of circuit	Reprogramming may significantly alter DFT
Tilt	Voltage drop on capacitor during shock	Usually 40–65%	Programmable in some devices; programming based on shock impedance	Reprogramming may significantly alter DFT
Pulse width	Duration of each phase of shock	For biphasic shock, typically 8–16 msec total	Based on shock impedance	Reprogramming may significantly alter DFT

* All programming must be individualized for each patient.

ATP = antitachycardia pacing; DFT = defibrillation threshold; EGM = electrogram; RX = ICD therapy; SVT = supraventricular tachycardia; VF = ventricular fibrillation; VT = ventricular tachycardia.

ICD Model: Gem DR 7271
Serial Number:

Nov 17, 2000 09:44:38
9960 Software Version 3.0
Copyright (c) Medtronic, Inc. 1997

Detection Report Page 1

Detection

	Enable	Interval (Rate)
VF	On	290 ms (207 bpm)
FVT	Off	320 ms (188 bpm)
VT	On	400 ms (150 bpm)

Number of Intervals to Detect

	Initial NID	Redetect NID
VF	18/24	12/16
VT	16	8

Sensitivity

Atrial	0.45 mV
Ventricular	0.3 mV

Dual Chamber SVT Criteria

AFib/AFlutter	On
Sinus Tach	On
Other 1:1 SVTs	On
SVT Limit	320 ms

Ventricular SVT Criteria

VT Stability	40 ms

Figure 10.2. Ventricular arrhythmia detection parameter report for the Medtronic model 7271 dual-chamber ICD. Up to three tachyarrhythmia detection zones are programmable based on ventricular rate. In this example, two zones are programmed: a VT zone is from 150 to 206 bpm, and a VF zone is over 207 bpm. An intermediate zone (fast VT, FVT) can also be programmed. This example shows the number of intervals to detection (NID) for the VT and VF zones. After initial detection, a redetect NID must also be satisfied before therapy delivery. Also shown are atrial and ventricular sensitivities and discriminator algorithms for supraventricular tachyarrhythmia.

tachyarrhythmia and ventricular tachycardia. The utility of using changing QRS morphology to differentiate between atrial fibrillation and ventricular tachycardia is shown in Figure 10.3.

With the incorporation of atrial sensing and bradycardia pacing in ICDs (here, dual-chamber ICDs), information from the atrial lead allows for further discrimination based on the relationship of atrial to ventricular activity. As demonstrated in Figure 10.4, the addition of an atrial electrogram is invaluable in proving ventriculoatrial dissociation, thus confirming the diagnosis of ventricular tachycardia. In some dual-chamber ICDs, discrimination between supraventricular tachyarrhythmia and ventricular tachycardia is based on stability of the atrial rate and whether the atrial rate is faster than the ventricular rate. Often, supraventricular tachyarrhythmia discrimination algorithms are subject to a sustained rate-duration limit that, once exceeded, triggers therapy. In Medtronic dual-chamber ICDs, the timing of atrial activity in relation to ventricular activity is determined (PR Logic, Medtronic, Inc., Minneapolis, MN). Certain patterns are associated with supraventricular tachyarrhythmias, atrial fibrillation, sinus tachycardia, far-field R wave sensing, and so on, and will inhibit therapy. Other patterns showing AV dissociation or retrograde conduction consistent with ventricular tachycardia will allow therapy. Generalized algorithms for arrhythmia detection using these discriminators in single and dual chamber ICDs are shown in Figure 10.5.

Table 10.2. Detection Enhancements in ICDs for Differentiation of SVT from VT

Parameter	What It Does	Potentially Useful For	Potential Problems
Stability	Suppresses therapy for tachyarrhythmias with variable ventricular rate	Atrial fibrillation	Underdetection of VT with irregular rate; failure to suppress therapy for SVTs with regular ventricular response
Onset	Suppresses therapy for tachyarrhythmias that slowly accelerate	Sinus tachycardia	Underdetection of gradually accelerating VT or VT onset during sinus tachycardia; failure to suppress therapy for sudden onset SVTs
Ventricular electrogram width	Suppresses therapy for tachyarrhythmias with narrow ventricular EGM correlated to narrow QRS complex	Potentially useful for differentiation of narrow complex SVT from VT	Limited specificity with bundle branch block; may prevent therapy for narrow complex VT
Ventricular electrogram morphology	Suppresses therapy for tachyarrhythmias with ventricular EGM morphology similar to that in sinus rhythm	Potentially useful for differentiation of SVT from VT	Limited specificity with bundle branch block
Sustained rate duration	Therapy for tachyarrhythmias finally delivered after this period of time, even if enhancements still met	Prevents indefinite inhibition of therapy for VT misdiagnosed as SVT	Therapy will eventually be delivered if the SVT continues after sustained rate duration expires
Atrial to ventricular ratio	Compares atrial to ventricular rate	Atrial fibrillation	Atrial undersensing can result in false diagnosis of VT
Atrial to ventricular timing	Evaluates the temporal relation of atrial electrogram to ventricular electrograms	Atrial fibrillation, 1:1 SVTs retrograde conduction	Variable A:V timing, long antegrade or retrograde AV conduction times

Note: Some detection enhancements are available only in certain models of ICD.
EGM = electrogram; SVT = supraventricular tachycardia; VT = ventricular tachycardia.

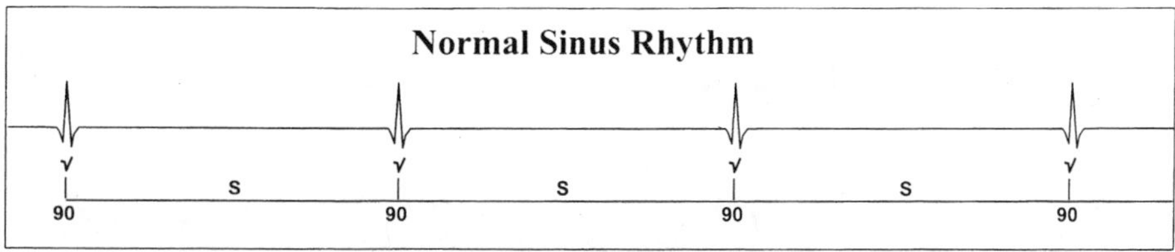

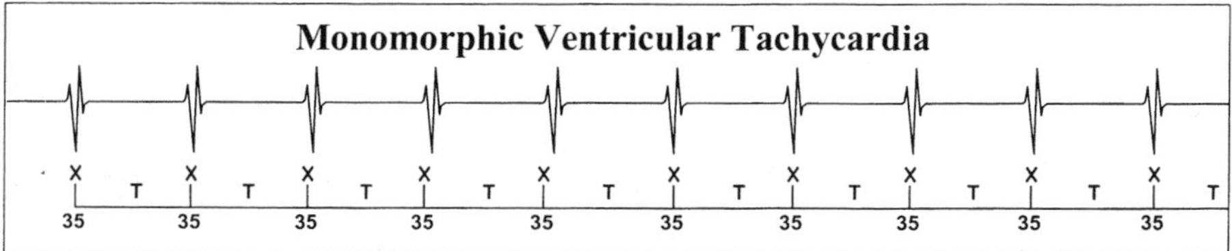

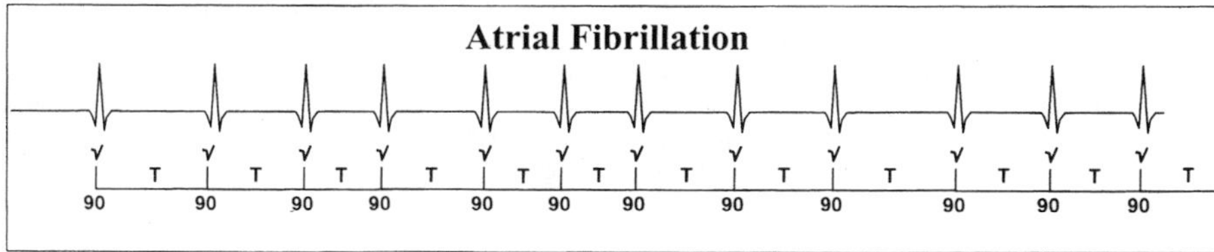

Figure 10.3. Schematic of electrogram morphology (EGM) discrimination between normal sinus rhythm, monomorphic ventricular tachycardia, and atrial fibrillation in a Ventritex (St. Jude) Angstrom single-chamber ICD. Notice how the ventricular electrogram morphology changes in ventricular tachycardia as compared to that of supraventricular rhythms. Each EGM complex is compared to a stored template that represents EGM morphology during sinus rhythm. The numbers below the EGM complexes are "morphology scores" denoting the percentage of template match agreement. If the morphology score is greater than the percent template match threshold, the EGM complex is marked with a "✓" and is presumed to be atrial in origin. If the EGM morphology score is less than the percent template match threshold, the EGM complex is marked with an "X" and is presumed to be ventricular in origin. "S" denotes sinus rhythm, whereas "T" denotes tachycardia.

Despite widespread implantation of dual-chamber ICDs in the past 6 years, the rate of inappropriate ICD discharges still approaches 20% or higher.[8] Clinical predictors of inappropriate therapy in ICD patients include New York Heart Association heart failure score (class I patients have a higher incidence of inappropriate shock) and history of atrial fibrillation.[9] Supraventricular tachyarrhythmias with sudden onset and a regular ventricular response (i.e., atrial flutter or macro-reentrant SVTs) where P waves fall in atrial channel-blanking periods are especially problematic for present generation ICDs. Although further programming to discriminate these arrhythmias could be done, it comes at the expense of decreased positive predictive value of the algorithm, with the potential for failure to sense ventricular tachycardia.

Ventricular Tachyarrhythmia Therapies: Programming of ventricular tachyarrhythmia therapies depends on the ventricular tachyarrhythmia rate,

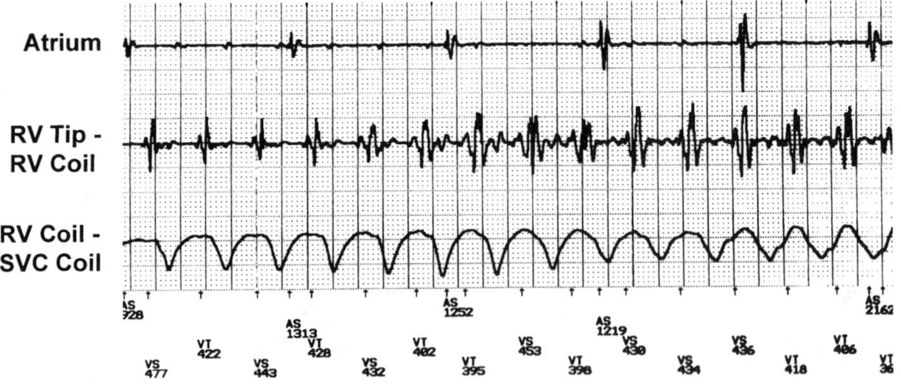

Figure 10.4. Ventricular tachycardia, as recorded by a Guidant Ventak AV dual-chamber ICD. AV dissociation is clearly demonstrated when comparing the atrial electrogram (Atrium, **top tracing**) to the ventricular electrogram (RV Tip–RV Coil, **middle tracing**), which is recorded from the distal tip electrode to the right ventricular defibrillation coil. The **bottom tracing** (RV Coil–SVC Coil) is a ventricular electrogram recorded from a coil on the portion of the ventricular lead that is in the superior vena cava to the distal coil located on the portion of the lead which is in the right ventricle. The marker channel annotations below the electrograms are AS = atrial sensed event; VS = ventricular sensed event; VT = ventricular sensed event meeting VT rate criteria. The numbers are the intervals in milliseconds between consecutive events.

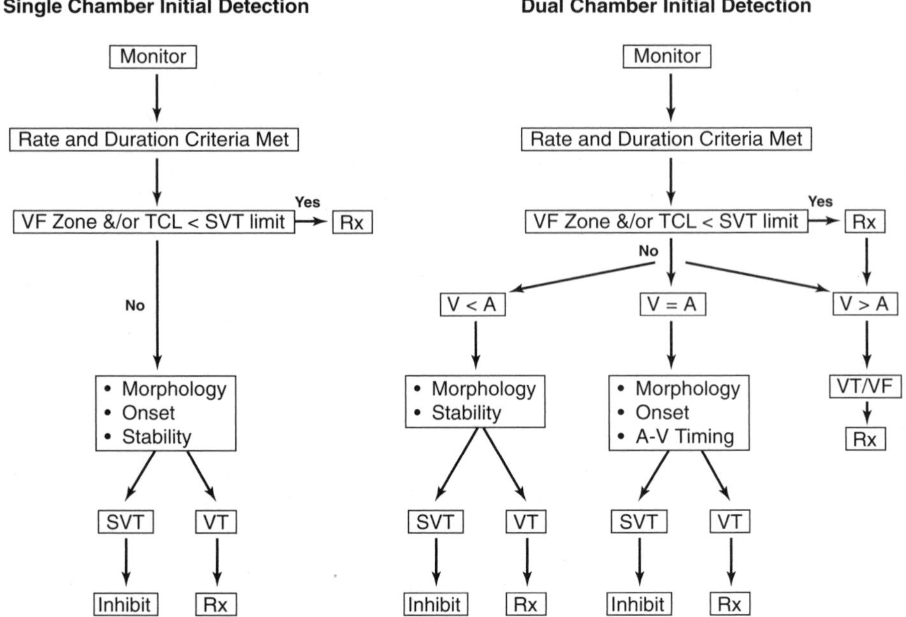

Figure 10.5. Generalized detection algorithms for single- and dual-chamber ICDs incorporating discrimination enhancement features. For the dual-chamber algorithm, a primary "decision point" is the difference between the atrial and ventricular rates. VF = ventricular fibrillation; TCL = tachycardia cycle length; Rx = ICD therapy; SVT = supraventricular tachycardia; VT = ventricular tachycardia; V = ventricle; A = atrial.

hemodynamic stability, and its response to therapy. For patients with hemodynamically tolerated ventricular tachycardia (generally <200 bpm), antitachycardia pacing (ATP) is the preferred choice for initial therapy because it has a greater than 90% success rate in terminating ventricular tachycardia.[10–12] The benefits of ATP are that it is painless to the patient and prolongs the ICD's battery life when compared to cardioversion. In patients who received an ICD for ventricular fibrillation, a VT detection zone with ATP as initial therapy should be empirically programmed because more than 50% of these patients will subsequently have ventricular tachycardia, which is terminated successfully with ATP.[12–14]

The risk of ATP accelerating initially stable ventricular tachycardia to a faster, hemodynamically unstable form is less than 1%.[15] Empiric programming of ATP as initial therapy for fast ventricular tachycardia up to 250 bpm has a 77% efficacy rate.[16] On the other hand, if a review of the stored episodes of ventricular tachycardia shows that ATP does not reliably terminate or possibly accelerates ventricular tachycardia, this therapy should be disabled and low-energy cardioversion (5 to 10 J) should be the initial therapy. Cardioversion energies less than 5 J should be avoided since they could precipitate atrial fibrillation.[17] Usually, up to six therapies are available for a VT zone, progressing from ATP and/or low-energy shocks to high-energy shocks. An example of programming multiple ventricular tachycardia therapies is shown in Figure 10.6.

ICD Model: Gem DR 7271
Serial Number:

Nov 17, 2000 09:41:33
9960 Software Version 3.0
Copyright (c) Medtronic, Inc. 1997

VT Therapies Report — Page 1

VT Therapies	Rx1	Rx2	Rx3	Rx4	Rx5	Rx6
VT Therapy Status	On	On	On	On	On	On
Therapy Type	Burst	Ramp	CV	CV	CV	CV
Initial # Pulses	8	10				
R-S1 Interval=(%RR)	91 %	84 %				
S1S2(Ramp+)=(%RR)						
S2SN(Ramp+)=(%RR)						
Interval Dec	10 ms	20 ms				
# Sequences	5	3				
Smart Mode	On	On				
Energy			5 J	15 J	35 J	35 J
Pathway			AX>B	AX>B	AX>B	AX>B
Anti-Tachy Pacing Minimum Interval		280 ms				

Figure 10.6. Review of therapies for the VT zone programmed for a Medtronic 7271 dual-chamber ICD. Up to six progressively more aggressive therapies (Rx) may be programmed. The initial therapy (Rx1) is a burst type antitachycardia pacing (ATP) with eight pulses being delivered in five sequences; each successive sequence pacing cycle length is decremented by 10 milliseconds. The second therapy (Rx2) is a more aggressive ramp ATP scheme. Therapies three to six (Rx3 to Rx6) are progressively higher energy shocks, up to the maximal output for the device (35 J). For all ICD therapy, each successive therapy should be more aggressive than the last.

Because defibrillation of ventricular fibrillation at any given shock energy is a probability function, the initial defibrillation energy for the VF zone should include an appropriate safety margin. What this margin should be is somewhat controversial, but programming a 10-J safety margin above the defibrillation threshold (DFT) energy is traditionally practiced. If the patient has a DFT of less than 10 J for VF at implant, an initial defibrillation of DFT + 10 J allows for a greater than 99% defibrillation success, a quicker charge time and time to therapy, and less battery drain than use of maximal energy.[18] A randomized study has demonstrated that safety margins of 4 to 6 J above carefully defined DFT at implant (DFT++) have the same efficacy in follow-up as full-output shocks.[19] If testing demonstrates that the DFT has increased over time, possible remedies include discontinuation of any drugs that could increase DFT (Box 10.1); addition of pure class III agents, such as sotalol, which can decrease the DFT; or revision of the ICD system, which may include repositioning or replacing the defibrillation lead, addition of a subcutaneous electrode array, or substituting another ICD with higher defibrillation energy output.

Some new devices allow for programmable energy pathways, waveforms, tilt, pulse width, and polarity to optimize the DFT noninvasively. Up to six progressively higher shock energies are usually available for VF zones, with maximal output mandatory for the final shocks.

Box 10.1. Drugs That May Elevate the Defibrillation Threshold

Class IA
- quinidine*
- procainamide*

Class IB
- lidocaine
- mexiletine*
- tocainide

Class IC
- flecainide*
- moricizine
- propafenone*

Class II
- propranolol

Class III
- amiodarone*

Class IV
- verapamil
- diltiazem

* Mixed data on effect of DFT.

PATIENTS WITH IMPLANTABLE CARDIOVERTER-DEFIBRILLATORS UNDERGOING PROCEDURES

All sources of electromagnetic interference (EMI)—including electrocautery, transcutaneous electrical neurologic stimulation units, radiofrequency ablation, lithotripsy, magnetic resonance imaging, radiation therapy—have the potential to trigger or inhibit ICD therapy or damage the ICD.

The ICDs of patients undergoing surgical procedures involving electrocautery are at particular risk of adverse events.

1. Sensing of cautery output by the ICD may either trigger therapy for presumed ventricular arrhythmias or inhibit pacing output.
2. Transmission of cautery current down the pacing/defibrillation leads to the heart may increase the pacing threshold.
3. The ICD may potentially be damaged or reprogrammed.

To prevent such problems, tachyarrhythmia detection/therapies should be disabled for the duration of the procedure. Ideally, this is done with the ICD programmer.

Alternatively, if it is determined that the ICD tachycardia therapies can be inactivated by magnet application, a magnet may be placed over the device by the anesthesiologist during surgery and removed at the conclusion of the procedure. The magnet can also be removed for needed therapy. Response of the ICD to a magnet is a programmable parameter in Guidant and St. Jude Medical devices and thus cannot be ascertained without knowing the programmed parameters. In Medtronic ICDs, tachyarrhythmia detection/treatment algorithms are inhibited while a magnet is applied and resume upon removal of the magnet. Bradyarrhythmia therapies are not inhibited by application of a magnet to ICDs. In some devices prolonged magnet application can turn therapies *off* until reactivation by repeat magnet application or with a programmer.

While tachyarrhythmia detections and therapies are turned off, the patient's electrocardiogram should be continuously monitored and external defibrillation should be readily available. Immediately following the procedure, the device should be interrogated and the pacing/sensing thresholds determined. All programmed parameters including activation of tachyarrhythmia detections/therapies should be confirmed.

The use of separate temporary or permanent bradycardia pacing systems in the ICD patient may cause a multitude of problems. Because the ICD cannot "blank" pacing stimuli from separate pacing units, these stimuli and subsequent R waves may be double-counted and trigger inappropriate therapies. An example of inappropriate double-counting in a patient with a single-chamber ICD and a separate dual-chamber pacing system is demonstrated in Figure 10.7A. In addition, the pacing unit may not be inhibited by ventricular fibrillation or ventricular tachycardia and continue to deliver pacing stimuli. Due to the sensing characteristics of automatic gain and automatic threshold sensing algorithms, ICDs may only count the pacing stimuli; this could lead to

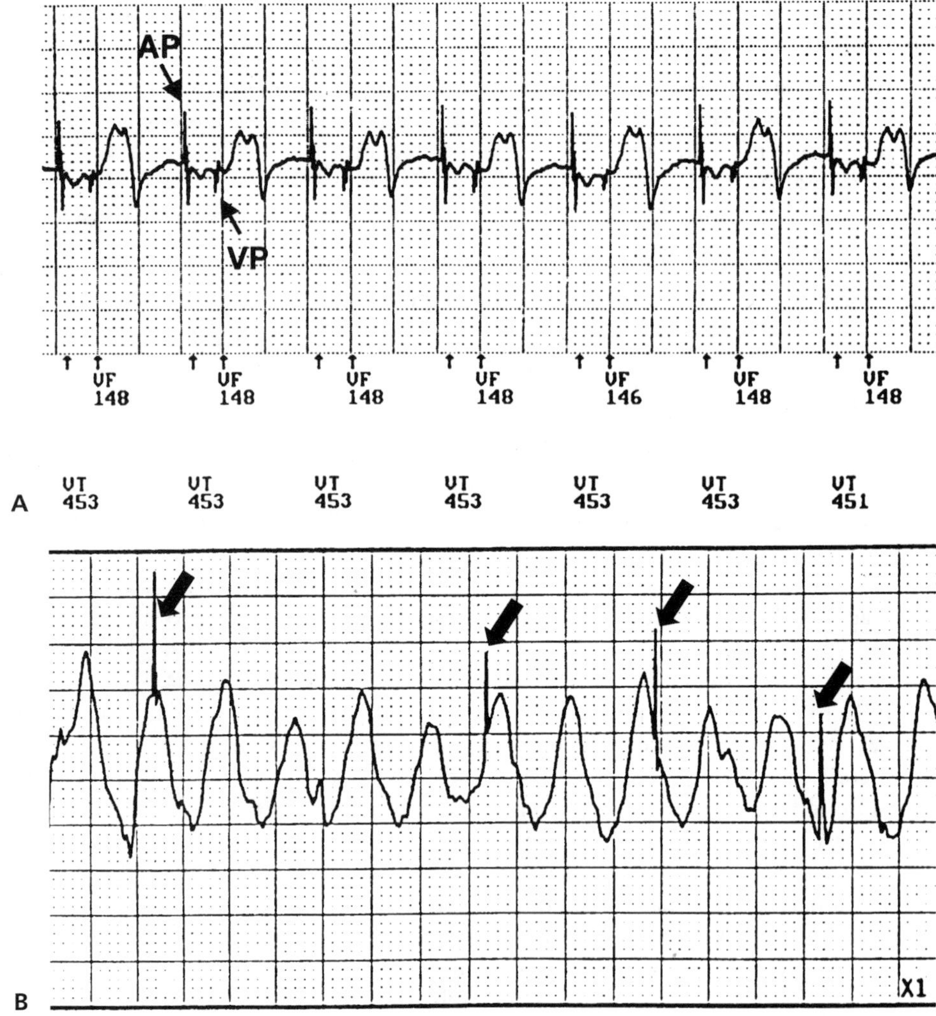

Figure 10.7. Problems with separate bradycardia pacing systems in patients with ICDs. **A:** Double counting of atrial and ventricular pacing artifacts from a dual-chamber pacemaker by a Guidant PRx single-chamber ICD. The ICD detects alternating ventricular cycle lengths of 148 and 453 milliseconds, which meet the rate criteria for tachycardia detection. **B:** Failure of a ventricular pacemaker to be inhibited by polymorphic ventricular tachycardia in a patient with an ICD. The surface ECG rhythm strip demonstrates polymorphic ventricular tachycardia and intermittent pacing spikes (*arrows*). The automatic gain control feature of the ICD decreased the sensing gain so that only the pacing artifacts and not the underlying polymorphic ventricular tachycardia were sensed. Because of this, therapy was never delivered by the ICD despite over 3 minutes of ventricular tachycardia.

underdetection of the ventricular arrhythmia and failure to deliver therapy, as shown in Figure 10.7B.

The procedure for elective cardioversion and external defibrillation in the ICD patient is similar to that for pacemaker patients described elsewhere in this text. Most ICDs are implanted in the left pectoral region, but older ICD systems may have been implanted in the left upper abdomen. For the ICD patient presenting with cardiac arrest, standard advanced cardiac lifesaving protocols for cardiopulmonary resuscitation (CPR) and external defibrillation should be followed as for any other patient. One should not wait for the ICD to deliver therapy, as malfunctions or ineffective therapies may have already occurred.

TROUBLESHOOTING IMPLANTABLE CARDIOVERTER-DEFIBRILLATORS

Troubleshooting ICD problems encompasses all aspects of bradycardia pacemaker malfunctions as well as evaluation of the appropriateness of therapies for ventricular tachycardia. Several scenarios with ICD patients demand sleuth work on the part of the follow-up physician. These scenarios include patients presenting with (1) bradycardia pacing malfunction, (2) single ICD discharge, (3) multiple ICD discharges, (4) syncope with no perceived ICD therapy, and (5) documented sustained ventricular tachycardia without ICD therapy. A careful history and physical examination, and inspection of the comprehensive data logs and stored electrograms often will provide answers to all of these scenarios. Further information can be obtained from the programmed device parameters, the device battery and capacitor status, and the lead performance.

Bradycardia Pacing by the Implantable Cardioverter-Defibrillator

Although most of the bradycardia pacing functions of the ICD are identical to a simple pacemaker, some features are necessarily different. Because of the high ventricular sensitivity and limited blanking periods needed to detect ventricular fibrillation, oversensing by the ICD may be more difficult to avoid or correct. Different parameters may be programmed for post-shock pacing and standard bradycardia pacing; unipolar pacing modes are not available in the ICD. As described previously, application of a magnet to an ICD inhibits tachycardia therapies but does not trigger the asynchronous bradycardia pacing mode. In some ICDs, prolonged magnet application will turn off tachycardia therapies (but bradycardia therapies are unaffected) until another magnet exposure occurs or the device is reactivated with the programmer.

Biventricular ICDs incorporate simultaneous left and right ventricular pacing for treatment of congestive heart failure caused by left ventricular dyssynchrony. Failure of either right or left ventricular pacing because of elevated pacing thresholds or lead dislodgment may change QRS morphology on the electrocardiogram. Double counting of conducted ventricular events could inhibit pacing.

Isolated Implantable Cardioverter-Defibrillator Discharge

Approximately 60% to 80% of ICD patients will receive a shock therapy within 5 years of implant.[20,21] Although ICD shocks are an expected occurrence, each event may frighten the patient, and these warrant careful evaluation by the physician. A flow diagram for the evaluation of ICD shocks is shown in Figure 10.8. Before they are discharged from the hospital after ICD implantation, patients should be educated about the procedures to follow after an ICD shock. Our practice is to have the patient call the office after the first shock is perceived. This allows us to assess the patient's level of anxiety, partially assess the appropriateness of the therapy, and provide reassurance. We interrogate the device electively within 1 to 2 days to ensure that the ICD is functioning appropriately. Thereafter, the patient may contact us for the infrequent shocks, depending on his or her level of comfort. We advise patients to call immediately when more than two shocks within 24 hours are experienced, as this may indicate failed device therapy or inappropriate shocks.

The goal of the physician presented with the patient who has had an ICD shock is to establish whether the therapy was appropriate. A full account of the events leading up to the shock should be elicited, including activities, medical compliance, use of new medications, syncope, palpitations, exposure to EMI, angina, and heart failure. Shocks preceded by syncope or presyncope are almost always appropriate. Shocks associated with heavy exertion, motion of the arm ipsilateral to the ICD, or exposure to electromagnetic current sources should raise suspicions of sinus tachycardia, lead noise, or EMI interference, respectively. Because approximately 40% of the shocks for ventricular tachycardia are asymptomatic, the absence of symptoms before the shock does not indicate a nonarrhythmic etiology.[22] Interrogation of the device therapy log is most useful in determining the cause of the shock. For ventricular tachycardia episodes, the stored electrograms will usually confirm the diagnosis by demonstrating AV dissociation or a change in the morphology compared to sinus rhythm. Otherwise, any noise, supraventricular tachyarrhythmia, or sinus tachycardia will be evident.

Regardless of the cause of the shock, hospitalization for an isolated ICD discharge is rarely warranted unless changes in the antiarrhythmic drug therapy are needed. Reassuring the patient that the device has functioned properly is always indicated. If the patient is particularly troubled by the shock, activating ATP therapy or initiating antiarrhythmic drug therapy may minimize recurrences. For an inappropriate shock, corrective measures must be taken. To avoid supraventricular tachyarrhythmias triggering inappropriate ICD therapy, activation of SVT discrimination algorithms, or antiarrhythmic or AV nodal blocking agents may be useful. Myopotential sensing may require reprogramming the device's sensitivity and performing follow-up testing for appropriate ventricular fibrillation detection. Noise should prompt a thorough search for a lead malfunction or any exposure to EMI.

Finally, some patients report ICD discharges when the ICD counters show no therapy being delivered. This phenomenon, called "phantom shocks," often

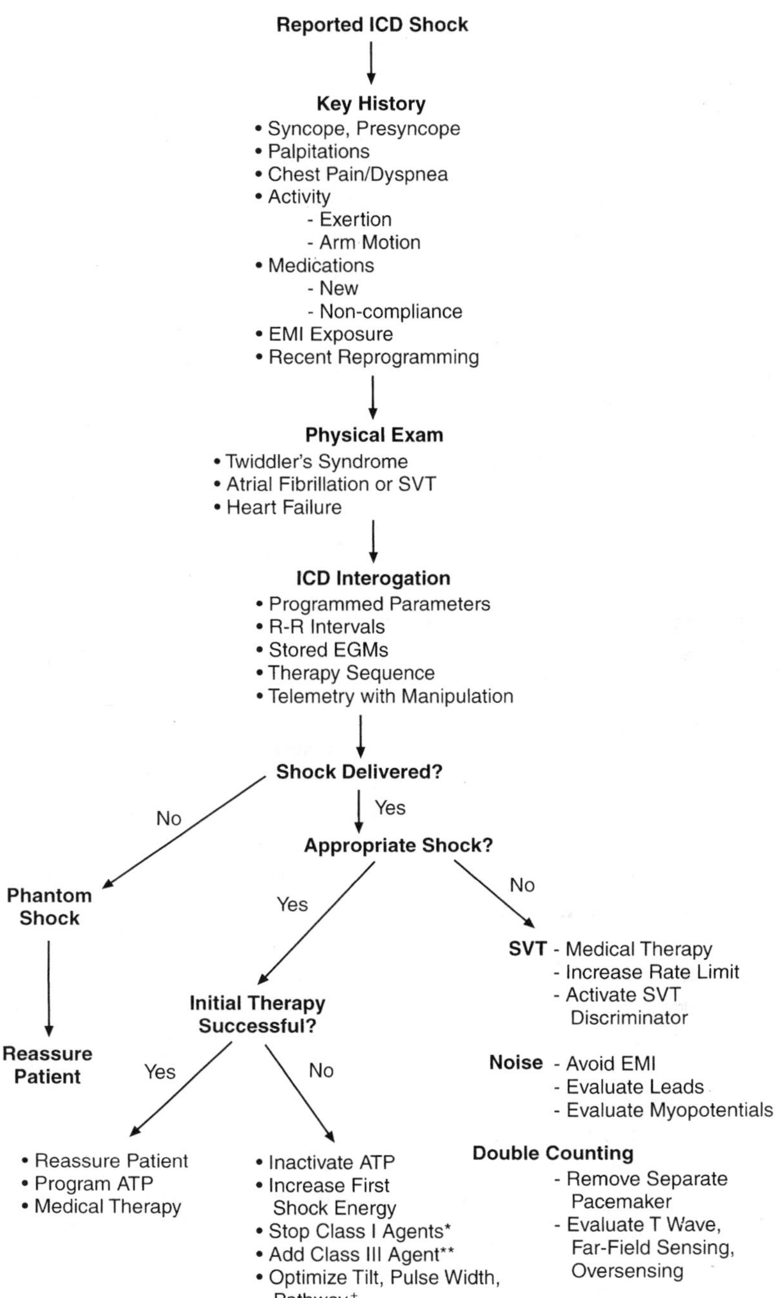

Figure 10.8. Flow diagram for evaluating ICD shocks. ATP = antitachycardia pacing; EGM = electrocardiograms; EMI = electromagnetic interference; SVT = supraventricular tachycardia. *See Box 10.1; **class III drugs include sotalol and dofetilide; not programmable in all devices.

occurs at night and may be due to anxiety, dream states, or hypnagogic contractures. Usually, reassurance is all that is needed but psychologic counseling is occasionally required.

Multiple Discharges

Multiple ICD discharges can be either appropriate or inappropriate. A differential diagnosis for multiple ICD discharges is included in Box 10.2. Because multiple ICD discharges often cause significant psychological stress to the patient, they should be considered a medical emergency.

Multiple Appropriate Discharges: Multiple appropriate discharges over minutes to days may result from incessant ventricular tachycardia, related to acute ischemia or infarction, electrolyte abnormalities, drug proarrhythmia, medical noncompliance, use of inotropic or pressor agents, or a spontaneous ventricular tachycardia "storm."[23,24] Examination of stored intracardiac electrograms will usually determine whether the shocks are appropriate.

Acute treatment of the patient with multiple appropriate ICD discharges should first focus on treating any underlying causes and/or initiating intravenous antiarrhythmic or beta blockade therapy.[23] If the patient is receiving multiple appropriate shocks for ventricular tachycardia, reprogramming to include ATP for ventricular tachycardia may diminish the number of shocks. Sometimes, the patient may benefit from a longer detection and confirmation time in the VT zone if most of the episodes of ventricular tachycardia are self-terminating. If multiple shocks result from ineffective therapies (i.e., ATP or a low-energy shock failing to convert the ventricular tachycardia), more aggressive initial therapy may diminish the total number of discharges the patient receives.

If initial therapies fail to terminate ventricular fibrillation, the DFT should be reevaluated, because it may rise over time. An important cause of increased DFT is drugs, as outlined in Box 9.1. DFT may also change after myocardial infarction, cardiac surgery, or lead/device movement. Occasionally, ICD system revision to change the current path, revise a lead, or install a high-output generator may be needed. Finally, catheter ablation of ventricular tachycardia foci may decrease the number of ventricular tachycardia episodes in drug refractory cases.[25]

Although this is rarely used today, some ICDs may still be programmed to "committed" mode in which therapy will be delivered after initial tachycardia detection criteria are met even if the arrhythmia spontaneously terminates. This mode of operation may result in frequent or multiple shocks for nonsustained ventricular arrhythmias. Some devices are capable of defibrillation therapy for atrial tachyarrhythmias. Multiple low-energy shocks are one strategy to terminate atrial fibrillation with these devices as an alternative or prelude to high energy therapy.

Multiple Inappropriate Discharges: In the case of repeated inappropriate discharges, the ICD should be promptly inactivated and the patient placed on telemetry with external defibrillation capabilities readily available. Most devices will have therapies inhibited as long as a magnet is in place over the generator. In some devices, prolonged magnet application will inactivate the device until the ICD is reactivated by the programmer or the magnet is applied again. Inappropriate ICD therapies may have many causes, but the most common cause is atrial fibrillation, as shown in Figure 10.9. Other atrial tachyarrhythmias including atrial flutter and sinus tachycardia may also trigger inappropriate ICD therapy. Once the device is inactivated, the atrial arrhythmia can be managed in a conventional manner. If the device cannot be immediately reprogrammed, chemical or electrical conversion of the atrial arrhythmia may be needed if ventricular rate control cannot be achieved. After initial control of the supraventricular tachyarrhythmia has been achieved, ICD tachyarrhythmia detection features for discrimination of supraventricular tachyarrhythmia from ventricular tachycardia may be useful in preventing further inappropriate therapies. Presently, it is unclear whether dual-chamber ICDs will decrease the number of inappropriate ICD therapies for supraventricular tachycardias (Fig. 10.10). Additionally, it is unclear whether the use of ventricular electrogram morphology algorithms will decrease inappropriate ICD therapies due to SVTs (see Fig. 10.10C). Ventricular electrogram morphology discrimination when used in conjunction with other SVT discriminators has a suboptimal sensitivity for atrial tachycardia.[26] SVTs with subtle rate-related changes in the QRS complex can also trigger inappropriate detection of ventricular tachyarrhythmias. Reprogramming of the percent template match to less rigorous criteria may improve

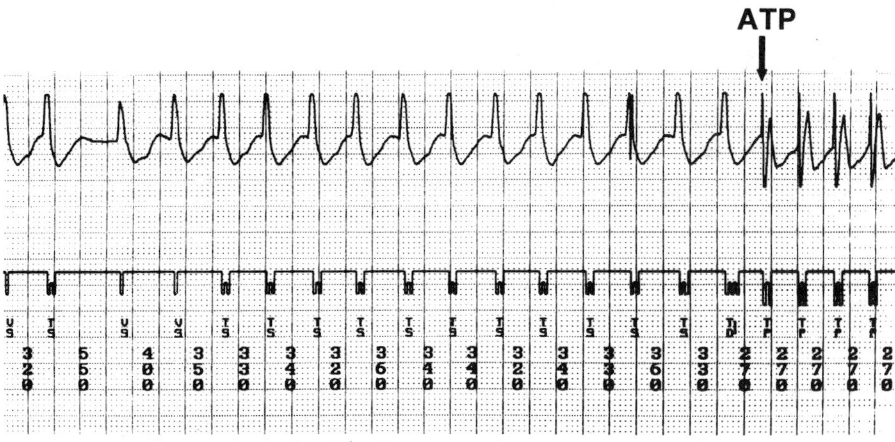

Figure 10.9. Atrial fibrillation and inappropriate therapy, as recorded by a Guidant Ventak Mini single-chamber ICD. Note the marked irregularity of the intracardiac ventricular electrogram **(top tracing)** and the ventricular cycle length, which varies between 290 and 500 milliseconds **(bottom tracing**, marker channel). The ventricular rate eventually falls into the VT zone (denoted by "TS" marker channel), and then ATP therapy is delivered (denoted by "TP" marker channel).

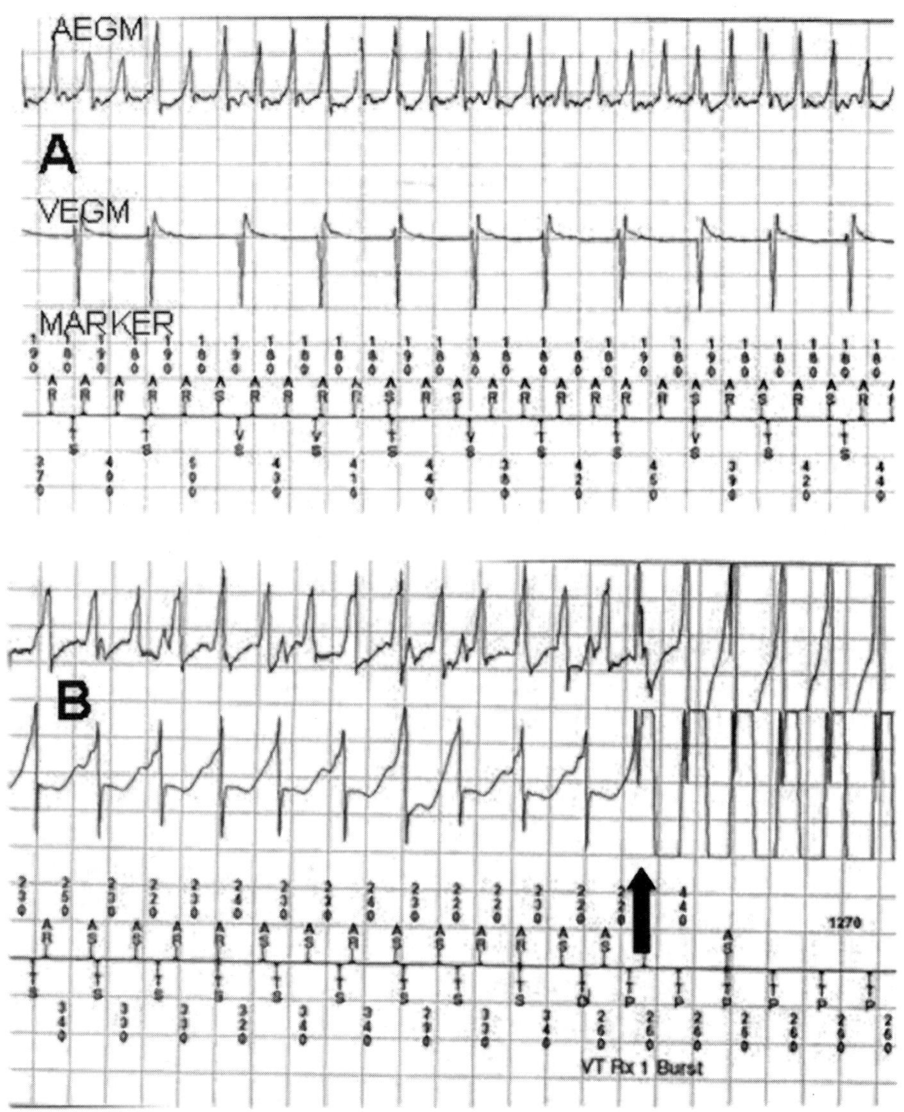

Figure 10.10. A: Atrial fibrillation with a rapid ventricular response leading to inappropriate therapy, as recorded by a Medtronic Gem DR dual-chamber ICD. Atrial electrogram (AEGM), ventricular electrogram (VEGM) and marker channel (MARKER) are shown. The patient is in atrial fibrillation with ventricular response from 370 to 500 milliseconds. The occasional long cycle lengths and irregularity prevent ventricular tachycardia detection. **Panel B:** With faster ventricular rate, the rhythm regularizes and no longer meets "unstable" rate criteria for diagnosis of atrial fibrillation in the VT zone. Antitachycardia pacing therapy is given as a result (*arrow*). **Panel C:** Failure of ventricular electrogram morphology discrimination in a St. Jude Photon dual-chamber ICD. The atrial and right ventricular (RV) channels show 1:1 conduction indicative of sinus tachycardia. Checks alternating with "X"s in the markers channel demonstrate an alternating match and mismatch with the stored ventricular electrogram template recorded in sinus rhythm. The poor match with the stored template probably results from misalignment of the electrogram with the template. The patient experienced inappropriate VT detection and ATP therapy.

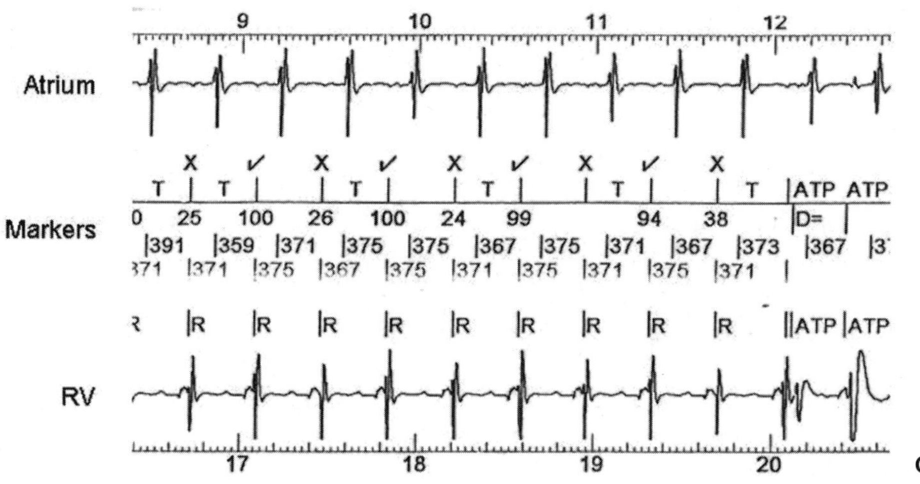

Figure 10.10. *Continued.*

SVT detection without adversely affecting sensitivity for VT detection. Some ICD patients who receive inappropriate shocks repeatedly for atrial fibrillation or atrial flutter require radiofrequency ablation of the AV node for definitive ventricular rate control.

Overcounting of ventricular events by the ICD is another important cause of inappropriate ICD discharge. An example of T wave oversensing in a patient with a ventricular lead with an integrated sensing bipole (right ventricular defibrillation coil and tip electrodes) is shown in Figure 10.11. This was corrected by decreasing the ventricular sensing and subsequent testing to confirm that ventricular fibrillation would be appropriately detected. In other cases, substitution of a lead with a true bipolar sensing electrode configuration or repositioning of the ventricular sensing lead may be needed. Double counting of atrial and/or ventricular pacing spikes on the ventricular lead is a potential problem when the ICD patient has a pacemaker as a separate device. This is remedied by reducing the output of the pacemaker or upgrading the ICD to a dual-chamber device with removal of the pacemaker.

Double counting of sensed ventricular events may occur in older biventricular ICDs (Guidant Contak, or conventional ICDs with right and left ventricular sensing/pacing electrodes connected via a Y-adapter), which sense from left and right ventricular tip electrodes to a right ventricular defibrillation coil or ring electrode. Such an example is shown in Figure 10.12. Decreasing ventricular sensitivity or increasing bradycardia pacing rate to assure continuous pacing may correct this problem. Often, the system must be revised with a biventricular device that senses only in the right ventricle.

In dual-chamber ICDs, far-field R wave sensing on the atrial lead can be interpreted as atrial fibrillation. In Figure 10.13, intermittent far-field R wave

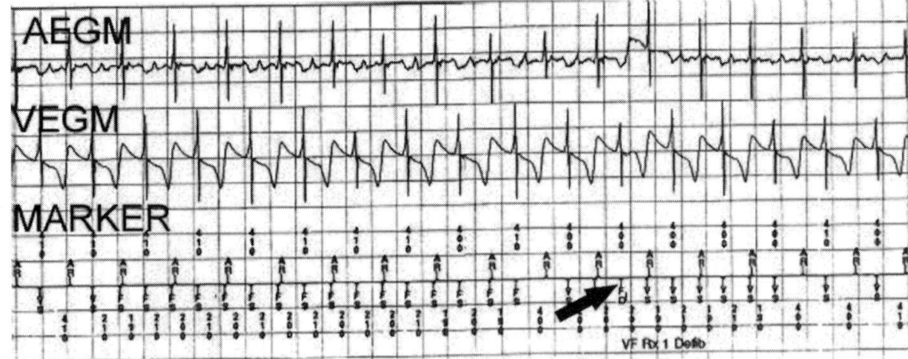

Figure 10.11. T wave oversensing causing double counting and inappropriate therapy for ventricular fibrillation in a Medtronic Gem DR dual-chamber ICD. The atrial channel **(top tracing)** shows a sinus tachycardia; the ventricular channel **(middle tracing)** shows large biphasic repolarization artifacts corresponding to the T wave after each high frequency ventricular electrogram. The T wave artifacts are detected as demonstrated by the marker channel ("FS," **bottom tracing**), leading to inappropriate detection of ventricular fibrillation.

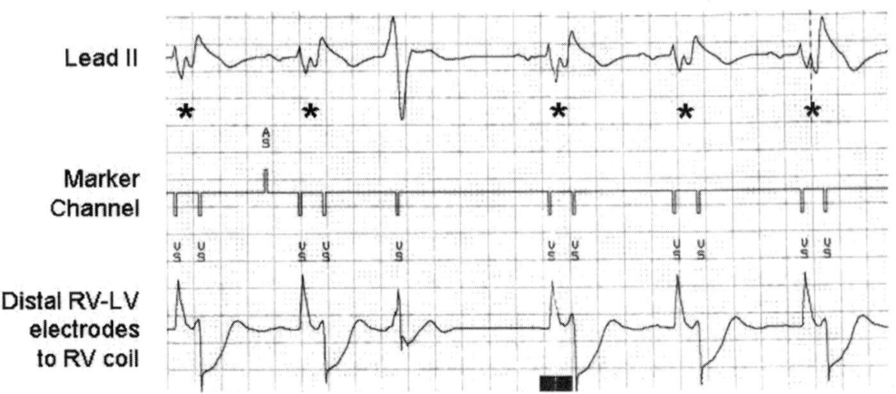

Figure 10.12. Double counting of intrinsic ventricular rhythm in a Medtronic biventricular device. A unipolar lead placed transvenously via the coronary sinus to a lateral cardiac vein was connected to the IS-1 connector of a right ventricular dedicated bipolar defibrillation lead using a Y adapter. The Y adapter was inserted in the IS-1 ventricular port of a conventional Medtronic dual chamber defibrillator. Both tip electrodes of the right and left ventricular leads served as the cathode and the proximal electrode of the right ventricular lead served as the anode, thus creating a large sensing dipole with resultant counting of both the right and left ventricular electrograms separately as shown on the marker channel (QRS complexes with double counting are noted by *). Such double counting in the setting of sinus tachycardia can trigger inappropriate therapy.

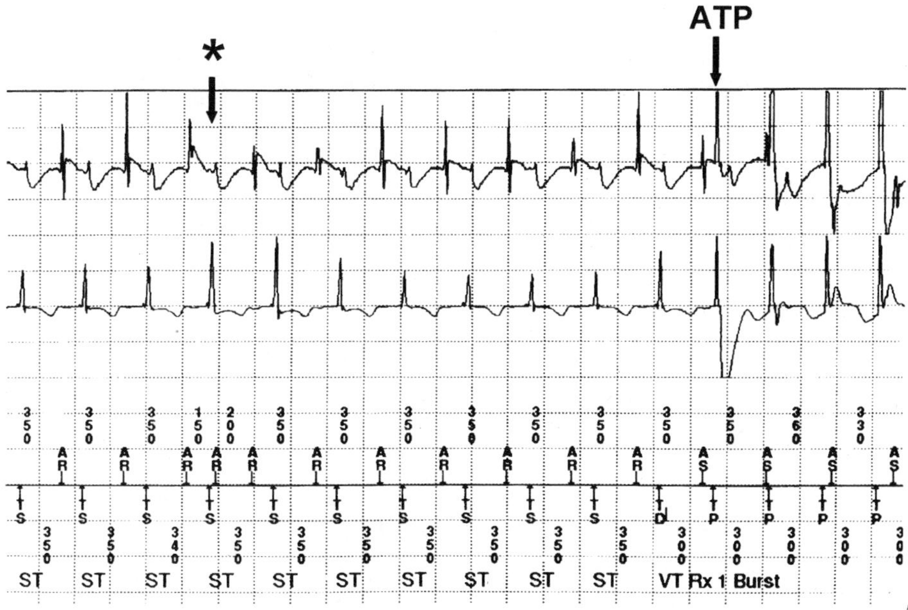

Figure 10.13. Inappropriate detection of a double tachycardia leading to therapy in a patient with a dual-chamber ICD. Far-field R waves are seen in the atrial electrogram **(top tracing)** during sinus tachycardia ("ST," marker channel, **bottom tracing**), are intermittently detected by the ICD (*), and are interpreted as atrial fibrillation. In the face of presumed atrial fibrillation being recorded on the atrial electrogram, the ICD assumes that the regular ventricular rhythm as recorded on the ventricular electrogram (middle tracing) is ventricular tachycardia, and it then initiates ATP therapy.

sensing during sinus tachycardia caused the ICD to misinterpret a double tachycardia (atrial fibrillation and ventricular tachycardia) for which therapy was delivered. In some cases this can be resolved by reprogramming atrial sensitivity. In other cases, the atrial lead must be repositioned to minimize far-field R wave sensing.

Extracardiac signals may be inappropriately sensed by the ventricular lead and can precipitate inappropriate ICD therapies. Diaphragmatic or chest wall myopotentials may be detected by some ICDs, especially those with automatic gain sensing (Fig. 10.14). Solutions include reprogramming of ventricular sensitivity, repositioning of the ventricular lead, or substitution of a true bipolar ventricular sensing lead. Another important source of inappropriate sensing is a conductor fracture or insulation failure in the ventricular sensing portion of the defibrillation lead. As shown in Figure 10.15, high frequency noise secondary to a lead fracture was interpreted by the ICD to be nonsustained ventricular fibrillation.

External EMI can also trigger ICD therapy. Potential sources include poorly shielded electrical equipment, welding devices, electrocautery, lithotripsy, com-

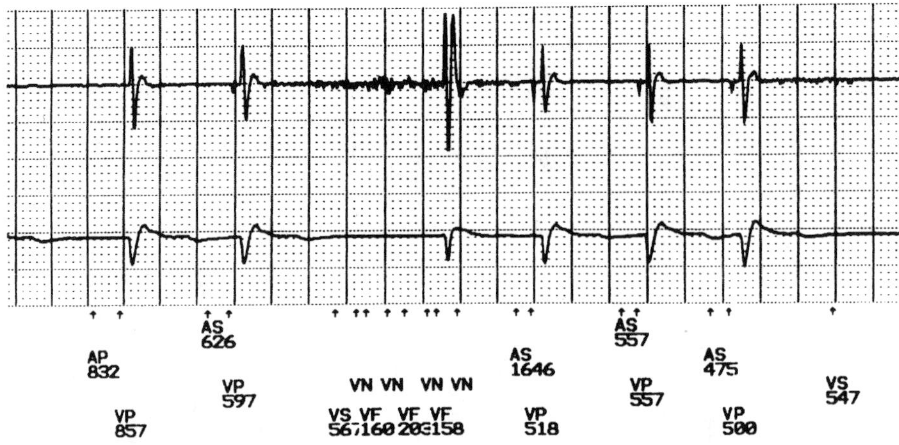

Figure 10.14. Myopotential sensing on the ventricular lead in a patient with a Guidant AV dual-chamber ICD. Routine interrogation of the ICD revealed multiple episodes of nonsustained ventricular fibrillation. A stored electrogram for one of these episodes reveals multiple R wave detections interpreted as ventricular fibrillation (marker channel, **bottom tracing**) while the ventricular electrogram (SVC coil to RV coil, **bottom tracing**) does not show any ventricular activity correlating to these marked ventricular fibrillation events. Examination of the intracardiac ventricular electrogram recorded between the distal ventricular lead tip to RV coil **(top tracing)** reveals low amplitude, high frequency myopotentials that are sensed (VS = ventricular beat sensed; VF = ventricular fibrillation sensed; VN = ventricular noise sensed; bottom marker channel). These high frequency components are not seen on the SVC to RV coil electrogram, which excludes the distal electrode.

mercial antitheft devices, and electric generators. Figure 10.16 depicts intracardiac electrograms recorded from a patient who was working on an alternator of a running car. The electrograms were interpreted as a "double tachycardia" (simultaneous atrial fibrillation and ventricular fibrillation), which triggered therapy. Obviously, treatment is avoidance of the EMI source.

Other potential causes of inappropriate sensing include interaction between the ventricular lead and guidewires inserted percutaneously into the venous system to allow for placement of central lines. Ventricular defibrillation leads could also interact unpredictably with other permanent transvenous pacing leads or catheters to cause inappropriate sensing.

Sustained Ventricular Arrhythmias Without Implantable Cardioverter-Defibrillator Therapy

The most common cause of no ICD therapy despite sustained ventricular tachycardia is because the ICD VT rate limit is set above that of the clinical ventricular tachycardia. Thus, the ICD does not detect the ventricular tachycardia. Slow ventricular tachycardia may present de novo in the patient who previously only had fast ventricular tachycardia or ventricular fibrillation, or may result from slowing of ventricular tachycardia by antiarrhythmic drugs (Fig. 10.17).

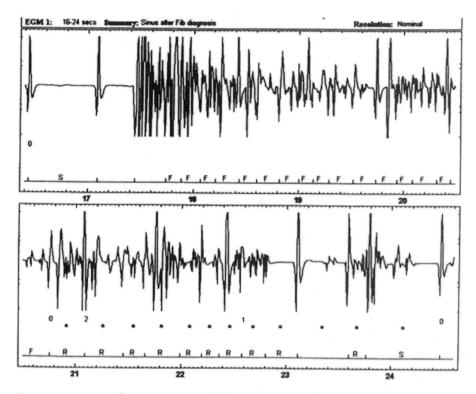

Figure 10.15. Lead fracture as recorded by a St. Jude Medical single-chamber ICD. The patient experienced shocks with motion of his arm ipsilateral to the device. In the clinic this detection was reproduced by the patient reaching over his head. Note the high-frequency signals that are detected as ventricular fibrillation ("F" on the marker channel) by the ICD.

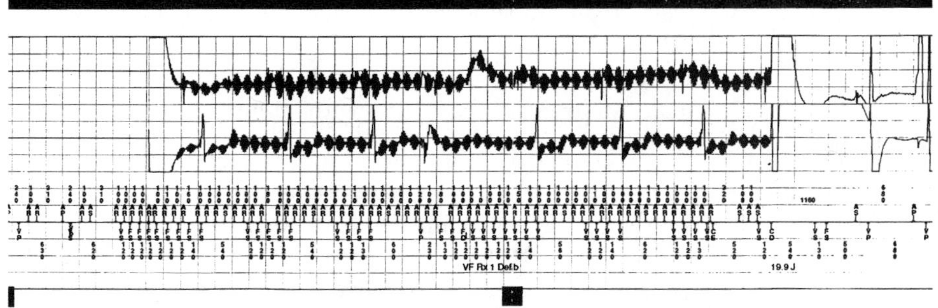

Figure 10.16. External high frequency electrical noise detected on both the atrial **(top)** and ventricular **(middle tracing)** channels of a Medtronic Gem DR dual-chamber ICD leading to inappropriate delivery of a 20-J shock for "ventricular fibrillation." The source of the electrical noise was an alternator on a running car on which the patient was working.

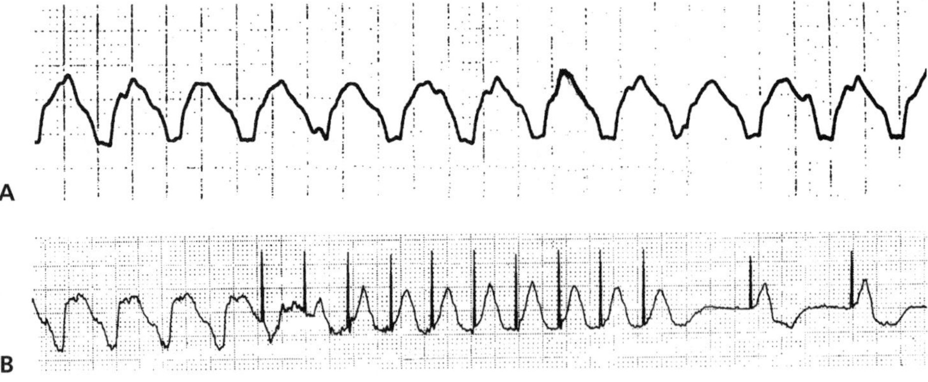

Figure 10.17. **A:** Failure to detect sustained ventricular tachycardia by an ICD due to a tachycardia rate slower than the programmed rate limit. The patient had received amiodarone therapy for 3 years before presenting with sustained ventricular tachycardia at 145 bpm. Because the VT detection rate limit was set at 160 bpm, the ICD did not identify ventricular tachycardia as being present. **B:** By reducing the rate limit to 130 bpm, the ventricular tachycardia was readily detected and terminated with a single burst of ATP.

Programming errors that may prevent therapy being delivered for ventricular tachyarrhythmias include:

1. Failure to reprogram tachyarrhythmia detections/therapies that have been temporarily suspended in patients undergoing surgery.
2. Only ventricular fibrillation therapies being programmed in the patient who previously has only had ventricular fibrillation but subsequently develops a slower ventricular tachycardia.
3. Overly aggressive supraventricular tachyarrhythmia discrimination schemes causing underdetection of ventricular tachycardia.
4. Intentionally very long initial detection algorithms for hemodynamically stable ventricular tachycardia.
5. Inadvertent device inactivation due to magnet exposure.
6. Low programmed ventricular sensitivity with failure to detect ventricular tachycardia/ventricular fibrillation.

System component failure is another important cause of delay or failure in delivery of effective therapy. This may include battery or capacitor failure causing prolonged charge times (Fig. 10.18). Lead problems contributing to failure to detect ventricular tachyarrhythmias or to deliver effective therapy include conductor fracture or insulation failure in either the ventricular rate sensing or high voltage circuits. Deterioration of the sensing characteristics of the ventricular lead over time can also result in failure to detect low amplitude electrograms during ventricular tachycardia or ventricular fibrillation.

```
TACHY EPISODE REPORT ---------------------------------- Page  2 of  2

THERAPY SEQUENCE
----------------
  VF  Rx 1:  Defib,  Energy(J):                0.0 - 20.0
                     Charge Time(sec):         20.60
                     Waveform:                 BIPHASIC
                     Pathway:                  AX>B
                     Delivered Energy (J):     19.5
                     Impedance(ohms):          45
```

Figure 10.18. Prolonged charge time causing a delay in therapy and syncope in a patient with a Medtronic 7221 ICD. Examination of the therapy sequence report from this patient reveals a charge time of 20.6 seconds to deliver a 20-J shock for ventricular fibrillation. This could result from capacitor or component failure, or from battery voltage near the end of the battery's life.

The ICD patient who presents with a sustained ventricular tachyarrhythmia should be promptly treated using accepted advanced cardiac life support protocols. The ICD should be inactivated until possible causes of malfunction have been explored (see Box 10.2).

Syncope with No Apparent Implantable Cardioverter-Defibrillator Discharge

Patients may present with a syncopal episode but no perceived ICD therapy. The patient workup should focus on whether the likely cause of syncope is due to a ventricular tachyarrhythmia. Box 10.3 lists a differential diagnosis for this scenario. If a ventricular tachyarrhythmia is the presumed cause of the syncope, a full device interrogation and lead testing will provide valuable clues as to whether system failure may have occurred. Often, a system failure has not occurred; rather, the patient has lost consciousness prior to ICD therapy. This may occur because of inappropriately long detection and redetection intervals or very complex tiered therapy schemes for ventricular tachycardia that may unnecessarily delay effective treatment. An example of a complex ventricular tachycardia therapy scheme that delayed definitive therapy for over 60 seconds is shown in Figure 10.19.

The patient may have symptomatic ventricular tachyarrhythmia episodes that are not registered by the ICD. Reasons for this include ventricular tachycardia slower than the programmed rate limits, supraventricular tachyarrhythmia discrimination algorithms preventing detection of ventricular tachycardia, and ventricular undersensing. If this situation is suspected, liberalization of detection criteria or activation of a slow VT zone may help to protect the patient until a definitive diagnosis can be made.

It should be remembered that not all syncope in the ICD patient is due to a ventricular arrhythmia. Bradyarrhythmias are also an important cause. Syncope may result from failure of bradycardia pacing in the pacemaker-dependent

Box 10.2. Causes for Multiple Implantable Cardioverter-Defibrillator Discharges

Appropriate Therapy

1. Electrical storm
2. Ineffective initial therapies
3. Incessant VT
4. Appropriate shocks for AF by atrial defibrillation functions

Inappropriate Therapy

1. Supraventricular tachycardias
   Atrial fibrillation
   Atrial flutter
   Sinus tachycardia
   Atrial tachycardia
   Reentrant SVT
2. Oversensing
   T wave
   Diaphragmatic/chest wall
   Other devices
   Lead dislodgment/double counting atrium and ventricle
3. Noise
   External electromagnetic noise (alternators/welding/cautery/lithotripsy)
   Loose set screw/extendable lead screw
   Lead fracture
4. Phantom shocks

#	Date/Time	Type	V. Cycle	Last Rx	Success	Duration
	Nov 21 11:23:30	VT	360 ms	VF Rx 1	Yes	1.1 min

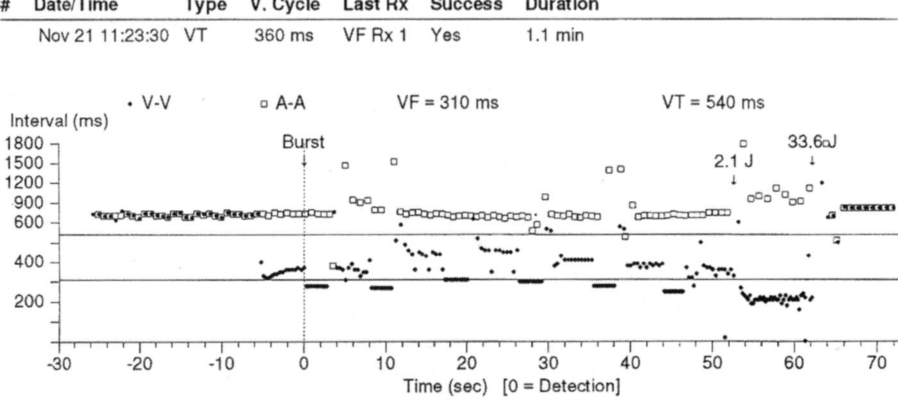

Figure 10.19. Graphical representation of sequential therapies appropriately delivered by a Medtronic Gem DR ICD. The time from detection Is shown on the horizontal axis. From left to right, VT with cycle length of 360 milliseconds is detected at time 0. Six bursts of ATP are delivered that change the VT rate but fail to terminate it. A 2.1-J shock accelerates VT, then a 33.6-J shock terminates the episode. More than 1 minute elapsed in VT before successful therapy was delivered (Duration).

Box 10.3. Syncope with Delayed or Absent Implantable Cardioverter-Defibrillator Therapy

1. **Ventricular tachyarrhythmias**
   - Device
     - Battery depletion
     - Capacitor failure
     - Other electronic failure
   - Lead related
     - Fracture of defibrillation circuit
     - Fracture of rate-sensing circuit
     - Lead dislodgment
   - Programming
     - Device inactivated
     - Detect and redetect intervals too long
     - SVT discrimination inhibits therapy
     - VT rate under rate limit
     - Initial therapies accelerate VT
     - Ineffective initial therapies
     - Undercounting due to signal size
   - Underlying substrate
     - Increased defibrillation threshold
       - Drugs
       - Congestive heart failure
       - Ischemia
       - Electrolyte abnormalities
2. **Non-arrhythmic causes of syncope**
   - Bradyarrhythmia and intolerance of ventricular pacing
   - Failure of bradycardia pacing
   - Seizure
   - Neurocardiogenic syncope
   - Orthostasis

ICD patient due to ventricular oversensing, loss of capture, lead malfunction, or ICD battery depletion. Other causes of syncope in the ICD patient include neurocardiogenic syncope, orthostatic hypotension, seizure, hypoglycemia, and psychogenic causes.

CONCLUSION

Patients who have ICDs need regular follow-up assessments to ascertain whether the ICD is functioning correctly. Follow-up assessments of the ICD encompass all aspects of pacemaker maintenance plus the complexities of automated tachyarrhythmia detection and treatment. In the case of suspected ICD malfunction, stored electrograms and noninvasive testing capabilities have simplified troubleshooting and help to determine the possible causes of malfunctions. Nevertheless, vigilance and a thorough understanding of ICD function remain essential to ICD follow-up assessments.

REFERENCES

1. Zucker MJ, Bloch GJ. Syncope and the law. In: Grubbs BP, Olshansky B, eds. Syncope: Mechanisms and Management. Armonk, NY: Futura, 1998:387–401.
2. Carnes CA, Mehdirad AA, Nelson SD. Drug and defibrillator interactions. Pharmacotherapy 1998;18:516–525.
3. Fletcher RD, Cintron GB, Johnson G, et al. Enalapril decreases prevalence of ventricular tachycardia in patients with chronic congestive heart failure: the V-HeFT II VA cooperative studies group. Circulation 1993;87(suppl 6):49–55.
4. Hjalmarson A. Prevention of sudden cardiac death with beta blockers. Clin Cardiol 1999;22(suppl 8):11–15.
5. De Sutter J, Tavernier R, De Buyzere M, et al. Lipid lowering drugs and recurrences of life-threatening ventricular arrhythmias in high-risk patients. J Am Coll Cardiol 2000;36:766–772.
6. Brodksy CM, Chang F, Vlay SC. Multicenter evaluation of implantable cardioverter defibrillator testing after implant: the Post Implant Testing Study (PITS). Pacing Clin Electrophysiol 1999;22:1769–1776.
7. Glikson M, Luria D, Friedman PA, et al. Are routine arrhythmia inductions necessary in patients with pectoral implantable cardioverter defibrillators? J Cardiovasc Electrophysiol 2000;11:127–135.
8. Kohlkamp K, Dornberger V, Mewis C, et al. Clinical experience with the new detection algorithms for atrial fibrillation of a defibrillator with dual chamber sensing and pacing. J Cardiovasc Electrophysiol 1999;10:905–915.
9. Nanthakumar K, Dorian P, Paquette M, et al. Is inappropriate implantable defibrillator shock therapy predictable? J Intervent Card Electrophysiol 2003;8:215–220.
10. Leitch JW, Gillis AM, Wyse DG, et al. Reduction in defibrillator shocks with an implantable device combining antitachycardia pacing and shock therapy. J Am Coll Cardiol 1991;18:145–151.
11. Naisir N, Pacifico A, Doyle TK, et al. Cadence Investigators. Spontaneous ventricular tachycardia treated by antitachycardia pacing. Am J Cardiol 1997;79:820–822.
12. Wood MA, Stambler BS, Damiano RJ, et al. Lessons learned from data logging in a multicenter clinical trial using a late-generation implantable cardioverter-defibrillator. J Am Coll Cardiol 1994;24:1692–1699.
13. Exner DV, Gillis AM, Sheldon RS, et al. Telemetry-documented, paceterminable ventricular tachycardia in patients with ventricular fibrillation. Am J Cardiol 1998;81:235–238.
14. Schaumann A, von zur Muhlen F, Herse B, et al. Empirical versus tested antitachycardia pacing in implantable cardioverter-defibrillators. Circulation 1998;97:66–74.
15. Gillis AM, Leitch JW, Sheldon RS, et al. A prospective randomized comparison of autodecremental pacing to burst pacing in device therapy for chronic ventricular tachycardia secondary to coronary artery disease. Am J Cardiol 1993;72:1146–1151.
16. Wathen MS, Sweeney MO, DeGroot PJ, et al. Shock reduction using antitachycardia pacing for spontaneous rapid ventricular tachycardia in patients with coronary artery disease. Circulation 2001;104:796–801.

17. Florin TJ, Weiss DN, Peters RW, et al. Induction of atrial fibrillation with low-energy defibrillator shocks in patients with implantable cardioverter defibrillators. Am J Cardiol 1997;80:960–962.
18. Kroll MW, Tchou PJ. Testing of implantable defibrillator functions at implantation. In: Ellenbogen KA, Kay GN, Wilkoff BL, eds. Clinical cardiac pacing and defibrillation. 2nd ed. Philadelphia: WB Saunders, 2000:540–561.
19. Gold MR, Higgins S, Klein R, et al. Efficacy and temporal stability of reduced safety margins for ventricular defibrillation. Circulation 2002;105:2043–2048.
20. Fogoros RN, Elson JJ, Bonnet CA. Actuarial incidence and pattern of occurrence of shocks following implantation of the automatic implantable cardioverter defibrillator. Pacing Clin Electrophysiol 1989;12:1465–1473.
21. Grimm W, Flores BT, Marchlinski FE. Shock occurrence and survival in 241 patients with implantable cardioverter-defibrillator therapy. Circulation 1993;87:1880–1887.
22. Hook BG, Callans DJ, Kleiman RB, et al. Implantable cardioverter-defibrillator therapy in the absence of significant symptoms. Rhythm diagnosis and management aided by stored electrogram analysis. Circulation 1993;87:1897–1906.
23. Nademanee K, Taylor R, Bailey WE, et al. Treating electrical storm: sympathetic blockade versus advanced cardiac life support-guided therapy. Circulation 2000;102: 742–747.
24. Wood MA, Simpson PM, Stambler BS, et al. Long-term temporal patterns of ventricular tachyarrhythmias. Circulation 1995;91:2371–2377.
25. Lauribe P, Shah D, Jais P, et al. Radiofrequency catheter ablation of drug refractory symptomatic ventricular ectopy: short- and long-term results. Pacing Clin Electrophysiol 1999;22:783–789.
26. Boriani G, Biffi M, Dall'Acqua A, et al. Rhythm discrimination by rate branch and QRS morphology in dual chamber implantable cardioverter defibrillators. Pacing Clin Electrophysiol 2003;26:466–470.

Follow-up Assessments of the Pacemaker Patient

Mark H. Schoenfeld and Mark L. Blitzer

11

THE GOALS OF PACEMAKER FOLLOW-UP ASSESSMENT

Pacemaker follow-up evaluations entail the repeated assessment of the pacing system and the patient to ensure appropriate and optimal pacer function and to detect and prevent pacemaker-related problems. The follow-up evaluation of a pacemaker patient begins in the immediate postimplantation period and extends throughout the patient's life, rather than throughout the life of the pacemaker system per se. The original indications for pacemaker insertion require periodic review, and new indications for modifications of the existing system also warrant continuing evaluation. The pacemaker physician needs to assess those symptoms not satisfactorily treated by the pacemaker as well as those symptoms potentially caused by the pacemaker. Systematic record-keeping is an important part of this process, particularly in following end-of-life parameters and in tracking patients whose systems may be subject to product recall or failure.

It remains a challenge to optimize the functioning and longevity of a pacemaker system in the face of constantly changing patient needs, whether those changes are in lifestyle, medical circumstances, cardiac function, or electrophysiologic milieu. The issue of who should perform pacemaker follow-up evaluations remains an ongoing debate—what is clear is that the relevant skills must be continuously and finely maintained.[1,2] This chapter explores these issues and examines the methodology of the pacemaker follow-up evaluation.[3–6]

THE IMMEDIATE POSTIMPLANTATION PERIOD

Following the implantation of a new pacemaker system, the patient is generally observed on a cardiac monitor for 24 hours to confirm adequate pacemaker function. The roles of ambulatory pacemaker implantation and shorter hospital stays remain controversial. Most patients receive prophylactic antibiotic coverage for at least 24 hours following pacer insertion. This practice is supported by the results of a meta-analysis.[7] Posteroanterior (PA) and lateral chest radiographs are obtained within 24 hours to confirm satisfactory positioning of the pacer lead(s) and to serve as a baseline for subsequent comparisons. Twelve-lead electrocardiograms both with and without pacing are obtained before discharge.

Most essential in the immediate postimplantation period is education of the patient. The importance of always carrying a pacemaker identification card must be stressed. Medical alert bracelets are often recommended as well. The patient is asked to refrain from vigorous activity involving the ipsilateral arm for a period of approximately 4 weeks to minimize the possibility of lead dislodgment. Also the patient should keep the incision completely dry for 5 to 7 days to minimize the chance of infection. One of the questions most commonly asked by patients prior to discharge is whether microwave ovens need to be avoided; with modern-day generators the answer is "no." Temporary driving restrictions may be appropriate for patients presenting with syncope until the follow-up assessment confirms that the pacemaker is functioning normally. Plans are then made for outpatient wound evaluation and suture or staple removal if needed, generally to occur within 2 to 4 weeks. Patients are asked to be attentive to any signs of fever or infection such as pain, redness, swelling, or drainage at the incision site.

THE FOLLOW-UP CLINIC AND RECORD-KEEPING

The personnel necessary to the pacemaker follow-up assessment includes a supervising physician, a pacemaker nurse or technician, and clerical staff for record-keeping and outpatient scheduling. Personnel directly involved in the pacemaker follow-up evaluation must be thoroughly familiar with all aspects of pacemaker function. The site of the pacemaker follow-up evaluation should allow history taking and patient examination and should be fully equipped to allow for analysis of pacemaker function (Box 11.1). This includes capabilities for 12-lead electrocardiography (with and without a magnet), radiography (and fluoroscopy, if possible), transtelephonic and ambulatory electrocardiographic monitoring, and availability of the programmers and physician's manual for every model of pacemaker encountered. The telephone numbers for technical support of all pacemaker manufacturers should be available. Depending on the number of different pacer models employed by the clinic, extensive familiarity with a wide variety of programming devices may be necessary because of the lack of universal programming.[8] A resuscitation cart, defibrillator, and transcutaneous pacemaker should be immediately available. The clinic staff should be capable of performing advanced life support.

Record-keeping is an indispensable component of a pacemaker clinic. Its purpose is to accurately record such patient demographics as name and address, to identify specifics of the pacer system used (model and serial numbers, implant values), to track patient symptoms and various parameters of pacemaker function (e.g., sensing and pacing thresholds, identified changes in magnet rate), and to update any changes in programmed parameters. Such records may be computer stored and allow for the generation of comprehensive updated reports.[9] Record-keeping also allows for organization and maintenance of strict sched-

Box 11.1. Pacemaker Clinic

Clinic Personnel
Pacemaker physician
Pacemaker nurse or technician
Clerical staff

Pacemaker and Patient Data
Patient's name, age, identification, address, phone number
Pacemaker generator data: model, serial number
Pacemaker lead(s): model, serial number
Operative note from implant with implant data
Complete follow-up records
Telephone numbers for pacemaker technical support

Equipment
Examination room
Pacemaker programmers
Physician manuals for each model pacer followed
ECG machine
External defibrillator and transcutaneous pacemaker
Code cart

Ancillary Requirements
X-ray and fluoroscopy
Tilt table
Blood chemistry laboratory
Holter/event monitoring

ules for patient follow-up assessments. This promotes identification of potential problems with pacer function well before they are actualized, rather than having patients drop in only after the problem has manifested.

The establishment of a federal pacemaker registry was mandated by Medicare guidelines, wherein specifics of pacer data such as patient demographics and model and serial numbers are reported at the time of implantation. This registry, coupled with manufacturer generated patient lists and accurate record-keeping by the pacer physician, should facilitate contacting patients if a systematic problem with a particular type of pacer system is identified or if a product advisory/recall is issued. If the physician has observed such a problem, such as premature battery depletion, the manufacturer can then be consulted to determine whether others may have made similar observations.

Independent of a formal recall, it is the responsibility of the pacer physician to decide whether corrective measures are warranted in a particular case. If a recall or advisory on a particular pacer product has been issued, the nature of the potential malfunction should determine the timing of the pacer-system revision, if required at all. If the reported component failure is random and unpredictable, then replacement should be undertaken more rapidly, especially in those patients who are deemed "pacer-dependent." Unfortunately, as of this writing, there is no manufacturer-independent, large-scale national device/lead database that allows physicians and their patients to be notified in a timely fashion of pacemaker system malfunctions.[10] Thus, the pacer physician must be ever vigilant as to trends of potential pacer malfunction in his or her practice as well as to reports from others, whether via other physicians or manufacturers' notifications.

THE OUTPATIENT VISIT

Even a routine pacemaker follow-up visit is a labor-intensive encounter with much to be accomplished in a timely manner including a brief history, examination, pacemaker evaluation, troubleshooting, reprogramming, and record-keeping. By keeping the goals of the visit in focus and maintaining an orderly approach to follow-up, the process can be made efficient (Fig. 11.1).

The first visit, approximately 2 to 4 weeks subsequent to implantation, is primarily directed toward evaluation of the healing wound. This is particularly important in diabetic patients prone to slower healing and patients requiring anticoagulation, in whom pocket hematomas can prove catastrophic.[11] Symptoms are reviewed as with any visit. Chest radiographs (PA and lateral) and electrocardiograms with and without pacing can be repeated at this time. Most problems arising within 2 weeks of implantation relate to either lead dislodgment, exit block, or healing of the incision or pocket. Arrangements for transtelephonic monitoring according to preset guidelines are made, as well as for the 3-month checkup. At that point, the inflammation associated with the tissue-electrode interface has generally resolved, allowing for assessment of chronic pacing and sensing thresholds. After the 3-month checkup, patients are generally seen twice yearly, or as otherwise dictated by their clinical needs (Table 11.1).

History

Subsequent visits should focus on device maintenance, optimization of function, and evaluation of patient complaints. The elicitation and evaluation of symptomatology requires careful sleuthing on the part of the pacemaker physician. Perceptions of pain, well being, or vigor may vary widely from patient to patient, depending on an individual's "threshold" for discomfort or malaise. These may also be a function of a patient's fears and expectations. If the patient does not feel "100% better" after pacer insertion, does this reflect malfunction, or were the patient's original symptoms multifactorial in etiology and not preventable by pacing alone? As such, it is sometimes difficult to distinguish symptoms that warrant only reassurance from those that may be subtle clues to underlying pacemaker malfunction, malprogramming, or "patient–pacer mismatch."

In pacer–patient mismatch, the pacer system may be functioning perfectly appropriately but fails to result in optimal patient functioning and indeed may even produce symptoms. For example, a previously vigorous patient who

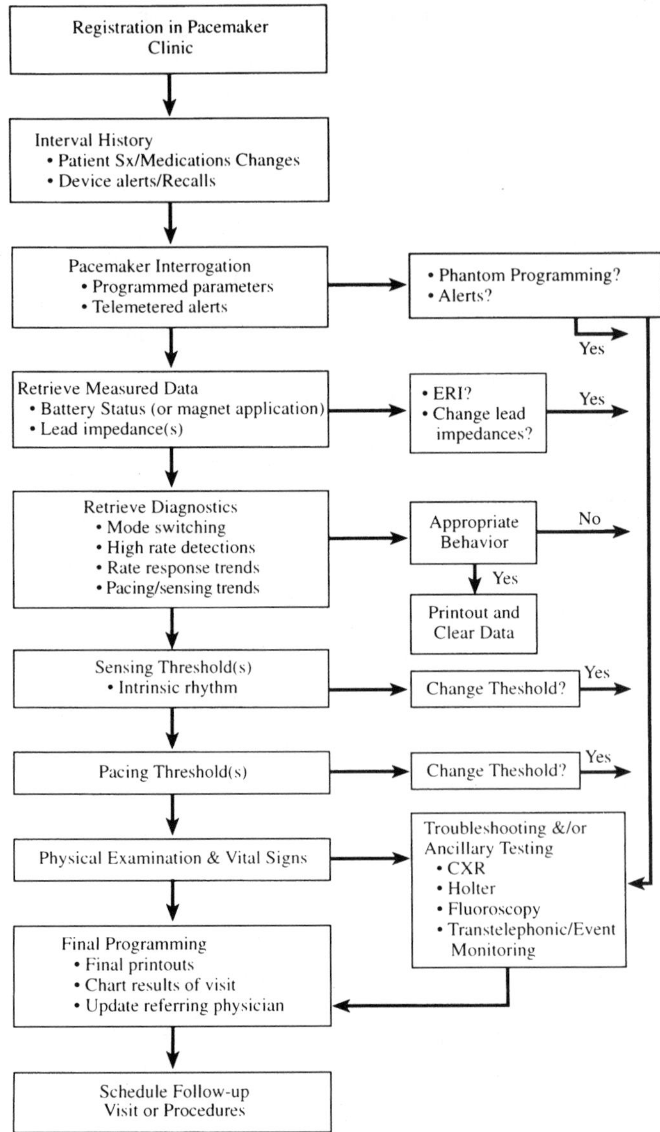

Figure 11.1. Flow chart for efficient pacemaker follow-up visit. Sx = symptoms; ERI = elective replacement indicators; CXR = chest radiograph.

Table 11.1. Schedules for Pacemaker Follow-up

	Outpatient Office Visit		Transtelephonic Monitoring	
	General Guidelines	**Medicare Guidelines**	**Medicare Guideline I**	**Medicare Guideline II**
Appropriate patients	All patients	All patients	Pacemakers with proven 5-yr longevity >90% and nonabrupt decline in output over ≥3 mo.	Pacemakers with inability to demonstrate 5-yr longevity >90% and nonabrupt decline in output over ≥3 mo (applies to most pacemakers).
Schedule	• 2–4 wk after implant • 3 mo after implant, then • Every 6 mo thereafter until approaching elective replacement indicators.	• Twice in first 6 mo. after implant, then *Single chamber* • Once every 12 mo. *Dual chamber* • Once every 6 mo.	*Single chamber* • First month: Every 2 wk. • 2nd to 36th mo: Every 8 wk. • Thereafter: Every 4 wk. *Dual chamber* • First month: Every 2 wk. • 2nd to 6th mo: Every 4 wk. • 7th to 36th mo: Every 8 wk. • Thereafter: Every 4 wk.	*Single chamber* • First month: Every 2 wk. • 2nd to 48th mo: Every 12 wk. • 49th to 72nd mo: Every 8 wk. *Dual chamber* • First month: Every 2 wk. • 2nd to 30th mo: Every 12 wk. • 31st to 48th mo: Every 8 wk. • Thereafter: Every 4 wk.

receives a dual-chamber system for complete heart block may be exertionally limited with an upper tracking rate of only 120 beats per minute (bpm), especially if electrical Wenckebach or 2:1 heart block develops at the pacemaker's upper rate limit (Fig. 11.2). Treadmill testing may, on occasion, be useful in assessing exercise tolerance, chronotropic competence, and maximal heart rates achievable, either independent of pacing or in the setting of specifically programmed parameters. In rate-adaptive systems it is particularly useful to assess activity-sensing thresholds as well as the rapidity of pacing rate increases and decreases with activity. For example, in an older patient who develops angina it may be important to make the system less sensitive to activity, lower the upper rate limit, and have a relatively quicker decline of pacing rate once activity ceases. Upper rate behavior in dual-chamber systems may also be appreciated with exercise testing (e.g., Wenckebach versus 2:1 block); exercise-induced arrhythmias potentially contributing to pacer-mediated tachycardias may rarely be observed.

Cardiac symptoms of angina or congestive heart failure may arise unrelated to the pacer, or to the arrhythmia that had prompted its original implantation. Pacer adjustments may, however, result in alleviation of these symptoms in some cases. The lower rate limit may be increased in patients with so-called "rate-limited cardiac output" to minimize their congestive heart failure. In contrast, patients with angina requiring increased time for diastolic coronary perfusion may benefit from a reduction in their rate limit or changes to their rate response parameters as discussed previously.

Symptoms reminiscent of the bradyarrhythmia for which a pacer was inserted may reappear, either because of pacemaker malfunction or, paradoxically, because of appropriate cardiac pacing that is poorly tolerated by the patient.[12] Reported symptoms may include dizziness, presyncope, or syncope, but may extend to more subtle concerns such as weakness, fatigability, and dyspnea. The appearance of these symptoms in the presence of a well-functioning pacer system may result from "pacemaker syndrome."[13–15] This

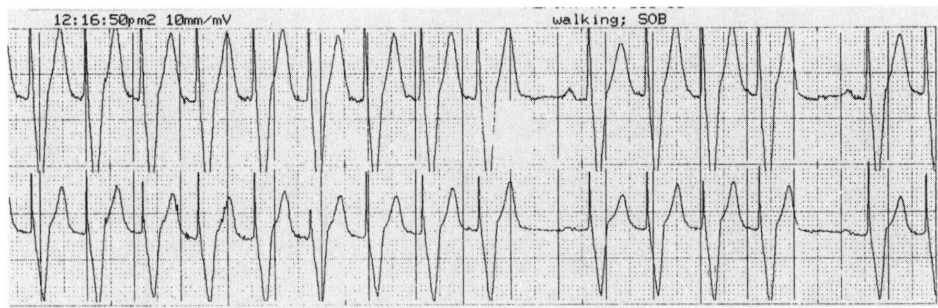

Figure 11.2. Holter transmission in a dual-chamber system with ventricular tracking at the upper rate of 120 ppm associated with electrical Wenckebach phenomenon. This vigorous patient reported exercise limitation and dyspnea in association with this upper rate limitation.

syndrome reflects the loss of atrioventricular synchrony during pacing and may produce systemic hypotension, atrioventricular valvular regurgitation, reduction in cardiac output, pulmonary congestion, and unpleasant neck pulsations (cannon A waves due to atrial contraction against a closed atrioventricular valve). In the worst-case scenario of atrioventricular dyssynchrony, retrograde 1:1 ventriculo-atrial conduction may occur with ventricular pacing. Retrograde VA conduction is observed in approximately 80% of patients with sick sinus syndrome and even in a small minority of patients (15%) with antegrade high-grade AV block.

A surprising number of patients may experience severe symptoms of pre-syncope, syncope, malaise, palpitations, or dyspnea from this "pacemaker syndrome." This phenomenon, commonly observed during single-chamber ventricular pacing, results in hemodynamic compromise from retrograde activation of the atria in some cases and from cyclic losses of synchrony between the atria and ventricles in other cases. The presence of retrograde ventriculoatrial conduction should be ascertained with electrocardiography, particularly in the inferior leads (e.g., II, III, and aVf) and/or telemetered intracardiac electrograms (Fig. 11.3). Blood pressure determinations should be made in the supine and erect positions with both ventricular pacing and during a nonpaced rhythm if possible. Rarely, cardiac output determinations may also be required to demonstrate hemodynamic compromise associated with ventricular pacing. If pacemaker syndrome is identified, consideration should be given to reprogramming the pacer to reduce pacer dependence (e.g., decrease the lower rate), but ultimately revision to a dual-chamber system may be required.

The patient with a pacer may occasionally report symptoms due to true pacemaker malfunction or inappropriate inhibition. This requires careful evaluation—namely, determination of sensing and pacing thresholds and consideration of the possibility of pacer inhibition by myopotentials or other electromagnetic interference. Other potentially symptomatic arrhythmias such as ventricular tachycardia, rapid atrial fibrillation, or other supraventricular tachy-

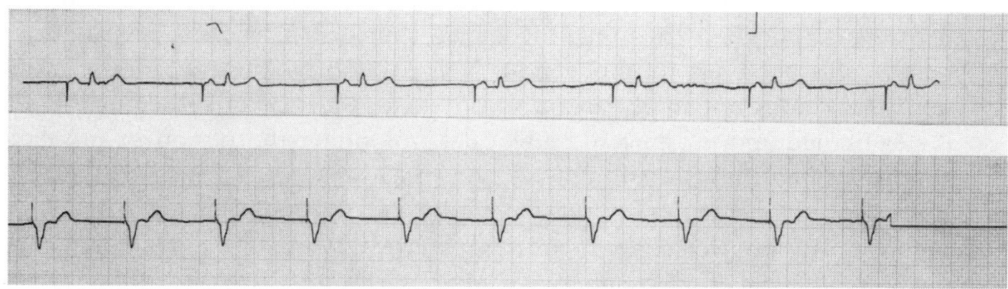

Figure 11.3. Top: The pacemaker is programmed to the DDD mode and there is 100% atrial pacing and no cardiac symptoms. **Bottom:** When the pacemaker was reprogrammed to the VVIR mode, the patient was dyspneic and became presyncopal despite rate-responsive pacing. Retrograde VA conduction is apparent with ventricular pacing. In some pacemakers with intracardiac electrograms, or marker channels, the VA conduction time can be measured at different heart rates.

cardias (SVT) need to be investigated as possibilities. Virtually all newer pacing systems have sophisticated diagnostics, often storing the actual electrogram from any such tachycardia. This greatly simplifies evaluation. Many pacemakers allow the clinician to attempt to terminate the SVTs with rapid atrial pacing if the patient were in persistent tachycardia at the time of a follow-up visit. Additionally, certain recent pacemakers even allow for the programming of atrial antitachycardia pacing to be automatically delivered for certain SVT. Pacemaker-mediated tachycardias may also arise and generate symptoms. Re-programming options to "defeat" PMT are addressed later in the chapter. Tilt testing may prove useful in revealing the presence of vasodepressor syncope. Under such circumstances, medical therapy with volume expansion, beta blockers or vasoconstrictors may prove useful. Pacemaker re-programming may also be beneficial. Increasing the lower pacing rate or activating certain specialized "rate-drop" algorithms may provide assistance. There is also early evidence that certain rate-adaptive sensors responsive to cardiac contractility may be particularly efficacious in minimizing recurrent vasovagal spells.[16] The extent that any pacing system can improve on vasovagal syncope, although this remains a source of controversy.[17]

Symptoms that are noncardiac but pacer-related may include myopectoral stimulation (most common in unipolar systems in which the generator case serves as the anode), concerns related to the pacemaker wound itself (pain, overt erosion) or diaphragmatic stimulation (reflecting pacing either through a thin right ventricular wall or via a lead in the vicinity of a phrenic nerve). The latter is clearly increasing in frequency with greater use of biventricular pacing systems where the LV lead is often in close apposition to and poorly insulated from the left phrenic nerve. A summary of commonly reported symptoms and their causes is given in Table 11.2.

Physical Examination

The physical examination is a critical aspect of pacemaker follow-up evaluations. Most attention will be directed toward the healing incision and pacer pocket, looking for erythema, tenderness, incipient or overt erosion, or pocket hematoma. Pocket hematomas occur in approximately 20% of patients who receive subcutaneous or intravenous heparin shortly postprocedure.[18] While a hematoma does not imply an infection exists, the risk of subsequent infection is heightened and most would advocate prolonging the period of prophylactic antibiotics until the hematoma has resolved. Conservative management is all that is usually required with temporary cessation of anticoagulants and more frequent follow-up to look for signs of pressure necrosis. Premature percutaneous aspiration of the pocket may actually be counterproductive diminishing the tamponading effect and increasing chances of further bleeding and infection.

Patients may note caudal migration of the generator or superficiality of the pacemaker leads, but these phenomena are infrequent and of concern only rarely. In a healthy pocket, the generator is freely mobile beneath the skin. An immobile generator especially when firmly adherent to the overlying skin raises the

Table 11.2. Common Symptoms in Pacemaker Patients

Symptom	Possible Causes
Swelling/pain at pacer site	Infection, hematoma, generator migration, Twiddler's syndrome, skin erosion, subclavian thrombosis, pectoral stimulation
Exercise intolerance, dyspnea on exertion	Pacemaker syndrome, low maximal heart rate settings, inadequate rate response settings, failure to capture, chronotropic incompetence
Dyspnea at rest	Pacemaker syndrome, pericardial effusion, failure to capture, pulmonary emboli from pacer leads
Palpitations	Atrial arrhythmias (tracked or conducted), pacemaker-mediated tachycardia, overly aggressive rate response settings, myopotential tracking, sensor-driven tachycardias, ventricular arrhythmias, pacemaker syndrome
Skeletal muscle/diaphragmatic stimulation	Pectoral muscle stimulation (unipolar), insulation failure, phrenic nerve stimulation, lead perforation, diaphragm stimulation through ventricle
Chest pain	Pericarditis, lead perforation, angina due to excessive rate response, pacemaker syndrome
Syncope, presyncope	Pacemaker syndrome, failure to capture, oversensing, crosstalk inhibition, EMI inhibition, ventricular arrhythmias, neurally mediated vasodepressor syncope
Edema	Loss capture, pacemaker syndrome, pericardial effusion, superior vena cava or subclavian vein thrombosis (upper extremities)

possibility of occult infection or pre-erosion. Erosion of a generator or a lead is potentially quite serious and may result in systemic infection (Fig. 11.4). A variety of approaches to "salvaging" an eroded system have been advocated, although ideally the entire system (including leads) should be explanted and replaced with a new system after an appropriate period of intravenous antibiotics. Swelling over the pulse generator may represent hematoma formation, seroma, or pocket infection. A fluctuant pocket should not be aspirated, as this may introduce infection into a sterile process and will not treat an infection if present. Suspected pocket infections should be surgically opened to confirm the diagnosis and to remove all hardware from an infected pocket. Pacemaker infections are *not* adequately treated by prolonged courses of antibiotics alone.

Myopectoral stimulation may be appreciated at the pocket site and is almost exclusively seen in unipolar systems. Certain generators are manufactured with one insulated side meant to be placed against the pectoral muscle. Rarely, myopectoral stimulation may be attributed to placement of such a generator can with the uninsulated side down against the pectoral muscle, leading to anodal stimulation of the underlying muscles; it may thus be corrected by inversion of

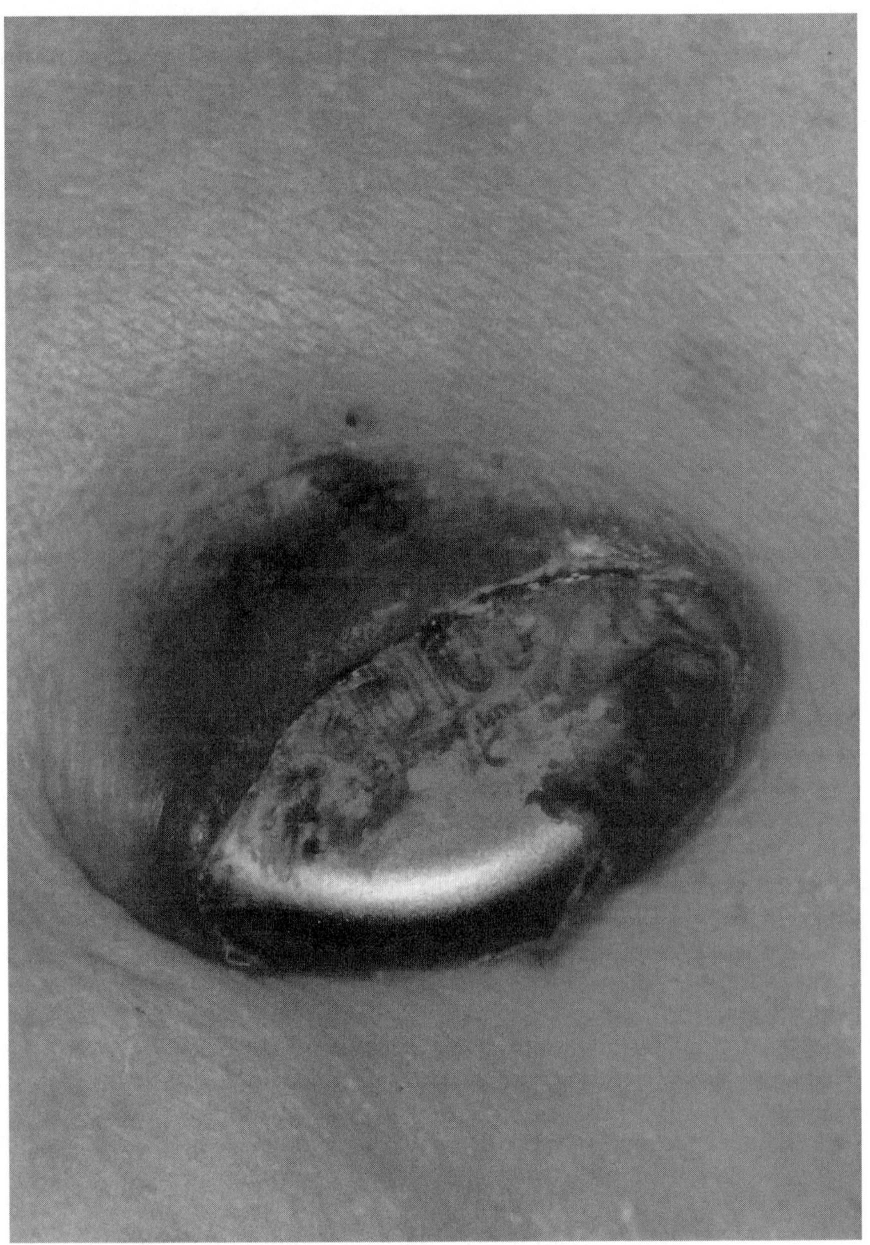

Figure 11.4. Pacemaker erosion.

the generator. It may also indicate lead or insulation fracture close to the muscle layer. Frequently no problem is identifiable, but the situation may be corrected by reprogramming to a lower output to avoid invasive revision to a bipolar system. Reduction of voltage is often effective in eliminating muscle stimulation—far more so than reduction of pulse width duration.

Diaphragmatic stimulation, if present, is usually apparent on physical examination but rarely requires fluoroscopy for confirmation. This problem is becoming more frequent with the use of biventricular pacing systems. As mentioned previously, it may indicate direct stimulation of the diaphragm through a thin ventricular wall, or, less commonly, through a perforated ventricle. In the former case, reduction of output may alleviate the problem. Another cause for diaphragmatic stimulation (right-sided) is phrenic nerve stimulation with a misplaced or dislodged atrial or ventricular lead. Depending on which lead is responsible, the corrective approach may entail inactivation of the atrial channel, reduction of atrial output, or re-positioning of the displaced lead.

Other important aspects of the physical examination include vital signs, with particular emphasis on pulse and blood pressure. The latter may vary significantly as a function of pacing mode (e.g., VVI versus DDD) or pacing rate. Neck veins should be evaluated for the presence of cannon A waves; cardiac examination should confirm paradoxical splitting of the second heart sound in most cases of right ventricular pacing, and should exclude the presence of a pericardial friction rub suggestive of cardiac perforation. The arm ipsilateral to the lead insertion site should be examined for edema, perhaps reflecting venous thrombosis which is usually a spontaneously resolving phenomenon and rarely responsible for thromboembolism. Arm elevation is often helpful while endogenous thrombolysis and recruitment of collateral circulation takes place. If symptoms are more marked, short-term anticoagulation with warfarin may speed the process. Edema coupled with inflammation may, less commonly, represent a gouty attack precipitated by the recent surgical implantation of a pacer system.

Physical manipulation of the pacer system should be undertaken to evaluate the integrity of the leads and their connections to the generator can. Rarely, inversion of the generator can lead to myopectoral stimulation and/or loss of capture in unipolar systems. This may result because the generator was implanted with the uninsulated side down or because the patient has reversed the can by "twiddling."[19]

In rate-adaptive systems dependent on sensing vibration, the can may be tapped to demonstrate increases in the pacing rate. Traction applied to the generator may expose a previously unsuspected malconnection or lead fracture and result in loss of capture or myopectoral stimulation. Confirmation of continued capture should be made with the patient in erect as well as supine position in cases where inadequate or insufficient lead "slack" may be present. Myopotential inhibition in single-chamber systems or myopotential triggering of ventricular pacing in dual-chamber systems may be elicited by various movements such as abduction of the arm ipsilateral to the generator. This is ordinarily an issue only for unipolar systems. The ability to observe real time intracardiac signals as well as the universal adaptation of marker channels has greatly eased this evaluation. If myopotential inhibition is elicited and clinically significant, reprogramming to a reduced sensitivity, to an asynchronous pacing mode, or to a triggered pacing mode may be undertaken to ensure continuous pacing in the pacer-dependent patient. Consideration of changing the unipolar system to a bipolar system is another option. Carotid sinus massage is another physical maneuver that may be employed to induce slowing to the lower rate limit, thereby confirming the ability of the pacemaker to capture. Rarely, carotid massage–induced slowing of the sinus node may be useful in dual-chamber systems to differentiate supraventricular tachycardia from physiological sinus tachycardia with ventricular tracking near the upper rate limit.

RADIOGRAPHY

The chest radiograph (posteroanterior and lateral using the dorsal spine technique) remains an important feature of the pacemaker follow-up evaluation, conveying a wealth of information.[20] Following implant, it serves to delineate lead positioning and screw-tip advancement in active fixation leads. Lead dislocation is rare beyond the first month after implantation. Subsequent radiographs may be scheduled on a periodic basis or only if specific questions are to be addressed.

In particular, lead conductor fractures may sometimes be identified in cases of lead failure in the setting of elevated lead impedance. These typically occur at sites of acute angulation or at sites of increased external stress such as the first rib-clavicular junction in leads placed via subclavian vein puncture or at anchoring sites if a protective sleeve was not applied at the time of implant. Fluoroscopy, in conjunction with traction on the lead and generator, may be required to delineate the fracture. Previously, a manufacturer's advisory on potential fracture of an inner J-shaped retention wire has recommended periodic cine-fluoroscopy to evaluate for fracture in certain active fixation J-shaped atrial leads (Telectronics Accufix series). The venous insertion site may be apparent on the film; jugular venous cutdown, for example, entails lead entry superior to the clavicle. Anatomic variants (such as persistent left superior vena cava) may also be appreciated. Clues to the polarity of the lead(s) may also be appreciated by analyzing either the distal tip for presence of a ring electrode or the header block, though whether the generator is actually programmed to bipolar or unipolar remains to be determined. Examination of the connector block may disclose retraction of the lead pin.

The generator may also be examined for position and, importantly, to identify the specific model in patients with an unknown system. Various radiographic identification codes exist that are manufacturer-specific and facilitate recognition of the specific device in question (Fig. 11.5). Comprehensive references exist to assist in this process.[21] Older systems not employing such radiographic codes may be identified on the basis of generator shape or battery configuration on the radiograph.

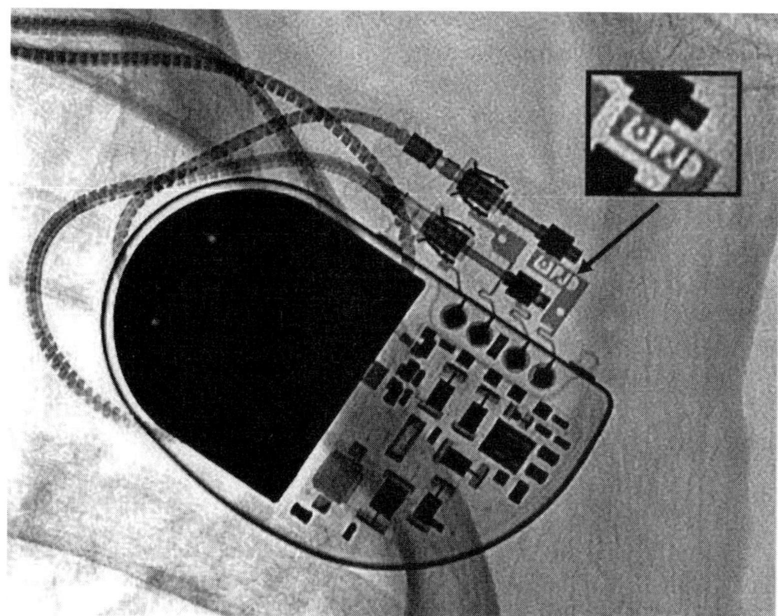

Figure 11.5. Radiographic identification of a pacer generator has been facilitated by the use of device-specific identification codes. The code appears horizontally in the right upper corner of the device. The code "PJD" following the Medtronic logo identifies the device as a Medtronic Sigma 303 pacemaker (insert).

ELECTROCARDIOGRAPHY AND MAGNET APPLICATION

It is beyond the scope of this chapter to provide a detailed discussion of pacemaker electrocardiography. Rather, a general approach to the use of electrocardiography in assessing pacemaker functioning will be addressed. The 12-lead electrocardiogram, both with and without pacing, is a useful tool in pacemaker follow-up assessments. Aside from confirming the pacer's ability to sense and capture, the electrocardiogram can provide important information on lead integrity and position.[22] For example, the typical morphology of a right ventricular paced complex is that of left bundle branch block, whereas right bundle branch block morphology may suggest left ventricular pacing, whether intentional (e.g., epicardial wires) or otherwise (e.g., perforation). A superior axis is common in leads in the RV apex while intermediate or inferiorly directed axis are suggestive of leads high on the septum or in the outflow tract.

Although multiprogrammability and telemetered data through the programmer have supplanted magnet application for detailed pacemaker analysis in most cases, magnet application remains an important aspect of pacemaker evaluation. In the absence of a programmer, magnet application with electrocardiographic monitoring confirms the ability to capture a cardiac chamber during asynchronous pacing. This may be otherwise inapparent if the patient's intrinsic rhythm inhibits pacer firing.

Magnet responses vary widely among manufacturers and even among various models of a single manufacturer (Table 11.3). For example, magnet application in single-chamber systems may result in asynchronous pacing at the standard rate or the programmed rate, ventricular demand pacing at a fast rate, or ventricular triggered pacing. Magnet application in dual-chamber systems may

Table 11.3. Pacemaker Magnet Application

Possible Responses to Magnet Application	Uses of Magnet Application
1. Asynchronous pacing • SSI to SOO • DDD to DOO with programmed or shortened AV delay • DDD to VOO 2. Triggered mode • SSI to SST 3. Rate change • Programmed rate • Faster rate than programmed 4. Threshold determination • Fixed percentage amplitude reduction over first few paced complexes • Vario function • Autothreshold search 5. Trigger electrogram storage 6. No change in pacer function • Programmable magnet response (on/off) • ICD	1. Device identification—some manufacturers or models have characteristic response. 2. Determination of single-chamber or dual-chamber pacing modes in patient with spontaneous rhythm that inhibits pacer output. 3. Elective replacement indicators—characteristic of each model. 4. Necessary for programming in some devices—reed switch actuation by magnet in programming head. 5. Threshold margin test in some devices. 6. Assesses pacing capture capabilities by asynchronous pacing. 7. Diagnosis of some problems related to oversensing, such as far-field signals, T-wave sensing, crosstalk inhibition. 8. Termination of pacemaker mediated tachycardias. 9. Underdrive pacing to terminate some arrhythmias, such as ventricular tachycardia. 10. Ensures pacing when electromagnetic interference may inhibit output, such as electrocautery. 11. Trigger electrogram storage. 12. Inactivates/activates certain ICDs, allows assessment of R-wave synchronization in certain ICDs ("beepogram"), asynchronous pacing does not occur with ICD magnet application.

result in dual-chamber asynchronous pacing at the programmed rate or at a standard rate, or at the programmed rate plus a fixed percent increment; or it may even result in asynchronous single-chamber ventricular pacing at a standard rate. Elective replacement indicators in some models may be elicited only in the magnet mode. In such instances, routine magnet application may be especially important for determining the need for replacement of a depleting pacer generator.

The application of a magnet over the generator is rarely associated with adverse effects. On occasion ventricular ectopy may result from asynchronous ventricular pacing, but this is seldom sustained. Caution is warranted if the patient has both a pacer and an implantable cardioverter-defibrillator; some implanted defibrillators may have tachycardia therapy inactivated by prolonged magnet exposure.

Because most devices respond to magnet application by asynchronous pacing, magnets may also be employed, both diagnostically and therapeutically, in cases where potential pacer malfunction is attributed to sensing problems (see Table 11.3). Magnet application can be therapeutic to terminate pacemaker-mediated tachycardia or to restore pacing in cases of oversensing. In cases of pacemaker dependence, rapid magnet conversion to asynchronous pacing may be critical in preventing asystole due to oversensing or crosstalk inhibition (particularly if the appropriate pacemaker programmer is unavailable). In some contemporary pacemakers; however, magnet application may trigger specialized pacemaker functions such as threshold search or electrogram storage rather than asynchronous pacing.

PACEMAKER DEPENDENCE

Pacemaker dependency connotes a condition in which cessation of pacemaker function may result in symptomatic bradycardia or ventricular asystole that endangers the patient. The term is problematic for a variety of reasons. First, it is often misused in cases when 100% pacing is observed. In this sense any pacer patient may be rendered "pacer dependent" by having the device programmed to a rate greater than her or his intrinsic heart rate. Second, in patients with conduction abnormalities such as atrioventricular block, the degree of impairment may vary from one point in time to another. That is, the ability to conduct 1:1 from atrium to ventricle may be somewhat "whimsical" and may also vary with the application of various medications that facilitate or depress conduction (Fig. 11.6). Lastly, with reprogramming of pacers to slower rates, gradual slowing of the pacer rate is more likely to allow the emergence of an escape rhythm than is a sudden cessation of pacing (Fig. 11.7).

In patients in whom gradual reprogramming of the generator to slower rates still results in 100% pacing at the slowest programmable rate, it is still possible to determine the presence (or absence) of an underlying rhythm if the

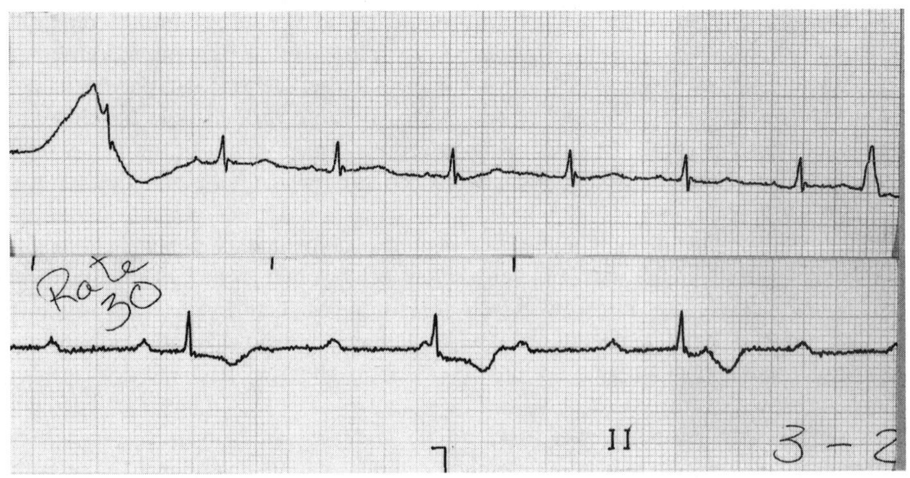

Figure 11.6. Top: Intact AV conduction in a pacer patient with resulting inhibition of pacer output. Pacemaker was originally inserted for complete heart block. **Bottom:** Underlying rhythm in the same patient several months later demonstrating recurrent complete heart block.

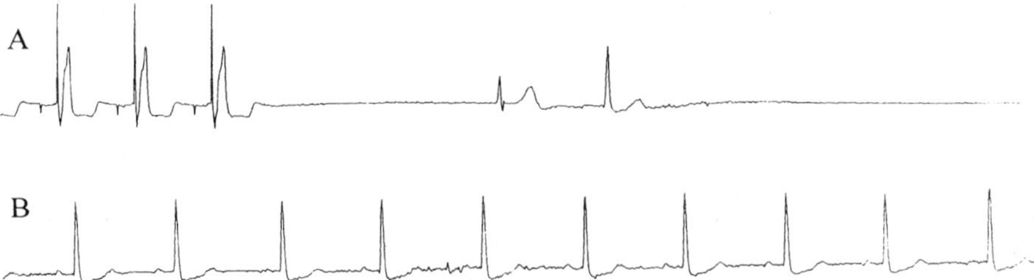

Figure 11.7. Emergence of escape rhythm in a 56-year-old woman 3 days after mitral valve replacement. **A:** The patient has been paced with temporary wires at 90 bpm since her surgery. Abrupt termination of pacing results in asystole lasting a total of 9 seconds. **B:** Hours after gradually decreasing the pacing rate to 50 bpm sinus rhythm at 70 bpm with normal AV conduction is noted. The patient was discharged from the hospital 2 days later without permanent pacing.

output is temporarily inhibited or programmed to subthreshold values. This practice may result in prolonged asystole during programming and should only be attempted if temporary programming is available that is rapidly reversible. Alternatively, chest wall stimulation may be applied with alligator clip cables from a temporary pacing device via skin electrodes (one situated directly over the generator can) in an effort to produce electromagnetic interference and thereby inhibit pacer output. This technique is particularly well suited to unipolar systems with limited programming capabilities for rate or output.

PROGRAMMERS

Pacemaker programmers are complex devices with which the pacemaker physician must be thoroughly familiar.[8] Pacemaker programmers enable both programmability and telemetry of a host of data including programming commands, administrative data, programmed data, measured data, and diagnostic data. All programmers, independent of the manufacturer, share certain architectural features. All modern programmers are computer based. There is an input section that allows operator interface with the computer programmer via a keyboard, light pen, and/or touch-sensitive screen. There is a telemetry interface associated with the programmer usually in the form of a handheld wand that transmits signals to and receives data from the pulse generator. The programmer is also associated with a printer for hardcopy printouts of pacemaker data. The printer may be physically integrated with the programmer or a separate component.

The three electromagnetic wave modalities that have enabled coupling between programmer and pacer generator have been magnetic coupling—application of a continuous or pulsed magnetic field that is detected by the generator's reed switch; inductive coupling—detection of pulsed magnetic fields through an antenna coil which then induces current flow that is detected as a coding scheme; and radiofrequency waves.[23] Radiofrequency energy allows for the most rapid transmission of a large amount of information through high frequency waves emitted by the programmer's antenna and received by the generator's antenna. The carrier frequencies depend upon the manufacturer.

Spurious programming remains a problem that may present in a variety of forms. "Phantom programming" refers to the reprogramming of a device by another physician unbeknownst to the original physician programmer. "Dysprogramming" is spurious programming due to an anomalous interference source such as electrocautery. "Misprogramming" is reprogramming of a pacer by a programmer in unanticipated fashion due to faulty program emission counts. Rarely, "cross-programming" may be observed as the unpredictable reprogramming of one manufacturer's pacemaker by another manufacturer's programmer. For this reason a pacemaker must only be interrogated and programmed with the specific manufacturer's programmer.

TELEMETRY, STORED AND REAL-TIME DATA

Pacemaker follow-up assessments can be performed efficiently using a systematic approach to interrogation and threshold testing (see Fig. 11.1). Even before any reprogramming is undertaken or thresholds are determined, the device should be interrogated to document the current programmed settings. All modern devices have such telemetry available. It should be emphasized that independent confirmation of such parameters as mode and rate should be made electrocardiographically after all interventions, because telemetry will not always reflect true programmed settings, although this is rare. This is particularly true in the case of pacer systems that have come into contact with extreme environmental noise (such as electrocautery or defibrillation) causing subsequent resetting of the device or pacer malfunction—in these cases, what you see (via telemetry) is not always what you get. The ability to undertake telemetry, as in the case of programming, is device-specific and requires manufacturer-specific programmers and/or modules. Inability to perform telemetry has several potential explanations including the wrong programmer has been used, the programmer is correct but lacks software updates to communicate with the present model, the device is an older model incapable of providing telemetry, the device has a circuit malfunction[24] or is at end of life.

The retrieval of stored and real-time data is an important part of each follow-up visit. When obtainable, real-time telemetry of measured data such as battery voltage or lead impedance may prove quite useful in diagnosing problems with impending battery depletion or lead integrity, respectively (Fig. 11.8).[25–31] A very low telemetered lead impedance may suggest problems with

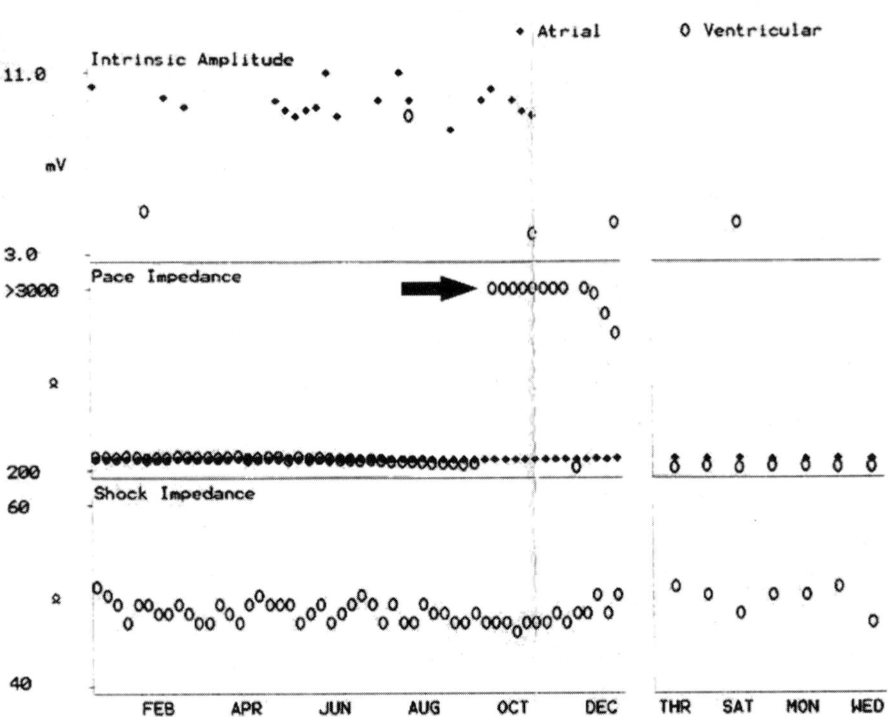

Figure 11.8. Graphic 6-month trend report of atrial and ventricular electrogram amplitudes, pacing lead and high voltage lead impedances in a Guidant ICD. From August to December, high ventricular lead impedances (open circle) were documented (arrow) but returned to normal at the time of the interrogation. The patient was demonstrated to have a fractured ventricular lead.

lead insulation, for example, whereas a very high telemetered impedance may indicate conductor fracture or a loose set-screw, which may not be apparent radiographically. With time, battery voltage declines and battery impedance rises, allowing projections of device longevity.

Historical information, such as initial implant values, may also be recorded in some systems and be available for recall via telemetry. Some models allow both programmers and generators to have actual times displayed, important in programming certain circadian features, as well as identifying when certain events, such as automatic mode switching, have occurred since the last interrogation.

Aside from identifying programmed settings and measured data, telemetry of event counters is usually possible with current systems. This data may assist in diagnosing certain problems reported by the patient and in optimizing pacer function. Histograms may be obtainable to demonstrate how often different rates occur during rate-adaptive pacing at a particular activity-sensing threshold. The determination of such events (or predicted events) may enable the physician to reprogram the device settings so as to achieve rates thought to be more appropriate or "physiologic" for the patient (sensor-indicated rate histogram) (Fig. 11.9).

Histograms of "event records" are available in many models, allowing for precise determination of when some event occurred, symptomatic or otherwise, and at what rate. In this fashion, episodes of tachycardia and other events, such as automatic mode switching or search hysteresis episodes, may be assessed in some models. Pacer generators may thus serve as their own mini-Holter monitors.

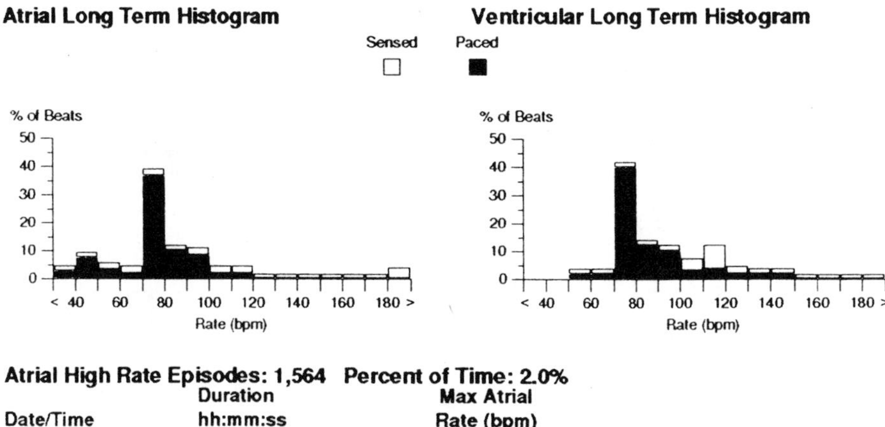

Figure 11.9. Telemetry of stored rate histogram for a patient with a rate-adaptive dual-chamber pacemaker. The histograms display long-term data for the atrial and ventricular paced and sensed rates.

Real-time intracardiac electrograms and marker channels may be available, depending on the system used; they facilitate the physician's ability to diagnose appropriate, or inappropriate, pacer function.[28] The size of the intracardiac electrograms may give the pacer physician a rough idea of the sensing capabilities of the system and may also delineate the strength of far-field signals. With some devices, the patient may freeze and store electrograms with external magnet application during symptomatic events or the device may automatically store electrograms in response to high heart rates (Fig. 11.10). This corresponds to an event monitor function of the device. The clinical utility of intracardiac electrograms includes identifying retrograde conduction, measuring ventriculoatrial conduction time, assisting rhythm identification, evaluating unusual sensing phenomena, evaluating lead connector integrity, assisting threshold determinations, and evaluating myopotential sensing.

Potentially more useful are marker channels, which denote when a particular channel (atrial or ventricular) is sensing activity or emitting a paced output (Fig. 11.11). By telling the physician what the pacer is "seeing and doing," certain phenomena, such as crosstalk inhibition, may be more easily defined. Event markers do, however, have their limitations. They describe pacer behavior but not its appropriateness; a stimulus output report does not necessarily imply capture.

SENSING AND PACING THRESHOLDS

For manual sensing threshold determination, the device should first be reprogrammed below the intrinsic rate to assess sensing. In single-chamber devices, ventricular sensing thresholds may be determined by then decreasing sensitivity (i.e., increasing the millivolt values) in the VVI mode to determine at what value

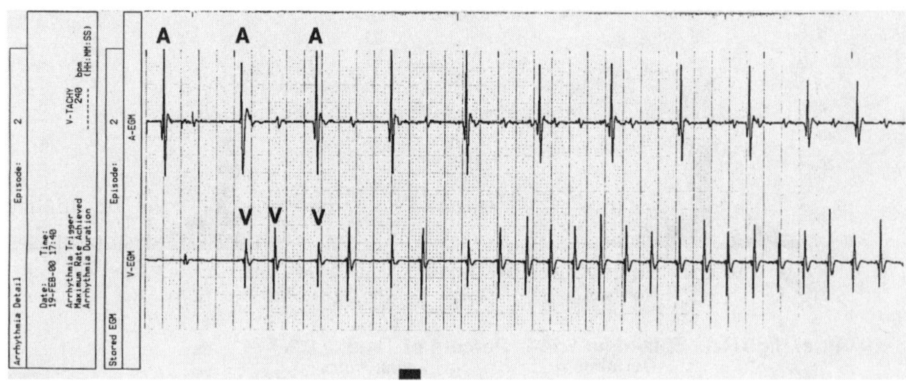

Figure 11.10. Stored atrial **(top)** and ventricular **(bottom)** electrograms from a pacemaker with automated electrogram capture triggered by a high ventricular rate. The patient experienced syncope at the time the electrograms were recorded. The documentation of AV dissociation is diagnostic of ventricular tachycardia.

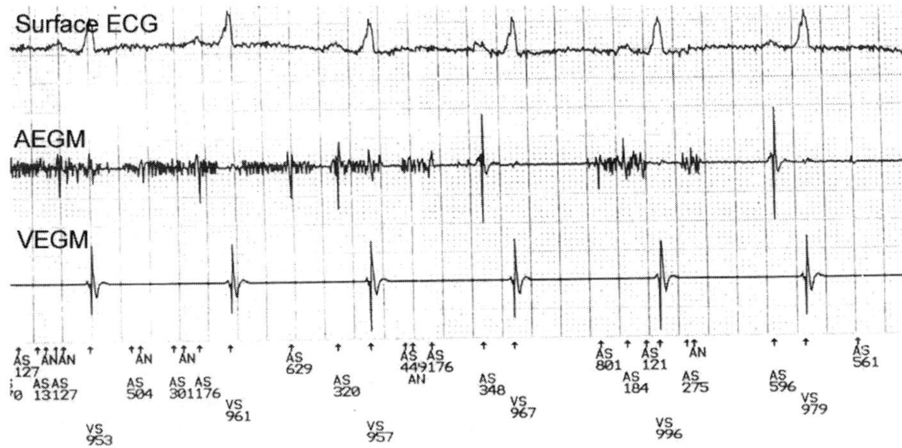

Figure 11.11. Surface ECG, atrial (AEGM) and ventricular (VEGM) intracardiac electrograms, and marker channel **(bottom)** demonstrating "noise" and oversensing on the atrial lead of a Guidant ICD. This resulted from an insulation break from subclavian crush.

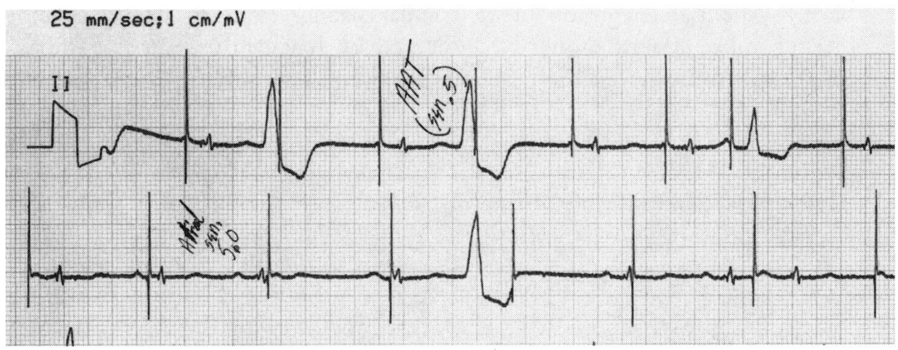

Figure 11.12. Atrial triggered pacing mode. **Top:** Maximal sensitivity of 0.5 mV atrial sensing is appropriate. **Bottom:** With reduction of atrial sensitivity to 5.0 mV there is a failure of atrial sensing with atrial spikes that do not coincide with native P waves.

pacer output is no longer inhibited. The same approach may be applied for establishing atrial-sensing thresholds. The triggered modes may also be used in their respective chambers to determine sensing thresholds. Failure to trigger a pacemaker spike at a given sensitivity value indicates undersensing (Fig. 11.12). Alternatively, triggered pacing by signals other than the P wave or QRS, such as T waves or myopotentials, indicate oversensing. In dual-chamber systems, atrial sensing can be confirmed by programming to a P-wave synchronous ventricular triggered mode, shortening the AV interval so as to trigger ventricular pacing, and reducing atrial sensitivity progressively until paced ventricular events no longer result. Ventricular sensing can either be checked in a VVI mode with the rate set lower than the intrinsic rate or alternatively in the DDD mode as long as the AV delay can be set sufficiently long to inhibit ventricular pacing. Newer devices provide other techniques to check sensing thresholds. Some automatically check atrial and ventricular electrogram amplitudes on a regular basis. The results are available for review upon interrogation. Others require running a sensing protocol that automates the process described above. Finally, in certain devices, the intracardiac signal can be printed on calibrated paper that allows direct reading of the size of the sensed signal. With this technique, small variations may exist compared with the signal measured by the device due to differences in filters between the telemetry circuit and the sensing circuit. In patients with atrial electrical standstill or complete heart block without a viable escape mechanism, sensing thresholds will not be obtainable.

For unipolar systems, particularly in pacemaker-dependent patients, the possibility of myopotential inhibition of ventricular output should be investigated. At increasing ventricular sensitivities, the patient is asked to perform isometric exercise using the arm ipsilateral to the generator, such as pushing the hands together in front of the chest (Fig. 11.13). One should look for "noise" on the surface lead and electrogram with inappropriate sensing of R waves on the marker channel and ventricular pacing inhibition. Likewise, the possibility of myopotential triggering of ventricular pacing from atrial oversensing in a dual-chamber system should be evaluated by having the patient perform deltopectoral isometric exercises at increasing atrial sensitivities. Atrial oversensing

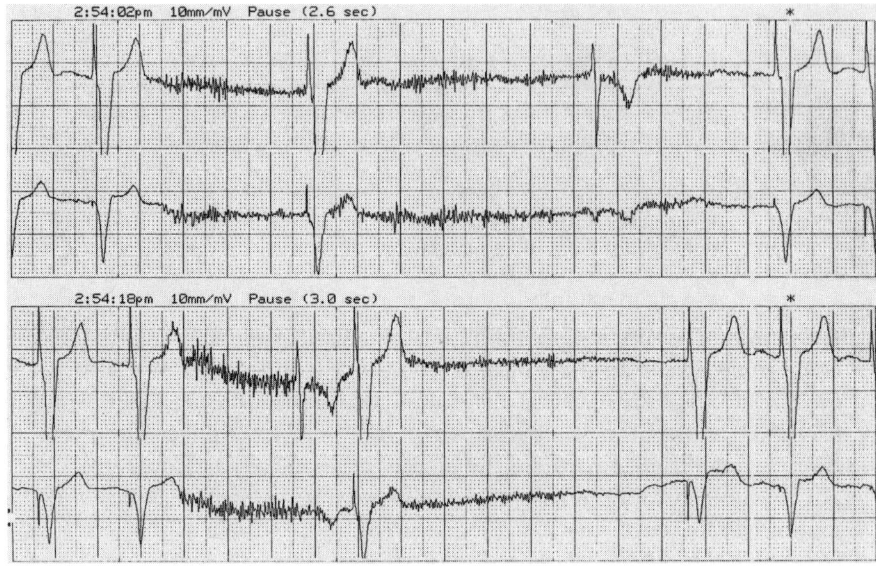

Figure 11.13. Two-channel Holter (simultaneous V_1 and modified V_5) showing symptomatic inhibition of pacing by myopotentials.

of myopotential or far-field R waves are frequent causes of inappropriate mode switching. In general, the chronic atrial and ventricular sensitivities settings should be set to a twofold to fourfold safety margin unless oversensing occurs (i.e., for an atrial sensing threshold of 2 mV, a sensitivity setting of 0.5 to 1.0 mV would be appropriate).

The pacing threshold determination is an important feature of pacer follow-up evaluations because generator longevity may be significantly enhanced if the output can be programmed to the lowest value that will provide an adequate safety margin for pacing. Particular longevity may be obtained if outputs can be programmed to 2.5 V, i.e., less than the lithium-iodine battery voltage of 2.8 V. At this output, the energy inefficient voltage doubling circuit can be avoided. Further decreases in output beyond this point provide diminishing energy savings. In practice, doubling the voltage threshold (at a pulse width of 0.4 or 0.5 milliseconds) or tripling the pulse width threshold (as long as less than 0.3 milliseconds) usually will provide an adequate safety margin. Energy consumption is directly proportional to the pulse width but increases with the square of voltage. If tripling the pulse width results in an interval less than 0.9 milliseconds, this is usually more energy efficient than doubling the voltage. Programming larger safety margins is typical immediately after implant to allow for the usual post-implant threshold increases. This process is almost always complete by 2 to 3 months allowing chronic thresholds to be programmed at that point. Programming larger safety margins should also be considered in the ventricular channel of pacemaker-dependent patients given the possibility of late unexpected threshold rises.[32]

Determination of pacing thresholds should be made for both chambers where applicable.[33] In patients with intact AV conduction, determination of atrial stimulation threshold is easiest measured in the AAI mode with the pacing rate set 10 to 20 bpm above the intrinsic rate. Atrial output (or pulse width) is progressively lowered until a QRS complex is "dropped" indicating loss of atrial capture. In patients with AV block, atrial capture must be measured in a DDD mode. The threshold may then be determined by noting the loss of a P wave on a surface tracing or the appearance of atrial sensed events on a marker channel or spontaneous atrial signal on an electrogram tracing. The latter two findings indicate return of spontaneous sinus node function after loss of atrial capture. Ventricular stimulation thresholds are most cleanly performed in VVI mode. DDD mode may also be used as an alternative particularly in patients who feel poorly with the loss of AV synchrony with VVI pacing. The AV delay must be set sufficiently short to "force" ventricular pacing and minimize fusion and pseudo-fusion which can obscure detection of loss of ventricular capture and result in falsely low perceived stimulation threshold. In pacemaker-dependent patients, loss of ventricular capture may result in asystole. Fortunately, most modern programmers permit rapid restoration of preprogrammed outputs with temporary pacing modes or automated threshold algorithms. The operator must remain vigilant though to terminate the test immediately after loss of capture is first noted.

Automaticity is a feature that has been applied to a number of pacemaker parameters to allow for device regulation without the need for continual clinician input. This is particularly the case with ventricular capture determinations. To date, auto-capture algorithms have been limited to the ventricle due to the relative ease of measuring the large evoked response with capture; however, devices capable of automatically measuring atrial capture are available as well. In some devices, the generator may be programmed to automatically determine the pacing threshold continuously or at periodic intervals and reset the output so as to ensure an adequate safety margin and simultaneously optimize device longevity. Certain devices which check capture on a beat-to-beat basis allow programming the output to as little as 0.25 V over the stimulation threshold. This option is being used increasingly to facilitate device follow-up.[34]

Programmability of polarity has become increasingly available in current pacemakers and, unfortunately, is not infrequently required. Problems with insulation defects in certain polyurethane leads subject to the "subclavian crush" syndrome, resulting in low impedance values, may be temporarily addressed by re-programming from bipolar to unipolar mode. This maneuver generally will increase the lead impedance in these situations and prevent loss of capture and possible undersensing, but will not prevent oversensing from make–break electrical transients arising from contact between the two conductors. Ultimately, lead replacement is required in the pacer-dependent patient. Occasionally, pacing or sensing thresholds will be significantly better in one polarity compared to the other. This may be helpful in the setting of marginal threshold values. General guidelines for chronic programming of common pacemaker parameters are given in Table 11.4.

THE ATRIOVENTRICULAR INTERVAL

Recent data[35] suggesting that right ventricular pacing may worsen symptoms of congestive heart failure in those with underlying cardiomyopathy has re-focused attention on appropriate programming of the AV interval. Certainly, in those with diminished LV function, one should make attempts to prolong the AV delay sufficiently to minimize RV pacing. This can be accomplished with programming a long fixed AV delay or programming "on" an AV search hysteresis feature which is being increasingly incorporated into new devices. With this feature, a backup AV interval is set as well as a further delay which is added to the programmed value allowing additional time to encourage native conduction. If no intrinsic R wave has been sensed by the end of the summed interval, the programmed "physiologic" AV delay will become active but with periodic searches for native conduction. Programming the device to DDI(R) mode is sometimes worthwhile as well. In contrast, patients with normal LV function are rarely able to distinguish between native conduction and P wave synchronous pacing. Nevertheless, the above techniques to minimize ventricular pacing may still be worthwhile if only to maximize battery duration. However, there is clearly an AV delay sufficiently long that the benefits of

Table 11.4. General Guidelines for Programming Common Pacemaker Parameters

Parameter	Situation	Chronic Setting	Comments
Lower rate limit	General	50–70 bpm	
	Minimal pacing desired	40–60 bpm	Use rate hysteresis
	Heart failure	70–90 bpm	Benefit of high rate pacing not proven
Upper rate limit	General	85% maximal predicted heart rate; [(220˜ age) × 0.85] bpm	Based on average levels of activity
	Children/athletes	(220˜ age) bpm	May require programming short refractory periods
	Coronary artery disease/angina	110–120 bpm	Approximates peak heart rates on maximal beta blockade
Pacing output	Fixed voltage	3–4× pulse width threshold	Minimizing voltage output is most efficient
	Fixed pulse width	2–3× voltage threshold	Use autothreshold functions
Sensitivity	Atrium	25–50% of threshold value	Need <1 mV setting for mode switching
	Ventricle	25–50% of threshold value	Evaluate oversensing in unipolar systems
AV delay	AV block	150–180 msec paced AV delay, sensed AV delay 25–50 msec < paced AV delay	Turn on rate adaptive AV delay in active patients
	Intrinsic AV conduction (no CHF)	Up to 220 msec	Longer AV delays may compromise hemodynamics, use AV interval hysteresis to promote intrinsic conduction
	Intrinsic AV conduction (CHF)	Often set even longer AV delays	Pacing induced desynchrony of very long AV delay
	Hypertrophic cardiomyopathy	Approximately 100 msec	Optimize by Doppler Use negative hysteresis to "force" ventricular pacing

inhibiting ventricular pacing are outweighed by the adverse hemodynamic effects which can result with marked first degree block. Much of this detrimental effect may be linked to atrial contraction occurring during or immediately after ventricular systole creating a "pseudo-pacemaker syndrome." Certain studies have demonstrated that this detrimental effect is seen with PR intervals of greater than 220 milliseconds.[36] In occasional patients who continue to complain of breathlessness after a pacemaker is implanted, an attempt at AV optimization using Doppler echocardiography or impedance cardiography may be warranted. Both AV as well as LV/RV optimization is a subject of particular interest in those with bi-ventricular pacemakers. Traditional mitral inflow and aortic outflow Doppler measurements as well as newer tissue Doppler techniques are being investigated.[37,38]

In contrast to the previous situations, there are also situations in which ventricular pacing is desired. This is particularly true when dual-chamber pacemakers are placed for symptom relief in those with hypertrophic obstructive cardiomyopathy. Programming a short fixed AV delay is one option although more sophisticated algorithms such as negative AV interval hysteresis can be quite effective in allowing for the longest AV interval that still provides 100% ventricular pacing. Patients with biventricular pacemakers represent another group where continuous ventricular pacing is desired. This is often difficult when these patients develop rapid atrial fibrillation. New algorithms are being developed to assist in this situation. One such algorithm automatically increases the ventricular pacing rate after every sensed ventricular event. Another provides a "triggered" mode where each sensed ventricular beat immediately results in LV pacing resulting in a fused QRS complex which is more synchronized than the intrinsic beat would be alone. Finally, in patients with a "traditional" dual-chamber pacemaker, underlying cardiomyopathy and a baseline right bundle branch block, biventricular pacing can often be simulated. To accomplish this, one carefully programs the AV delay so as to create fusion between the RV paced complex and the native QRS (which, due to the RBBB, is activating the left ventricle first) and thus, create some measure of re-synchrony.

A differential AV delay is now incorporated into virtually all modern pacemakers. This allows for programming of a shorter AV delay for the sensed AV interval (SAV) compared with the paced AV interval (PAV). This accounts for the fact that the pacemaker does not recognize a sensed atrial event (and start the SAV timer) until atrial depolarization is well under way. The differential AV delay thus keeps the time between atrial and ventricular contraction constant regardless of the presence of atrial pacing. A differential value of 25 to 40 milliseconds is considered appropriate. Most pacemakers also now have a rate responsive AV delay feature. This provides for a shortening of the AV interval during exercise mimicking the normal positive dromotropic effect seen in those with normal AV conduction. This feature provides a hemodynamic benefit as well as allow for the programming of a higher maximum tracking rate. This feature should ordinarily be programmed "on" in those with AV conduction disturbances.

SPECIAL CONSIDERATIONS IN DUAL-CHAMBER SYSTEMS

In dual-chamber systems several problems may require evaluation during follow-up evaluations as the clinical situation arises. The possibility of cross talk; that is, inappropriate sensing of the atrial pacing artifact on the ventricular channel resulting in ventricular pacing inhibition can be assessed by programming the ventricular channel to highest sensitivity and the atrial output to its highest value (Fig. 11.14). The programmed rate should exceed the native rate so as to require continuous atrial pacing, and the programmed AV interval should be shorter than the native PR interval. The absence of cross talk inhibition at maximal atrial output and maximal ventricular sensitivity suggests that this problem is not likely to be encountered at usual settings. Fortunately, cross talk is much less of a problem with modern pulse generators that incorporate various techniques to minimize this problem such as ventricular blanking periods and cross-talk sensing windows. Assessment of this phenomenon should be undertaken cautiously in patients with heart block, because ventricular asystole may occur. Identification of cross talk warrants re-programming, when possible, to lower atrial output or ventricular sensitivity, prolongation of ventricular blanking period, or consideration of another mode such as VDD.

The propensity for pacemaker-mediated tachycardia (PMT) in the DDD mode may be explored by shortening the postventricular atrial refractory period

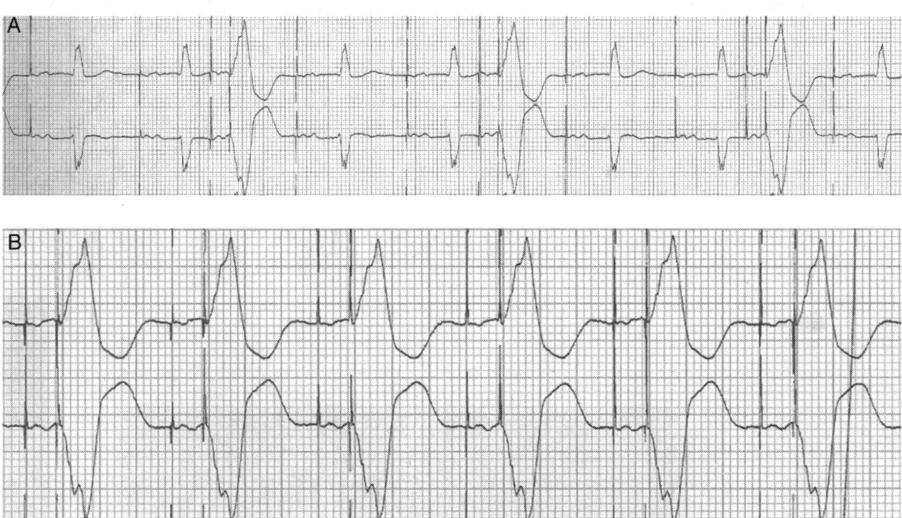

Figure 11.14. Cross talk in a unipolar dual chamber pacemaker. **Panel A:** This patient was referred for loss of capture on the ventricular lead. The ECG shows atrial pacing consistently but ventricular output on only the first cardiac cycle. Telemetry showed ventricular sensing within 40 to 60 milliseconds of the pacing output that inhibits ventricular pacing. After reducing atrial sensitivity from 2.8 to 5.6 mV inhibition of ventricular output was corrected. This device did not have programmable postatrial pacing ventricular blanking intervals or safety pacing that would have also resolved the cross talk.

(PVARP) to its minimum and programming atrial output to subthreshold levels. If retrograde ventriculoatrial conduction is present, PMT may be observed if it is triggered by a spontaneous PVC or if loss of atrial capture occurs. In the latter case, the AV sequential paced rhythm fails to capture the atrium but captures the ventricle, with retrograde conduction leading to activation of the atrium and setting up PMT. PMT may be managed by decreasing the upper ventricular tracking rate, extending the PVARP (which may limit the desired upper tracking limit), changing to a nonatrial tracking mode such as DDI or activating PMT intervention algorithms. These can include an increase in the PVARP after a PVC which will minimize the chance of initiating a PMT or periodically "dropping" a ventricular paced beat with any tachycardia near the upper rate limit. This will terminate the tachycardia if it is indeed a PMT but only create a brief pause if the rhythm were an intrinsic atrial rhythm that the pacemaker was tracking, i.e., sinus tachycardia. Many devices allow programming of a rate-adaptive PVARP that shortens the PVARP at more rapid rates permitting a long PVARP at rest without unduly imposing limits on the upper rate.

Not infrequently, a patient with a dual-chamber device will present with new onset atrial fibrillation or flutter. The atrial fibrillation or flutter waves may be sensed and trigger rapid ventricular responses, often irregularly (Fig. 11.15). Automatic mode switching is a very important feature incorporated into many dual-chamber pacemakers for the management of atrial arrhythmias (Fig. 11.16). It allows reversion from dual-chamber pacing to single-chamber ventricular pacing (or to a non-atrial tracking mode such as DDI(R)) when atrial arrhythmias are recognized, and a return to dual-chamber mode when sinus rhythm has been restored. In general, this algorithm works well, but occasional undersensing of fibrillatory waves may result in frequent switches back to DDD mode

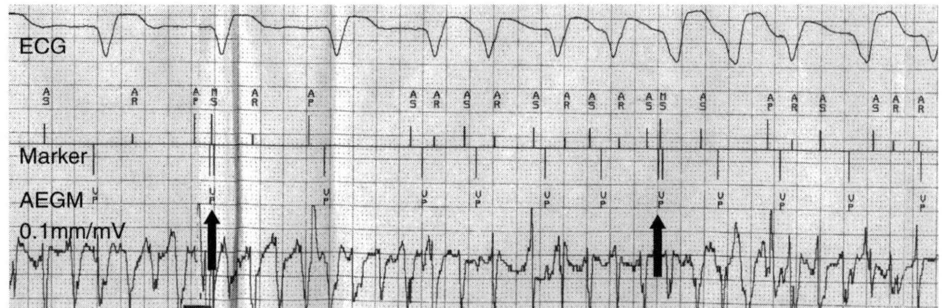

Figure 11.15. Rhythm strip showing intermittent ventricular tracking of atrial flutter/atrial fibrillation resulting in irregular ventricular pacing near the upper rate limit in the DDD mode. At the start of the tracing, the device is in mode switch non-atrial tracking mode with a slow paced ventricular rate. At the *first arrow*, the device exits mode switching to DDD mode because of atrial undersensing (MS on marker annotations). The *second arrow* identifies re-activation of mode switch behavior due to consistent atrial sensing with brief tracking at the upper rate limit. AEGM = atrial electrogram.

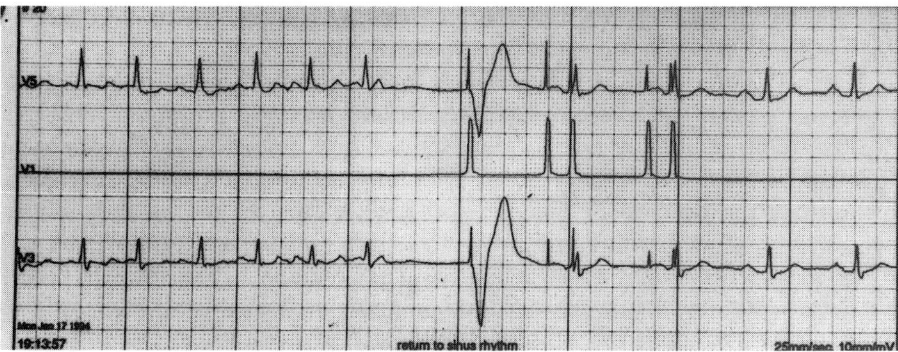

Figure 11.16. Reversion from non-atrial tracking mode during paroxysmal atrial fibrillation to dual-chamber pacing once the sinus mechanism has returned, in a pacer programmed to allow automatic mode switching.

for several seconds before re-recognizing the atrial dysrhythmia and again mode-switching. This often results in the reporting of hundreds or even thousands of mode-switch events corresponding to a single or just a few more sustained episodes of atrial fibrillation. In non–mode-switching devices, the upper tracking rate limit may be reduced to minimize rapid ventricular tracking, but it is often more effective to reprogram the device to a DDIR or VVIR mode. The DDIR mode works particularly well for patients with significant sinus node dysfunction but intact AV conduction who spend much of their time in sinus rhythm with atrial pacing. In some devices, atrial flutter may be converted to sinus rhythm by temporary burst pacing from the atrial channel manually or as part of automated atrial antitachycardia pacing therapies. Guidelines for chronic programming of basic dual-chamber pacemaker parameters are shown in Table 11.4.

OUTPATIENT MONITORING

A variety of electrocardiographic techniques enable ambulatory determinations of pacemaker function between clinic visits. The most important of these is transtelephonic monitoring of the patient's free-running and magnet rates.[29,30] This technique does not supplant the direct outpatient visit with the pacer physician. It does, however, reduce the frequency of outpatient visits, which may be particularly burdensome for patients who are frail, in nursing homes, or are unable to travel. Guidelines for transtelephonic and office follow-up schedules are listed in Table 11.1.

Deviations from the recommended schedules may be needed for pacemaker dependent patients, devices under recall or alert, or for changes in the patient's clinical condition. Despite its limitations, transtelephonic monitoring enables the pacer physician to determine changes in free-running or magnet pacing rates indicative of battery depletion and may indicate problems with pacemaker sensing or capture. Patients experiencing symptoms potentially related to pacer function or malfunction are encouraged to transmit their rhythm when they are symptomatic, independent of the above scheduling guidelines.

As an extension of this approach, 24-hour Holter monitoring may be useful for uncovering problems with pacer malfunction that are potentially responsible for a patient's symptoms (Fig. 11.17).[31] The approach is limited by sampling error in patients with infrequent symptoms, as no abnormalities may be identified if the patient is "having a good day." Rather, the technique is more often useful in demonstrating previously unsuspected and asymptomatic malfunctions, such as intermittent undersensing or myopotential triggering. Activity-related rate trends warranting reprogramming, particularly with dual-chamber or rate-adaptive pacing, may be observed with Holter monitoring.

Presently, all manufacturers of pacemakers and ICDs have recently released or will shortly release enhanced outpatient monitoring devices. These devices often take advantage of newer wireless technologies and the Internet. These systems can "interrogate" the implanted device and provide information equivalent to that when interrogating a device in the office including stored electrograms from high rate events in pacemakers as well as printouts from VT/VF events in defibrillators.[39] Some monitoring devices can be placed on a nightstand in a patient's bedroom and will communicate with the device wirelessly without the need for any patient involvement. Transmission can be automated to occur at pre-ordained times or in response to trigger signals sent out by the device after specific events like defibrillator shocks or ERI being reached. Other monitoring systems require the patient to hold the unit near their device. The physician can receive this information either via fax or on a secure website over the Internet.[40] While the technology is already available for the physician to remotely re-program the device, safety concerns limit access to this feature presently. Similar to stand-alone programmers, manufacturers are using proprietary technology and thus the chance for universal equipment appears remote.

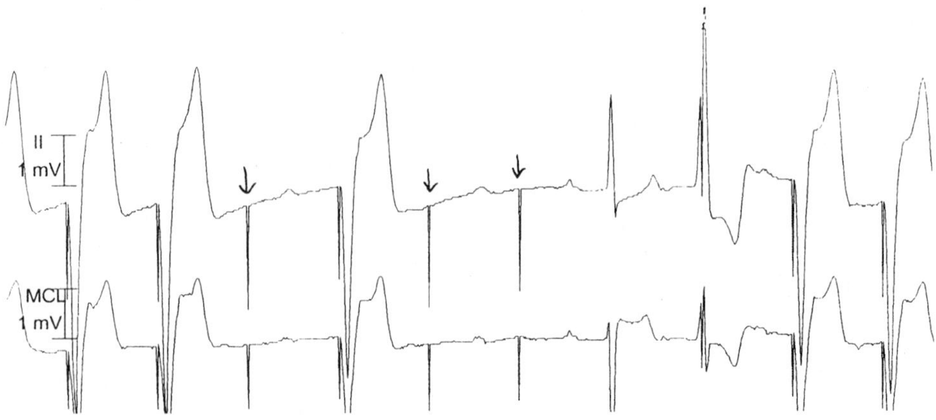

Figure 11.17. Intermittent loss of ventricular capture documented on ambulatory Holter monitoring.

ELECTIVE REPLACEMENT INDICATORS

The behavior of pacemakers approaching battery depletion is highly variable among different manufacturers and even among different models from the same maker. It is important to distinguish end-of-life (EOL) from ERI. The former connotes gross pacemaker malfunction or lack of function; the latter strives to indicate a time when generator replacement should be considered well in advance of end of life.[41,42] ERIs should be reached in the absence of patient symptoms or electrocardiographically demonstrated abnormalities in free-running pacer function. Indeed, changes in behavior, such as in magnet rates, may occur years in advance of true end of life. ERIs are used to recommend generator change within a period of a few weeks to months. They are device-specific and may be found by consulting with the manufacturer or the physician's manual. When it is available, real-time telemetry of available battery voltage and impedance may be useful in confirming battery depletion, particularly as progressive increases in battery impedance are observed. In most systems, however, changes in pacing rate are the predominant indicators of the need for elective replacement.

As the lithium iodine battery discharges, the internal impedance of the battery to current flow increases. At or near EOL, transient high current drain from the battery may further reduce the output voltage. This may result in temporary or persistent loss of device function (Fig. 11.18). If near ERI, the reduced ouput voltage may drop battery voltage below ERI levels, tripping the ERI behavior. Some devices will revert from the ERI mode (unlatched behavior) once battery voltage has recovered. If the behavior is latched, the ERI mode can be canceled only by reprogramming the device. True ERI or EOL behavior must be distinguished from "power on reset" (POR) mode that results from

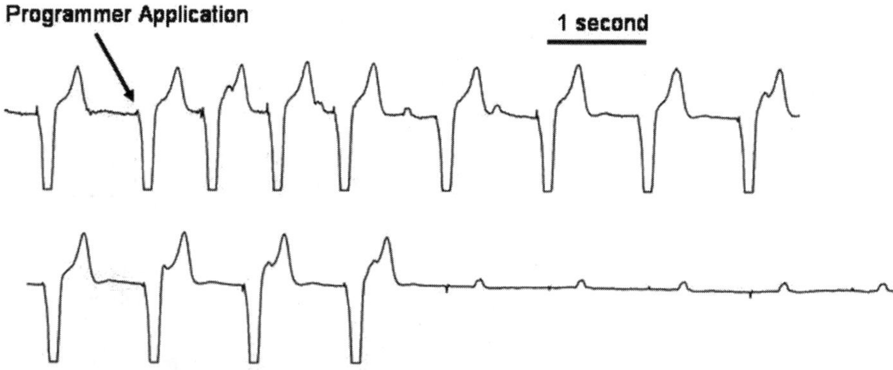

Figure 11.18. Loss of capture during programmer head (magnet) application in a pacemaker at end of battery life. The pacemaker telemetry was non-functional. Three paced beats at 100 bpm denote magnet application. With continued application of the programming head capture was lost due to increased current demand on the battery. A temporary pacemaker was in place anticipating such an occurrence.

loss or corruption of the pacemaker's volatile electronic memory. POR mode is a simple backup pacing mode (typically VVI or VOO) that is stored in non-volatile, read-only memory and allows the device to function after loss of programmable memory. The POR mode and ERI modes and rates of operation may or may not be identical for a given device. If identical, POR may be distinguished from ERI by a satisfactory battery voltage in POR and a low battery voltage in ERI. POR mode can be latched or unlatched. If battery voltage is not available but POR is unlatched, the device may be reprogrammed to continuous pacing at high output for 30 minutes ("battery stress test"). If ERI has occurred, the device will again revert to ERI; if POR has occurred, the programmed function will continue.

A summary of pacemaker behavior throughout the stages of battery life is shown in Table 11.5.

SPECIAL SITUATIONS ENCOUNTERED BY THE PACEMAKER PATIENT

The pacer physician is often asked to evaluate a pacemaker patient before surgery. In addition to obtaining details from the history and physical examination outlined previously, it is most essential to establish the degree of pacer dependence and, via telemetry, the current programmed settings. Operating room personnel including the surgeon, nursing staff, and anesthesiologists all need to be aware of the presence of the device, the potential EMI encountered in the operating room, and corrective techniques. An external defibrillator with transcutaneous pacing capabilities should be easily accessible. Electrocautery, often required intraoperatively, may result in a variety of pacemaker phenomena. Electrocautery may cause transient inhibition of pacer output because of oversensing of electromagnetic interference. If pacer dependence has been demonstrated preoperatively, the device may be programmed to either an asynchronous mode or a triggered mode to preempt undue inhibition of pacer output. If such programming is not possible, then a magnet may be taped over the generator during the period of cautery. However, by activating the reed switch, magnet application may make certain older pacemakers vulnerable to spurious re-programming. It is ideal to avoid electrocautery entirely if possible, especially near the pacer generator. The cautery grounding pad should be placed as far as possible from the generator and in a location where the vector from the electrocautery tip to the pad moves directly away from the pacemaker generator. In addition, short bursts of cautery and use of bipolar cautery are recommended. The major issue with an implantable cardiac defibrillator is the risk of oversensing noise resulting in inappropriate defibrillator shocks.

Both electrocautery and defibrillation can produce irreversible damage to the generator. This is more likely in older devices that lack protective mechanisms such as zener diodes, which shunt energy away from the delicate device circuitry. They may also result in resetting of the generator to a backup or noise-reversion mode. Pacemaker interrogation with pacing and sensing thresholds should be performed before and after the surgical procedure. Recommendations

Table 11.5. Pacemaker Behavior by Battery Status for Lithium–Iodine Cell

	BOL	ERI	EOL	POR
Cause	No significant battery use	Voltage reduced but still able to support basic or all pacer functions	Voltage unable to support basic or any pacer functions	Loss or corruption of volatile memory controlling pacer function
Voltage	Approx. 2.8 V	Approx. 2.1–2.4 V*	≤approx. 2.1 V*	>approx. 2.4 V*
Battery impedance	<1 k ohms	≤approx. 5–10 k ohms*	≥approx. 5–10 k ohms*	<approx. 5–10 k ohms*
Behavior	As programmed	• Percent or fixed decrease in free-running rate or magnet rate • Increase in pulse width duration • Change to simpler mode: DDDR to VVI, VVIR to VVI/VOO	• Cessation of all pacer function • Failure to communicate or reprogram • Change to simplest mode: DDDR to VOO, VVI to VOO	• Change to simpler mode: DDDR to VVI, VVIR to VVI • Change to unipolar lead polarity • Percent or fixed change in free-running rate or magnet rate
Diagnosis	High voltage, low battery impedance, BOL magnet/free running rate	Battery voltage reduced, elevated battery impedance, restricted programmability, ERI free running or magnet rate (after 60-second magnet application), telemetered advisory	Failure to communicate or program, failure to pace sense, very low battery voltage, very high	Battery voltage >ERI, battery impedance <ERI, telemetered advisory, exposure to EMI, perform battery "stress test"
Correction	None needed	Generator change in weeks to months	Immediate generator change	Reprogram generator

* Specific values will vary from manufacturer to manufacturer.
BOL = beginning of life; EOL = end of life; ERI = elective replacement indicators.

for perioperative management in those with implantable devices are discussed in Table 11.6.

Transient undersensing and both acute and chronic rises in pacing threshold have also been observed with defibrillation and cardioversion (Fig. 11.19).[43] Some of this may relate to transmission of current down the lead(s) causing a burn at the tissue-electrode interface resulting in the potential for exit block. The majority of problems seen after electrical cardioversions are encountered with unipolar pacemakers implanted in the right pectoral fossa. To minimize these types of phenomena, cardioversion or defibrillation should be performed via anteroposterior rather than anteroapical paddles. Minimizing the defibrillating energy by using more efficient biphasic defibrillators is desirable. In addition, pacing and sensing thresholds should be checked following external defibrillation. Finally, equipment for temporary pacing should be nearby, especially for a pacemaker-dependent patient.

Other sources of electromagnetic interference encountered in the hospital setting are magnetic resonance imaging (MRI), extracorporeal shock-wave

Table 11.6. Intra-Operative Management of Devices

Intra-Operative Problem	Solution
Cautery-induced pacing inhibition	Program device to asynchronous mode (best) or Place and tape magnet over device with pacemaker dependent patients Place grounding pad away from device Limit electrocautery to short bursts with pauses between bursts Bipolar preferable to monopolar electrocautery Coagulation mode preferable to cutting Use lowest effective power output Monitor telemetry for pacemaker inhibition Monitor pulse with second means; i.e., arterial line or oximetry tracing in case of cautery-induced artifact on telemetry
Cautery-induced inappropriate ICD shocks	Turn off tachy detection on device via the programmer (best) or Place and tape magnet over the device
Inadvertent device re-programming or device malfunction	Interrogate the device post-operatively to assess for threshold rises, reset modes, or changes in tachy mode Have backup transcutaneous pacer and defibrillator readily accessible. Staff should know make and model number of device as well as device settings and pacer dependency

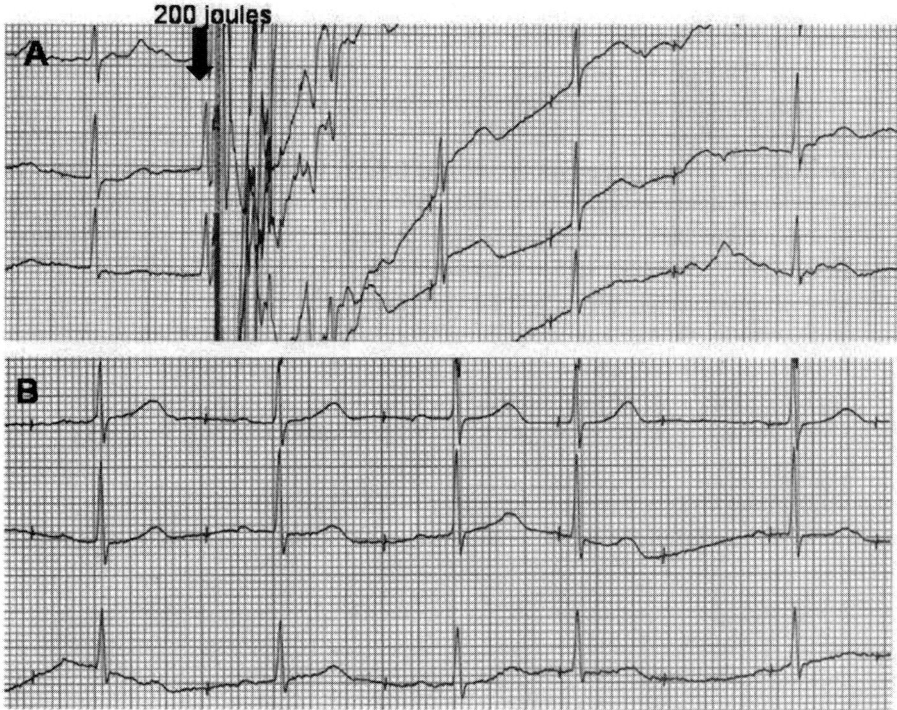

Figure 11.19. Loss of capture in a VVI pacemaker following DC cardioversion for atrial fibrillation **(Panel A)**. **Panel B** was obtained 3 minutes after the shock showing persistent loss of capture at the paced rate of 60 bpm. The threshold increased transiently from 0.6 to 3 V, but returned to baseline within 10 minutes.

lithotripsy, radiofrequency ablation, and radiation therapy. MRI presents a particularly noxious environment for cardiac devices. Potential interactions include reed switch closure, pacing inhibition, inappropriate ICD discharges, and rapid pacing. The latter can be initiated either from the pulse generator or, independently, by the induction of current flow along the lead. Lead dislodgment or the induction of torque on the generator itself remain possible, but with diminishing amounts of ferrous material in recently constructed systems there is much less rotational and translational forces brought to bear.[44] In general, the presence of a pacemaker or ICD should be considered a contraindication to MRI. Before device placement, the implanter should give careful thought to the potential need for MRI and, when feasible, complete the imaging before implant. In very rare situations, use of an MRI may be considered but only with close coordination and discussion among electrophysiologist, radiologist, and patient. Factors that may decrease the likelihood of complications include use of less powerful MRI machines, imaging of extremities (i.e., device not within gantry), careful re-programming of device, thoughtful selection of appropriate spin sequences, periprocedural monitoring, and restriction of scans to non–pacemaker-dependent patients.[45]

In the case of lithotripsy, distancing of the pacer from the focal point of the lithotripsy is recommended to avoid potential problems with undue inhibition of pacer output or irregular sensing.[46] This is particularly true in activity-sensing devices dependent on piezoelectric crystals. These crystals may be capable of oversensing shock waves and result in increased pacing rates; alternatively, they may be susceptible to damage (e.g., crystal is shattered) from the shock waves. Current recommendations in this procedure are:

1. Patients with piezoelectric activity-sensing rate-responsive pacemakers should not undergo lithotripsy if the device is implanted in the abdomen.
2. Patients with activity-sensing rate-adaptive pacemakers implanted in the thorax should have their rate-responsive features turned off.
3. The pulse generator must not be submerged below the water level in the tank.
4. Patients with implanted dual-chamber devices should be programmed to the VVI mode before lithotripsy.

Radiofrequency ablation is often undertaken in the EP lab to effect permanent cure of various atrial and ventricular tachyarrhythmias. This energy can at times result in reprogramming the device to a reset mode, or transiently cause asynchronous pacing due to noise reversion or pacemaker inhibition.[47] The latter can be particularly relevant in the patient undergoing AV node catheter ablation, which results in complete heart block and pacemaker dependency (Fig. 11.20). Re-programming the device to an asynchronous mode will prevent this issue from arising. RF energy can result in spurious shocks in those with ICDs. Antitachycardia therapies should be programmed "off." Rarely, threshold rises may be observed.

Radiation therapy (e.g., for breast or lung cancer) to the chest may be unavoidable in certain patients with pacemakers. Ionizing radiation can result in random component failure and premature battery depletion. To minimize this risk, appropriate methods of shielding the generator and limiting the field of radiation should be discussed with the radiation therapist. Damage may result in sudden loss of output, alterations in programmed parameters, and rate runaway. In rare instances, a newly placed contralateral system or generator repositioning using lead extenders should be considered. If included in the radiation field, the device should be interrogated after each treatment, however, delayed malfunctions may still occur.

It has also been recognized increasingly that cellular telephones may interfere with the function of implanted devices. In one study, the potential for any type of interference was 20%, with associated symptoms in 7.2%, when the telephone was placed over the generator.[48] The most common pacemaker interactions include tracking interference on the atrial channel followed by asynchronous pacing and ventricular inhibition. Potential ICD interactions include reed switch activation leading to VT under-detection and erroneous

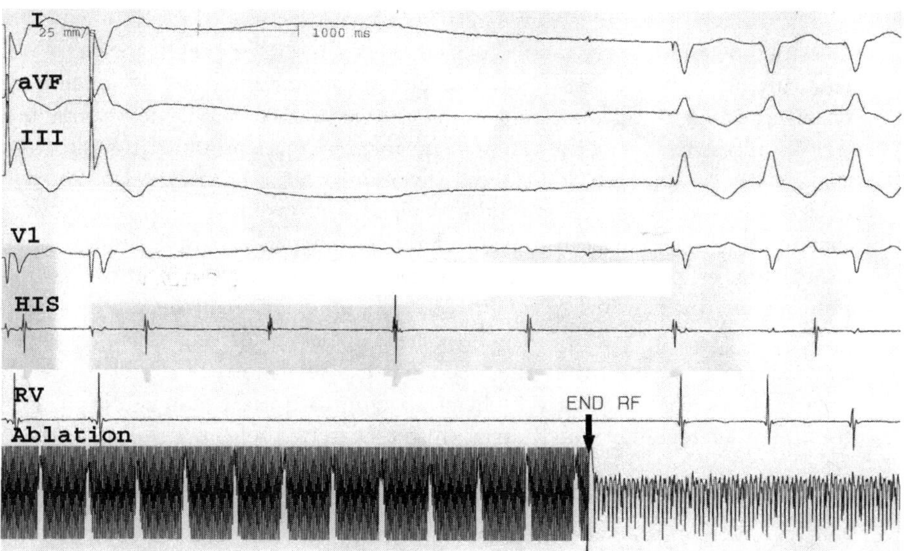

Figure 11.20. Multi-channel recording of a patient with a single lead ICD undergoing RF ablation of the AV node. The ablation is successful but the RF energy results in ventricular oversensing with resulting inhibition of ventricular pacing and CHB without escape. When the RF delivery is stopped, ventricular pacing resumes.

shock therapy, although latter reports have been extraordinarily rare. Interference was more common in older devices without feed-through filters. Interestingly, the incidence of interaction is similar between unipolar and bipolar devices. A reasonable recommendation would be to avoid placing cellular telephones in the breast pocket over the device.[49] Some advocate holding the telephone over the ear contralateral to the device. Particular care should be exercised with high-powered fixed cellular devices such as those in cars and boats.

Anti-theft surveillance systems are becoming ubiquitous in retail centers. Several different technologies are used to detect metal alloy-containing tags on merchandise. These have also been observed to potentially interact with implanted devices, resulting in inappropriate device triggering or, in the case of implanted defibrillators, inappropriate discharge.[50] In these situations, we observed one patient whose device reverts from dual-chamber pacing to single-chamber ventricular pacing with resultant pacemaker syndrome. These interactions appear to be clinically infrequent, particularly with diminishing use of acousto-magnetic technology. Patients should be told to walk through the store threshold without either lingering or leaning directly against the gates.[51,52] Similarly, patients may pass through security metal detectors without lingering but will trip the detector. Patients with implanted devices should notify security staff of the presence of the device. The metal-detecting wand may be passed over the device quickly in a single stroke. Repeated back-and-forth motions over the device are to be avoided.

Transcutaneous electronic nerve stimulation units (TENS) do not readily interfere with modern bipolar pacemakers. In pacemaker-dependent patients particularly with unipolar leads, the electrocardiography (ECG) tracing should be monitored during treatment or re-programmed to an asynchronous mode.[53] TENS units have clearly resulted in inappropriate defibrillator shocks (Fig. 11.21).[54] Patients with ICDs who absolutely require TENS should have the marker channel observed with the device in a "monitor-only" mode with the first treatment to rule out any interference. Electroconvulsive therapy is safe in the pacemaker patient. Medical diathermy should be avoided in the area of the pulse generator. A summary of EMI/Device interactions is shown in Table 11.7.

The pacer physician may be called upon to terminate tachyarrhythmias acutely, preferably without the need for cardioversion or defibrillation. Some devices allow for temporary high-rate pacing to greater than 300 ppm, allowing for the pace termination of atrial flutter. Rarely, application of a magnet with resultant asynchronous pacing may be successful in terminating a tachyarrhythmia. Re-programming the device to faster rates for overdrive pacing, or using the triggered mode with chest wall stimulation to "program in" extra stimuli, may also prove useful. Some devices allow for programmed stimulation in either chamber using the programmer. In all cases, the intervention should be undertaken cautiously with defibrillator backup.

The diagnosis of myocardial ischemia/infarction in the pacemaker patient is complicated by the left bundle branch block pattern imposed by right ven-

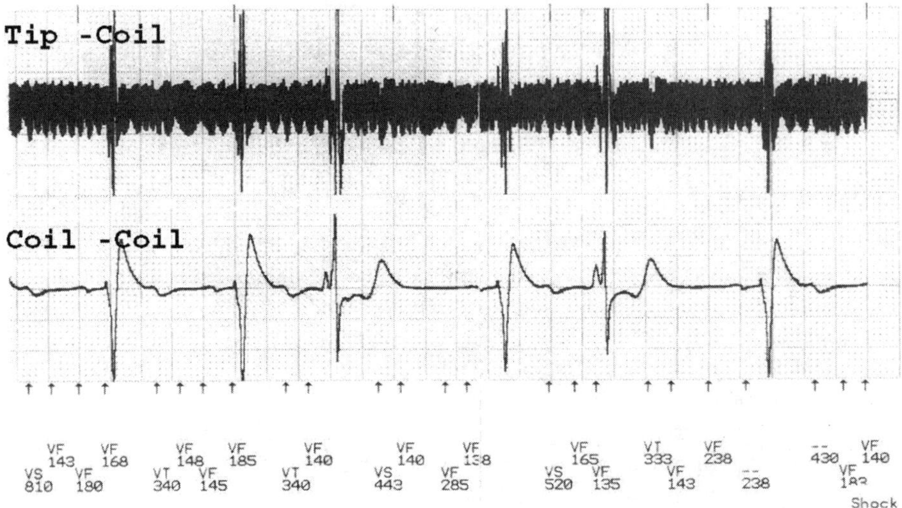

Figure 11.21. Intracardiac electrogram from a patient with a single lead ICD undergoing TENS. In hopes of achieving better pain relief, the patient independently turned up the output to maximum. This resulted in inappropriate detection of VF and high output shock delivery.

Table 11.7. Solutions to EMI/Device Interactions

Source of EMI	Solutions
Cellular telephones	Keep telephone out of breast pocket over device Use contralateral ear Keep fixed high-output telephones; i.e., car or boat phones at least 6 inches away from device
Electronic surveillance equipment	Walk through entranceway without pause
MRI	Avoid with pacemaker or ICD unless extreme circumstance
Airport Metal Detector	Inform security personnel of device; walking through detector will not harm implantable device but may trigger detector; request hand or wand search. Wand should not be held directly over ICD
DC Cardioversion	Place pads in anteroposterior position at least 5 cm away from generator. Backup transcutaneous brady pacing should be available in pacer-dependent patients. Use of biphasic shocks to minimize required energy device should be interrogated post shock
Household appliances (microwave ovens, television, toasters)	No specific concerns, avoid electrical shocks
Transcutaneous nerve stimulation (TENS)	Consider magnet use or re-programming to an asynchronous mode with unipolar pacemakers or with pacer-dependent patients ICD patients should proceed with caution and consider having the device monitored with the first session to assure no inappropriate detections
Radiation therapy	Discuss treatment with radiotherapist. Shield device particularly with treatment of thoracic tumors. Continuous EKG monitoring during treatment in pacemaker-dependent patients receiving high-dose treatment. Rarely, the device will need to be moved using lead extenders. Increase frequency of device monitoring
RF ablation	Re-program to asynchronous mode in pacemaker-dependent patients Turn "off" tachytherapy in ICDs Interrogate the device post-procedure

tricular pacing and the classic findings of ischemia are frequently obscured. In the setting of continuous ventricular pacing, acute infarction may produce subtle findings on electrocardiography. These findings may include development of small Q waves, alterations in the amplitude of the paced QRS complexes, new

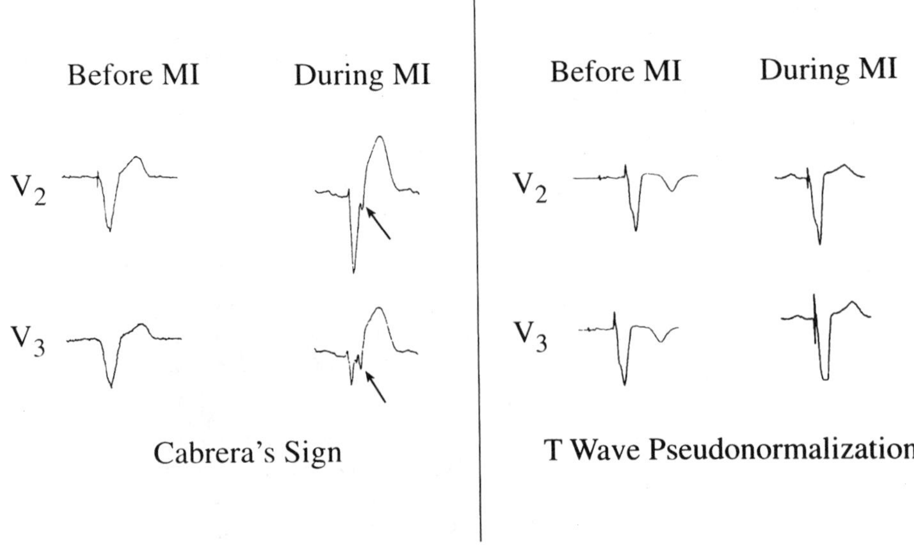

Figure 11.22. Diagnosis of myocardial ischemia in the setting of continuous ventricular pacing. **Left panel:** Precordial leads V_2 and V_3 before and during a documented acute anterior myocardial infarction. The late terminal notching of the ascending limb of the paced QRS complex is known as "Cabrera's sign" (*arrow*). Also note the increased ST segment elevation in these leads during infarction. **Right panel:** Pseudonormalization of the T waves in leads V_2 and V_3 during an acute infarction.

ST-segment elevation, T-wave changes or pseudonormalization, or notching of the terminal part of the paced QRS in the precordial leads (Cabrera's sign, Fig. 11.22).[55] All of these changes are best appreciated by comparing a current ECG with those previously recorded. Inhibition of the pacemaker with a programmer or asynchronous pacing during magnet application may reveal the patient's intrinsic QRS for a clearer diagnosis of ischemia. T-wave changes alone should be interpreted with caution in this setting because ventricular pacing may produce T-wave abnormalities, which are persistent after the discontinuation of pacing (T-wave memory). However, these post-pacing repolarization changes do not produce ST-segment elevation or depression.

REFERENCES

1. Schoenfeld MH. Quality assurance in cardiac electrophysiology and pacing: a brief synopsis. Pacing Clin Electrophysiol 1994;17:267–269.
2. Schoenfeld MH. Manpower concerns in cardiac electrophysiology and pacing. Pacing Clin Electrophysiol 1995;18:1977–1979.
3. Furman S. Cardiac pacing and pacemakers: VIII. Am Heart J 1977;94:795–804.

4. Griffin JC, Schuenenemyer TD, Hess KR, et al. Pacemaker follow up: i detection and correction of pacemaker system malfunction. Pacing (physiol 1986;9:387–391.
5. Furman S. Pacemaker follow-up. In: Furman S, Hayes DL, Holmes DR, eds. A Practice of Cardiac Pacing. 2nd ed. Mount Kisco, NY: Futura, 1989.
6. Levine PA. Proceedings of the policy conference of the North American Society of Pacing and Electrophysiology on programmability and pacemaker follow-up programs. Clin Prog Pacing Electrophysiol 1984;2:145–191.
7. DaCosta A, Kirkorian G, Cucherat M, et al. Antibiotic prophylaxis for permanent pacemaker implantation: a meta-analysis. Circulation 1998;97:1796–1801.
8. Schoenfeld MH. A primer on pacemaker programmers. Pacing Clin Electrophysiol 1993;16:2044–2052.
9. MacGregor DC, Covvey HD, Noble EJ, et al. Computer-assisted reporting system for the follow-up of patients with cardiac pacemakers. Pacing Clin Electrophysiol 1980;3:568–588.
10. Schoenfeld MH. Recommendations for implementation of a North American multicenter arrhythmia device/lead database. Pacing Clin Electrophysiol 1992;15: 1632–1636.
11. Byrd CL, Schwartz SJ, Gonzalez M, et al. Pacemaker clinic evaluations: key to early identification of surgical problems. Pacing Clin Electrophysiol 1986;9:1259–1264.
12. Hoffman A, Jost M, Pfisterer M, et al. Persisting symptoms despite permanent pacing. Incidence, causes, and follow-up. Chest 1984;85:207–210.
13. Ausubel K, Furman S. The pacemaker syndrome. Ann Intern Med 1985;103: 420–429.
14. Ellenbogen KA, Thames MD, Mohanty PK. New insights into pacemaker syndrome gained from hemodynamic, humoral and vascular responses during ventriculoatrial pacing. Am J Cardiol 1990;65:53–59.
15. Kenny RS, Sutton R. Pacemaker syndrome. BMJ 1986;293:902–903.
16. Deharo JC, Brunetto AB, Bellocci F, et al. DDDR pacing driven by contractility versus DDI pacing in vasovagal syncope: a multi-center, randomized study. Pacing Clin Electrophysiol 2003;26:447–450.
17. Connolly SJ, Sheldon R, Thorpe KE, et al. Pacemaker therapy for prevention of syncope in patients with recurrent severe vasovagal syncope: Second Vasovagal Pacemkaer Study (VPS II): a randomized trial. JAMA 2003;289:2224–2229.
18. Michaud GF, Pelosi F Jr, Noble MD, et al. A randomized trial comparing heparin initiation 6 h or 24 h after pacemaker or defibrillator implantation. J Am Coll Cardiol 2000;35:1915–1918.
19. Saliba BC, Ghantous AE, Schoenfeld MH, et al. Twiddler's syndrome with transvenous defibrillators in the pectoral region. Pacing Clin Electrophysiol 1999;22:1419–1421.
20. Steiner RM, Morse D. The radiology of cardiac pacemakers. JAMA 1978;240: 2574–2576.
21. Morse D, Parsonnet V, Gessman L, et al. eds. A guide to cardiac pacemakers, defibrillators, and related products. North Carolina: Droege Computing Services; 1991.
22. Mugica J, Henry L, Rollet M, et al. The clinical utility of pacemaker follow-up visits. Pacing Clin Electrophysiol 1986;9:1249–1251.
23. Schoenfeld MH. Pacemaker programmers: an updated synopsis. Cardiac Electrophysiol Rev 1999;3:20–23.
24. Blitzer ML, Marieb MA, Schoenfeld MH. Inability to communicate with ICDs: an underreported failure mode. Pacing Clin Electrophysiol 2001;24:13–15.

25. Levine PA, Sholder J, Duncan JL. Clinical benefits of telemetered electrograms in assessment of DDD function. Pacing Clin Electrophysiol 1984;7:1170–1177.
26. Sanders R, Martin R, Fruman H, Goldberg MK. Data storage and retrieval by implantable pacemakers for diagnostic purposes. Pacing Clin Electrophysiol 1984;7: 1228–1233.
27. Sholder J, Levine PA, Mann BM, et al. Bidirectional telemetry and interrogation. In: Barold SS, Mugica J, eds. Cardiac pacing. The third decade of cardiac pacing. Mount Kisco, NY: Futura, 1982:145–166.
28. Duffin EG Jr. The marker channel: a telemetric diagnostic aid. Pacing Clin Electrophysiol 1984;7:1165–1169.
29. Strathmore NF, Mond HG. Noninvasive monitoring and testing of pacemaker function. Pacing Clin Electrophysiol 1987;10:1359–1370.
30. Zinberg A. Transtelephonic follow-up. Clin Prog Pacing Electrophysiol 1984;2:177.
31. Famularo MA, Kennedy HL. Ambulatory electrocardiography in the assessment of pacemaker function. Am Heart J 1982;104:1086–1094.
32. Danilovic D, Ohm OH. Pacing threshold trends and variability in modern tined leads assessed using high resolution automatic measurements: conversion of pulse width into voltage thresholds. Pacing Clin Electrophysiol 1999;22:567–587.
33. Luceri RM, Hayes DL. Follow-up of DDD pacemakers. Pacing Clin Electrophysiol 1984;7:1187–1194.
34. Schoenfeld MH, Markowitz HT. Device follow-up in the age of automaticity. Pacing Clin Electrophysiol 2000;23:803–806.
35. Wilkoff BL, Cook JR, Epstein AE, et al. Dual-chamber pacing or ventricular backup pacing in patients with an implantable defibrillator: the Dual Chamber and VVI Defibrillator (DAVID) Trial. JAMA 2002;288:3115–3123.
36. Vardas PE, Simantrakis EN, Parthenakis FL, et al. AAIR versus DDDR pacing in patients with impaired sinus node chronotropy: an echocardiographic and cardiopulmonary study. Pacing Clin Electrophysiol 1997;20:1762–1768.
37. Meluzin J, Novak M, Mullerov AJ, et al. A fast and simple echocardiographic method of determination of the optimal atrioventricular delay in patients after biventricular stimulation. Pacing Clin Electrophysiol 2004;27:58–64.
38. Sogaard P, Egeblad H, Pedersen AK, et al. Sequential versus simultaneous biventricular resynchronization for severe heart failure. Circulation 2002;106:2078–2084.
39. Theuns DA, Res JC, Jordaens LJ. Home monitoring in ICD therapy: future perspectives. Europace 2003;5:139–142.
40. Schoenfeld MH, Compton SJ, Mead RH, et al. Remote monitoring of implantable cardioverter-defibrillators: a prospective analysis. Pacing Clin Electrophysiol (in press).
41. Barold SS, Schoenfeld MH. Pacemaker elective replacement indicators: latched or unlatched? Pacing Clin Electrophysiol 1989;12:990–995.
42. Barold SS, Schoenfeld MH, Falkoff MD, et al. Elective replacement indicators of simple and complex pacemakers. In: Barold SS, Mugica J, eds. New perspectives in cardiac pacing. 2nd ed. Mount Kisco, NY: Futura, 1991:493–526.
43. Levine PA, Barold SS, Fletcher RD, Talbot P. Adverse acute and chronic effects of electrical defibrillation and cardioversion of implanted unipolar cardiac pacing systems. J Am Coll Cardiol 1983;1:1413–1422.
44. Gimbel JR, Johnson D, Levine PA, et al. Safe performance of magnetic resonance imaging on five patients with permanent cardiac pacemakers. Pacing Clin Electrophysiol 1996;19:913–919.

45. Sommer T, Vahlhaus C, Lauck G, et al. MR imaging and cardiac pacemakers: In vitro evaluation and in vivo studies in 51 patients at 0.5 T. Radiology 2000;215:869–879.
46. Cooper D, Wilkoff B, Masterson M, et al. Effects of extracorporeal shock wave lithotripsy on cardiac pacemakers and its safety in patients with implanted cardiac pacemakers. Pacing Clin Electrophysiol 1988;11:1607–1616.
47. Pinski SL, Trohman RG. Interference in implanted cardiac devices, Part 1. Pacing Clin Electrophysiol 2002;25:1367–1381.
48. Hayes DL, Wang PJ, Reynolds DW, et al. Interference with cardiac pacemakers by cellular telephones. N Engl J Med 1997;336:1473–1479.
49. Blitzer ML, Schoenfeld MH. Effects of electromagnetic interference on implanted cardiac devices. In: Raviele A, ed. Cardiac arrhythmias 2003. Milan: Springer-Verlag Italia 2004:911–918.
50. Groh WJ, Boschee SA, Engelstein ED, et al. Interactions between electronic article surveillance systems and implantable cardioverter-defibrillators. Circulation 1999; 100:387–392.
51. McIvor ME, Reddinger J, Floden E, Sheppard RC. Study of pacemaker and implantable cardioverter defibrillator triggering by electronic article surveillance devices (SPICED TEAS). Pacing Clin Electrophysiol 1998;221:1847–1861.
52. Goldschlager N, Epstein A, Friedman P, et al. Environmental and drug effects on patients with pacemakers and implantable cardioverter defibrillators. Arch Intern Med 2001;161:649–655.
53. Eriksson M, Schuller H, Sjolund B. Hazards from transcutaneous nerve stimulation in patients with pacemakers. Lancet 1978;1:1319.
54. Philbin DM, Marieb MA, Aithal KH, Schoenfeld MH. Inappropriate shocks delivered by an ICD as a result of sensed potentials from a transcutaneous electronic nerve stimulation unit. Pacing Clin Electrophysiol 1998;21:2010–2011.
55. Barold SS, Falkoff MD, Ong LS, et al. Electrocardiographic diagnoses of myocardial infarction during ventricular pacing. Cardiol Clin 1987;5:403.

Index

A

AAIR pacing, 156

Ablation techniques, radiofrequency catheter, 42. *See also* Radiofrequency ablation

Accelerometers, 108, 109*f*
- advantage of, 112
- body motion detected by, 111
- in rate-adaptive pacing systems, 109–110, 109*f*

Accufix J lead, 248

Accufix wire fragment retrieval, for lead extraction, 257, 257*f*

Activity sensors
- compared with accelerometers, 111–112
- limitations of, 110–111
- and minute-ventilation sensing, 114
- in rate-adaptive systems, 109

Adolescents, pacing for, 27–29

Advanced life support, in pacemaker clinic, 501

AEI
- defined, 266*b*
- in ventricular-based timing system, 292, 294, 295*f*

Afterdepolarizations, 77–78

Air embolism
- avoidance of, 234*b*
- as implantation complication, 234

Alkalosis, ventricular capture in, 178

American College of Cardiology (ACC)
- guidelines of, 201, 259
- pacemaker criteria of, 4
- pacing codes introduced by, 266

American Heart Association (AHA)
- guidelines of, 201, 259
- pacemaker criteria of, 4
- pacing codes introduced by, 266
- on temporary pacing, 40

Amplitude of pacing stimulation, malfunction of, 331

Analgesia, for elective generator replacement. *See also* Pain

Anatomy
- in cardiac pacing, 2–3, 2*t*
- coronary venous, 426, 426*f*–428*f*

Anesthesia, for implantation procedures, 198, 215

Angina, in follow-up assessment, 506

Angioplasty, temporary pacing during, 41

Antiarrhythmics
- and pacemaker malfunction, 330
- and stimulation threshold, 61
- and ventricular thresholds, 178

Antibiotic prophylaxis, for pacemaker implantation, 205

Antibiotic therapy, recurrence of sepsis after, 245

Anticoagulation
- in cardiac perforation, 236
- and pacemaker implantation, 204–205

Antitachycardia pacing (ATP), 400, 401*f*
- burst and ramp, 401
- compared with low-energy cardioversion, 400, 402*f*
- risk of, 479

Antitachycardia therapies, 536

Arrhythmias. *See also specific arrhythmias*
  detected by ICDs, 397–399, 399*f*
  as lead placement complication, 234–235, 235*b*
Artifacts, recording, 337*f*, 338*f*, 350, 356–358
Aspiration, with transesophageal pacing, 187
ATP interval, in ICD programming, 474*t*
Atrial antitachycardia (AAI) pacemakers, 73
Atrial-based pacing, compared with ventricular pacing, 157–158
Atrial capture threshold test, 316I*f*
Atrial fibrillation
  alternating with bradycardia, 16*f*
  and inappropriate ICD therapy, 487*f*, 488*f*–489*f*
  intermittent ventricular tracking of, 528*f*
  morphology score for, 477*f*
  prevention algorithm in, 305
Atrial flutter
  electrograms during, 397*f*
  intermittent ventricular tracking of, 528*f*
  temporary pacing for, 42
Atrial flutter response (AFR), 304–305, 306*f*
Atrial lead implantation, 221–223
Atrial-only defibrillators, 407
Atrial pacing
  appropriate, 521*f*
  hemodynamic evaluation of, 139*t*
  synchronous (AOO), 268
Atrial refractory period (ARP), 281
Atrial sensing window (ASW), 277
Atrial synchronous (P-tracking) pacing, 277–278, 279*f*
Atrioventricular (AV) block
  acquired, 5
    differential diagnosis of, 10, 11*b*
    ECGs in, 5*f*, 6*f*, 8*f*, 9*f*
    escape rhythm in, 5, 6*f*, 10
    indications for permanent pacing in, 7–10, 8*f*, 9*f*, 10*f*
  AV sequential *vs.* VVI pacing for, 33*t*–34*t*
  common medications causing, 17*b*
  ECG in, 37*f*
  high-grade
    during acute MI, 39
    causes of, 11*b*
    escape rhythm in, 6*f*
  programming for, 56
  strength-duration relation in, 51*f*
  temporary pacing for, 36
Atrioventricular (AV) conduction, and mode selection, 155, 155*f*, 156
Atrioventricular (AV) delays, and optimal hemodynamics, 136
Atrioventricular (AV) interval, 283–289, 283*f*–285*f*, 287*f*, 288*f*
  appropriate programming of, 524–526
  atrial sensed *vs.* atrial paced, 137, 138*f*, 139
  differential, 286–288, 287*f*
  Doppler studies for, 137, 137*f*, 138*f*
  effects of, 136–137
  hemodynamics of short, 421, 421*f*
  hysteresis, 288–289
  and left ventricular performance, 422, 422*f*
  rate-adaptive, 288, 288*f*
Atrioventricular (AV) junction, ablation of, 423
Atrioventricular (AV) node
  anatomy of, 1, 2*t*
  physiology of, 3–4
Atrioventricular (AV) pacing
  atrial *vs.*, 139–140, 139*t*
  hemodynamic evaluation of, 124, 125*t*, 139*t*
  sequential, 178
Atrioventricular (AV) sequential asynchronous (DOO) pacing, 268, 269*f*
Atrioventricular (AV) synchronous pacing, ventricular pacing compared with, 136
Atrioventricular (AV) synchrony
  advantages of, 123–136, 135–136
  and atrial pressures, 130–135, 130f–135*f*
  benefits of, 126, 127*f*
  blood pressure in, 123–126, 123*f*–125*f*
  and cardiac output, 126–129
  hemodynamics of, 122–123
  in higher heart rates, 153
  and mode selection, 155, 157
  and pacemaker syndrome, 140
  and rate modulation, 153, 154*f*, 155
  and stroke volume, 151
Atrioventricular optimization, 421, 422*f*
Atrioventricular sequential, non-P-synchronous pacing
  with dual-chamber sensing, 276, 277*f*, 278*f*
  rate-modulated with dual-chamber sensing, 276–277

Atrioventricular sequential, ventricular inhibited (DV), 273, 274*f*
Atropine, in bradycardia, 36, 37
Automated capture features, 79–82, 80*f*
Automaticity, in follow-up assessment, 524
Automatic sensing alogorithm, 341
Autosensing functions, 82
AVID study, 381
A waves
  absense of, 419*f*
  giant, 133, 135
  in PCW pressures, 132–133
Axillary vein, thrombosis of, 239
Axillary vein approach, to pacemaker implantation, 211–212*f*, *213*

B
Back pain, with transesophageal pacing, 186
Bacteremia, in temporary pacing, 183
Bacterial endocarditis, temporary pacing in, 41–42
Bandpass filtering, signal processing with, 104–105, 105*f*
Base rate behavior
  atrial-based timing in, 295–296, 296*f*
  atrial fibrillation prevention algorithms in, 305
  atrial flutter response, 304–305, 306*f*
  automatic mode switch, 298
  and battery status, 533*t*
  comparison of atrial-based and ventricular-based systems, 296–298, 297*f*
  mode switching, 302–304, 303*f*, 305*f*
  rate smoothing, 306
  sensor input, 298
  and sinus preference, 305
  upper rate, 298–302, 299*f*, 300*f*
  ventricular-based timing, 292–294, 295*f*
  ventricular rate regularization, 306
Batteries
  decay characteristics of, 101, 101f
  depletion of, 467
  and elective replacement indicators, 469
  lithium-iodine, 98, 99–102, 99*f*
  longevity of, 100–101
  and pacemaker behavior, 533*t*
Beta blockers
  and ICD therapy, 383
  and stimulation threshold, 61
Bifascicular block
  in asymptomatic patients, 10–11
  indications for pacing in, 10–14
Bipolar leads
  insulation defects in, 331
  in minute-ventilation pacemakers, 115
Bipolar pacing
  advantages of, 65
  stimulation threshold in, 58–59
Bipolar split cathodal configuration, 65, 66*f*
Bipolar systems, pacing stimulus in, 325, 326*f*
Biventricular device implants, 157
Biventricular pacing, 65–67
  in advanced heart failure, 25
  complications of, 245
  in HOCM, 147
  and intrinsic conduction delay, 432, 434*f*
  12 lead ECGs of, 449*f*
  long-term benefits from, 149
  with loss of capture, 363
  polarities for, 434, 435*f*
  pulse generator configurations for, 434, 436*f*
  and ventricular hemodynamics, 148*f*
Biventricular pacing systems
  diaphragmatic stimulation in, 511
  growth in, 408
Blanking period, 106, 281
Bleeding
  as implantation complication, 243
  during pacemaker implantation, 234
Blood pressure
  and AV synchrony, 123–126, 123*f*–125*f*
  in follow-up clinic, 507
  as function of pacing mode, 511
Bradyarrhythmias
  percussion pacing for, 188
  temporary pacing for, 163
Bradyasystolic arrest, 189
Bradycardia
  in children, 27–28
  in sinus node dysfunction, 15
  temporary pacing for, 36
Bradycardia pacing, 402*f*
  by ICD, 483
  problems with, 482*f*
  and syncope, 495–496
"Buddy" wire, 256

Bundle branches
  anatomy of, 2*t,* 3
  physiology of, 2*t,* 4

C
CABG Patch trial, 383
Cabrera's sign, 540, 540*f*
Canadian Implantable Defibrillator Study (CIDS), 381–382
Canadian Trial of Physiologic Pacing (CTOPP), 32
Capacitance
  calculating, 100
  and defibrillation efficacy, 404
Capture, cardiac
  and functional noncapture, 339, 340*b*
  initiating and sustaining, 178
  in transcutaneous pacing, 164–165
Capture, failure to
  pacing stimuli absent with, 345
  stimuli present with, 325–339, 327*t*
Capture, loss of, 535*f*
  atrial, 353–354, 354*f*
  biventricular rhythms with, 363
  evaluation of, 326
  and exit block, 329
  and high thresholds, 329
  and lead dislodgment, 326, 328
  during magnet application, 531*f*
  pacing stimulus present with, 352–354, 352*f*–354*f*
  during transvenous pacing, 179*t*
  ventricular, 352–353, 353*f*
Capture thresholds
  high, 330
  in ventricular lead positioning, 221
Cardiac arrest, electrical capture in, 167
Cardiac contractility modulation, non-excitatory, 460
Cardiac index
  in paired stress testing, 152
  ventricular function curves for, 129*f*
Cardiac output
  and AV synchrony, 126–129
  in exercise physiology, 149–150
  in follow-up assessment, 506
  in transcutaneous pacing, 167
Cardiac resuscitation, cough-induced, 188
Cardiac resynchronization therapy (CRT), 65, 157
  ACC/AHA/NASPE Guidelines for, 451*b*
  clinical trials, 455–457, 456*t*
  clinical trials of, 455
  for dilated cardiomyopathy, 415–420
  functional mitral regurgitation in, 423
  fundamental premise of, 420
  implementation of, 423
  and incidence of heart failure, 415
  left ventricular and right ventricular capture, 444–445, 445*f*–450*f*
  mechanisms of, 421–423, 421*f,* 422*f*
  optimal LV lead placement in, 432–433, 433*f*
  pacemaker electrocardiography, 444–445, 445*f*–450*f*
  pacing systems for
    biventricular or univentricular stimulation in, 437–438
    leads and electrodes in, 433–437, 435*f*
  patient selection for, 450–455
  programming considerations in
    atrioventricular optimization, 440–442, 442*f*–443*f*
    interventricular timing, 444
    pacing modes, 438
    pacing outputs, 442, 444
    ventricular double-counting in, 439–440, 440*f,* 441*f*
  responders and nonresponders, 446–448, 450*f*–451*f*
  stimulation at LV free wall site in, 448, 451*f*
  surgical approach to LV lead placement, 431, 431*f*
  transvenous left ventricular lead placement in, 424–430, 424*f*–430*f*
Cardiac transplantation, orthotopic, 29–30
Cardiomegaly, 7
Cardiomyopathy. *See* Dilated cardiomyopathy; Hypertrophic obstructive cardiomyopathy
Cardiopulmonary resuscitation (CPR)
  for ICD patient, 483
  and transcutaneous pacing, 189
Cardioversion
  in ICD patient, 483
  intraprocedural, 235
  loss of capture during, 535*f*

Cardioverter defibrillators. *See* Implantable cardioverter defibrillators
Carditis, in Lyme disease, 42
Carotid sinus massage, 512
Carotid sinus syndrome
  hypersensitive, 20
  indications for pacemaker implantation in, 21–22
Catecholamines, and stimulation threshold, 61
Catheterization, cardiac, 40–41
Catheter placement
  confirmation of, 175–176
  with electrocariography, 175, 176*f*
  in transvenous pacing, 171
Catheters
  balloon-tipped, 175, 425*f*
  bipolar configuration of, 169
  placement of, 171–172
  pulmonary artery, 169, 171*f*, 172*f*
  transesophageal pacing, 185*f*
  in transvenous pacing, 169, 170*f*, 172, 173*f*, 174*f*
Cellular telephone
  pacemaker interactions with, 536
Central venous access, 196
Cephalic vein approach
  to lead extraction, 251–253
  to pacemaker implantation, 213–214, 214*f*
Chest pain
  in follow-up assessment, 509*t*
  with transesophageal pacing, 186
Chest radiographs
  of cardiac perforation, 237*f*
  displacement of terminal pin on, 335*f*
  following implantation, 324
  in follow-up assessment, 500
  insulation defect on, 334, 334*f*
  lead fracture on, 332*f*
Children, pacing for, 27–29
Chronaxie, on strength-duration curve, 50–51, 51*f*, 52
Chronotropic assessment exercise protocol (CAEP), 152, 152t, 153
Chronotropic competence
  in follow-up assessment, 506
  and mode selection, 155, 155*f*
Chronotropic incompetence, 225
  diagnosis of, 151–152
  and recurrence of symptoms, 350–351
  in sinus node dysfunction, 16, 17
Circadian response, 279
Classification, for pacemaker implantation, 4–5
  for adolescents, 28–29
  AV block, 7–10, 8*f*, 9*f*, 10*t*
  bifascicular and trifascicular block, 14
  for children, 28–29
  in dilated cardiomyopathy, 25
  following AMI, 30–31
  in hypersensitive carotid sinus syncope, 22
  in hypertrophic cardiomyopathy, 24
  in neurogenic syncope, 22
  orthotopic cardiac transplantation, 29
  sinus node dysfunction, 17–18
  in tachycardia, 27
Classification, for temporary pacing, 40
Clavicle, in venous access, 206, 208*f*
Clinic, follow-up, 501–503, 502*b*. *See also* Follow-up assessment
Clinical trials, CRT
  COMPANION, 408, 452, 457, 458*t*, 459
  CONTAK cardioverter-defibrillator, 457, 458*t*
  MIRACLE ICD, 448, 456*t*, 457, 458*t*
  M-PATHY study, 23–24
Code, pacing, 266–268
Committed AV sequential pacing, 275, 275*f*
COMPANION clinical trial, 408, 452, 457, 458*t*, 459
Complications, implantation
  acute, 231*b*
  air embolism, 234
  bleeding, 234
  costs of, 231
  delayed, 232*b*
  incidence of, 231
  infection, 244
  lead placement associated with, 234
  of upgrading, 232
  of venous access, 232–234
Conduction system
  anatomy of, 2–3, 2*t*
  histology of, 2*t*, 3
  myocardial fibrosis and, 49–50
  physiology of, 2*t*, 3–4
  temporary pacing for, 38–39

Conductors
braided, 89, 90f
coaxial, 91, 92f
coiled, 89, 90f
design of, 89
fracture, 334, 336
Congestive heart failure, in follow-up assessment, 506
Connectors, lead
bipolar, 96f
design of, 96–98
varieties of, 97f
Consultation, for pacemaker implantation, 198
CONTAK cardioverter-defibrillator, 457, 458*t*
Contrast solution, in pacemaker implantation, 210
Cook Extraction Registry, 249
Cook stylet, 252*f*
Coronary artery disease, DCM associated with, 415
Coronary sinus
cannulation of, 424*f*
venous anatomy of, 426, 426*f*–428*f* (*see also* Venography)
venous tortuousity of, 427, 429*f*
Corticosteroids. *See also* Steroids
and pacing thresholds, 58
and stimulation threshold, 61
Cough
cardiac resuscitation induced by, 189, 191
in neurally mediated syncope, 18–19
Coupling interval, in ICD programming, 473*t*
Crosstalk, 274
and blanking period, 106
defined, 357
evaluation of, 357–359, 357*f*–359*f*
FFRW, 358
in follow-up assessment, 527*f*
sensing window in, 286
and ventricular blanking period, 275
Crosstalk detection window, 358*f*
Crosstalk sensing window, 286

D
DAVID study, 387, 400
DDD pacing mode, selection of, 32
DDDR pacing mode
and cardiac indices, 152
differentiating fusion from capture in, 81
Death, cardiac
in bifascicular block, 11
incidence of, 455
prevention of sudden, 380
Decrement, in ICD programming, 473*t*
Defecation, in neurally mediated syncope, 18–19
Defibrillation
achieving, 400–401, 403
external, 483
and generator damage, 532, 534
shock polarity in, 403
tilt monophasic shock, 403, 403*f*
Defibrillation success curve, 390*f*, 391
Defibrillation threshold (DFT)
and anatomic position, 405–406
effect of drugs on, 480*b*
high, 406*t*
and implantation safety margin, 406
measurement of, 407
and pulse generator size, 404
testing for, 389, 391*t*, 392, 392*f*, 393
in triad configuration, 404–405
Defibrillation threshold testing, 471
Defibrillation waveforms, 401, 403, 403*f*
Defibrillators, in pacemaker clinic, 501. *See also* Implantable cardioverter-defibrillator
DEFINITE study, 383
Deltopectoral groove, in venous access, 206, 208f
Dependency, pacemaker, 515–516, 516*f*
Detection, in ICD programming, 472*t*
Detection enhancements, for ventricular tachyarrhythmia, 476*t*
Device behavior, features affecting, 266, 267*b*. *See also* Base rate behavior
Dexamethasone. *See also* Steroids
in electrode design, 85
and pacing thresholds, 58
Diagnostics, pacemaker, 363
electrograms, 366, 368–369*f*
event counters, 367, 369, 370*f*, 371*f*, 372, 373*f*, 374
event markers, 366

measured data, 364, 366
stored data, 367
Diaphragmatic stimulation
in follow-up assessment, 508
on physical examination, 511
Diathermy, electrical interference from, 72
Digital sampling, and recording artifacts, 336, 338*f*
Dilated cardiomyopathy, 24–25
abnormal electrical timing in, 415–420
and AV sequential pacing, 178
biventricular pacemaking in, 196
heart failure associated with, 415
indications for pacing in, 25
Dilator, in pacemaker implantation, 210
Dilator-sheath technique, 209
DINAMIT study, 383
Discharges, ICD
isolated, 484, 486, 487*f*
multiple appropriate, 486, 495, 496*f*
multiple inappropriate, 486–492, 487*f*–492*f*, 496, 496*f*
Dislodgment
in follow-up visit, 503
in transvenous pacing, 179
Documentation
of implant procedure, 323
importance of, 258–259
Doppler analysis
for AV interval, 136, 137f, 138*f*
for CRT patients, 453
in CRT programming, 440
mitral inflow patterns, 417, 418*f*
transmitral blood flow, 441, 442*f*, 443*f*
Double counting
due to loss of atrial tracking, 439, 440*f*
example of, 489, 490*f*
prevention of ventricular, 440, 441*f*
"Double tachycardia," 492
Driving restrictions, in ICD follow-up, 467
Drugs. *See also* Medications; *specific drugs*
defibrillation threshold elevated by, 480*b*
toxicity, 8
transient bradycardia caused by, 17*b*, 42
Dual Chamber and VVI Implantable Defibrillator (DAVID), 143. *See also* DAVID study
Dual-chamber ICD systems, evolution of, 386–387, 387*f*, 398–400
Dual-chamber pacemakers, 143
AP chest radiograph of, 207*f*
preservation of AV synchrony using, 156
Dual-chamber pacing
acute hemodynamic effects of, 23, 23*f*
advantages to, 31–32
afterdepolarizations in, 78
hemodynamic benefit of, 24
potential adverse effects of, 400
rate-modulated, 142–143
and sensing with inhibition and tracking, 278–279, 280*f*, 281
with single lead, 74
vs. backup pacing, 143
Dual-chamber pacing systems
correct lead connection in, 242
discrimination enhancement features in, 478*f*
and pacemaker syndrome, 141
revision of, 226*f*
ventricular lead positioning in, 217–221
Dual-chamber rate-modulated (DDDR) pacing
risks of, 156
and timing cycles, 307–313, 307*f*–312*f*
Dual-chamber systems
evaluation of crosstalk in, 357–359, 357*f*–359*f*
in follow-up assessments, 527–529
malfunction evaluation of
classes of, 351–352
with sensing problems, 355–357
stimulus present with loss of capture, 352–354, 352*f*–354*f*
myopotential triggering of ventricular pacing in, 511
pacemaker-mediated tachycardias in, 359–363, 361*f*, 362*f*
Dyspnea, in follow-up assessment, 507, 507*f*, 509*t*

E

Echocardiogram, in cardiac perforation, 237*f*
Edema, in follow-up assessment, 509*t*, 511
Ejection fraction
and AV synchrony, 125t, 135
in biventricular pacing, 149
Elective replacement indicators (ERIs), 469, 531

Electrical cycle, events of cardiac, 417*f*
Electrical timing. *See* Disordered electrical timing
Electrocardiogram (ECG)
  after pacemaker implantation, 229
  from DDDR pacemaker, 308*f*
  during lead placement, 235
  paced, 265
  during pacemaker implantation, 200
  perforated pacing catheter on, 182*f*
Electrocardiographic guidance, for catheter placement, 175, 176*f*
Electrocardiography, CRT, 444–445, 445*f*–450*f*
Electrocautery
  complications with, 242
  effect on ICD of, 481
  and generator damage, 532, 534
  interference from, 72
  in lead extraction, 251
Electrode-myocardial interface
  inflammatory reaction at, 344
  injury at, 329
Electrodes
  active fixation leads for, 86–89, 87*f*, 88*f*
  capacitance of, 67
  chemical composition of, 84
  in CRT pacing systems, 433–437, 435*f*
  design of, 83
  epimyocardial, 95
  fixation mechanism of, 86, 87*f*
  microdislodgement of, 62–63
  orthogonal, 74
  permanent transvenous pacing, 87*f*
  and QRS morphology, 177, 177*t*
  shape of, 83
  steroid-eluting, 84–86, 85*f*
  surface structure of, 83–84
  in transesophageal pacing, 186
Electrogram (EGM)
  after implantation, 324
  atrial, 488*f*
  bipolar atrial, 368*f*–369
  diagnostics with, 366–367
  far-field R wave on cardiac, 73, 73*f*, 74
  lead dislodgment on, 328
  low amplitude, 342*t*
  stored, 396–397, 397*f*, 398*f*
  transesophageal cardiac, 186, 187*f*
  unipolar, 175, 176*f*, 177
  ventricular, 488*f*
Electrogram (EGM), intracardiac
  bipolar, 72
  characteristics of, 69–71
  high-pass filtering of, 70
  intrinsic deflection in, 69, 70*f*
  telemetry of, 107
  time-related changes in, 78
Electrogram morphology (EGM), 477*f*
Electromagnetic interference (EMI), 345
  device interactions with, 539*t*
  effect on ICD, 481
  ICD therapy triggered by external, 491–492
  sources of, 534–535
  susceptibility to, 244
Emergencies
  equipment for, 200
  single-chamber pacing in, 177–178
  transcutaneous pacing in, 164
  transvenous pacing in, 175, 189
Emphysema, and transcutaneous pacing thresholds, 165–166
End-diastolic volume index (EDVI), 129*f*
Endless-loop tachycardia (ELT), 314–317, 360, 361*f*
  in atrial capture threshold test, 316, 316*f*
  automatic termination of, 360, 362*f*
  in biventricular pacing, 361
Endocardial activation maps, electroanatomic, 453*f*
Endocarditis
  pacemaker associated, 244–245
  temporary pacing in, 41–42
Epicardial pacing, 183, 184*f*
Epicardium, pacing leads sutured to, 95, 95*f*
Epinephrine, and ventricular thresholds, 178
Erb's dystrophy, 7, 8
Erosion
  of generator, 509
  pacemaker, 510*f*
  of pacing hardware, 242–243, 243*f*
Escape rhythm, after mitral valve replacement, 516*f*
Esophageal lead, 354
Evaluation, outpatient pacemaker, 324. *See also* Follow-up assessment

Event counters
subsystem performance, 369, 371*f*, 372*f*
time-based system performance, 369, 372, 373, 373*f*
total system performance, 367, 369, 370*f*
Event logs, in device interrogation, 469, 470*f*
Event markers, function of, 366
Event rercords, histograms of, 519, 519*f*
Excitability, property of, 47
Excitable tissues, characteristics of, 48
Exercise
accelerometers during, 111–112
and QT interval, 115
and rate-adaptive pacing systems, 110–111
rate adaptive response to, 114
as work, 150
Exercise intolerance, in follow-up assessment, 509*t*
Exercise physiology, and rate modulation, 149–151, 150*f*
Exercise test, in sinus node dysfunction, 16
Exercise tolerance
in follow-up assessment, 506
in sinus node dysfunction, 15, 16–17
Exertional intolerance, 151
Exit block, 61, 61*f*, 329
Extracardiac signals, inappropriately sensed, 491, 491*f*–493*f*
Extraction Registry, 249

F
Faradic resistance, 69
Far-field R wave (FFRW), 358, 491*f*
Fatigue, in sinus node dysfunction, 15, 16
Femoral approach, to lead extraction, 253–257, 258*f*–*259f*
Fibrosis, myocardial, 49
Fibrous capsule
development of, 56–57
surrounding electrode, 56, 57f
Fibrous tissue, and lead maturation, 329
Fick principle, 150
Fixation technologies
active, 86–89, 87*f*, 88*f*
in CRT, 425
passive, 86
Flecainide, and stimulation threshold, 61
Fluoropolymers, as lead insulators, 386
Fluoroscopy
digital capabilities for, 199
during generator insertion, 225
in lead extraction, 250, 252
in lead implantation, 217
in pacemaker implantation, 211, 212*f*, 213
in patient follow-up, 501, 502*b*
requirements for, 197
in transvenous pacing, 171–172, 173f, 174f
ventricular lead extraction with, 255*f*
Follow-up after ICD placement
device interrogation, 468–469
history in, 468
immediate, 467
physical examination in, 468
procedures during, 481–483
programming and, 471–480, 472*t*–474*t*
system component testing, 469–480
Follow-up assessment
atrioventricular interval in, 524, 525
common symptoms in, 509*t*
dual-chamber systems in, 527–529
elective replacement indicators in, 531–532, 531*f*
electrocardiography in, 513–515
immediate postimplantation period, 500–501
outpatient monitoring in, 529–530, 530*f*
pacemaker dependence in, 515–516, 516*f*
physical examination in, 508–509, 511–512
programmers in, 517
radiography in, 512, 513*f*
sensing threshold determination in, 520–524, 521*f*, 522*f*
telemetry in, 517–520, 518*f*–520*f*
Framingham study, 415

G
Generator/defibrillator, transcutaneous pacing, 163, 164*f*
Generators. *See also* Pulse generators
compatibility with leads of, 227, 229*t*
complications associated with, 231*b*
esophageal pacing, 185
implantation of, 214–215
indications for changing, 227
insertion of, 225–229
magnet-related pacing rate of, 102

miniaturization of, 196
problems with, 241–244, 242*f*
radiographic identification of, 513*f*
registration of, 230
temporary external transvenous pacing, 172*f*
temporary pacing, 169
transcutaneous pacing, 163, 164*f*
transesophageal pacing, 185–186, 185*f*
Glucocorticoids, and ventricular thresholds, 178
Glucose, and ventricular thresholds, 178
Guidewires, 424*f*

H
Heart block
and pacemaker dependence, 516*ff*
risk score for, 39
transcutaneous pacing during, 166f
Heart block, congenital
pacing for, 27–29
permanent pacing in, 28
Heart failure
abnormal electrical timing in, 415–420
cardiac contractility modulation for, 460
early detection of, 408
incidence of, 415
indications for pacing in, 25
and right ventricular pacing, 142–143, 158
Heart rate
in exercise physiology, 150, 151
histogram, 290*f*
and minute ventilation, 114
and response to exercise, 154f
and treadmill testing, 114
and VA conduction, 507*f*
Heart transplantation. *See* Cardiac transplantation
Hematoma
as implantation complication, 243
pocket, 503, 508
Hemodynamics
of alternative site right ventricular pacing, 141–142
of atrioventricular synchrony, 122–1434
in hypertrophic obstructive cardiomyopathy, 144–149
Hemothorax, as implantation complication, 233
Heparin, low-molecular-weight, 204. *See also* Anticoagulation
His bundle
anatomy of, 1, 2*t*, 3
physiology of, 2*t*, 3–4
recordings
in AV block, 13*f*
in chronic bifascicular block, 12, 12*f*
Histograms
of event records, 519, 519*f*
heart rate, 290*f*
Holter monitor
inhibition of pacing on, 522, 522*f*
insulation defect on, 332–333
loss of ventricular capture on, 530*f*
Wenckebach phenomenon on, 506*f*
Hormonal levels, and ventricular pacing, 136
Hydration, for pacemaker implantation, 204
Hyperglycemia
stimulation threshold during, 60
ventricular capture in, 178
Hyperkalemia
and pacemaker malfunction, 330
stimulation threshold during, 60
and ventricular thresholds, 178
Hypertensive heart disease, and AV sequential pacing, 178. *See also* Blood pressure
Hypertrophic cardiomyopathy, 128, 129
and AV sequential pacing, 178
indications for pacing in, 22–23
obstructive (HOCM)
dual-chamber pacing in, 144–145
impact of AV sequential pacing on, 145, 146f–147f
permanent pacing for, 24
Hypotension
rationale for pacing in, 126
in ventricular pacing, 126
Hypoxemia, stimulation threshold during, 60
Hypoxia
in sleep apnnea, 8
ventricular capture in, 178
Hysteresis
pauses associated with, 350
programming of, 289–292, 290*f*, 291*f*
refinement of search, 289, 292
types of, 289

I
Impedance
calculating, 66–67
defined, 62
determination of, 62
evolution of, 63
high atrial lead, 518*f*
measurement-to-measurement changes in, 330
in minute-ventilation sensing, 113, 113f, 114
polarization, 63, 64f, 79
sensing, 78–79
tripolar transthoracic, 113, 113f, 114
Implantable cardioverter-defibrillators (ICDs)
arrhythmia detection of, 397–399, 399*f*
atrial defibrillators, 407
clinical trials with, 481–484
evolution of, 380
indications for, 380–384, 381*b*
intra-operative management of, 532, 534, 534*t*
lead systems for, 385 (*see also* Lead design)
longevity of, 409
primary function of, 408
pulse generators for, 384 (*see also* Pulse generators)
rate sensing in, 394–397, 394*f*–395*f*, 397*f*
remote monitoring of, 409
stored electrograms in, 396–397, 397*f*, 398*f*
Implantable cardioverter-defibrillator (ICD) therapies, 143
arrhythmia discrimination in, 408
defibrillation, 400, 401, 403–407
evolution of, 409
pacing, 398–400
Implantation, ICD, 387. *See also* Follow-up
defibrillation testing in, 388–389, 390*f*–391*f*
follow-up after, 393
principles of, 387–388
venous access for, 388
Implantation, pacemaker, 196
approaches to
axillary vein, 211–212*f*, *213*
cephalic vein, 213–214, 214*f*
subclavian, 209
causes of arrhythmia during, 235*b*
complications of, 231–249
cost-effectiveness of, 202
decision process for, 203f
documentation of, 323–324
ECG during, 200
epicardial and transmyocardial lead placement in, 223–224
generator insertion, 225–229
inflammatory response to, 57, 57f
lead insertion in, 215–217
atrial implantation, 221–223
ventricular positioning, 217–221
logistical requirements for, 198–200
medical-legal aspects of, 258–259, 259*b*
pacemaker pocket in, 214–215
patient assessment for, 200–202, 203f
patient preparation for, 205–206
physician qualifications for, 197–198
post-procedure management of, 229–230
preimplantation orders, 204–205
procedure for, 206–214
single-lead VDD pacing, 224–225
sites for, 205, 206, 208f, 483
surface landmarks for, 208f
team approach to, 197
Infection
as complication, 244–245
in temporary pacing, 183
Inflammatory response, to pacemaker implantation, 57, 57f
Informed consent, 201, 202
Insulation
failure, 342*t*
lead
defects in, 330–334, 341, 344
evolution of, 386
for permanent pacing, 91
polyurethane, 93, 93t, 94, 94f
silicone rubber, 91, 93t
Internet, and patient monitoring systems, 530
Interrogation, device
event logs, 469, 470*f*
programmed parameters for, 468–469
system data in, 469
Interventricular delay
defined, 418
in dilated cardiomyopathy, 416–419
Interventricular refractory period (IVRP), 77
Intravascular hemodynamic monitors, 408
Intraventricular conduction disorders, temporary pacing for, 38–40

delay, 419–420

on threshold, 61
de pointes, 43
and ventricular thresholds, 178

J
J retention wire, 89, 199
J-shaped active-fixation lead, 222, 222*f*

K
Kearns-Sayre syndrome, 7, 8

L
Laboratory tests, pre-implant, 204
Lead conductor fractures, 512
Lead design, 82
 conductors in, 89–91
 connectors in, 96
 electrodes, 83–89
 insulation in, 91–94
Lead-extraction kit, 250
Lead placement
 complications associated with, 231*b*, 234–244
 dislodgment rates and, 238–239
 indications for replacement, 348*t*
 left ventricular
  optimal, 432–433, 433*f*
  surgical approach to, 431, 431*f*
  transvenous approach to, 424–425, 424*f*, 425*f*
 parameters for, 221t, 223
 transvenous left ventricular, 425*f*, 426–430, 426*f*–430*f*
Leads. *See also* Atrial lead implantation; Ventricular lead positioning
 abandonment of, 258
 characteristics of, 216b
 coaxial, 336
 compatibility with generators of, 227, 229*t*
 components of, 82
 in CRT pacing systems, 433–437, 435*f*
 discontinued styles, 227
 dislodgment of, 326, 328, 342*t*
  atrial, 222*f*
  incidence of, 231
  and undersensing, 344
 epicardial placement, 223
 epimyocardial, 95, 95f
 extraction of
  Accufix wire fragment retrieval, 257, 257*f*
  cephalic approach, 251
  complications of, 247
  coronary venous leads, 258
  documentation for, 258–259
  femoral approach to, 253–257, 258*f*–*259f*
  indications for, 246*b*, 247–249
  information for, 250*b*
  principles of, 245–247
  risk of death from, 249
  technique for, 249–251, 254*f*
  thoracotomy for, 258
  tools for, 251–258, 252*f*, 254*f*
 failure of, 248, 512
 fracture of, 89, 238, 493*f*
  diagnosis of, 332*f*
  in follow-up assessment, 518*f*
 implantation of, 215–217
 registration of, 230
 transmyocardial placement, 223, 224*f*
Lead systems
 evolution of, 385
 insulation for, 386
 triad configuration for, 404
 types of, 385*f*, 386
 unipolar configuration for, 404
Left bundle branch block
 biventricular sensing in, 439, 439*f*
 complete, 10
Left ventricle
 dysfunction, 7
 filling velocities for, 418*f*
 and prolonged native AV conduction, 416, 419*f*
 pumping function of, 423
Left ventricular pacing
 hemodynamics of, 145–149
 and intrinsic conduction delay, 432, 434*f*
Left ventricular stimulation thresholds, high, 427–430, 429*f*, 430*f*
Left ventricular systolic dysfunction, 24–25. *See also* Cardiomyopathy, dilated
Left ventricular systolic pressure, in transcutaneous pacing, 167
Lithium-iodine batteries, 98, 99–102, 99f
 advantage of, 99–100
 decay characteristics of, 101, 101f

pacemaker behavior with, 531–532, 533*t*

Lithotripsy
effect on ICD of, 481
procedure, 536

Lyme disease, 8, 42

M

MADIT II (clinical trial), 143, 382, 384

Magnesium, in torsades de pointes, 43

Magnet application
for detailed pacemaker analysis, 513–515, 514*t*
tachycardia therapies inactivated by, 481, 515

Magnetic resonance imaging (MRI)
effect on ICD of, 481
EMI from, 534–535

Magnet pacing, transtelephone monitoring of, 505*t*, 529–530

Malfunction, pacemaker
diagnosis of, 322
end-of-life, 531
in follow-up assessment, 507
manufacturer notification for, 503
misinterpretations of, 324

Malfunction evaluation
baseline data for, 323–324, 323*b*
differential diagnosis in, 375
of dual-chamber systems
classes of, 351–352
crosstalk, 357–359, 357*f*–359*f*
pacemaker-mediated tachycardias, 359–363, 361*f*, 362*f*
with sensing problems, 355–357
stimulus present with loss of capture, 352–354, 352*f*–354*f*
high thresholds in, 328–330
of single-chamber systems, 324–325
and recurrence of symptoms, 350–351, 351*f*
stimuli absent with failure to capture, 345–350, 346*f*, 347*f*, 348*t*
stimuli present with failure to capture, 325–339, 327*t*
stimuli present with failure to sense, 339–345

Maximum sensor rate (MSR), 308, 310
pacing at, 315*f*
rate response of DDR pacemaker at, 309*f*
and timing systems, 313

Maximum tracking rate (MTR), 308–312
exceeding, 309–120, 311–312
graphical presentation of, 76
rate response of DDR pacemaker at, 309*f*
ventricular tracking at, 302

Measured data, 364, 366

Mechanical pacing systems, 188–189

Medial subclavicular musculotendinous complex, and malfunction, 331

Medicare
ICD approval of, 383
registry mandated by, 502

Medications. *See also* Drugs; *specific medications*
defibrillation threshold elevated by, 480*b*
transient bradycardia caused by, 17*b*, 42

Meta-analysis, of prophylactic antibiotics, 500

Metal detectors
electrical interference from, 72
and inappropriate device triggering, 537

Microdislodgment, of electrodes, 62–63

Microprocessor based pacemaker, implantation of, 196

Microwaves, electrical interference from, 72

Micturition, in neurally mediated syncope, 18–19

Minute ventilation, 108
defined, 112
sensors, 112–115

MIRACLE implantable cardioverter-defibrillator, 448, 456*t*, 457, 458*t*

Misinterpretation, of normal function, 350

Mitral regurgitation
assessment of, 468
reduction in functional, 423

Mitral valve replacement, temporary pacing in, 516*f*

Mixed venous oxygen saturation sensors, 116

Modes, pacing, 317–318
atrial inhibited pacing, 270–271, 270*f*, 271*f*
atrial synchronous, 268, 277–278, 279*f*
AV sequential, non-P-synchronous, 276, 277*f*, 278*f*
AV sequential, ventricular inhibited, 273, 274*f*
AV sequential asynchronous, 268, 269*f*
committed AV sequential pacing, 275, 275*f*
in CRT, 438

dual-chamber, 278–279, 280*f*, 281
and patient assessment, 201
rate-modulated pacing, 272–273
single-chamber triggered-mode, 271–272
unsafe, 244
ventricular asynchronous, 268, 268*f*
ventricular inhibited pacing, 269, 269*f*, 270*f*
and ventricular refractoriness, 275
Mode selection
guidelines for, 157
in ventricular pacing, 155–158
MOde Selection Trial (MOST), 142
Mode switching, 302–304, 303*f*, 305*f*
automatic, 529*f*
functions, 155–156
programming and, 528*f*
Monitoring
home based remote, 469, 470*f*
during postimplantation surgery, 481
transtelephonic, 503, 505*t*
Morphology scores, 477*f*
M-PATHY study, 23–24
MSR. *see* Maximum sensor rate
MTR. *See* Maximum tracking rate
MTR interval, 299, 300, 300*f*
Multicenter Investigation of Limitation of Infarct Size (MILIS) study, 39
Multisite pacing, 434, 435*f*
Muscular atrophy, peroneal, 7, 8
Muscular dystrophy, myotonic, 8
MUSTT trial, 382
Myocardial infarction
and AV sequential pacing, 178
in continuous ventricular pacing, 540*f*
ECG in, 37*f*
high-grade AV block during, 39*t*
large anteroseptal, 31*f*
in pacemaker patient, 538–540
permanent pacing after, 30–31
temporary pacing for, 32, 35
Myocardial ischemia
in pacemaker patient, 538–540
ventricular capture in, 178
Myocardial stimulation
effects of pacing rate on, 59–60–60*f*
electrophysiology of, 47–50
elements of, 47
stimulation threshold in, 50–59
Myocardium, inflammatory reaction of, 329
Myopectoral stimulation, in follow-up assessment, 508
Myopotentials
from diaphragm or pectoral muscles, 396
pacing inhibited by, 522*f*
reducing sensitivity to, 347
sensing on ventricular lead, 492*f*
Myotomy-myectomy, in hypertrophic cardiomyopathy, 24

N
Na+-K+ ATPase exchange pump, 47–48
Native signal, change in, 340
Neck turning, presyncope associated with, 20, 21*f*
Needle's eye device, 253, 256
Neurocardiogenic syncope. *See also* Syncope
cardiac pacing for, 19–21
forms of, 18
indications for pacemaker implantation in, 21–22
Neurologic stimulation units, effect on ICD of, 481
Noise, from insulation break, 521*f*
Noise mode operation, 345
Noise mode response, 281
Noise reversion circuits, 105
Nomenclature, pacing, 266–268
Noncapture, functional, 339, 340*b*
Noncompetitive atrial pacing (NCAP), 317
North American Society of Pacing and Electrophysiology (NASPE), guidelines of, 259

O
Open-heart surgery, temporary pacing for, 41
Orthostatic hypotension, rational for pacing in, 22
Orthotopic cardiac transplantation, 29–30
Outpatients, monitoring, 529–530, 530*f*. *See also* Follow-up assessment
Outpatient visits
history-taking in, 503, 506–508
Medicare guidelines for, 505*t*
physical examination in, 508–509, 511–512
planning, 504*f*
scheduling for, 503, 505*t*

Oversensing
- causes of, 346–347, 349
- defined, 346
- diaphragmatic, 349
- with dual-chamber pacing, 356–357, 356*f*
- and false signal, 347–348
- from insulation break, 521*f*
- pacing system malfunction due to, 346*f*
- reducing sensitivity in, 347
- repeated ventricular, 333, 333*f*
- during transvenous pacing, 180t

Oxygen consumption
- in exercise physiology, 150
- and minute ventilation, 114
- in transcutaneous pacing, 167

P

Paced AV interval (PAV), 526
Pacemaker insertion, indications for, 500. *See also* Implantation, pacemaker
Pacemaker-mediated tachycardia (PMT), 314, 315–316, 359–363, 361*f*, 362*f*. *See also* Endless-loop tachycardia
Pacemaker pocket
- placing, 214–215
- revision of, 227–229

Pacemaker-programmer system, documentation for, 324
Pacemakers
- atrial antitachycardia, 73
- components of, 322
- early, 114
- eccentricities of, 363
- migration of, 242

Pacemakers, permanent. *See also* Temporary pacing
- as constant-voltage generators, 54
- indications for, 4–5
- mode selection for, 31–32
- stimulus amplitude of, 56

Pacemaker Selection in Elderly (PASE) study, 231
Pacemaker syndrome, 178
- causes of, 140–141
- evaluation of, 350
- and mode selection, 156
- prevention of, 141
- symptoms of, 507

Pacemaker therapy, delayed, 232*b*
Pacer-patient mismatch, 503–506
Pacing
- indications for, 201
- preoperative, 41
- transcutaneous cardiac, 163–168
- transvenous, 169–183

Pacing in Cardiomyopathy (PIC) study, 24
Pacing stimuli, absent, 347, 348*t*
Pacing system analyzers (PSAs), 200, 201*f*
- for baseline data, 323–324
- filtering characteristics of, 340, 342–343*f*
- pacing pulse delivered by, 67

Pacing system malfunction, tools for evaluation of, 322–323. *See also* Malfunction evaluation
Pacing systems, 322–323
- baseline data for, 323–324, 323*b*
- capability of, 149
- epicardial, 183, 184*f*
- mechanical cardiac, 188–189
- physiologic property of, 149
- rate-adaptive, 109–112
- rate-modulating, 152
- transesophageal, 183–187

Pacing thresholds
- in follow-up assessment, 523
- in follow-up testing, 470–471

Pain
- generator associated with, 242
- in transcutaneous pacing, 167, 168*t*

Palpitations, in follow-up assessment, 509*t*
Paroxysmal atrial arrhythmias, mode selection for, 32
PASE study, 32
PATCH-CHF II studies, 432, 433*f*, 452, 452*f*, 454
Pathway/polarity, in ICD programming, 474*t*. *See also* Polarity
Patient education, for immediate postimplantation period, 501
Patients, ICD
- and CRT, 446–448, 450*f*–451*f*
- separate temporary systems in, 481, 482*f*, 483

Pauses, differential diagnosis of, 347, 348*t*
Perforation, myocardial, 231
- during lead placement, 236–237
- signs and symptoms of, 181, 182*t*
- in temporary pacing, 182*t*

Pericardial effusion, and transcutaneous pacing thresholds, 165–166
Pericardiocentesis
  in cardiac perforation, 236
  emergency, 200
Pericarditis, with perforated catheters, 181
Peroneal muscular atrophy, 7, 8
"Phantom programming," 517
"Phantom shocks," 484, 485
Phrenic nerve stimulation, high, 427–430, 429*f*, 430*f*
Physiologic pacing, 122
Pneumothorax
  avoiding, 171
  documenting absence of, 226
  as implantation complication, 233
  incidence of, 231
  treatment of, 233
Pocket hematomas, 508
Polarity
  in biventricular pacing, 434, 435*f*
  in ICD programming, 474*t*
  independent programming of, 67
  programmability of, 524
  sensing of, 77–78
Polarization effect, at electrode-myocardial interface, 64*f*
Polyurethane, for lead insulation, 93, 93*t*, 94*f*, 386
Post AV Nodal Ablation Evaluation (PAVE) Trial, 149
Postventricular atrial blanking (PVAB) period, 304
Postventricular atrial refractory period (PVARP)
  automatic extension of, 315
  in CRT devices, 74*f*
  and ELT, 360
  in follow-up assessment, 527–528
  in functional undersensing, 362
  and timing systems, 314
Power on reset (POR) mode, 531–532
Premature ventricular contraction (PVC)
  inhibition of atrial tracking by, 75*f*
  and loss of atrial tracking, 74*f*
  and PMT, 360
  with retrograde P wave, 317*f*
Presyncope
  in AV block, 6
  classic triggers associated with, 20, 21*f*
  in follow-up assessment, 509*t*
Procainamide, and stimulation threshold, 61
Programmers, pacemaker, 517
Programming
  and crosstalk, 527*f*
  and dyspnea, 507, 507*f*
  of pacemaker, 230, 525*t*
Programming, ICD
  basic parameters for, 472*t*–474*t*
  electrogram morphology (EGM) in, 477*f*
  ventricular tachyarrhythmia detection, 471, 475–477, 475*f*, 476*t*, 477*f*, 478*f*
  ventricular tachyarrhythmia therapies, 477–481
Prolonged AV delay, in dilated cardiomyopathy, 416, 418*f*, 419*f*
Prolonged QRS duration (QRSd), in chronic DCM, 417
Prolonged QT syndrome
  ECG in, 26*f*
  permanent pacing for, 25
Prophylactic antibiotics, 500
Pseudofracture, 334*f*
Pseudomalfunction
  defined, 363
  functions associated with, 365*b*
Pulmonary artery catheters, 169, 171*f*, 172*f*
Pulmonary capillary wedge (PCW) pressure
  during AV-synchronous pacing, 130, 130*f*
  phasic changes in, 132–135, 134*f*–135*f*
  during ventricular pacing, 130–131, 130*f*–133*f*
Pulse duration
  independent programming of, 67
  programming of, 52
Pulse generators, 398. *See also* Generators; Pacemakers
  active pectoral, 404
  for biventricular pacing, 434, 436*f*
  component malfunction of, 349–350
  components of, 322
  in CRT pacing systems, 434, 436*f*
  data logging capabilities in, 396
  of early ICDs, 380
  evolution of, 384
  functional elements of, 98
  lithium-iodine battery for, 98, 99–102, 99*f*

microprocessors, 107–108
multisite pacing, 434, 435*f,* 437
and noise reversion circuits, 105
output circuits for, 102–104
output pulse waveforms of, 103–104, 104*f*
power source for, 98–102
programmability of, 384–385
replacement of, 226–229
sensing circuits of, 104–106
size of, 274, 384, 408
telemetry circuits, 107
timing circuits of, 106–107

Pulse oximetry, during pacemaker implantation, 200
Pulses, in ICD programming, 473*t*
Pulse width, in ICD programming, 474*t*
Purkinje fibers
action potential of, 48*f*
forming His bundle, 1, 2*t,* 3
PVARP. *See* Postventricular atrial refractory period
P wave
and AV delay, 317*f*
in lead dislodgment, 328

Q

QRS complex
in AV block, 7, 8, 8*f*–9*f, 10,* 36
in CRT pacemaker electrocardiography, 444, 448*f*
electrocardiographically paced, 177
during LV free wall pacing, 447*f*
in pacemaker programming, 526*f*
during RV pacing, 446*f*
and RVS pacing, 142
in torsades de pointes, 42–43
during ventricular pacing, 445*f*
QRS prolongation, pacing both ventricles simultaneously in, 145
QT interval
and exercise, 115–116
prolongation of, 25
QT-sensing pacing systems, potential advantages of, 115, 116
Quality of life
and mode selection, 156
and rate-modulated systems, 153
Quinidine, and stimulation threshold, 61

R

Radar, electrical interference from, 72
Radiation therapy
effect on devices, 536
effect on ICD of, 481
EMI/device interactions in, 539*t*
temporary pacing in, 42
Radiofrequency ablation
development of new techniques, 42
effect on ICD of, 481
and EMI/device interactions, 539*t*
for reentrant SVT arrhythmias, 27
ventricular oversensing caused by, 537*f*
Radiographic evaluation. *See also* Chest radiograph
of cardiac placement, 175
conductor fracture on, 336
Radiographic identification, of pacemaker systems, 512, 513*f*
RAM (random access memory), of pulse generators, 98, 107–108
Rate-adaptive pacing systems, 109–112
with minute-ventilation-sensing, 112–115
motion-sensing, 109–112, 109*f*
signal processing in, 110
Rate-adaptive sensors, designing, 108–109
Rate drop response (RDR), 289
diagrammatic representation of, 291*f*
nominal values for, 292, 293*f*
Rate-modulated pacing
single-chamber, 272–273, 272*f*
single-chamber and dual-chamber, 273
Rate modulation
advantage of, 151–155, 152*t,* 153*f*–154*f*
and AV synchrony, 153, 154*f,* 155
and exercise physiology, 149–151, 150*f*
hemodynamic benefits of, 153, 154*f,* 155
and mode selection, 155
need for, 149
Rate-responsive AV delay (RRAVD), and timing systems, 314
Rate sensing, 394–397, 394*f*–395*f,* 397*f*
Rate smoothing, 302*f,* 306
introduction of, 301
maximal sensor-driven, 310
Recalls, for pacer products, 502
Recording artifacts
common, 350

in malfunction evaluation, 336–338, 337*f*, 338*f*
Redetection, in ICD programming, 472*t*
Refractory periods, 279, 280*f*, 281–183, 282*f*
function of, 279, 281
sensing, 106
Removal, indications for pacemaker, 243
Repetitive non-reentrant ventriculo-atrial synchronous (RNRVAS) rhythm, 361*f*, 362
Resuscitation, cough-induced cardiac, 189
Resuscitation cart, in pacemaker clinic, 501, 502*b*
Resynchronization, in prolonged QRS complexes, 145, 146*f*. *See also* Cardiac resynchronization therapy
Retrograde VA conduction, in pacemaker syndrome, 140
Rheobase, on strength-duration curve, 50–51, 51*f*
Right bundle branch block (RBBB)
during cardiac catheterization, 40
and left anterior hemiblock, 10 (*see also* Bifascicular block)
and left posterior hemiblock, 10 (*see also* Bifascicular block)
during temporary ventricular pacing, 177
Right ventricular d*P*/d*t* peak endocardial acceleration, 116
Right ventricular outflow tract (RVOT)
hemodynamics of, 141–142
lead positioned in, 218, 219*f*
Right ventricular pacing
alternative site, 141–142
effects of continuous, 142–144
Right ventricular septal (RVS) pacing, 142
Risk factors, for erosion, 243
ROM (read only memory), of pulse generators, 98, 107–108

S

Safety margins
and automated capture features, 79–82, 80*f*
based on DFT method, 389, 391*t*, 392
and defibrillation threshold, 406
for pacemaker-dependent patients, 56
programming of, 523
SCD HeFT study, 383, 384, 408
Sedation
for implantation procedures, 198
for pacemaker implantation, 205
Seldinger approach, 209
Sensed AV interval (SAV), in follow-up assessment, 526
Sensing. *See also* Oversensing; Undersensing
and automated capture features, 79
and autosensing functions, 82
and bipolar *vs.* unipolar leads, 64–65
in cardiac resyncrhonization tube devices, 74–77, 74*f*–76*f*
electrogram, 67, 69
in follow-up testing, 469–470
impedance, 78–79
and intracardiac electrograms, 69–71
of polarization, 77–78
potential difficulties with, 395
unipolar and bipolar, 72–74
Sensing circuits, 104–106
Sensing failure
functional undersensing, 345
pacing stimuli present with, 339–345
Sensing thresholds, in follow-up assessment, 520–524, 521*f*, 522*f*
Sensors, minute ventilation, 112–115
Sepsis
complications of, 244–245
in temporary pacing, 183
Sheath-dilator, in pacemaker implantation, 210
Shocks
cautery-induced ICD, 534*t*
evaluation of ICD, 484, 485*f*, 486
Sick sinus syndrome, 14. *See also* sinus node dysfunction
AV sequential *vs.* VVI pacing for, 33*t*–34*t*
DDDR pacing in, 152–153, 153*f*
in follow-up assessment, 507
mode selection in, 32
Silicone rubber, for lead insulation, 91, 93*t*, 386
Single-chamber systems
discriminaiton enhancement features in, 478*f*
in emergencies, 177–178
malfunction evaluation of, 324–325
and recurrence of symptoms, 350–351, 351*f*

stimuli absent with failure to capture, 345–350, 346*f*, 347*f*, 348*t*
stimuli present with failure to capture, 325–339, 327*t*
stimuli present with failure to sense, 339–345
myopotential inhibition in, 511
Single-chamber triggered-mode pacing, 271–272
Single-lead VDD pacing, 224–225
Sinoatrial (SA) node
anatomy of, 1, 2*t*
physiology of, 3, 4
Sinus node dysfunction
cardiac pacing for, 16
common medications causing, 17*b*
ECG in, 15*f*
etiologies of, 14
pacemakers implanted for, 16
pacing mode appropriate for, 17
symptoms of, 14–15
temporary pacing for, 35–36
Sleep, stimulation threshold during, 60
Spectranetics stylet, 252*f*
Split cathodal configuration, and impedance, 66
Staphylococcus aureus, 244
Stenting, in thrombosis complication, 241
Steroids
for exit block, 239
and high thresholds, 329
Stimulation threshold
bipolar, 58–59
defined, 50
determination of, 52
metabolic effects on, 60–61
pharmacologic effects on, 61
rate-dependence of, 60
and strength-duration curve, 51*f*, 52, 53*f*
and strength-duration relation, 50–53
strength-interval relation in, 58–59, 59*f*
time-dependent changes in, 54–58
typical evolution of, 54–56, 55*f*
Stimulus amplitude
independent programming of, 67
programming of, 52, 56
Stokes-Adams attacks, 5
Strength-duration curves
for constant-current stimulation, 53–54, 54*f*
for constant-voltage stimulation, 51*f*, 53–54, 54*f*
factors influencing, 52–53
in threshold testing, 52, 53*f*
Stroke volume
and AV synchrony, 151
in exercise physiology, 150, 151
and response to exercise, 154*f*
ventricular function curves for, 128*f*
Stylets
in atrial lead implantation, 221–222, 223
for lead insertion, 216
locking, 251–252, 252*f*
in ventricular lead positioning, 217–218
Subclavian method, of pacemaker implantation, 209–211
Subclavian venous puncture, complications associated with, 232–234
Subclavian venous system
anatomy of, 212*f*
occlusion of, 199, 199f
thrombosis of, 239
Superior vena cava, occlusion of, 241
Supraventricular tachyarrhythmias (SVTs)
conditions precipitating, 435–436
differentiation of, 476*t*
episodes of, 436
inappropriate ICD therapies for, 487, 488*f*–489*f*
Surgeons, for lead extraction, 249
Surgery
intraoperative management of devices, 534*t*
preoperative pacer evaluation for, 532
temporary pacing in, 42
and transcutaneous pacing thresholds, 165
Surgical instruments, for pacemaker implantation, 200
Surveillance systems
and inappropriate device triggering, 537
Suture sleeve, and malfunction, 331
SVT discriminators, in ICD programming, 473*t*
Swallowing, in neurally mediated syncope, 18–19
Swelling, in follow-up assessment, 509*t*
Syncope. *See also* Neurocardiogenic syncope
in bifascicular or trifascicular block, 12–13
carotid sinus, 20–21
causes of, 18

- with delayed or absent ICD therapy, 494, 495, 495*f*, 497*f*
- in follow-up assessment, 509*t*
- neurally mediated, 18–22
- in pacemaker syndrome, 140
- troubleshooting, 495, 496*b*, 496*f*, 497*b*
- in ventricular pacing, 126
- in ventricular tachycardia, 520*f*

System data, in device interrogation, 469

T

Tachyarrhythmias. *See also specific tachyarrhythmias*
- during lead placement, 235
- and mode selection, 155, 155*f*
- permanent pacing for, 27
- prevention and termination of, 25–27

Tachy-brady syndrome, 16, 16*f*

Tachycardia
- endless-loop, 314–317, 316*f*
- inappropriate detection of, 490–491, 491*f*
- and magnet application, 515
- pacemaker-mediated, 359–363, 361*f*, 362*f*
- temporary pacing for, 42–43

Tamponade, in cardiac perforation, 236

Telemetry
- atrial electrogram, 353
- battery depletion on, 531, 531*f*
- in follow-up assessment, 517–520, 518*f*–520*f*
- with inactivated ICD, 486–487
- mean hourly heart rate on, 290*f*
- of stored rate histogram, 519*f*

Telemetry circuits, 107

Telephone
- EMI/device interactions with cellular, 536
- transtelephonic monitoring, 505*t*, 529

Temporary pacing
- comparison of techniques for, 190*t*
- complications of, 181
- for extended periods, 171
- indications for, 32–40, 35*b*
- in infections, 41–42
- myocardial perforation in, 182*t*
- optimal technique for, 189–191, 189*t*
- during revision of systems, 227
- during surgery, 41
- thromboembolic events from, 181–182

Testing, system component
- of defibrillation threshold, 471
- pacing thresholds in, 470–471
- sensing in, 469–470

Thoracotomy
- in lead extraction, 250, 258
- for lead placement, 431, 431*f*

Threshold stimulation, bipolar *vs.* unipolar, 63–65

Thromboembolic events, from temporary pacing, 181–182

Thrombolytics, in cardiac perforation, 236

Thrombolytic therapies, and subsequent heart block, 39

Thrombosis, as lead placement complication, 239–241, 241*f*

Thrombus, in lead dislodgment, 328

Tilt, in ICD programming, 474*t*

Tilt testing
- cardioinhibitory response in, 20*f*, 21*f*
- in neurocardiogenic syncope, 19
- vasodepressor response to, 19*f*

Timing cycles, 275–276
- abbreviations used for, 265–266, 266*b*
- atrioventricular interval in, 283–289, 283*f*–285*f*, 287*f*, 288*f*
- components of, 317
- DDDR, 313–314, 313*f*
- effect of dual-chamber rate-modulated pacemakers on, 307–313, 307*f*–312*f*
- hysteresis programming in, 289–292, 290*f*, 291*f*
- refractory periods in, 279, 280*f*, 281–183, 282*f*
- and sinus preference, 305
- undersensing in, 339–340
- variations in, 265

Timing system, effects of, 313–314

Torsades de pointes
- causes of, 26*b*, 43
- temporary pacing for, 42–43

Total atrial refractory period (TARP), 75, 282

Transcutaneous electronic nerve stimulation units (TENS), 538, 539*t*

Transcutaneous pacing
- complications related to, 167–168
- disadvantages to, 163
- failure of, 167, 168*t*
- during heart block, 166*f*
- initiation of, 163–164, 165
- painful, 167, 168*t*

for prophylactic use, 191
thresholds in, 165–166
ventricular capture with, 167
Transesophageal pacing
catheters and electrodes for, 183, 185, 185*f*
generators for, 185–186, 185*f*
indications for, 183–187
Transtelephonic monitoring, schedule for, 505*t*, 529
Transvenous pacing
catheter electrodes in, 169, 170*f*
catheter placement in, 172, 173*f*, 174*f*
in clinical practice, 169
complications of, 181
loss of capture during, 179*t*
loss of sensing during, 180*t*
malfunction of, 178–179, 179*t*
oversensing during, 180*t*
QRS morphology in, 177
surgery for, 197
Treadmill testing, in follow-up assessment, 506
Trendelenburg positioning, 200
Trifascicular block, indications for pacing in, 10–14
Troubleshooting
baseline data for, 323–324, 323*b*
extracardiac signals, 491, 491*f*–493*f*
of isolated ICD discharge, 484, 485*f*, 486
schematic for, 374, 374*f*
Troubleshooting, ICD, 483
of bradycardia pacing, 483
double counting of ventricular events, 489, 490*f*
far-field R wave sensing, 489, 491, 491*f*
for multiple discharges, 486–492, 487*f*–492*f*
overcounting of ventricular events, 489, 490*f*
sustained ventricular arrhythmias, 492–495, 494*f*, 495*f*, 496*b*
syncope, 495, 496*b*, 496*f*, 497*b*
T waves, 347
Twiddler's syndrome, 238

U
Ultrasound, during pacemaker implantation, 200
Undersensing
atrial, 355
and component malfunction, 344
defined, 339, 341*f*
with dual-chamber pacing, 355–356
etiology of, 340
functional, 345, 345*b*, 362
inappropriately programmed sensitivity in, 341, 342*t*
lead dislodgment, 344
transient, 534
ventricular, 356
of ventricular fibrillation, 394*f*, 395, 396
Unipolar leads, insulation defects in, 331
Unipolar pacing
cathodal stimulation during, 175
compared with bipolar pacing, 63–64
Unipolar split cathodal configuration, 65–66, 66f
Unipolar systems, pacing stimulus in, 325, 325*f*
Univentricular pacing, 12 lead ECGs of, 449*f*
Upper limit of vulnerability (ULV), 392
Upper rate behavior, 298–302, 299*f*, 300*f*

V
Vagotonic block, 9*f*
VAI
and timing systems, 314
Vascular resistance, and AV symchrony, 135
Vasovagal syndrome, in neurally mediated syncope, 18–19
Venography
anterior interventricular vein on, 426, 427*f*
femoral approach to retrograde coronary, 425*f*
large lateral marginal veins on, 427, 428*f*
lead positioning on, 430, 430*f*
in pacemaker implantation, 211, 212*f*
subclavian, 199, 199*f*
Venous access
approaches for, 197
complications associated with, 231*b*, 232–234
for pacemaker implantation, 206–209
for transvenous pacing, 169
Venous thrombosis
as lead placement complication, 239–241, 241*f*
silent, 240–241
Ventricular arrhythmias
detection report for, 475*f*

without ICD therapy, 492–495, 494*f*, 495*f*, 496*b*
Ventricular asynchronous (VOO) pacing, 268, 268*f*
Ventricular-based timing, 278*f*, 292–294, 295*f*
Ventricular blanking period, 275, 285
Ventricular capture
in complete heart block, 166*f*
ECG assessment of, 448, 450*f*
intermittent loss of, 530*f*
with transcutaneous pacing, 598
in transesophageal pacing, 186
in transvenous pacing, 178
Ventricular dyssynchrony
CRT for, 450
incidence of, 457
Ventricular ectopy, and magnet application, 515
Ventricular fibrillation
inappropriate delivery of shock for, 492, 493*f*
multiple episodes of nonsustained, 491, 492*f*
with percussion pacing, 189
with transvenous pacing, 181
undersensing of, 394*f*, 395, 396
Ventricular function curves, 127–128, 128*f*, 129, 129*f*
Ventricular inhibited (VVI) pacing, 269, 269*f*, 270*f*
AV sequential *vs.*, 32
selection of, 32
Ventricular lead positioning, 217–221
apical, 217–218
ECG in, 220*f*
radiographic views, 219, 219*f*
in right ventricular outflow tract, 218
threshold parameter testing in, 220–221
Ventricular pacing
in AV conduction, 144, 144*f*
AV synchronous pacing compared with, 126–127, 136
blood pressure in, 124, 125f, 126
compared with atrial-based pacing, 157–158
effect of transcutaneous pacing on, 166
ejection fraction in, 135
in follow-up assessment, 526
hemodynamic compromise associated with, 507*f*
hemodynamic evaluation of, 124, 125*t*
minimizing, 155–158
and pacemaker syndrome, 140–141
PCW pressure in, 130–131, 130*f*–133*f*
physical signs related to, 140
QRS axis in, 445*f*
A waves in, 135
Ventricular rate regularization, 306
Ventricular resynchronization, 421, 422
Ventricular sensing, evaluation of, 355–356
Ventricular sensitivity, in ICD programming, 472*t*
Ventricular tachyarrhythmia
failure to detect, 494, 495*f*
ICD detection of, 471, 475–477, 475*f*, 476*t*, 477*f*, 478*f*
Ventricular tachyarrhythmia therapies, 477–481
Ventricular tachycardia
antitachycardia pacing termination of, 400, 402*f*
AV dissociation in, 478*f*
detection enhancements for, 476*t*
in follow-up assessment, 520*f*
ICD failure to detect, 492, 494*f*
inappropriate detection of, 76
and inappropriate ICD therapies, 487, 488*f*–489*f*
morphology score for, 477*f*
in transcutaneous pacing, 168
Ventriculoatrial (VA) conduction, 126, 507*f*
VF zone, in ICD programming, 472*t*
VT zone
in ICD programming, 472*t*
therapies programmed for, 479*f*
ventricular rate in, 487*f*

W

Waveforms, biphasic, 404
Wedensky effect, 52–53
Wenckebach interval, calculation of, 300
Wenckebach phenomenon, on Holter transmission, 506*f*
Wilkoff chronotropic assessment exercise protocol (CAEP), 152, 152*t*, 153
Wilkoff stylet, 252*f*
Work, exercise as, 150